# OMICs
# TECHNOLOGIES
## TOOLS FOR FOOD SCIENCE

# OMICs

## TECHNOLOGIES
### TOOLS FOR FOOD SCIENCE

EDITED BY
## NOUREDDINE BENKEBLIA

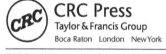

**CRC Press**
Taylor & Francis Group
Boca Raton London New York

CRC Press is an imprint of the
Taylor & Francis Group, an **informa** business

CRC Press
Taylor & Francis Group
6000 Broken Sound Parkway NW, Suite 300
Boca Raton, FL 33487-2742

First issued in paperback 2016

© 2012 by Taylor & Francis Group, LLC
CRC Press is an imprint of Taylor & Francis Group, an Informa business

No claim to original U.S. Government works

Version Date: 20111215

ISBN 13: 978-1-138-19924-8 (pbk)
ISBN 13: 978-1-4398-3706-1 (hbk)

### Library of Congress Cataloging-in-Publication Data

Omics technologies : tools for food science / editor, Noureddine Benkeblia.
    p. ; cm.
Includes bibliographical references and index.
ISBN 978-1-4398-3706-1 (hardcover : alk. paper)
I. Benkeblia, Noureddine.
[DNLM: 1. Biotechnology. 2. Food Technology. 3. Food. 4. Genomics. 5. Nutritional Physiological Phenomena. WA 695]

610.28--dc23                                           2011046674

**Visit the Taylor & Francis Web site at**
**http://www.taylorandfrancis.com**

**and the CRC Press Web site at**
**http://www.crcpress.com**

*To my beloved family: My wife Leila, my daughter Zahra, and my son Mohamed*

*"Strength is temporary, Generosity is Endless."*

# Contents

# Preface

Since the 1970s, biological and life sciences have seen considerable progress. Subsequently, the emergence of new biotechnologies, including OMICs, has had a positive impact on all disciplines in the biological and life sciences. With new discoveries in molecular biology and analytical chemistry and biochemistry, new tools are being developed that will likely revolutionize the study of food science and nutrition. Prior to these discoveries, food science and nutrition, as well as other food science disciplines, relied on classic chemistry and biochemistry techniques, and these techniques remained relatively unchanged for decades. More recently, however, new advances in the field, resulting in "Omics" technologies, have explored the areas of genomics, transcriptomics, proteomics, metabolimics, ionomics, nutrigenomics, nutriproteomics, etc., revealing many fundamental pathways and biochemical processes that drive food science and nutrition. Because Omics technologies help to better visualize the changes that occur when the genetic, environment, or nutrition of living organisms is altered, targeted analysis would be a key component of the food assessment paradigm in which nutrient qualities, anti-nutritional factors, allergens, or other components of potential biological activity to living organisms will be quantitatively and qualitatively analyzed and assessed. Although classic targeted compositional analysis provides the evidence needed to assess food nutrients and their impact on health, Omics technologies can add more value to food quality and safety assessment processes. Modern agriculture, including transgenic crops, GMOs, and disease biocontrols, has raised a number of issues, and new Omics technologies can be counted on to solve these issues and to show the way to sustainable and environment-friendly agriculture. This book, which provides comprehensive information on Omics and food science and nutrition, is a reliable reference in understanding the role of new emerging technologies in the area of food science and nutrition.

**Noureddine Benkeblia**

For MATLAB® and Simulink® product information, please contact:

The MathWorks, Inc.
3 Apple Hill Drive
Natick, MA, 07160-2098 USA
Tel: 508-647-7000
Fax: 508-647-7001
E-mail: info@mathworks.com
Web: www.mathworks.com

# Editor

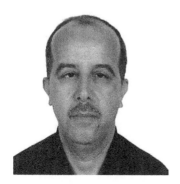

**Dr. Noureddine Benkeblia** is a professor of crop science. His area of specialization is food science, with a focus on postharvest food-plants' biochemistry and physiology. His work is mainly devoted to the metabolism of the carbohydrate fructooligosaccharides (FOS) during plant development and storage periods. Dr. Benkeblia introduced the new concept of systems biology—metabolomics—to investigate the mechanisms of biosynthesis and the accumulation of FOS in liliaceous plants. He received his BSc, MPhil, and DAgrSc from the Institut National Agronomique, and his DAgr from Kagoshima University. After serving as a teacher in Algeria for a few years, he joined Institut National de la Recherche Agronomique (INRA), Avignon (France), as a postdoctoral scientist in 2001. From 2002 to 2007, he worked as a visiting professor at the University of Rakuno Gakuen, Ebetsu (Japan). Dr. Benkeblia joined the Department of Life Sciences at the University of the West Indies (Jamaica) in 2008, continuing his work on the physiology, biochemistry, and metabolomics of fructan-containing plants in Jamaica. He also works on the postharvest physiology and biochemistry of local fruits.

# Contributors

**Noureddine Benkeblia**
Department of Life Sciences
University of the West Indies at Mona
Jamaica, West Indies

**Joan W. Bennett**
School of Environmental and Biological
    Sciences
Rutgers University
New Brunswick, New Jersey

**Deepak Bhatnagar**
United States Department of
    Agriculture/Agricultural Research
    Service
Southern Regional Research Center
New Orleans, Louisiana

**Claudio Bonghi**
Department of Environmental
    Agronomy and Crop Science
University of Padua
Padua, Italy

**Roberta Bordoni**
Institute of Biomedical Technologies
National Research Council
Milan, Italy

**Anthony R. Borneman**
The Australian Wine Research Institute
Adelaide, South Australia, Australia

**Silvia Braglia**
Faculty of Agriculture
University of Bologna
Reggio Emilia, Italy

**Allan Brown**
Department of Horticultural Science
Plants for Human Health Institute
North Carolina State University
Kannapolis, North Carolina

**Bianca Castiglioni**
Institute of Agricultural Biology
    and Biotechnology
National Research Council
Milan, Italy

**Gu Chen**
College of Light Industry and Food
    Sciences
South China University of Technology
Guangzhou, China

**Alejandro Cifuentes**
Laboratory of Foodomics
Institute of Food Science
    Research (CIAL)
National Research Council
    of Spain (CSIC)
Madrid, Spain

**Thomas E. Cleveland**
United States Department of
    Agriculture/Agricultural Research
    Service
Southern Regional Research Center
New Orleans, Louisiana

**Clarissa Consolandi**
Institute of Biomedical Technologies
National Research Council
Milan, Italy

**Paola Cremonesi**
Institute of Agricultural Biology
    and Biotechnology
National Research Council
Milan, Italy

**Carlos H. Crisosto**
Department of Plant Sciences
University of California
Davis, California

**Abhaya Dandekar**
Department of Plant Sciences
University of California
Davis, California

**Roberta Davoli**
Faculty of Agriculture
University of Bologna
Reggio Emilia, Italy

**Gianluca De Bellis**
Institute of Biomedical Technologies
National Research Council
Milan, Italy

**Virginia Garcia-Cañas**
Laboratory of Foodomics
Institute of Food science
    Research (CIAL)
National Research Council
    of Spain (CSIC)
Madrid, Spain

**Béatrice Godard**
Faculty of Medicine
Department of Social and Preventive
    Medicine
Université de Montréal
Montréal, Quebec, Canada

**Ruth M. Hamill**
Teagasc
Ashtown Food Research Centre
Dublin, Ireland

**Miguel Herrero**
Laboratory of Foodomics
Institute of Food science
    Research (CIAL)
National Research Council
    of Spain (CSIC)
Madrid, Spain

**Kristin Hollung**
Nofima AS
Ås, Norway

**Klasien Horstman**
Department of Health, Ethics
    and Society
School for Primary Care and Public
    Health (CAPHRI)
Maastricht University
Maastricht, the Netherlands

**Thierry Hurlimann**
Faculty of Medicine
Department of Social and Preventive
    Medicine
Université de Montréal
Montréal, Quebec, Canada

**Elena Ibañez**
Laboratory of Foodomics
Institute of Food science
    Research (CIAL)
National Research Council
    of Spain (CSIC)
Madrid, Spain

**Sarada Krishnan**
Director of Horticulture
Denver Botanic Gardens
Denver, Colorado

**Li Li**
Robert W. Holley Center for Agriculture
    and Health
Agricultural Research Service
United States Department of
    Agriculture
and
Department of Plant Breeding
    and Genetics
Cornell University
Ithaca, New York

**George A. Manganaris**
Department of Agricultural Sciences,
  Biotechnology and Food Science
Cyprus University of Technology
Lemesos, Cyprus

**Begonya Marcos**
Teagasc
Ashtown Food Research Centre
Dublin, Ireland

**Federico Martinelli**
Department of Plant Sciences
University of California
Davis, California

**Anne Maria Mullen**
Teagasc
Ashtown Food Research Centre
Dublin, Ireland

**William C. Nierman**
J. Craig Venter Institute
Rockville, Maryland

and

Department of Biochemistry and
  Molecular Biology
The George Washington University
  School of Medicine
Washington, District of Columbia

**Andrew H. Paterson**
Plant Genome Mapping Laboratory
University of Georgia
Athens, Georgia

**Gary Payne**
Department of Plant Pathology
North Carolina State University
Raleigh, North Carolina

**Clelia Peano**
Institute of Biomedical Technologies
National Research Council
Milan, Italy

**Bart Penders**
Department of Health, Ethics
  and Society
School for Public Health and Primary
  Care (CAPHRI)
Maastricht University
Maastricht, the Netherlands

**Isak S. Pretorius**
Australian Wine Research Institute
Adelaide, South Australia, Australia

**Dilip K. Rai**
Teagasc
Ashtown Food Research Centre
Dublin, Ireland

**Tom A. Ranker**
Division of Environmental Biology
National Science Foundation
Arlington, Virginia

**Marco Severgnini**
Institute of Biomedical Technologies
National Research Council
Milan, Italy

**Carolina Simó**
Laboratory of Foodomics
Institute of Food science
  Research (CIAL)
National Research Council
  of Spain (CSIC)
Madrid, Spain

**Raphaelle Stenne**
Faculty of Medicine
Department of Social and Preventive
  Medicine
Université de Montréal
Montréal, Quebec, Canada

**Corine S.C. Ting**
Australian Wine Research Institute
Adelaide, South Australia, Australia


**Eva Veiseth-Kent**
Nofima AS
Ås, Norway


**Rein Vos**
Department of Health, Ethics
    and Society
School for Primary Care and Public
    Health (CAPHRI)
Maastricht University
Maastricht, the Netherlands

**Jiujiang Yu**
United States Department of
    Agriculture/Agricultural Research
    Service
Southern Regional Research Center
New Orleans, Louisiana

**Paolo Zambonelli**
Faculty of Agriculture
University of Bologna
Reggio Emilia, Italy

**Xuewu Zhang**
College of Light Industry and Food
    Sciences
South China University of Technology
Guangzhou, China

# 1 Nutrition Science and "Omics" Technologies
## Ethical Aspects in Global Health

*Béatrice Godard, Thierry Hurlimann,
and Raphaelle Stenne*

## CONTENTS

## 1.1 INTRODUCTION

Nutrition science has broadened into a full range of interests, activities, and knowledge. Nutrigenomics is one of the extents covered by nutritional science. It allows a deeper understanding of metabolism, disease pathophysiology, and health that ultimately could be used to prevent or treat the most common chronic diseases in the world, such as, for instance cancer, cardiovascular disease, and diabetes. Many promises have been made regarding the potential outcomes of nutrigenomics research, and the scope of such applications is actually striking: Nutrigenomics information is going to be relevant not only for patients but also for healthy individuals and populations. However, it remains unclear and controversial whether nutrigenomics studies and their current or potential applications will actually benefit populations, in particular vulnerable and underserved populations. Different forces may drive the choice of research priorities and shape the claims that are made when communicating the goals or the results of nutrigenomics studies and applications. Moreover, the assessment of the scientific evidence linked to nutrition, genetics/genomics, and health claims is difficult. The complexity of global health governance and of potential prevention measures in public and global health based on nutrigenomics knowledge, but also ethical issues relating to social justice and to the risks of stigmatization and discrimination are major challenges both in developed and emerging countries. Moreover, the development of nutrigenomics along with "personalized medicine" may also alter our relation to food, medicalizing food choices and eating behaviors and blurring boundaries between health and disease, and between food and drugs.

In terms of global health, nutrigenomics is more than premature claims and much debated promises about personalized nutritional interventions on individuals. Beyond questionable commercial claims, nutrigenomics is also knowledge about, and recognition of, the considerable impacts of underfeeding and malnutrition on genome (and epigenome) integrity and stability. As such, nutrigenomics research offers a valuable opportunity to give strength to the debate about the unacceptable consequences of hunger and malnutrition worldwide and to support a newly and potentially significant convergence in research priorities that could benefit both developed and developing countries. One may hope that if so managed by stakeholders as to take seriously the major ethical issues it generates, nutrigenomics could be placed on the global agenda that aims to improve population health (Godard and Hurlimann 2009).

## 1.2   NUTRITION SCIENCE AND "OMICS" TECHNOLOGIES

Since the completion of the Human Genome Project, nutrition science has undergone a fundamental, molecular transformation (Lévesque et al. 2008, Omic-Ethics Research Group 2011, Ozdemir and Godard 2007). New bioinformatics tools and genomics biotechnologies have enabled researchers to analyze the complex interplay of metabolism, gene expression and function, and, more broadly, genetic diversity within and between human populations. Nutrition science has branched out with the advent of a new discipline: nutrigenomics. The premise is that nutrigenomics applications will provide individuals with tools to help customize their diet so as to help prevent disease and promote their well-being. Nutrigenomics is often described as one of the latest applications of genomics technologies in the field of personalized health interventions. Yet nutrigenomics goes beyond personalized health interventions. It covers disparate fields of nutrition science, which may each pursue different goals and thus may have multiple facets.

Nutrigenomics aims to understand gene–diet interactions and the latter's influence on individual responses to food on disease susceptibility, as well as on population health. Nutrigenomics information is expected to be relevant for treatment and also for prevention in the general population. Nutrigenomics research focuses on the bidirectional study of genetic factors influencing host (individuals' or populations') responses to diet as well as the effects of bioactive constituents in food on host genome and gene expression (Omic-Ethics Research Group 2011, Ozdemir and Godard 2007). This bidirectional approach to the study of genome–diet interaction creates a dual avenue for tangible nutrigenomics applications, as shown in Figure 1.1.

The public health focus of nutrigenomics research, and the day-to-day importance of food in peoples' lives, may create unrealistic expectations and may raise

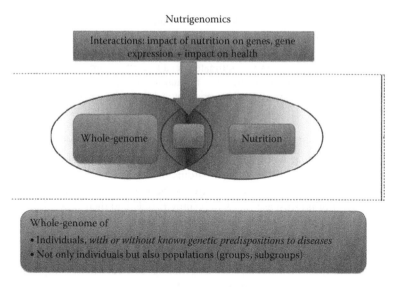

**FIGURE 1.1** Bidirectional nature of food genome interactions.

unexpected ethical and social issues. These expectations can exceed the threshold for biohype if not approached in an evidence-based manner. In fact, if (nutri) genomics may inform our understanding of population differences in disease distribution by focusing on new insights into the global pattern of human genetic variation, different factors play a role in health outcomes: socioeconomic status, cultural practices (e.g., diet), discrimination, and access to health care. For instance, there is overwhelming evidence for the existence of disparities in health when American ethnic minority groups are compared to their white counterparts. There are a number of health disparity diseases that result from an interplay between genetic and social influences. A health disparity disease such as Type 2 diabetes is a good example of the interplay of genetic and social factors. For nutrigenomics research to maintain its present pace and momentum, sponsors, investigators, and health professionals cannot neglect the significance of socio-ethical factors in the uptake of innovation and adoption of new health technologies. And although the benefits of considering genomic and social factors that contribute to health disparities, if ethical principles are not factored in, the health of nations may deteriorate while the economy prospers, especially in the case of developing and emerging nations (People's Health Movement 2010). Risks to global health include limited sources of health commodities, commercial exploitation of health delivery, industry contribution to poor health (tobacco, junk food), and jeopardized food security. The field of nutrition is not immune to these risks: Imbalanced diets account for a substantial portion of preventable morbidity and mortality in all countries. Obesity has become a global epidemic and in certain countries occurs simultaneously with micronutrient deficiencies. Inadequate diets, hunger, and malnutrition continue to be critical problems in developing countries. The mere "putting in place" of ethical principles could somehow counter the massive economic forces that underlie inequality and malnutrition.

Addressing ethical and social issues related to nutrigenomics could pave the way to a more equitable adoption of genomics technologies in nutritional sciences. It is said that

> the adoption of nutrigenomics will ultimately lead to further market segmentation as this knowledge will identify 'at risk' patients and provide guidance for dietary regimens and lifestyles to have a positive impact on public health and overall quality of life (Barton 2010)

Research findings clearly indicate expected benefits in terms of understanding the link between nutrition, genome damage, and health; improvement of outcomes in the treatment of diseases; the prevention of chronic diseases in healthy individuals with or without any genetic predisposition; the treatment of genetic susceptibilities through the identification of pre-disease states in healthy people and their prevention through personal dietary interventions; the development of functional foods and the engineering of tailored foods with optimal concentrations of micronutrients; as well as public and individual health promotion, disease prevention, and the reduction of health care costs (Kaput and Rodriguez 2004). Research findings also reveal the complexities and uncertainties related to nutrigenomics science itself; of potential applications to public and global health, such as some of the limitations of population prevention strategies that could result from nutrigenomics (such as the prevention paradox, i.e., "a preventive measure which brings much benefit to the population [yet] offers little to each participating individual" (Rose 1985)); of the research environment, which involves many actors, public and private interests, the transition to clinical applications (Mohan and Deepa 2007); of the complexity of communication processes; and, finally, of the complexity of the ethical issues associated with nutrigenomics research and its potential applications (Godard and Hurlimann 2009). The latter are notably about the medicalization of food and genetic reductionism (Bergmann et al. 2008), responsibility for health and consequent risks of discrimination of individuals who would not comply with personalized dietary recommendations, stigmatization of at-risk and healthy people, individual access to nutrigenetics tests and services or to specific foods and nutriments, risks of biohype, risks linked to the direct commercialization of this technology, and, last but not least—well before potential applications in clinics and daily life—unfairness and inequity in research participation (Hurlimann et al. 2011). In this regard, an unfair exclusion of specific population groups increases their risk of discrimination, but also impacts on the generalizability of research findings and thus on the efficacy of potential public and global health applications. Such exclusions from nutrigenomics research could lead to unrealistic or premature claims about the scope and benefits of research findings. In such a context, the question arises: How best to promote nutrigenomics research that would benefit all populations and how to translate nutrigenomics research findings into more effective health services and products?

## 1.3 ETHICS CORE AS THE BEST ASSISTANCE

Biomedical research ethics consists of analyzing ethical issues raised when people are involved as participants in research. It aims (1) to protect research participants; (2) to promote research while ensuring that research is conducted in a way that serves the interests of individuals, groups, and/or society as a whole; and (3) to examine specific research activities for their ethical soundness, looking at issues such as risk management, protection of privacy, the process of informed consent, and so on. Biomedical research ethics rests on three basic principles: first, respect of individuals, which is given a concrete expression by the use of informed consent, that is, subjects must be given the opportunity to choose what shall or shall not happen to them; second, beneficence and, consequently, nonmaleficence, which require an assessment of the nature and scope of risks and benefits in a systematic manner, with research aiming to maximize possible benefits and minimize possible harms. And, third, justice, which requires a fair selection of subjects, the benefits and risks of research having to be distributed fairly. Many guidelines have been developed by different organizations to help researchers and Institutional Review Boards respect these ethical principles in biomedical research (The Council for International Organizations of Medical Sciences 2002, World Medical Association 2008). Despite their merits, these guidelines have been criticized for representing Western values with limited utility and application in different sociocultural contexts, in spite of their apparent universality. For instance, criticisms of liberalism led a shift from addressing narrow issues such as cultural differences in informed consent practices toward a greater emphasis on development and social justice (Benatar et al. 2003, 2005, Singer and Benatar 2001). While recognizing the universality of the basic principles mentioned earlier, a more cautious approach aims to recognize that there are core moral norms. A pluralistic perspective (rather than a relativistic approach, in the nihilistic sense that everything would be permitted) is increasingly being promoted in research ethics. It seeks to promote an international dialog with a view to understanding the differences, avoiding the predominance of any one particular value system, and rather to search for community values.

In the context of global health where the goals are promoting and protecting the health of the public, improving well-being in communities, and contributing to social justice, the limits of Western approaches are more obvious. Moreover, a lack of institutional review boards and training, as well as a dependency on industry are significant in many emerging countries. As noted by Hellsten, "in terms of global bioethics, there is the recognition of the global context, particularly the economic disequilibrium and the potential for exploitation of those already most vulnerable and disadvantaged." It then appears important to address ethical issues in a global context, taking into account many factors—economic, social, political, religious, and cultural—and adopting various ethical methodologies in a search for global solutions (Hellsten 2008).

The quest for equity is a fundamental value for global health. How does the research address inequality and who will benefit from the results? In other words, how to counteract the "10/90 gap" where over 90% of global research dollars are spent on health problems that affect only 10% of the world? The risk that research reinforce disparities rather than diminish them, or the risk of ethical relativism, that is, changing ethical values or priorities according to the situation, or to accommodate lesser values (e.g., consent, standard of care, etc.) are all pressing ethical issues that require global solutions with a particular attention to poorer, vulnerable, and underserved populations. Therefore, the role of international organizations, such as the World Medical Association or the Council for International Organizations of Medical Sciences, is critical. It is also essential to involve communities in order to move from a "semicolonial relationship" to a true partnership, with the knowledge created being held communally (Pinto and Upshur 2009). In fact, if multidisciplinary approaches and the participation of multiple stakeholders are key in research ethics, the foundations of global health ethics rest largely on communitarian approaches to health interventions, where constructing a "good society" should be a stated goal, based on a philosophy of health and human rights where all should enjoy a minimal standard of health and health care. These approaches form the basis to move forward in exploring global health ethics and formulating principles to use in research and clinical work, including nutrigenomics.

In addition to three basic ethical principles in biomedical research ethics—respect, beneficence, justice—humility, introspection, solidarity, and social justice are also important principles for global health ethics (Benatar et al. 2003, Pinto and Upshur 2009). According to the authors, humility, in connection with beneficence, calls for recognizing the Western limitations within the setting of global health work and for seeking direction from the host community as to their needs, their experience and their perspective on etiologies and solutions. Introspection or antidiscriminatory analysis is also important for ensuring that the research addresses the gap between knowledge and practice. Acting out of solidarity allows that the goals and values be aligned with those of the community and prevent its marginalization, while working in a social justice perspective implies that global health work should concern itself with diminishing inequity.

## 1.4 GLOBAL HEALTH ETHICS: MANY WORLDS, ONE ETHICS?

Ethics deals with the "right thing to do," and provides some reasons for standards of behavior. Therefore, it requires a detailed analysis of any situation, the motives present, and an understanding of other people's positions. In terms of global health, research priorities, and justice, we face an increase of chronic diseases, a double burden of under- and overnutrition in emerging countries, inequalities between countries, but also within countries, as well as an increase of the costs of health technologies, including genomics technologies. How then to promote nutrigenomics research that would benefit communities and populations? As in biomedical research ethics in general, fairness and equity in research participation, as well as the appropriate inclusion of subjects should be prerequisites. Several guidelines refer to the principle of distributive justice, "which requires the equitable distribution of both the burdens and benefits of participation in research" (The Council for International Organizations of Medical Sciences 2002). This principle implies that no group should be deprived of its fair share of the benefits of research, short term or long term; such benefits include the direct benefits of participation as well as the benefits of the new knowledge that the research is designed to yield (The Council for International Organizations of Medical Sciences 2002).

The Council for International Organizations of Medical Sciences points out that "sponsors of research or investigators cannot, in general, be held accountable for unjust conditions where the research is conducted, but they must refrain from practices that are likely to worsen unjust conditions or contribute to new inequities" (The Council for International Organizations of Medical Sciences 2002). Guideline 12, *Equitable distribution of burdens and benefits in the selection of groups of subjects in research*, stipulates that "groups or communities to be invited to be subjects of research should be selected in such a way that the burdens and benefits of the research will be equitably distributed. The exclusion of groups that might benefit from study participation must be justified" (The Council for International Organizations of Medical Sciences 2002). In the past, groups of persons were excluded from participation in research for what were then considered good reasons. As a consequence of such exclusions, information about the diagnosis, prevention, and treatment of diseases in such groups of persons were and might be still limited. This has resulted in serious injustices and it became a moral principle that researchers should be inclusive in selecting research participants. It is now acknowledged that

> researchers shall not exclude individuals from the opportunity to participate in research on the basis of attributes such as religion, culture, ethnicity, race, gender, age, language, linguistic proficiency, disability or sexual orientation, unless there is a valid reason for the exclusion (The Interagency Advisory Panel on Research Ethics 2010).

The policies of many national governments and professional societies recognize the need to redress these injustices by encouraging the participation of previously excluded groups or communities in biomedical research.

Conversely, there has been a perception, sometimes correct, that certain groups of persons, such as socioeconomically disadvantaged groups, but also entire communities, have been overused as research subjects. This has been particularly likely to occur in countries or communities with insufficiently developed systems for the protection of the rights and welfare of human research subjects. As expressed by the Council for International Organizations of Medical Sciences,

> such overuse is especially questionable when the populations or communities concerned bear the burdens of participation in research but are extremely unlikely ever to enjoy the benefits of new knowledge and products developed as a result of the research (The Council for International Organizations of Medical Sciences 2002).

There is no doubt that the overuse of certain groups or communities is unjust for several reasons. Yet even as these groups should not be excluded from research protocols, it would not be unjust to selectively recruit them to serve as subjects in research designed to address problems that are prevalent in their group—malnutrition, for example.

In nutrigenomics research, why would such exclusions constitute an ethical issue? First, depending on the geographic location of research participants, the generalizability of results may be limited: Micronutrient contents and accessibility of food may vary considerably from one region to another; methods of diagnosis and management of diseases studied in nutrigenomics also vary between countries, and one must bear in mind the cultural differences in eating habits. These variations have led some authors to consider that nutrition trials should not only include ethnic minorities and vulnerable populations, but indeed target them (Myser 2003). Second, limitations in the representativeness of the population diversity may have a considerable impact on the generalizability of results: Ethnicity, race, and ancestry are important concepts in genomics and public health research, important for addressing stratification and study design issues in complex traits, especially for heterogeneous populations (Indian Genome Variation Consortium 2008). Although we do not have distinct biological types of "races," we do note differences in the frequency of genetic markers across human ancestral groups. These differences, which for the most part describe continental populations (geographical distance), are believed to harbor the answers to why some individuals and groups may be more susceptible or resistant to diseases and may also hold the key to understanding why human groups respond differently to medications (Indian Genome Variation Consortium 2008). Third, there are other exclusion criteria based on practical considerations that are questionable, such as the difficulties experienced by some research participants to fill out food questionnaires, their noncompliance to interventions' studies, or when potential research participants were not enrolled in previous studies. For instance, difficulties in filling out questionnaires may originate in cultural differences that are ignored if questionnaires are not adapted to the ethnicity and cultural/dietary habits of participants. Such exclusions may impact on the fairness of participants' eligibility and on the generalizability of findings as well as on the efficacy of potential applications in public and global health. They may increase the stigmatization of or discrimination against specific groups or communities, possibly leading to unrealistic claims of nutrigenomics research.

## 1.5  WHAT ARE REALISTIC AND ACHIEVABLE PROMISES OF NUTRIGENOMICS FOR GLOBAL HEALTH?

In addition to the complexity of genomics association studies, nutrigenomics research must tackle the complexity of diets, food components, and the multiple targets and effects that different nutrients in varying amounts may have in the human body. Thus, the assessment of the scientific validity of research protocols, of the scope of research results, and of the efficacy of potential nutrigenomics applications in public and global health is challenging. A lack of any concrete scientific standard of evidence, the uncertainty about the potential efficacy of public health measures based on nutrigenomics applications, a lack of appreciation of the complexity of nutrigenomics, its potential impacts, and the context in which it occurs may create a fertile ground for biohype, namely for unrealistic promises, excessive publicity, and premature claims in advertising materials. It also raises major issues about the way research results are communicated to the public or used by firms to sell nutrigenetics tests to consumers. The debate about the commercialization of nutrigenetics tests and the validity of such tests has widened considerably. The barriers and facilitators to the uptake of nutrigenomics research findings are summarized in Figure 1.2.

Noting that nutrigenomics raises many hopes and expectations (while not immune to biohype), noting that research in nutrigenomics is complex and that the interpretation of results remains a challenge, noting that personalized nutrition and many applications of nutrigenomics, despite commercial marketing and claims, are still considered premature, and noting that there are many ethical issues both in research

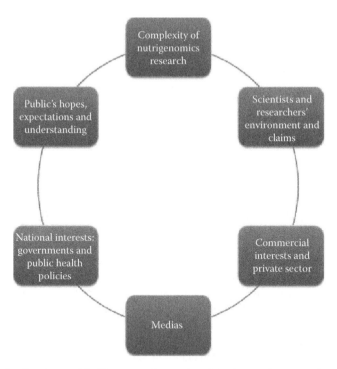

**FIGURE 1.2** Barriers and facilitators to the uptake of nutrigenomics research.

and potential clinical applications, the communication of these issues to a broader audience would be desirable so as to increase the awareness of the ethical and scientific issues at stake. Ethical issues surrounding nutrigenomics (at both clinical research and clinical application levels) should be raised, their existence be brought to the attention of all actors involved in this field, including the lay public, various communities, and populations, should be provided with appropriate and easily accessible information regarding these issues.

It is important to engage with the various stakeholders in order to work out how the ethics dimension can be of the best assistance and what the most important ethics and policy issues for the dissemination of research findings in nutrigenomics are anticipated to be. Indeed, as nutrigenomics involves different research disciplines, scientific efforts to understand the complexity of nutrition/genetics bidirectionality raise myriad ethical questions (Kaput and Rodriguez 2004). Inadequate diets and malnutrition continue to be critical problems worldwide. Imbalanced diets account for a substantial portion of preventable morbidity and mortality. Obesity has become a global epidemic, while in certain countries it co-occurs with micronutrient deficiencies. It is said that "nutrigenomics could be an important part of reining in global healthcare expenditures, as governments continue to seek alternative ways to address diseases and conditions" (Barton 2010). To that end, better standards of evidence in the field of nutrigenomics are needed. The scientific validity of existing nutrigenomics tests has to be demonstrated, despite the claims of specialized commercial firms or promises such as can be found in the media.

This underscores the need for a more comprehensive view of ethical issues, possible only by integrating a "working alliance" between researchers, research participants, patients, health care providers, and ethics experts from both Western and emerging countries as the basis for effective and high quality health care that protects the interests of research participants, patients, and populations (Fuertes et al. 2007, Morley and Williams 2006). Being involved in this debate will offer an opportunity to highlight important gaps in our understanding of a number of ethically relevant aspects of nutrigenomics and their potential impact on global health.

## 1.6   POTENTIAL IMPACT OF A DEBATE WITH STAKEHOLDERS

Engaging in a debate is a way of contributing to the exchange, synthesis, and ethically sound application of nutrigenomics research findings in the context of an intricate set of interactions among researchers and knowledge users while easing the complexity of public health decision making. In this dynamic, the role of research sponsors and scientists is paramount, but so is the role of institutional review boards and health professionals. Studies have shown the merits of a heightened awareness of the ethical and scientific issues regarding chronic diseases, especially where different stakeholders within a focused community of practice attempted to address the impact of such diseases. According to Henry (2008), various levels of success have been demonstrated when there is exchange, synthesis, and an ethically sound application of research findings within an elaborate set of interactions among researchers and knowledge users. Like Henry, it is critical to accelerate the operationalization of research benefits for all individuals with a view to more effective and responsive services and products, in turn leading to improved health (Henry 2008). There is a growing debate about the need for regulations that would frame the access to and the supply of genetic tests. The way information is marketed and communicated in this field impacts both public and professional attitudes. As a consequence, it also impacts public and global health (Glauser 2010).

Many research projects in nutrigenomics focus on an individual approach, whereas personalized nutrition will likely not solve public and global health problems, inequalities, and so on. But is such an approach a sufficient reason to claim that nutrigenomics cannot be of benefit for global health? When millions lack access to basic nutrition, how to promote nutrigenomics research that would benefit them? Nutrigenomics will not address the immediate food needs of poor people or entire populations in emerging countries, nor will it put in place high-priority policy measures necessary to improve access to basic nutrition.

## 1.7   CONCLUSION: A SHIFT IN THINKING

Nutrigenomics raises many hopes and expectations but is still in its infancy. Research in nutrigenomics is complex and the interpretation of results remains a challenge. Medical, cultural, and ethical aspects should be considered to ensure a sound development of this new field of science. Fairness and equity in research participation should be strengthened, otherwise major problems might occur in terms of global health and justice. Nutrigenomics could favor people and countries that are well-off, increasing health inequalities. Emerging economies are now coping with a double burden of under- and overnutrition. Simultaneously, potential benefits from nutrigenomics, whether in fighting malnutrition or chronic diseases, should not be overlooked. Emphasis should not be put solely on genetic solutions and other more accessible, social, and political measures should not be neglected.

The complexity of global health governance and of potential prevention measures in public and global health based on nutrigenomics knowledge, but also ethical issues relating to social justice and to the risk of stigmatization and discrimination are major challenges both in developed and emerging countries. Additional requirements of research in emerging countries such as the benchmarks established by Emmanuel et al. (2000) might be necessary to counteract the "10/90 gap," but also to counteract the risk of ethical relativism, that is, changing ethical values or priorities according to the situation or to accommodate "lesser" values. According to the CIOMS,

> the ethical requirement that research be responsive to the health needs of the population or community in which it is carried out calls for decisions on what is needed to fulfil the requirement. It is not sufficient simply to determine that a disease is prevalent in the population and that new or further research is needed: The ethical requirement of "responsiveness" can be fulfilled only if successful interventions or other kinds of health benefits are made available to the population (The Council for International Organizations of Medical Sciences 2002).

With regard to nutrigenomics, this implies that future research should include multidisciplinary assessments of realistic options for investigators to address the issue of exclusion, clarify the use of ethnic categories in health research and identify the barriers and facilitators to the involvement of different population groups in research. This calls for a shift in thinking: If the scientific community, in particular experts in ethics, hope to contribute to major contemporary social and ethical debates, they will need to contribute to the critical exploration of an emerging transnational global health research/ethics.

## REFERENCES

Barton, C.L. 2010. *The Future of Nutrigenomics: New Opportunities in Personalized Nutrition and Food-Pharma Collaboration.* Business Insights, England, U.K.

Benatar, S., Daar, A., and P. Singer. 2003. Global health ethics: The rationale for mutual caring. *Int Aff* 79:107–138.

Benatar, S., Daar, A., and P. Singer. 2005. Global health challenges: The need for an expanded discourse on bioethics. *PLoS Med* 2:587–589.

Bergmann, M.M., Görman, U., and J.C. Mathers. 2008. Bioethical considerations for human nutrigenomics. *Annu Rev Nutr* 28:447–467.

Emmanuel, E., Wendler, D., and C. Grady. 2000. What makes clinical research ethical? *JAMA* 283:2701–2711.

Fuertes, J.N., Mislowack, A., Bennett, J. et al. 2007. The physician–patient working alliance. *Patient Educ Couns* 66(1):29–36.

Glauser, W. 2010. Standardization of genetic tests needed. *Can Med Assoc J* 19(Oct.):182.

Godard, B. and T. Hurlimann. 2009. Nutrigenomics for global health: Ethical challenges for underserved populations. *Curr Pharmacogenomics Pers Med* 7:205–214.

Hellsten, S.K. 2008. Global bioethics: Utopia or reality? *Dev World Bioeth* 8(2):70–81.

Henry, J.L. 2008. The need for knowledge translation in chronic pain. *Pain Res Manag* 13:465–476.

Hurlimann, T., Stenne, R., Menuz, V., and B. Godard. 2011. Inclusion and exclusion in nutrigenetics clinical research: Ethical and scientific challenges. *J Nutrigenet Nutrigenomics* (in revision).

Indian Genome Variation Consortium. 2008. Genetic landscape of the people of India: A canvas for disease gene exploration. *J Genet* 87:3–20.

Kaput, J. and R.L. Rodriguez. 2004. Nutritional genomics: The next frontier in the postgenomic era. *Physiol Gen* 16:166–177.

Lévesque, L., Ozdemir, V., Gremmen, B., and B. Godard. 2008. Integrating anticipated nutrigenomics bioscience applications with ethical aspects. *OMICS* 12:1–16.

Mohan, V. and M. Deepa. 2007. Measuring obesity to assess cardiovascular risk—Inch tape, weighing machine, or both? *J Assoc Physicians India* 5:617–619.

Morley, S. and A.C. Williams. 2006. RCTs of psychological treatments for chronic pain: Progress and challenges. *Pain* 121:171–172.

Myser, C. 2003. Differences from somewhere: The normativity of whiteness in bioethics in the United States. *Am J Bioet* 3:1–11.

Omic-Ethics Research Group. 2011. What is nutrigenomics? http://www.omics-ethics.org (accessed January 26, 2011).

Ozdemir, V. and B. Godard. 2007. Evidenced-based management of nutrigenomics expectations and ELSIs. *Pharmacogenomics* 8:1051–1062.

People's Health Movement. 2010. Right to Food and Nutrition Watch. Land Grabbing and nutrition. Challenges for Global Governance. FIAN International, Heidelberg, Germany. http://www.fian.org (accessed October 2, 2011).

Pinto, A. and R. Upshur. 2009. Global health for students. *Dev World Bioeth* 9:1–10.

Rose, G. 1985. Sick individuals and sick populations. *Int J Epidemiol* 14:32–38.

Singer, P. and S. Benatar. 2001. Beyond Helsinki: A vision for global health ethics. Improving ethical behaviour depends on strengthening capacity. *BMJ* 322:747–748.

The Council for International Organizations of Medical Sciences. 2002. International Ethical Guidelines for Biomedical Research Involving Human Subjects. WHO, Geneva, Switzerland.

The Interagency Advisory Panel on Research Ethics. 2010. *TCPS 2—Tri-Council Policy Statement: Ethical Conduct for Research Involving Humans*. Ottawa, Ontario, Canada.

World Medical Association. 2008. *Declaration of Helsinki Ethical Principles for Medical Research Involving Human Subjects*. WHO, Geneva, Switzerland.

# 2 Array Platform for Food Safety and Quality

*Clarissa Consolandi, Paola Cremonesi,*
*Marco Severgnini, Roberta Bordoni, Clelia Peano,*
*Gianluca De Bellis, and Bianca Castiglioni*

## CONTENTS

## 2.1 INTRODUCTION

The safety of foods and ingredients for human alimentation or animal feeding has always been a great concern. On the one hand, control over the presence of potentially harmful pathogens and contaminants has historically been one of the most exploited sectors for the development and commercialization of diagnostic tests. Although infections of food-borne pathogens have been controlled, the prevalence of food-borne diseases is substantial. Hundreds of outbreaks of food-borne infection cases occur around the world (Bresee et al. 2002) and up to 30% of the population in industrialized nations suffers from food-borne illness each year. On the other hand, since the first introduction of genetically modified (GM) tobacco in 1998, the detection of genetically modified organisms (GMOs) has increasingly gained importance over the years: several organizations, including the Food and Agriculture Organization (FAO) of the United Nations and the World Health Organization (WHO), have provided specific guidelines for the safety assessment of GM foods.

More generally, the presence of many varieties of each agricultural and livestock product, together with the increased attention of the customer community, is suggesting the development of reliable methods for assessing and certifying the origin of food, feed, and ingredients, which is of primary importance for the protection of consumers, in particular for fraud prevention (Woolfe and Primrose 2004). In today's global economy, this requires complete traceability, defined as the ability to trace and follow food, feed, and ingredients through all stages of production, processing, and distribution (Raspor 2005). Moreover, the improvements made in molecular techniques, combined with classical methodologies, are allowing the discovery of new markers and parameters for defining the optimal characteristics of a product, on the basis of its organoleptic and nutritional aspects, as well as its consequent potential effects on human health. Among the available and emerging techniques that can be applied on this area related to food safety and quality assessment, molecular methods and, in particular, microarray-based assays are gaining importance and are establishing themselves as a reliable alternative to existing methods. In the last decade, traditional methods for evaluating food safety and quality have been integrated by innovative technologies based on array approaches.

This chapter is presented in four main parts:

1. An overview of the microarray platforms, either commercial or academic, which have been applied in the field.
2. An alternative molecular method, namely the ligation detection reaction, associated to a universal array-based hybridization (LDR–UA).
3. The description of the results obtained by optimizing LDR–UA–based assays onto four chosen applications, covering some of the most common sectors related to food and feed production.
4. A look at the newly discovered and promising DNA-based technologies, which are emerging as potentially interesting for the further development of the food safety/quality area.

## 2.2  OVERVIEW OF EXISTING ARRAY PLATFORMS

The principle of the microarray relies on the key insight, made already over a quarter of a century ago, that labeled nucleic acid molecules can be exploited to probe other nucleic acid molecules attached to a support, thanks to the well-known property of DNA strands to recognize and bind their complementary sequences. Each microarray consists of a solid surface (often glass) upon which is deposited (printed) a large number of discrete aliquots of known nucleotide sequences (probes), which can recognize their target via base complementarities (Ramsay 1998).

Microarrays can be distinguished based upon characteristics such as the nature of the probe, the support type used, and the specific method used for probe addressing and/or target detection. Moreover, thanks to the advances in fabrication, robotics, and bioinformatics, microarray technology has continued to improve in terms of efficiency, discriminatory power, reproducibility, sensitivity, and specificity.

The main applications in food safety/quality field, in which this technology has been developed and employed, are described in detail in the following.

### 2.2.1 GENETICALLY MODIFIED ORGANISM DETECTION IN FOOD

The presence of GM material in food, feed, and food products is governed by European Regulation 1829, which insists on a labeling standard for all products containing GM-based materials. Specifically, materials delivered either directly to the consumer or via a third party must be labeled if their production has involved the use of GM materials, even if the product itself contains no DNA or protein originating from a GMO (as is the case for highly refined products, such as oil or starch). Labeling is required where the content of any authorized GM ingredient exceeds 0.9% of the food or feed product; in this case, the term "genetically modified" must appear in the list of ingredients immediately following the relevant ingredient. Below this threshold, the presence of GM material is considered to be accidental or technically unavoidable, and the product can be sold without labeling. For non-authorized GM ingredients, the threshold is set at 0.5%, provided that the source GMO has been pre-evaluated, and that an appropriate detection method for its presence is available. For seed, the threshold is 0% (i.e., all GM seeds must be labeled) according to 2001/18/EC.

The GM components of a food or feed are considered by some legislation as contaminants (Hemmer 1997), resulting in a considerable demand for analytical methods capable of detecting, identifying, and quantifying the presence of either GM DNA or protein, at the farm gate, the processor, and the retailer levels. Very often, however, the extraction and purification of DNA from the sample is a particularly critical step, in terms of both yield and quality (Cankar et al. 2006, Peano et al. 2004), and requires a careful choice and optimization among the available extraction methods.

Most current detection methods rely either on the polymerase chain reaction (PCR) to amplify transgene sequence(s) or on immunological methods (primarily ELISA, the enzyme-linked immunosorbent assay) to bind to a transgene product. Although specific DNA sequences can be detected by hybridization, it is PCR in its various formats (qualitative PCR, end-point quantitative PCR, and quantitative real-time PCR) that has been generally accepted by the regulatory authorities (Marmiroli et al. 2003). All PCR assays require a minimum number of target DNA sequences to be present in the template and that the sequence of the target DNA is known. Refinements introduced in PCR technology made it the only reliable method to detect the presence of a specific DNA sequence from samples containing little and/or poor quality DNA. PCR-based tests for the presence of GM material have

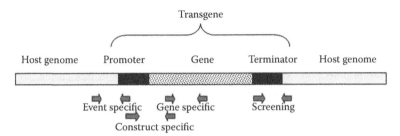

**FIGURE 2.1** Schematic of a typical transgene construct. The host DNA is genomic DNA of the GM crop; the transgene consists of a promoter, the gene itself, and a terminator. Primer pairs targeting particular sequences around and within the transgene integration site are indicated.

been classified according to their level of specificity (Holst-Jensen et al. 2003) into those whose targets are (a) widely used sequences, such as P-35S (CaMV 35S promoter), T-35S (CaMV 35S terminator), T-Nos (terminator of the nopaline synthase gene), bla (β-lactamase), and nptII (neomycin phosphotransferase II); (b) sequences within a specific transgene; (c) sequences that are construct-specific, an example being the junction between the promoter sequence used to drive the transgene and the transgene itself; and (d) sequences that are event-specific, such as the transgene integration site (Figure 2.1). A number of suitable primer pairs have been developed over the last decade, but some of these have a rather limited application range. An increasing number of event-specific assays are now present in GM crops, for example, Roundup Ready™ (RR) in soybean (Taverniers et al. 2001), MON810 (Hernandez et al. 2003a), Bt11 (Holst-Jensen et al. 2003), Starlink (Windels et al. 2003), NK603 (Huang and Pan 2004), and MON863 (Yang et al. 2006) in maize, and MON1445 and MON531 (Yang et al. 2007) in cotton. Some methods based on oligonucleotide arrays, suitable for the detection of "unknown events," have been presented (Tengs et al. 2007).

Moreover, since both the number of authorized transgenic events and the cultivation area of GM crops are rapidly increasing, there is a need to accelerate the methods for GM detection, as well as to be able to identify several transgenes in a single reaction. One approach takes advantage of multiplex PCR, in which several primer pairs are included in the PCR to permit the simultaneous detection of multiple target sequences.

As a result, multiplex PCR has become the prime tool for GM detection (Xu et al. 2007). Multiplex PCR is expected to save considerable time and work in GMO detection by decreasing the number of reactions required. Several studies have shown multiplex PCR to be a rapid and convenient assay for GMO detection (Hernandez et al. 2003b). Matsuoka et al. (2001) developed a multiplex PCR system to distinguish five commercial lines of GM maize. James et al. (2003) described three qualitative multiplex PCR systems for soybean, maize, and canola. A commercially available kit, the Biosmart Allin 1.0 GMO Screening System (Promega, Madison, WI), permits the nested multiplex PCR detection of GMOs containing the CaMV 35S promoter; the kit also detects sequences from soybean and corn and sequences of an internal positive control (i.e., chloroplastic gene).

As the level of multiplexing necessarily rises, it will become evermore difficult to distinguish between the various PCR products on the basis of their amplicon length. To overcome the fact that the outcome of PCR is not always completely unambiguous, some post-PCR control is necessary to confirm sequence identity. The development of a more flexible discriminating tool than conventional electrophoresis is, therefore, of some priority if an ever-broader range of GM crop varieties have to be efficiently genotyped. Thus, microarray technology has the potential to combine detection, identification, and quantification of effectively an unlimited number of GM events in a single experiment (Aarts et al. 2002). In the context of GM detection, a number of features have been derived from transgene sequences, so the hybridization patterns (both qualitative and quantitative) can reveal both whether the analyte represents a GM variety, and which GM events are present.

A new microarray tool was developed by Tengs et al. (2007). The method is PCR independent and applies direct hybridization of total genomic DNA. Using custom-designed microarrays (NimbleExpress arrays, Affymetrix, Santa Clara, CA), they analyzed GM lines of *Arabidopsis thaliana* and *Oryza sativa* showing that, without prior knowledge about the transgene sequence, fragment(s) ($\geq$140 bp) of the element(s) used in the genetic transformation can be identified. These arrays were designed to have 25 bp probes tiled throughout 235 vector sequences downloaded from GenBank. This approach gave good results in detecting specifically and in a very sensitive way the presence of transgene sequences and gave sufficient information for further characterization of unknown genetic constructs in plants. The only requirements were (a) access to a small amount of pure transgene plant material, (b) genetic construct above a certain size (here $\geq$140 bp), and (c) construct showing some degree of sequence similarity with published genetic elements.

Microarray technology can be combined with multiplex PCR, for instance, to assess the content of various transgenic maize events in samples of food and feed by using the multiplex PCR amplicon as the analyte to hybridize onto a DNA array carrying transgenic features (Rudi et al. 2003). A low-density array allowing the parallel detection of nine GM events, including P-35S, T-Nos, and nptII, used biotin labeled amplicons, which were detected colorimetrically (Leimanis et al. 2006). A further low-density array that detects P-35S and T-Nos has been described, as well as corn invertase and soy lectin genes. This array employed a microporous, hydrophobic polyester cloth as a solid support. Similarly, an array containing features based on 8 structural genes has been demonstrated to be informative for the identification of RR soybean (Xu et al. 2005), and has recently been extended to include 20 genetic elements (Xu et al. 2006). This system not only tells whether the sample is made of GMOs, but it can also distinguish which kind of plant it belongs to and which characteristics it has, like insect and herbicide resistance. Specific transgene integration junction sequences were exploited as features to identify one commercial GM-soybean and six GM-maize events (Xu et al. 2007).

A commercial kit, DualChip® GMO, has been developed by Eppendorf Array Technologies (EAT, Namur, Belgium) by coupling multiplex PCR assays to microarray hybridization. The system detects and identifies GM events by screening simultaneously multiple genetic elements. The experimental design consists of four sets of multiplex PCR using biotinylated primers, specific for the amplification of screening elements, species reference elements, and control elements. After multiplex amplification, the PCR products are hybridized on one single microarray containing capture probe sets that are specific for the sequences present in Bt176 maize, MON810 maize, Bt11 sweet maize, MON531 cotton, GA21 maize, and Roundup Ready soya (RRS™) GMO events. The detection of the biotinylated sequences is done using the Silverquant colorimetric detection.

Peptide nucleic acids (PNAs) have been proposed to be superior to oligonucleotides as a basis for microarray features, because their hybridization characteristics are more robust (Weiler et al. 1997). Several PNA-based arrays have been used to identify DNA mutations (Song et al. 2005), and, recently, a PNA chip has been developed for the parallel detection of five transgenes and two plant species in both raw material and processed food (Germini et al. 2005). The protocol for attaching the PNA probes to the slide was modified from that used for oligonucleotides, with spacers added to distance the features from the slide surface. The combination of this array platform with multiplex PCR appears to represent a reliable analytical means for GMO detection in the food chain (Germini et al. 2005, Peano et al. 2005b).

## 2.2.2  FOOD-BORNE PATHOGEN DETECTION

Food-borne outbreaks are infections caused in humans by the consumption of a common contaminated foodstuff. Food-borne illness can also manifest as an intoxication from the consumption of food with preformed toxins and can occur even if viable pathogens are no longer present (i.e., when heating is not required or if the temperature is not sufficient to inactivate the toxins) (Bresee et al. 2002). The major pathogens implicated in this illnesses are *Bacillus cereus*, *Clostridium botulinum*, and *Staphylococcus aureus*, which produce emetic toxin, botulinum toxin, and enterotoxins, respectively (Balaban and Rasooly 2000). Bacteria such as *Escherichia coli* 0157:H7, *Listeria monocytogenes*, and *Campylobacter jejuni* are just few examples of food-borne pathogens associated with meat, cheese, or raw milk, which can cause severe symptoms to children and elderly people. *Salmonella enteritidis* is the most common serovar, and eggs or products thereof are the most frequently implicated foodstuffs.

To minimize the prevalence of food-borne diseases and reduce microbial contaminations in food supplies, effectively monitoring the occurrence and distribution of bacterial pathogens in food is essential. While the risk of contracting such diseases may be in some way reduced by careful food handling procedures in child and elder clinical care facilities, yet the most successful strategy would be to ensure an outstanding food quality and safety along all the food chain, literally "from farm to fork."

Genome sequences are now available for many of the microbes that cause food-borne diseases. This information provides a tool for the rapid detection and identification of such organisms by microarray technology. A pathogen detection array typically consists of many discretely located pathogen-specific detector sequences that are immobilized on a solid support, such as glass slides, to create a microarray. For signal amplification, in general, the target DNA to be tested is amplified using consensus primers that target a genomic region containing the pathogen-specific sequences and is labeled simultaneously or subsequently. In this way, it may be possible to differentiate a large number of organisms using a single PCR, provided that sufficient discriminatory potential exists within the region that is used. Subsequently, labeled amplicons are hybridized to the array under stringent conditions.

To select a common gene fragment for identification of multiple pathogens, such gene must contain conserved regions common to all these pathogens, and, on the other hand, must have sufficient sequence diversity for species identification (Wong et al. 2000). The ribosomal DNA genes contain alternating areas of high conservation and high variability: (1) the variability allows classification over a wide range of taxonomic levels, sometimes even below the species level; (2) the conservation, on the other hand, makes them suitable for identification of different species or genera of bacteria (Wang et al. 2002a, 2002b). Closely related microbial species often differ in a single (single-nucleotide polymorphism, SNP) or in a few bases in such genes. Although the number of mutations in the 16S–23S rRNA spacer region is big, this region very often results too short to identify certain species of bacteria. The mutation rate of 23S rRNA DNA fragment is even larger than that of 16S–23S rRNA DNA spacer region, making it more suitable for bacteria identification. In literature, the 16S rDNA (Helps et al. 1999, Matar et al. 1999, Siqueira et al. 2000, Smith et al. 1996), 23S rDNA (Frahm et al. 1998, Straub et al. 1999, Tesfaye and Holl 1998), and 16S–23S rRNA DNA spacer regions (Gu et al. 1998, Hamid et al. 2002, Madico et al. 2000, Sasaki et al. 2001) have been reported for the identification of bacteria.

Currently, some DNA array technologies have been described as suitable methods to detect multiple food-borne pathogens using a single PCR assay on 16S rRNA region. By using an array of specific oligonucleotides, Chiang et al. (2006) were able to detect strains of *Bacillus* spp., *E. coli*, *Salmonella* spp., *Staphylococcus* spp., and *Vibrio* spp. (which may cause food-borne outbreaks or sporadic cases) at the genus level. A rapid (<4 h) detection method that used universal PCR primers to amplify the variable regions of bacterial 16S rRNA DNA, followed by reverse hybridization of the PCR products to 15 oligonucleotidic selected probes on the chip was developed; 179 out of 182 randomly selected strains were correctly identified with no nonspecific cross-reactions (detection rate >98%). Another 16S-based approach was employed by Eom et al. (2007) for the simultaneous analysis of seven selected food-borne pathogenic bacteria through strategic optimal design of capture probes from characteristic regions of this ribosomal sequence. A statistical criterion on the *p*-value calculation was used to distinguish each target pathogen. A different single PCR approach, based on a mutation-rich region of the 23S rRNA gene was selected as the discrimination target from 14 species and genera of bacteria causing food-borne infections and 2 unrelated bacterial species by Hong et al. (2004). Bacterial DNA was PCR amplified through 23S universal primers and then hybridized onto an oligonucleotide array. Results indicated that 10 species (*Staph. aureus*, *E. coli*, *C. jejuni*, *Shigella dysenteriae*, *Vibrio cholerae*, *Vibrio parahaemolyticus*, *Proteus vulgaris*, *B. cereus*, *L. monocytogenes*, and *C. botulinum*) showed high sensitivity and specificity, whereas 2 others (*Salmonella enterica* and *Yersinia enterocolitica*) gave weak cross-reaction with *E. coli*, but no positive results were obtained on *Clostridium perfringens* and *Streptococcus pyogenes*.

Although the ribosomal genes have been used in a number of diagnostic microarray assays, the presence of highly conserved regions in the 16S rRNA DNA gene and the short and incomplete data of the 16S–23S intergenic spacer and the 23S rRNA DNA gene, respectively, sometimes make these target genes unsuitable for the identification of certain bacteria.

Specific serotype or virulence markers can be used to develop accurate identification and subtyping methods for use in food-borne pathogens microarray, providing a more sensitive, rapid, and informative detection. One of the first applications of this strategy was an oligonucleotide microarray developed for discrimination among strains of *E. coli* and other pathogenic enteric bacteria, using genus- or species-specific virulence genes as targets (Chizhikov et al. 2001). The presence of six genes (*eaeA, slt-I, slt-II, fliC, rfbE*, and *ipaH*) encoding bacterial antigenic determinants and virulence factors of bacterial strains was monitored by multiplex PCR followed by hybridization. To achieve multiplex amplification, relaxed annealing conditions were used, but the limitation of the primer pairs used in multi-PCR system restricted its potential applications in the automated identification and characterization of bacterial pathogens. For the identification of three Vibrio species (*Vibrio vulnificus, V. cholerae*, and *V. parahaemolyticus*) a gene-specific DNA microarray coupled with a multiplex PCR was needed (Panicker et al. 2004), helping to reduce false-negative identification during testing of a complex matrix such as shellfish tissue. Another application of multiple-target array was described by Volokhov et al. (2003) for the identification of four *Campylobacter* species (*C. jejuni, C. coli, C. lari*, and *C. upsaliensis*). This assay relies on the PCR amplification of specific regions in five target genes (*fur, glyA, cdtABC, ceuB-C*, and *fliY*) in separate tubes, followed by one-tube synthesis of all ssRNA transcripts from the T7 promoter and hybridization of the RNA probes to the microarray.

Moreover, in the characterization of 15 serotypes of *Shigella* and *E. coli*, a multiplex PCR approach was used to generate templates for a DNA microarray targeting 3 glycosyltransferase encoding genes (Li et al. 2006). The custom microarray generated by Sergeev et al. (2006) was composed by 19 probe sets, consisting of 5 probes each, on 19 different markers and tested on bacterial strains of *Bacillus* group, obtaining a resolution at species level, with characterization of different strains based on toxicity genes. More recently, Wang et al. (2007) described a composite 16S rRNA, *invA* and *virA* oligonucleotide microarray to identify 22 common pathogenic species, combining PCR amplification and a reverse hybridization of the products to species-specific oligonucleotide probes; 20 out of the 22 bacteria species were successfully identifiable by their 16S rRNA sequence, whereas the remaining 2, *Shigella* spp. and *Salmonella* spp., needed the amplification of *virA* and *invA*, respectively. Thanks to this experimental design, authors obtained a multiple phylogenetic resolution, focusing on species and family/genus level. Although the sensitivity of this microarray assay was 100 CFU/mL on spiked *E. coli* sample, five false negatives out of seven contaminated food samples were detected. The aim of the study by Giannino et al. (2009) was the validation of an oligonucleotide array for the simultaneous detection of a variety of microorganisms in raw milk. In this assay, both universal primers and a specific multiplex PCR were used for the rapid differentiation of bacterial species at low concentrations. The hypervariable regions V3 and V6 of 16S rRNA gene, a variable region of 23S rRNA genes and several genes specific for virulence factors were selected to detect 14 widespread bacterial species, including lactic acid bacteria (LAB) and food-borne pathogens. The differentiation of dominant species in a complex microbial community, such as raw milk, was achieved by the application of short discriminating probes differing by few nucleotides. Finally, a low-density microarray, using 14 species-specific gene targets, was applied to simultaneously detect 4 important pathogens (*E. coli* O157:H7, *S. enterica*, *L. monocytogenes*, and *C. jejuni*) causing food-related human illnesses worldwide (Suo et al. 2010). Targeting 14 species-specific and 2 toxin genes, the resolution of the array was at species level and a detection sensitivity of $10^{-4}$ ng (approximately 20 copies) of each genomic DNA was obtained by hybridizing the 14-plex PCR products amplified. In order to reliably detect low abundant pathogens in food, selective enrichment of the target pathogens for at least 8 h was considered to be necessary for most detection methods.

A last strategy to select target sequences involves the screening of random parts of the genome to find diagnostic sequences. Nevertheless, since the location of possible useful sequences in the genome is a priori unknown, there are few sequence data available for comparison to other organisms in order to guarantee specificity. As a consequence, extensive screening is required to ensure specificity of a potential marker. In Perreten et al. (2005), detection of up to 90 antibiotic resistance genes in gram-positive bacteria was successfully performed by hybridization of genomic DNA onto the commercial ArrayTubes platform (Clondiag Technologies, Jena, Germany). Each antibiotic resistance gene is represented by two specific oligonucleotides chosen from consensus sequences of gene families, except for nine genes for which only one specific oligonucleotide could be developed. In this way, the microarray was composed of a total of 137 oligonucleotides. However, antibiotic resistance due to single-base mutations of the target genes could not be considered, since highly stringent annealing temperatures would be necessary to obtain a specific hybridization. Furthermore, Kim et al. (2008) fabricated a specific 70-mer oligonucleotide array by comparing the genomic sequence of each target pathogen with the genomic sequences of other nonpathogenic bacteria, including those of some closely related to food-borne pathogens. The microarray that targeted 16 bacterial species, was composed of 112 probes, including positive and negative control oligonucleotides and showed a resolution at species level.

### 2.2.3   FARM ANIMAL GENOTYPING FOR FOOD QUALITY ASSESSMENT

Farm animal populations harbor rich collections of mutations with phenotypic effects that have been purposefully enriched by breeding. In livestock, the identification of genes that control growth, energy metabolism, development, appetite, reproduction and behavior, as well as other traits that have been manipulated by breeding are of particular interest. The majority of these economically important traits are complex, continuously distributed phenotypes, which are influenced by multiple polygenes located at quantitative trait loci (QTL), dispersed across the genome. Genome research in farm animals adds to our basic understanding of the genetics a deeper control over these traits; the results will be applied in breeding programs to reduce the incidence of disease and to improve product quality and production efficiency (Andersson 2001).

Substantial advances have been made over the past decades through the application of molecular genetics in the identification of genes and chromosomal regions that contain loci affecting traits of importance in livestock production (Andersson 2001). This has enabled opportunities to enhance genetic improvement programs in livestock by direct selection of genes or genomic regions that affect economic traits through marker-assisted selection (Dekkers and Hospital 2002). The reason for the current vital interest in SNPs is the hope that they could be used as markers to identify genes associated with QTLs. To verify the practical usability of candidate SNPs in marker-assisted selection applied to local population, there is a need for a uniform and cost-effective methodological platform, allowing for simultaneous genotyping of many SNPs.

In cattle, several SNPs were found as candidate polymorphisms linked to QTLs (Schwerin 2001). For example, more than 95% of the proteins contained in ruminant milk are coded by six well-characterized structural genes (Martin et al. 2002): two for the main whey proteins α-LA and β-LG (LALBA and LGB genes), and four for the CN, αS1-CN, αS2-CN, β-CN, and κ-CN (CSN1S1, CSN1S2, CSN2, and CSN3, respectively), which are tightly linked in a 250 kb cluster (Ferretti et al. 1990, Threadgill and Womack 1990) on chromosome 6 (Hayes et al. 1993, Popescu et al. 1996). A recent revision of milk protein nomenclature considering only protein polymorphisms (Farrell et al. 2004) includes 8 αS1-CN, 4 αS2-CN, 12 β-CN, 11 κ-CN, 11 β-LG, and 3 α-LA variants within the genus *Bos*. In addition to the effects of milk protein variants on milk composition and cheese-making properties (Di Stasio and Mariani 2000, Martin et al. 2002), statistically significant associations with several milk production traits have also been identified for sites of polymorphism within noncoding regions in the CN complex (Martin et al. 2002). This is the case of a polymorphism within the short interspersed nucleotide element Bov-A2 in the second intron of CSN3, described by Damiani et al. (2000), and of the polymorphisms of the CSN1S1 promoter, described by Prinzenberg et al. (2003). Thus, the CN cluster polymorphisms have to be considered as a whole complex in which expression sequence polymorphisms could help explain the productive implications of the different CN loci and the results obtained from the detection of CN gene effects on productive traits at the haplotype level (Boettcher et al. 2004, Braunschweig et al. 2000, Ikonen et al. 2001).

The importance of going deeper into the knowledge on milk protein polymorphisms in cattle is, therefore, evident. The availability of a fast method that allows the simultaneous typing of a great number of mutations affecting milk protein structure and composition could help researchers, as well as breeding associations, to identify the genetic milk protein variations. Microarray technology offered the potential of opening new doors in the study of genome complexity, thanks to the extreme degree of parallelization (Ramsay 1998).

Arrays can be used to study DNA, with the primary aim being the identification and the genotyping of genetic polymorphisms. Hybridization and hybridization plus enzymatic processing were the two diverse approaches available to discriminate among different alleles when using microarray technology (Hacia 1999,

Kurg et al. 2000, Pastinen et al. 2000). As an example applied to animal characterization, an oligonucleotide microarray based on the arrayed primer extension technique was described by Kaminski et al. (2006), allowing for the parallel genotyping of many SNPs located in genes involved in cow milk protein biosynthesis to identify those associated with milk performance traits.

This oligonucleotide microarray was used to identify which of the 16 candidate SNPs were associated with milk performance traits in Holstein cows. Four hundred cows were genotyped by the developed and validated microarray, finding significant associations between four single SNPs, namely DGAT1 (acyloCoA:diacylglycerol acyltransferase), LTF (lactoferrin), CSN3 (κ-casein), and GHR (growth hormone receptor) and fat and protein yield and percentages. Many significant associations between combined genotypes (almost two SNPs) and milk performance traits were found. For example, the associations between the combined genotypes DGAT1/LTF and DGAT1/LEPTIN analyzed traits were well studied.

The use of SNP markers in candidate genes that are thought to be associated with certain QTLs is the only choice for genomes for which no whole genome SNP database is available, providing the presence of a good number of SNPs dispersed in many publicly available resources. In the pig genome, for example, good candidates for such approaches are SNPs within genes associated directly, indirectly, or potentially, with pork yield and quality. So far, most functional effects of polymorphisms have been evaluated for single SNPs. To date, candidate SNPs have been genotyped individually by different methods (RFLP, SSCP, DGGE, and sequencing). Further exploration of the variation of pork traits should combine data on as many candidate SNPs as possible. In the near future, gene interaction studies will give better insight into the genetic basis of pork qualities. It is thought that the simultaneous genotyping of many informative SNPs in a uniform population will lead to a better understanding of the genetic background of pork traits.

Recently, a microarray allowing for simultaneous genotyping of 85 SNPs located in 81 candidate genes involved in pork traits of potential interest in pig-breeding programs was developed. SNiPORK is an oligonucleotide microarray based on the APEX technique cited earlier, allowing genotyping of SNPs in genes of interest for pork yield and quality traits (Kaminski et al. 2008). For the 85 selected SNPs, 100% repeatability was proved by double genotyping of 13 randomly chosen boars. The primary application of the SNiPORK chip was the simultaneous genotyping of dozens of SNPs to study gene interaction and, consequently, better understand the genetic background of pork yield and quality. The chip may prospectively be used for evolutionary studies, evaluation of genetic distances between wild and domestic pig breeds, traceability tests, as well as the starting point for developing a platform for identification and paternity analysis.

### 2.2.4 OLIVE OIL TRACEABILITY AND AUTHENTICITY

Olive (*Olea europaea* L.) cultivation and olive oil production are important economic activities in the Mediterranean basin. Olive oil consumption is increasing throughout the entire world, especially due to its beneficial health effects. Depending on the extraction procedure, olive oil may be classified as extra-virgin, virgin, refined, or olive-pomace oil (International Olive Council 2006). Extra-virgin oil is considered of the highest quality, with regard to both organoleptic and health aspects. However, even among extra-virgin oils, quality varies depending on the cultivars and on the employed environmental conditions of growth. To help consumers in distinguishing these oils on the basis of their characteristics and origins, the European Union has established awards such as Protected Designation of Origin (PDO), Registered Designation of Origin (RDO), Protected Geographical Indication (PGI), and Traditional Speciality Guaranteed (TSG) (article 2 of EU Reg. 2018/92). In recent years, increased attention to food safety has stimulated the interest in the authenticity of food products. Traceability is of fundamental importance for extra-virgin olive oils, especially those claiming PDO, RDO, or PGI status.

DNA markers have been used to identify olive cultivars, and they are increasingly being applied to solve traceability and provenance issues (Consolandi et al. 2008). Food DNA analysis may represent an attractive and alternative choice to the more classical analytical methods, because DNA, compared to other macromolecules and metabolites, is less influenced by environmental and processing conditions and provides an opportunity for direct comparison of different genetic material (Martins-Lopes et al. 2008, Pafundo et al. 2005, 2007, Pasqualone et al. 2007). However, Claros et al. (2000) gave evidence that soil and climate (indirectly related to the geographic origin) had significant influence on cultivar differentiation during the years. In addition, Breton et al. (2004) found that the genetic diversity of olive cultivars was strongly dependent on the region and country of origin.

Since the discovery of amplifiable DNA from olive oil, different genetic markers have been used to target DNA in an attempt to recognize the cultivar employed for the production. The genetic markers are amplified fragments of DNA, the most useful of which are randomly amplified polymorphic DNA (RAPD), sequence characterized amplified region (SCAR), amplified fragment length polymorphism (AFLP), inter-simple sequence repeat (ISSR), and microsatellites or simple sequence repeat (SSR). The most important uses of these genetic markers can be summarized in three aspects. First, genetic markers can be used to distinguish olive tree cultivars, extracting the DNA from the olive leaves (Gemas et al. 2004, Sanz-Cortes et al. 2003). This usually includes a clustering or discriminant analysis to perform a classification of the olive varieties studied. Moreover, in some discriminant analyses, the geographical influence of the growing location of the olive trees was shown (Gemas et al. 2004).

Second, genetic markers can be used to distinguish olive varieties when DNA is extracted directly from the olive oils (Breton et al. 2004, Martins-Lopes et al. 2008, Muzzalupo et al. 2007, Pasqualone et al. 2007). This procedure has some limitations because oil DNA is highly degraded and many interferences exist. In this sense, microsatellites, which consist of a specific sequence of DNA bases or nucleotides that contains mono-, di-, tri-, or tetra-tandem repeats, were used by Breton et al. (2004), allowing the main cultivar used for an elaborated olive oil to be distinguished.

Finally, the traceability from olive leaves to olive oils was the aim of some researchers (Doveri et al. 2006, Muzzalupo et al. 2007, Pafundo et al. 2005, 2007), which found a high degree of concordance between DNA extracted from olive leaves and the DNA extracted from olive oils, when the DNA extraction procedure for both samples was well established. However, DNA extracted from olive oil was highly degraded and contaminated with inhibitors of PCR reactions, which limited the applicability of DNA genetic markers to internal olive oil traceability (Montemurro et al. 2008, Pafundo et al. 2007). Two reasons were the main factors affecting the reproducibility of this traceability method. On the one hand, the amount of DNA extracted from leaf, flesh, embryo, and paste samples was variable because DNA was recovered more from leaves than from any other material (Doveri et al. 2006). On the other hand, the quantity and quality of DNA extracted from the olive leaves or the olive oils had a great influence on the PCR conditions and provided low reproducibility for the genetic markers used (Claros et al. 2000). For this reason, the methods used for DNA extraction in olive leaves or olive oils are varied. The cetyltrimethylammonium bromide (CTAB) method (Murray and Thompson 1980) has been the most used for DNA extraction. CTAB is a cationic detergent, which solubilizes membranes and forms DNA complexes.

In general, the comparison of DNA extracted from leaves and oils is difficult. For example, Montemurro et al. (2008) used AFLP markers, DNA sequences that allow the simultaneous screening of a large number of specific locations (loci) without any preliminary sequence knowledge, to obtain the AFLP electrophoretic patterns of leaf and oil DNAs. Since patterns showed differences in the band intensity between the two agarose gels, the authors suggested that results depended on the different quality of DNA extracted in the studied samples. Doveri et al. (2006) found a high degree of nonconcordance between commercial monovarietal olive oil DNA and DNA from a reference leaf. They concluded that the commercial monovarietal olive oils could contain up to 5%–10% of oil deriving from other cultivars.

As a consequence, to date, the only array platform for olive oil quality assessment is the one developed by Consolandi et al. (2007, 2008), which will be described in detail in Section 2.4.2.

In conclusion, olive oil traceability is gaining importance due to the development of olive oils with specific characteristics. Consumers demand high-quality olive oils, including those with PDO labels or coupage/monovarietal oils with certain properties characteristic of the olive variety from which they are elaborated. It is necessary to find new traceability markers less influenced by the environmental conditions, fruit ripening, and extraction technology than compositional markers and more easily obtainable than DNA markers.

The investigation of other biomacromolecular components present in olive oils as novel traceability markers could be promising for establishing the botanical origin of olive oils because they may present a high differentiation potential due to their own molecular complexity.

## 2.3   PCR–LDR–UA PLATFORM

Homemade assays were developed with the specific aim of overcoming the limits generally related to "very high density" arrays, such as low flexibility and multiplexing. However, standard hybridization protocols, although simpler than other assays, often suffer from reproducibility issues and nontrivial optimizations due to the probes' melting temperatures, hybridization buffers, washing solutions stringencies, etc.

Thus, a new brand of assays based on the properties of specific enzymes was developed: they can be classified on the basis of their molecular principle or on the interface type between the molecular species. Conventional solid-phase arrays, operating on a solid–liquid interface, have some important disadvantages. One is that the analyte solution is static on the array during hybridization and each arrayed spot actually samples only from its immediate or near-immediate environment. Second, the high concentration of DNA present at each feature can generate steric hindrance during the hybridization reaction. Several alternative array systems have been developed in the attempt to overcome these shortcomings. An example is the Nanogen system (www.nanogen.com/technologies/microarray) in which the probability of successful hybridization events is enhanced by attaching a negative electric charge to the analyte, and providing the features with a positive charge. In gel-based DNA chips, steric hindrance is reduced because the surface over which hybridization occurs is three dimensional. A rather different approach dispenses altogether with the concept of a solid support, and instead attaches the probes to microspheres, which are held in a liquid suspension (e.g., suspension array technology (Nolan and Sklar 2002) and bead array counter (Edelstein et al. 2000)). The large numbers of features presented on the microarray imply a large data output, so the design and provision of adequate data analysis instrumentation are becoming increasingly important. This is an active area of product development, driven by the interest in gene expression profiling, where analysis of large datasets is already routine (Miraglia et al. 2004).

Among the available liquid-phase assays, based on different molecular alternative molecular approaches, we chose to apply a PCR–ligation detection reaction combined with universal arrays (PCR–LDR–UA) technique, which was developed to uncouple the probe/target recognition and annealing from the microarray hybridization, reducing costs and conferring higher flexibility and selectivity. This method appears to be a scalable and robust protocol, applicable in all the aforementioned fields.

### 2.3.1 DESCRIPTION OF THE MOLECULAR MECHANISM

The PCR–LDR–UA was introduced in the late 1990s by Gerry et al. (1999). This molecular array approach relates to the detection of nucleic acid sequence differences using, upstream, a PCR amplification reaction of a target region using specific primers, and, then, a ligation, a hybridization capture, and a detection phase (Figure 2.2).

The *amplification step* (Figure 2.2A) is performed through PCR on a single or multiple target(s), in order to increase the quantity of the specific DNA fragments within a sample, as well as reduce its molecular complexity; this technique allows the subsequent molecular reactions to be performed with higher specificity and sensitivity.

The *ligation phase* (Figure 2.2B) utilizes a LDR between one oligonucleotide probe that has a target sequence-specific portion and an addressable array-specific portion, called common probe (CP), and a second oligonucleotide probe, called discriminating oligo (DS), having a target sequence-specific portion and a detectable label. This step requires a sample containing one or more nucleotide sequences with

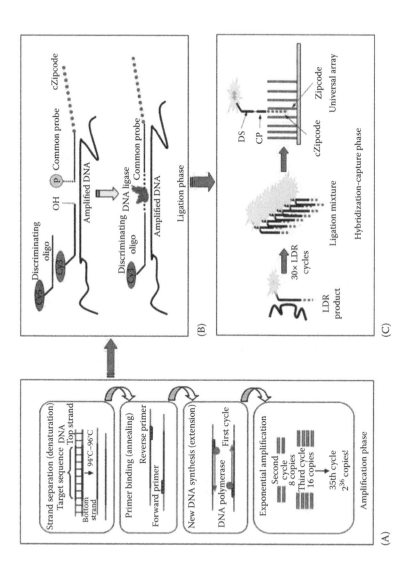

**FIGURE 2.2** Description of the PCR–LDR–UA molecular mechanism. The approach is composed of: (A) specific PCR amplification, in which the target DNA is amplified and the complexity of the sample reduced; (B) ligation step, in which a thermostable ligase seals together the CP and the DS, the presence of a perfect match between the template and the probe pair; and (C) hybridization-capture phase, in which the fluorescent molecules are hybridized on the UA and addressed to specific positions through zipcode sequences.

a plurality of sequence differences. These two oligonucleotide probes in a particular set are suitable for ligating together when hybridized adjacent to one another on a corresponding target nucleotide sequence. However, they have at least one mismatch that interferes with such ligation when hybridized to another nucleotide sequence present in the sample. The method relies on the high selectivity of a thermostable DNA ligase enzyme, which requires perfect complementarity of dsDNA structure to successfully catalyze the covalent joining of two adjacently hybridized probes. The DNA ligase enzyme seals the nick between the two adjacent oligonucleotides (the CP and the DS), annealed to a complementary target, only if the oligonucleotides are perfectly base-paired, in particular, at the junction site. The sample, the plurality of oligonucleotide probe sets, and the ligase are blended to form a mixture that is subjected to more ligase detection reaction cycles comprising a denaturation treatment and an annealing treatment. The denaturation treatment involves separating any annealed oligonucleotides from the target nucleotide sequences, so that target DNA could act as a template for other molecules in further cycled ligation reactions.

The next phase of the process is the *hybridization-capture phase* (Figure 2.2C), which needs a solid support with capture oligonucleotides immobilized at particular known sites. The capture oligonucleotides are complementary to the addressable array-specific portions of the CPs. The mixture, after being subjected to the ligation phase, is contacted with the solid support under conditions effective to hybridize the addressable array-specific portions to the capture oligonucleotides in a base-specific manner. As a result, the addressable array-specific portions are captured on the solid support at the site with the complementary capture oligonucleotides.

The presence of a specific target is determined by hybridizing the content of a LDR to an addressable DNA UA, on which every single spot contains oligonucleotides with a unique zipcode (Chen et al. 2000). Zipcodes are oligonucleotides, 24 bases in length, that have been designed to have closely matched melting temperature values ($T_m = 70°C–82°C$) and minimal sequence homology with the natural genome. Each zipcode sequence is composed of 6 tetramers: the 256 ($4^4$) possible combinations in which the 4 bases can be arranged as tetramers were reduced to a set of 36; these were chosen such that the tetramer differed from all others by at least 2 bases. These 24-mers hybridize specifically to molecules containing sequences that are complementary to the zipcodes. A unique zipcode complement is affixed to the 3′ end of each CP. By linking the zipcode complements to fluorescent primers via a tandem PCR–LDR strategy, zipcode microarrays can be used to assess the presence of mutations in biological specimens. During hybridization, the cZipcode drives the LDR product to the corresponding zipcode on the chip surface. Detection of a hybridized LDR product is accomplished by the visualization of specific fluorophores, either Cy3 or Cy5, attached to the 5′ end of the discriminating primers. Because the zipcodes represent unique artificial sequences, zipcode microarrays can be used as a "universal platform" for molecular recognition, by simply changing the gene-specific sequences linked to the zipcode complements.

The last experimental phase is the *detection step*. During this step of the process, the reporter labels of the ligated product sequences are captured on the solid support at particular sites. When the presence of the fluorophore bound to the solid support is detected, usually via an image acquisition (i.e., scanning) of the arrays with lasers set at proper wavelengths, the respective presence of one or more specific nucleotide sequences in the sample is indicated.

This molecular mechanism contains a number of advantages over prior systems. Using the UA, it is possible to overcome one of the major limitations of DNA microarray approaches based on hybridization. Optimal hybridization conditions are difficult to determine for large sets of different probes, which need to be hybridized on a DNA chip at the same time. Other array-based SNP genotyping methods exist, such as single base primer extension (Pastinen et al. 2000) and arrayed primer extension (Kaminski et al. 2005, Kurg et al. 2000), but optimal probes must be designed for each SNP and multiplexing may be difficult or impossible. In the UA-based approach, the optimization of hybridization conditions for each probe set is not required. The LDR–UA platform is particularly interesting for its need of only an initial optimization. During the hybridization reaction, the cZipcode sequences appended to the CPs hybridize with the complementary zipcodes of the UA. Inasmuch as the zipcodes were already designed for this purpose, it is unnecessary to set new hybridization conditions, and new probe pairs can be added to the array without further optimization, thus reducing costs and setup time. Furthermore, problems due to secondary structures of the target DNA or steric hindrances of differently sized nucleic acid hybrids formed on the microarrays after hybridization are minimized. However, this method requires an extra step (the ligation) with respect to DNA microarray approaches based on hybridization. Furthermore, this platform can be used to carry out multiplex analyses of complex genetic systems: it is possible to target several PCR amplicons at the same time in a single ligation reaction (multiplexing). As a result, a large number of nucleotide sequence differences in a sample can be detected at one time.

## 2.3.2 Strategies for Probe Design

In all DNA array-based technologies, the recognition mechanism is accomplished through exploiting the capability of nucleic acid single strands to recognize their complementary sequences. Thus, the discriminative power (i.e., sensitivity and specificity) of each assay is largely dependent on the DNA sequences actually used as probes and their ability to selectively hybridize on their target complement. For this reason, the probe design step is one of the most critical and important of each experiment.

Many different applications of microarray technology in food safety field have been developed. In the scientific community, the determination of a common strategy for approaching the probe design step and which can be employed in all (or in the majority) of them is nearly impossible. Bacterial databases themselves are constantly and frequently upgraded, often undergoing changes of classification, thus making an exhaustive and definitive design of the best probes very hard. Moreover, the so-called resolution of the assays can vary according to the different phylogenetic levels of bacterial taxonomy, focusing on either species level, within a limited number of families, or on subspecies, on a single or very few species.

Many differences are due to the different molecular techniques adopted in any application; many others, on the other hand, to inter-lab variability, related mainly to the different pipelines that groups working on microarray have established in their multiyear experience. Each one tends to approach this step according to what they have, experimentally and empirically, determined as the best strategy. Anyway, the main features that have to be accomplished in any probe design can be summarized in the following:

1. Maximize the specificity of the probes to the interesting species ("positive set") and reduce the nonspecific signal due to interaction of the probes to all other species present in a sample ("negative set").
2. When dealing with probes designed at different phylogenetic level (i.e., interrogating different species/families), minimize the possibility to have undesired cross talk that obfuscates the discrimination.
3. Have a nearly identical response during hybridization of the DNA target, via similar melting temperatures for all the probes.
4. Preserve the accessibility of the probes to the target, avoiding the formation of secondary structures (i.e., hairpins, self-match, etc.).

Designing reliable oligonucleotide probes on bacterial genomes is not a trivial task, due to their generally low GC content, their low sequence complexity, or many repeats leading to cross-hybridization. For this reason, oligonucleotides with length in the range of 20–80 nt are usually preferred in current microarray detection applications. Advantages and drawbacks of short and long oligonucleotide probes have been discussed and pointed out in previous works (Chou et al. 2004, Relogio et al. 2002), whose conclusions can be summarized as follows: shorter oligonucleotide probes (~25 nt) are characterized by a higher sensitivity, detecting even a minor genetic variant (i.e., single nucleotide mismatch) between the template and the probe in a bacterial population; second, they allow multiple probe design per each target, decreasing the possibility of false-positive calls. On the other hand, longer (~70 nt) probes seem to be characterized by higher specificity and stronger fluorescent signals of the hybridized targets.

In any case, to achieve optimal results, it is fundamental that the starting set of sequences is carefully selected: many sequences with low-similarity regions in the initial dataset bias the probe design by badly aligned subsequences. Sequences of off-target or distantly related species could negatively act in the process of multiple alignment, as well, leading to poorly aligned datasets and erroneous designs. On the other side, using sequences nearly identical to each other can cause the opposite behavior, in which no discriminating positions can be determined. When the number of species to be targeted is too high and/or the difference between the selected genomic regions is too low, a critical grouping of the context-specific sequences in clusters can be performed. This operation maximizes the detection power and minimizes the possibility of cross talk between the probes. Moreover, standard molecular procedures, like PCR amplification, can help in enriching the sample, discriminating the subsets of sequences that constitute the actual database from those completely unrelated to the biological context. The actual strategy for implementing the probes depends strongly on the molecular techniques adopted in the detection assay. Hybridization-based probes are certainly the most popular and commonly used in microarray detection experiments: mutations are identified on the basis of the higher thermal stability of the perfectly matched probes as compared to mismatched probes. When used for probe design in detection application, the strategies based on internal mismatches, or on unique stretches of nucleotides, rely upon a decreased melting temperature of mismatched duplexes rather than on a perfectly matched base pair between the probe and the target.

This choice, although reasonable and cost saving, undergoes a series of drawbacks, which have to be considered carefully, especially when dealing with high-complexity samples: in order to have the maximum available sensitivity in detecting mismatches, where possible, multiple mutations are desirable to discriminate between target and nontarget sequences; this represents a hindrance for the usually short length of the probes and also imposes a series of optimizations in the thermo-dynamic parameters of the candidates, which should possess similar or nearly identical melting temperatures, apart from not being subjected to secondary structure formations during hybridization. A careful *in silico* check of the candidate probes is necessary for excluding any possible undesired match with nontarget sequences. BLAST alignment tool (Altschul et al. 1990) has been employed for this purpose in a wide number of published applications (Sergeev et al. 2006, Suo et al. 2010, Wang et al. 2007). Moreover, many available software performing probe designs base their specificity checks on BLAST or on extensive specificity checks (Vijaya Satya et al. 2008), even when it implies a huge number of comparisons and computations.

Although very complete, this procedure is actually inapplicable for experiments on a reduced number of species or in which the complexity has been reduced by means of molecular procedures, since the time and the instrumentation required for running the program are disproportionate to the final result, making it too computationally intensive and unnecessary for the scope. Therefore, for analytical and diagnostic purposes, hybridization is generally combined with some other selection or enrichment procedures. Enzyme-mediated methods, on the other hand, rely on interrogation of a mutation by combining the action of specific oligonucleotides to enzymes capable of a fine discrimination at base level. In this case, the search is for a single base that characterizes a species against all the others in a group of interest. The presence of a point mutation is assessed by correct enzyme-mediated base pairing.

Ligase-based methods rely upon the discriminative power of ligases or polymerases–ligases mixtures for assessing genotype in specific positions of the selected genomic target. Probe design, in this case, is characterized by fewer problems connected to specificity, provided there is a dataset as complete as possible. Moreover, the use of thermally stable enzymes allows the reactions to occur at relatively high temperatures, avoiding many of the problems related to secondary structures, which are less likely to occur at typical LDR annealing temperatures (i.e., around 65°C) than the majority of microarray hybridization temperatures (i.e., around 45°C).

Among the available software, a few of them have implemented probes for molecular techniques other than hybridization: PathogenMIPer (Thiyagarajan et al. 2006) works on molecular inversion assays, starting with a selection of unique sequences on a reduced dataset and, then, with a global comparison to all non-target genomes; ProbeMaker (Stenberg et al. 2005), instead, is a multi-application framework, which takes a set of target sequences and a number of so-called tag sequences as input. These tag sequences are multipurpose targets for a plethora of applications (e.g., restriction sites, binding sites for amplification primers, or fluorescent detection probes).

In a recent application of the PCR–LDR–UA technique to the identification of 15 major food-borne and disease-related bacteria in milk samples (Cremonesi et al. 2009), we employed ORMA (oligonucleotide retrieving for molecular applications) (Severgnini et al. 2009), a bioinformatic tool, specifically designed for searching and determining discriminating positions among sets of highly homologous sequences. A graphical representation of this concept is depicted in Figure 2.3. The software allowed the creation of 15 consensus out of the 752 constituting the initial dataset of milk pathogens 16S rRNA gene sequences and the design of 392 candidates, which were ranked according to the ORMA-calculated scores and selected one per target species. This design tool is especially valuable in analyzing sequences coming from genomic regions, like those of 16S rRNA gene, which are characterized by both highly conserved and highly mutating regions. ORMA searches specifically for regions having one or more bases specific to the desired target and not to any other sequence possibly involved into the design. Optionally, sequences can be grouped together to form homogeneous clusters on which a consensus sequence can be calculated. The software was implemented as a network of MATLAB® scripts, designed to perform an accurate search of all the positions able to specifically discriminate sequences belonging to the positive set among all those constituting the negative set. A series of filters and scores are calculated in order to give a rank to the candidate probes and select high-quality oligonucleotide probes to be used in molecular applications. The intra-group and the inter-group scores are used to retrieve a list of probes covering the highest number of species of the positive set (intra-group score) and having the lowest interaction (inter-group score) with those of the negative set. Provided that the initial database of sequences is accurate, updated, and as complete as possible, ORMA can determine discriminating positions and specific probes on any set of sequences, in any gene or genomic region. Its implementation, in fact, is not based on an internal database of sequences, which are, instead, retrieved and loaded from external resources. The multiple alignment step needed for using the tool can be performed according to one of the many available software and formats, such as fasta files, formatted multiple sequence files (.msf) and Clustal-like aligned files (.aln). Due to its modular structure and the straightforwardness of other applications from the already implemented one, probe set retrieval and filtering methods could be easily added, extending ORMA for the use in other molecular applications: the design of probes for mini-sequencing application would imply the determination of one probe with its 3′ end one base before the variation, whereas the design of a reporting probe for a TaqMan real-time PCR assay would mean the determination of one oligonucleotide with the single base variation in the middle of the sequence.

The LDR application represents an extreme complexity reduction procedure for making the probe design and specificity check easier on GMO detection in soybean and maize (Peano et al. 2005a). The five tested varieties, in fact, underwent a specific primer design to amplify the junction regions of the recombinant DNA constructs; thus, the fragment used for subsequent detection, is one of the specific constructs of

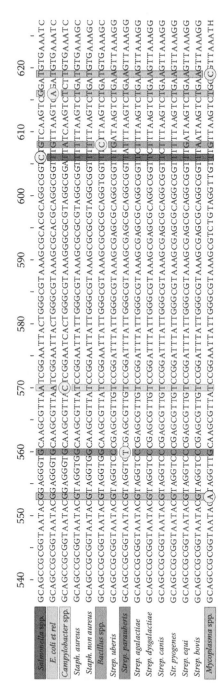

**FIGURE 2.3** Partial alignment of group-specific 16S rRNA consensus sequences belonging to a milk pathogen detection assay and an example of the probe design using ORMA for *Salmonella*, *E. coli et rel*, *Campylobacter*, *Bacillus*, *Strep. Parauberis*, and *Mycoplasma*. The positions of interest for each bacterial group are indicated by boxes of different shades of gray, and the discriminating base is circled.

that variety and represents a unique sequence on which the LDR probe pairs have to be built on. Primers were optimized in order to generate short-length amplicons (maximum length 241 bp) and to perform multiplex PCRs without generating excessive quantities of primer dimers. The LDR oligonucleotide probes were designed on these unique amplified sequences, with length giving similar thermodynamic features.

Probe design for microarray-based assays for food quality assessment is basically different from the procedure used for pathogen or GMO detection. In fact, in this kind of application, the positions to be tested are, usually, known *a priori*, thus avoiding the need to search for discriminating bases. Considering the case of bi-allelic polymorphisms, each point can assume only one out of three possible values (homozygosis AA or BB or heterozygosis AB). Given a certain number of samples (or varieties) and their haplotype on a group of molecular markers, the design pipeline should accomplish the following tasks:

1. Determine the minimum number of polymorphisms needed to correctly discriminate between the different varieties under analysis.
2. Design a set of probes insisting on the selected polymorphisms according to chosen molecular approach.
3. Test the specificity of the designed probe pair against the negative-set database.

For example, in the application reported in Chessa et al. (2007), a total of 22 SNP markers in 8 fragments of cattle genome have been selected, since they have been recognized as playing an important role in the bovine milk protein production. Similarly to the GMO detection experiment, although applied on a two-color array, the assay was based on a multiplex PCR that simultaneously amplified all the fragments containing the selected SNPs. Thus, the LDR probe pairs were selected to insist on those positions, with optimizations needed to have nearly identical melting temperatures. Each allele of the polymorphism was associated with a discriminating probe fluorescently labeled in either Cy3 or Cy5. For the two deletions present in the CSN1S1 promoter, two CPs were designed. Due to the lack of a negative set, the specificity of the absence of homology with other sequences was checked in the GenBank database using BLAST. Similarly, in Consolandi et al. (2008), the fragments containing the 17 SNPs for the characterization of 49 monovarietal oils were preamplified through a multiplex PCR. Thus, the probe design was based on those known positions, with no particular difficulty, provided there is an in silico specificity check via BLAST. While the steps indicated as points 2 and 3 are common to all probe designs and have been described in detail for detection assays in the previous paragraphs, point 1 represents an important and nontrivial procedure. Although, conceptually, the task is apparently simple (i.e., determine which is the minimum set of polymorphisms needed to discriminate among a given number of varieties), this is easier said than done when it has to be implemented via an algorithm in an automated way. A recent addiction we made to ORMA is a procedure for reducing the complexity of an assay to the essential SNPs, through the iterative exclusion of one polymorphism at a time. Basically, given $n$ as the number of varieties and $m$ as the number of SNPs, the algorithm tests if, discarding one polymorphism, the $m - 1$ remaining are still sufficient to grant a unique molecular fingerprint of all the *n* varieties. If such, the procedure is iterated until two or more varieties could not be distinguished any more. Since the minimum set can be dependent on the order on which the SNPs are iteratively excluded from the analysis, a series of permutations are performed, testing all permutations (in case of less than 6 polymorphisms, i.e., 720 permutations, equal to *n*!) or a maximum of 1000 random shifts of the data. The new reduced set of SNPs is used to design the candidate probes for each of the varieties under analysis.

### 2.3.3 DATA ANALYSIS

Data analysis in microarray detection experiments in food safety contexts depends largely on the laboratory experience in microarray data analysis and on the software used, as happens with probe design strategies. Actually, there is no already established pipeline or a unique way to deal with the data. However, the common task of all the strategies employed in all the applications in the field is to determine, for each probe, whether its signal is significantly different from both the background and the nonspecific signal. One of the most common and simplest strategies is based on calculating a ratio of the specific and the background signal, assigning then a threshold for flagging the found ratio as significant for the presence of a probe or not. The threshold, very often, is arbitrary, let us say 3 or 10 times the background (Sergeev et al. 2006, Wang et al. 2007) or its standard deviation (Ahn and Walt 2005); sometimes, an internal negative control is considered as the reference for the comparison (Suo et al. 2010). When multiple probes are used for assessing the presence of a target, even lower thresholds (e.g., PM/MM ratio >1.5 in Wilson et al. (2002), based on Affymetrix arrays) can be used. Multiple probe correction accomplished through replicates of the same probe can be used to increase the robustness of each call and reduce the occurrence of false positives and negatives. Usually, three or four replicates are averaged or requested to be consistently present (Sergeev et al. 2006, Suo et al. 2010). The influence of local background phenomena is taken into account by background subtraction from the signal, in order to consider only the part of the fluorescent intensity directly associated with the hybridization of the labeled molecules to the probe features and not aspecifically lying on the microarray surface. In Peano et al. (2005a), local background was subtracted from the mean intensity of each feature and mean and standard deviation for quadruplicate samples were calculated. The hybridization fluorescence intensities from nonspecific zipcodes were calculated and averaged. A signal-to-noise ratio, calculated as the ratio between the average intensity of specific and nonspecific signals, was obtained. A threshold of three was used to determine if this ratio indicated a specific hybridization signal or an unspecific one.

More recently, some other groups, on the other hand, adopted statistical concepts in order to have a more robust estimation of which targets are really present and which only possess a weak signal, possibly due to nonspecific hybridization. In Volokhov et al. (2003), signals that differed from the average background at a statistically significant level ($P < 0.01$) were considered positive; similarly, in Cremonesi et al. (2009), for each oligonucleotide, we required the population of all the replicates to be above the intensity of "blank" spots (i.e., with no oligonucleotide spotted), plus two times their standard deviations by applying a one-sided Student $t$-test ($P < 0.01$). Typically, each zipcode population was made by quadruplicate spots, whereas the null distribution of the "blanks" was made up by six. In any case, in order to have a consistent estimation of the real amount of target immobilized on the probes, a filter for excluding outlier values was applied, such that features whose intensity resulted 2.5-fold above or below the average were discarded. Similarly, filters can also be applied on the basis of the population coefficient of variation (ratio between the standard deviation and the mean of the replicates), to exclude outlier features in test populations varying more than 100% of the average, or on having a certain number or replicates above the local background.

The procedure described earlier is applicable to all contexts in which the aim of the experiment is to determine the presence of a certain molecular species in a given sample. Usually, in these kinds of assays, the quantitative aspects needed for accomplishing standard safety rules are analyzed on the basis of the sensitivity of the initial PCR by determining the detection limit, that is, the minimum amount of pathogen or heterologous DNA that can be detected by the amplification. The LDR and hybridization assays can be only semiquantitative, since the fluorescence intensity of the probes results proportional to the relative amount of DNA of a given target within a single sample. The comparative analysis of multiple samples needs a calibration, through the normalization of the data to a common standard, present in all the initial samples. However, the absolute estimation of the starting DNA quantity is strongly biased by the PCR step, which is, at the moment, not avoidable.

In genotyping experiments, on the other hand, in which the quantitation of the presence of each allele in each SNP is fundamental, the steps to be accomplished by the analysis are at least two: (a) determine if a marker is present in the sample and, thus, if its quantification is a reliable estimation of the real amount of molecules hybridized on each probe and (b) estimate the relative amount of each of the alleles tested. If the first step presents no aspects different from those described for the pathogen or GMO detection assays cited earlier, the latter implies normalization and a relative estimation of the allele 1/allele 2 ratio. In Chessa et al. (2007), each zipcode, firstly, underwent a local background correction and an averaging on all the replicates. An artificial ligation control, made up by a two DS + one CP trio of probes, insisting on a synthetic template synthesized with equimolar quantities of two alleles differing by the discriminating base of the DS was used for normalization purposes. The ratio between the average intensity of the Cy3 and Cy5 channels was used for correcting the fluorescence imbalance (and other channel-related biases) of average Cy3 intensity for a given zipcode to obtain a corrected fluorescent intensity (cFICy3). To define the genotype for each SNP, the allelic fraction (AF), which estimates the relative amount of allele 1 (Cy3) with respect to allele 2 (Cy5) by using the equation: $AF = cFICy3/(cFICy3 + FICy5)$, was calculated. The same procedure, with a further averaging on triplicate experiments and a filter on inter-experiments coefficient of variation (<5%), was applied also in Consolandi et al. (2008). The AF values of each SNP were plotted simultaneously to analyze their distribution as a function of the three possible genotypes, and clustering techniques (e.g., $k$-means clustering method) were used to assign each calculated AF to one of the three theoretical groups, which correspond to AFs of 1, 0.5, and 0 (Consolandi et al. 2008).

## 2.4 ACTUAL APPLICATIONS OF OUR TECHNOLOGY

The starting point of the entire PCR–LDR–UA procedure is the DNA extraction from fresh samples, followed by amplification of the target genes using specific primers for the region of interest. After the purification of the PCR amplicons, the ligation reaction is carried out in liquid phase and the LDR products are hybridized onto UA for the identification of DNA variations. The fluorescence signals are acquired by means of a laser scanner and the images collected are quantified using appropriate software. A statistical data analysis is performed in order to find which nucleic acid sequence differences are present (Figure 2.4). We report a couple of applications for both detection and quality assessment macroareas in the following. Within each group, we assessed an application on products of vegetable origin and one on animal-derived products. In particular, we describe PCR–LDR–UA assays for (a) GMO detection in flours and bakery products through targeting of the main existing transgenic targets; (b) monovarietal olive oil characterization through the genotyping of certain number of SNPs sufficient to discriminate the main varieties cultivated in the Mediterranean area; (c) milk pathogen detection in milk, targeting the specific polymorphisms of some pathogens of interest, linked to bovine mastitis

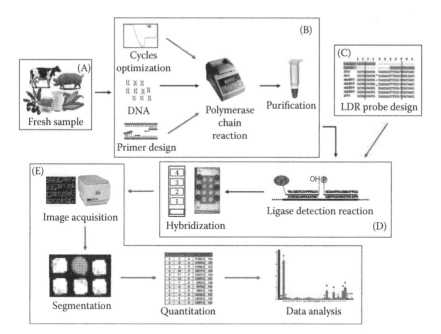

**FIGURE 2.4** Flowchart of the PCR–LDR–UA assay. Starting from food sample (A), a PCR reaction is performed with specific primers, optimal thermal cycles, and a suitable quantity of DNA is extracted from the sample (B). LDR assay is designed on the basis of probe pairs capable of discriminating the species or the alleles under analysis (C); then, the cyclic reaction is performed and the obtained products are hybridized onto the UA array (D). Finally, image acquisition is performed, followed by feature segmentation (i.e., assigning each pixel of the image as belonging to the feature or the background), quantitation, and data analysis (E). Black arrows in the figure represent "wet" steps, whereas gray ones represent "in silico" steps.

and/or food-borne intoxication; and (d) casein typing in bovine milk, with association to the aplotype effects on milk composition and cheese production.

Comprehensive applications of the PCR–LDR–UA assays in food safety/quality
field can be seen in Table 2.1.

## 2.4.1 GMO DETECTION

To assess the applicability of this technology to GMO screening, two different multiplex
PCR assays (mPCR1 and mPCR2), for the simultaneous screening of different GMO
events in the same reaction, were developed. In particular, multiplex PCRs were
optimized to amplify, at the same time, five different transgenic targets: RRS™,
maize MON810, GA21, Bt176, and Bt11, and two endogenous genes, one specific
for soybean (lectin gene) and one for maize (zein gene), included as internal control
targets. These transgenic events were preferentially targeted after an accurate evaluation of the GMOs most widely diffused on the market.

A major difference between mPCR1 and mPCR2 assays was in the design of
PCR primers. In the mPCR1 assay, several primer pairs targeted internal parts of the
exogenous DNA sequences, which were taken from literature and, then, individually tested for their selectivity and efficiency in amplifying their targets (Germini
et al. 2004). In the mPCR2 assay, instead, the junction regions within the transgenic
constructs were specifically targeted. The sequences of the junction regions were
derived from the transgenic sequences available in databases, specific primers were
designed to target these regions and the amplicons obtained after their amplification
were directly sequenced; their sequences have been deposited in GenBank (Peano
et al. 2005a). This second mPCR represents a substantial improvement, because of
the absolute specificity of the sequences targeted, considering the discrepancies that
can be found in the sequences reported in literature and in databases for the same
type of transgenic constructs.

Moreover, these multiplex PCRs were designed in order to produce short amplicons to trace transgenic DNA even in processed foods, in which technological
treatments could have led to significant DNA degradation, thus avoiding the risk of
false-negative results.

These two multiplex PCRs have constituted the basis for the development of an
efficient LDR platform for GMO traceability based on microarray technology. To
evaluate the specificity of LDR probes of both mPCR1 and mPCR2 assays, and to
investigate probe interference, mPCR reactions were performed on DNA prepared
from standard flours (containing known percentages of individual GMOs) and from
mixtures of DNA representing from two to five GMOs.

Considerable differences between mPCR1 and mPCR2 in terms of molecular
specificity of the selected LDR probes were observed. For mPCR2–LDR–UA assay,
it was demonstrated that only the expected spots lit up after array hybridization and
scanning and no signal was detectable in the negative control. This could be relevant
when trying to detect a minimal amount of GMO material in the presence of a large
excess of molecular background, like wild-type maize and soybean. For mPCR1–
LDR–UA assay, instead, only some LDR probes were specific, with the presence of
some "contamination," which has been individuated already at the multiplex PCR level,

**TABLE 2.1**
**Overview of the Main Applications of PCR–LDR–UA Assay**

| Application | Target Genes | PCR Type | No. of Probes | Assay Type | Detection Limit | Food Matrix | Reference |
|---|---|---|---|---|---|---|---|
| GMO detection | RRS<br>MON810<br>GA21<br>Bt176<br>Bt11<br>Lectin<br>Zein | Multiplex (7-plex) | 7 | 1 color | 0.2%, 0.4% for Bt11 | Flours, biscuits, commercial foodstuff | Peano et al. (2005a) and Germini et al. (2004) |
| Olive oil traceability | Stearoyl-ACP desaturase<br>Fatty acid desaturase<br>Cycloartenol synthase<br>Lupeol synthase<br>Chalcone synthase<br>Anthocyanidin synthase<br>Calcium binding protein<br>Clone SRAP-5<br>Phenylalanine ammonia lyase | Multiplex (13-plex) | 17 | 2 color | NA | Monovarietal oil | Consolandi et al. (2008) |

(continued)

**TABLE 2.1 (continued)**
**Overview of the Main Applications of PCR–LDR–UA Assay**

| Application | Target Genes | PCR Type | No. of Probes | Assay Type | Detection Limit | Food Matrix | Reference |
|---|---|---|---|---|---|---|---|
| Bovine milk protein genotyping | CSN1S1 exon 17<br>CSN2 exon 6<br>CSN2 exon 7<br>CSN3 exon 4<br>LGB exon 3<br>LGB exon 4<br>CSN3 intron 2<br>CSN1S1 promoter | Multiplex (8-plex) | 22 | 2 color | NA | Bovine milk | Chessa et al. (2007) |
| Milk pathogen detection | 16S rRNA | Single-plex | 16 | 1 color | 6 fmol, 12 fmol for *Staph. aureus* | Bovine, ovine, caprine milk | Cremonesi et al. (2009) |

The table reports data on target genes employed by each assay, PCR type (single or multiplex), the number of specific probes selected, the assay type (one/two color), sensitivity of the assay (when available), and food matrix under analysis.

as shown in capillary electrophoresis analysis. Because the two multiplex PCRs are different in the primers design approach, it was assumed that the amplification of junction regions is more specific than the amplification of the internal parts of the transgenic construct.

After testing the molecular specificity of the two mPCR–LDR–UA assays, their sensitivity was assessed in order to evaluate if these two molecular tools were suitable for GMO traceability in the range of GMO percentages relevant to the regulations of the European Community.

Multiplex PCR of different amplicons is well known to introduce a bias in the original composition of the target sequences (Gerry et al. 1999). PCR products obtained from DNA extracted from standards containing different percentages of GMOs do not maintain the original ratio between the transgenic content and the effective soybean and maize content (in terms of gene copy number transgene vs. lectin or maize genes). After normalization of signal intensity, the bias introduced by PCR amplification was further confirmed in LDR–UA assay: the amplified product does not maintain the original ratio between the transgene and the reference gene, because one target was amplified better than the other one and the amplicons had different concentrations with respect to the original situation. The LDR assay, nevertheless, confirmed the results obtained from amplification reaction and evidenced in the capillary electrophoresis analysis, reproducing faithfully all the situations analyzed.

Then, the limit of detection of the LDR–UA platform was evaluated, using mPCR2 performed with different DNA mixtures at decreasing percentages (from 20% to 0.2%) of each of the five GMOs analyzed. The results demonstrated that it is rather complex to define an absolute limit of detection for LDR–UA approach. For some events, such as MON810, RRS, and GA21, the limit could be below 0.2%, but for Bt176 the limit was above 0.2% and for Bt11 it was above 0.4%. Given the variability of these results, the level of sensitivity of the mPCR2–LDR–UA approach is suitable for food analysis, according to the European Union normative, where the maximum level of GMO contamination permitted has been set at 0.9%.

The mPCR–LDR–UA approach was also applied on traceability of GMO in processed material, such as biscuits made from 80% commercial wheat flour and 20% laboratory prepared soybean flour containing known concentration of RRS (from 0.1% to 2%). This analysis has been performed also on the flours used for preparation of the biscuits, in order to evaluate if the baking process could determine the degradation of genomic DNA. The limit of detection in the case of mPCR–LDR–UA analysis of DNA extracted from biscuits was 0.1% of RRS content and this result fits well with the previously determined limit of detection of the LDR–UA approach.

Finally, the mPCR–LDR–UA approach was tested on real samples to evaluate the matrix effect. Six commercially available foodstuffs containing maize or soybean, previously analyzed with mPCR1 assay, were submitted to LDR in presence of the entire set of oligonucleotide probes. After hybridization onto the UA, the signal intensity reflected the composition of the multiplex amplified material as highlighted by electrophoresis analysis. Soybean and maize, through their lectin and zein reference genes, were correctly identified in accordance with the composition of each commercial sample. These results confirmed the reliability of the mPCR–LDR–UA analysis for GMO detection, also on real food matrixes.

### 2.4.2 Olive Oil Traceability

Single nucleotide polymorphisms have recently been reported as suitable for resolving traceability issues; compared to other commonly used genetic markers, they occur more frequently in the genome, are stably inherited, and can exist in coding regions, occasionally leading to aminoacid changes in the encoded polypeptides (Brookes 1999). Thus, since they are abundant and uniformly distributed within the genome, a panel of SNPs can be assessed to discriminate numerous similar subspecies.

Single nucleotide polymorphisms, located in different genomic sequences of olive cultivars commonly used for oil production in the Mediterranean area were previously identified (Consolandi et al. 2007). On the basis of 17 SNPs, 49 olive varieties were discriminated. A previous work employed genomic DNA extracted and amplified from fresh olive leaves; thus, the aim of the study was to develop a DNA extraction method that allowed the retrieval of genomic DNA of sufficient quality (from a reasonable quantity of starting oil sample) to extend the microarray assay to the more difficult analysis of DNA extracted from monovarietal olive oils. A new DNA extraction protocol from olive oil was developed and evaluated in terms of yield, speed, and reliability compared with currently available protocols. Different studies have demonstrated that it is possible to extract DNA from olive oil in a quantity and quality suitable for PCR analysis (Breton et al. 2004, Busconi et al. 2003), but all these methods required large volumes of olive oil sample, and none appeared to be really applicable on routine analysis in commercial analytical laboratories. The new method was designed to disrupt neutral micelles by addition of the surfactant Tween 20 after solubilization with hexane, and, thereby, recover DNA from the oily, rather than from the aqueous, phase. The use of this surfactant was the biggest difference with the other published methods, which used different organic solvents to separate the oily phase from the aqueous and pellet phases.

The second step of this research was to implement, as a time- and cost-saving step, a multiplex PCR in which all 13 DNA sequences containing the 17 SNP loci under study would be simultaneously amplified in a single reaction. Thirteen primer pairs were ex novo designed in order to amplify the genomic regions containing the 17 SNPs previously described in Consolandi et al. (2007). Quality controls performed on the amplified products revealed the suitability of the protocol to amplify up to 11 out of 13 DNA fragments, with variable but reasonable yields. The method for DNA extraction, followed by a multiplex PCR–LDR–UA procedure, was entirely validated in a test for the discrimination of 8 different monovarietal olive oils, demonstrating how it may be used to genetically identify oils from 49 common olive cultivars (Consolandi et al. 2008). A supervised *k*-means clustering performed on the estimated allelic frequencies for each sample, allowed the identification of three nonoverlapping clusters, centered around the theoretical optimal frequencies (i.e., 0, 0.5, and 1). Multiple determinations on 12 experiments confirmed the reproducibility and the very low variability of the genotyping assignments. Moreover, a hierarchical clustering demonstrated that the 11 fragments are enough to assess the aplotype of up to 49 olive varieties.

### 2.4.3 BOVINE MILK PROTEIN GENOTYPING

A fast method for typing the main mutations of bovine milk protein genes by using an approach based on the LDR and a UA was developed and validated by Chessa et al. (2007). Polymorphisms in both the coding and noncoding sequences of αS1-casein, β-casein, κ-casein, and β-lactoglobulin genes were considered because of their well-known effects on milk composition and cheese production. A total of 22 polymorphic sites, corresponding to 21 different variants, were included in the diagnostic microarray.

Milk was chosen as a matrix for the DNA extraction because it is particularly suitable for the routine genetic analyses that could be performed by means of the LDR–UA assay. In fact, milk is more suitable, accessible, and easily recovered than blood or hair in dairy cattle for the screening of milk protein loci in the female population by means of the DNA chip developed. A multiplex PCR was developed to amplify all the DNA target sequences simultaneously and LDR allowed targeting several PCR amplicons, at the same time, in a single ligation reaction. Moreover, the use of a multiplex PCR reaction for the simultaneous amplification of eight different fragments allowed for increasing throughput and lowered time and costs.

The LDR–UA assay was validated by analyzing 100 Italian Friesian DNA samples, which were also genotyped by conventional methods, both at the protein level, by means of milk isoelectrofocusing, and at the molecular level using PCR–RFLP and PCR single-strand conformation polymorphism techniques.

The genotypes obtained using the LDR–UA approach were in full agreement with those obtained by the conventional analyses. Further, an important result of the LDR–UA assay was a more accurate genotyping of the different milk protein alleles than was found with conventional typing methods. At the κ-casein gene, in fact, four samples were heterozygous (three reference samples and one validation sample) for an allele coding for Thr136 and Ala148. This variant, which can be considered as the wild type of the genus *Bos*, is not usually identifiable by the conventional typing methods used.

Another innovative result was the successful use of two different fluorophores for the deletion genotyping. As pioneered by Gerry et al. (1999) and Favis et al. (2000), the LDR–UA platform also allowed insertion and deletion polymorphisms to be genotyped. For the *CSN1S1* promoter, this approach was applied by designing two CPs, differing at their 3′-nucleotide, to detect two deletions at the *CNS1S1* promoter.

The whole procedure, from DNA extraction to signal analysis, required almost 10h for the typing of 24 samples. The LDR–UA technology offered the power of a microarray format, facilitating the genotyping of different genomic regions, which could be investigated for phylogenetic and association studies, for the evaluation of genetic distances among cattle breeds and the domestication history of bovine species, and for dairy cattle identification and parentage control. In selection, the chip could also be used to analyze CN haplotypes, instead of single loci, which would help to exploit the effects of the entire CN cluster on milk yield and component traits. Interrogation of known SNPs, compared with the most popular DNA markers (microsatellites), is attractive, because of their genetic stability and amenability to high throughput with automated technology. They are considered a realistic alternative in livestock identification, kinship analysis, and linkage studies. The multiplex PCR–LDR–UA technology could become a powerful tool for their detection and exploitation in animal breeding.

### 2.4.4 Milk Pathogen Detection

A new DNA chip based on the use of a PCR–LDR–UA assay was developed and validated by Cremonesi et al. (2009) to detect, directly from milk samples, microbial pathogens known to cause bovine, ovine, and caprine mastitis, to be responsible for food-borne intoxication or infection, or both. Specific probes were designed on the 16S rRNA gene and employed for the identification of 15 different bacterial groups at different phylogenetic levels: *Staph. aureus*, *Streptococcus agalactiae*, non-aureus staphylococci (NAS), *Streptococcus bovis*, *Streptococcus equi*, *Streptococcus canis*, *Streptococcus dysgalactiae*, *Streptococcus parauberis*, *Streptococcus uberis*, *Strep. pyogenes*, *Mycoplasma* spp., *Salmonella* spp., *Bacillus* spp., *Campylobacter* spp., and *E. coli* and related species.

The bacterial pathogens on the assay panel were chosen to include (a) the organisms most frequently isolated from mastitis samples, such as *Staph. aureus*, *Strep. agalactiae*, *Strep. uberis*, and some NAS; (b) those that have been recently described as a contagious cause of subclinical mastitis, such as *Mycoplasma* spp. (Fox et al. 2005); and (c) those potentially dangerous for human health, such as *E. coli* and related species (Bottero et al. 2004), *Salmonella* spp. (Jayarao et al. 1999), *Staph. aureus* (De Buyser et al. 2001), *B. cereus* (Wong et al. 1988), and *Strep. equi* spp. *Zooepidemicus* (Bergonier et al. 1999).

The specificity of the probe pairs was tested separately with the 16S rRNA products on a total of 22 ATCC or isolated bacterial strains. Generally, the presence of typical endogenous microflora might mask the detection of food-borne pathogens; thus, in order to determine the ability of the PCR–LDR–UA assay to identify pathogens in mixed bacterial populations, we prepared and analyzed artificially unbalanced DNA mixtures of different microbial species, obtaining efficient and highly specific detections. The designed probes correctly differentiated the *Streptococcus* spp. causing mastitis; to determine the prevalence of different species in dairy herds, one probe was designed for the following species of the *Streptococcus* group: *Strep. agalactiae*, *Strep. equi*, *Strep. dysgalactiae*, *Strep. uberis*, *Strep. parauberis*, *Strep. bovis*, *Strep. canis*. The PCR–LDR–UA assay allowed for discrimination between *Strep. uberis* and *Strep. parauberis* on the basis of a single PCR on the 16S rRNA gene, avoiding the use of species-specific PCR primers (Hassan et al. 2005). Probe pairs for *Strep. equi* and *Strep. dysgalactiae* were designed to identify any of the two subspecies of each; thus, the discrimination of *Strep. equi* spp. *zooepidemicus* from *Strep. equi* spp. *equi* and *Strep. dysgalactiae* spp. *equisimilis* from *Strep. dysgalactiae* ssp. *dysgalactiae* was not possible with the present set of LDR probe pairs. Moreover, strains of *Mycoplasma bovis*, *Mycoplasma agalactiae*, *Mycoplasma arginini*, *Mycoplasma capri*, *Mycoplasma capricolum*, and *Mycoplasma mycoides* could be clearly identified as belonging to the *Mycoplasma* genus by the specific probe pair in the PCR–LDR–UA assay, providing an improved diagnostic method for this pathogen.

To test the sensitivity of the method and the correlation between signal intensity and template concentration, the assay was evaluated by separate LDR on serial dilutions from 50 to 6 fmol of *M. bovis, Strep. agalactiae, Strep. pyogenes*, and *Staph. aureus* 16S rRNA-PCR products. Considering a threshold p-value of 0.01 on the one-sided *t*-test, for significance of the presence of a probe, *M. bovis, Strep. agalactiae*, and *Strep. pyogenes* revealed a detection limit of 6 fmol, whereas *Staph. aureus* was limited to 12 fmol, which is, anyway, below the limit imposed by the European Community of 500 cfu/mL (corresponding to approximately 150 fmol) (EC 2073/2005).

Finally, the performance of the LDR probe pairs was evaluated using DNA extracted from 50 milk samples, 47 of which were from mastitic animals. The LDR results obtained from the analysis of these samples revealed a good correlation with those obtained from the microbiological assays, also showing the presence of *Bacillus* spp. in two mastitic milk samples and specifying the presence of *Strep. uberis* (8 samples), *Strep. agalactiae* (6), *Strep. dysgalactiae* (3), *Strep. equi* (2), *Strep. bovis* (4), and *Strep. canis* (3) for the *Streptococcus* spp., and NAS (7) for the *Staphylococcus* spp. Nine samples were positive for *Staph. aureus*, whereas 11 were positive for *Mycoplasma* spp. Three samples were negative with both bacteriological and LDR analyses and acted as negative controls. The PCR–LDR–UA assay, including DNA extraction, PCR amplification, LDR, and data analysis, could be completed in less than 7 h.

## 2.5   EMERGING TRENDS

### 2.5.1   LAB-ON-CHIP

Nanotechnology and microfluidic principles are being applied to the design of microdevices and microsystems for analytical purposes (Baeumner 2003). Both food safety and quality can be addressed with these technologies, especially in the context of arrays of sensors aimed at the simultaneous detection of multiple targets. In channels with a diameter of a few micrometers, fluid flow is governed by properties that can be exploited for analytical purposes (separations coupled to mass spectroscopy, high-throughput screening in drug development, bioanalyses, examination and manipulation of samples consisting of a single cell or a single molecule) (Whitesides 2006). The generic requirements for these devices are a system to inject reagents and samples, a system to move and mix them, and a set of detectors (and/or components for the purification of particular products). Proper mixing is particularly important, because the laminar flow of fluids in a microchannel is turbulence free. The effectiveness of LabChip technology (Agilent Technologies, Santa Clara, CA) combined with the Agilent Bioanalyser 2100 system to detect GM content in soybean has been compared with conventional electrophoresis and with capillary electrophoresis. While both the latter techniques were reliable, the LabChip approach gave more reproducible results (Birch et al. 2001). The advantages of biosensors in food analyses are that they can measure different targets in parallel; moreover, they are versatile, highly sensitive, and specific; they can operate in real time and *in situ*; they can be miniaturized and assembled into arrays to make portable devices; and they do not require highly trained personnel for their operation. Several innovative approaches are currently under development for rapid and automatic detection of biological warfare agents, such as disease organisms. The development of portable instruments for real-time PCR and for microarrays based on microfluidics will likely benefit the food industry, since all these systems can be adapted to detection of food ingredients and contaminants, including GMOs, simply by changing the probes employed (Ivnitski et al. 2003).

### 2.5.2 Deep Sequencing

In recent years, many innovative sequencing technologies, such as Roche GS FLX and Illumina Genome Analyzer platforms, have been implemented; both are high-throughput methods that made possible the collection of new genetic information or the confirmation of the existing datasets. 454 Life Sciences (Margulies et al. 2005) exploits pyrosequencing, whereas Illumina employs a four-color DNA sequencing-by-synthesis technology. The amount of data in food-associated projects has grown up dramatically, but there is still the need for an increase of this information. Although the number of drafts or completed bacterial genomes has undergone a huge increase from 35 total (Abee et al. 2004) in 2004 to 121 complete + 359 drafts in 2010, there is still a lack of genetic information, which makes high-throughput sequencing a valuable technique in the characterization of potential threats to human health. Massive genome sequencing can provide a more detailed real-time assessment of genetic traits characteristic of the outbreak strains than those that could be achieved with routine typing methods. The possibility of horizontal transfer of genetic traits between different species makes this type of technology, capable of following bacteria evolution, particularly valuable.

Roche GS FLX platform was employed for the high-throughput pyrosequencing of two subtypes of *L. monocytogenes*, which caused a nationwide outbreak of listeriosis in Canada in 2008 (Gilmour et al. 2010). Whole genome sequencing enabled a characterization of virulence factors and genetic diversity (in particular, SNP and indels mutations) within a natural *L. monocytogenes* population. Recent advances in technology and experimental techniques, together with computational methods, are essential also for discovering new molecular markers (SNPs) for food quality evaluation; in particular, the advent of ultra-massive sequencing technologies has made possible the whole sequencing of complex plants genomes and transcriptomes.

The parallel analysis of transcriptional and metabolic profiles is at the forefront of systems biology and the most used technologies, up to now, are a combination of GC-MS and microarray (Urbanczyk-Wochniak et al. 2003). However, the varietal identification and traceability with technologies based on DNA molecular polymorphisms analysis, such as RFLP, AFLP, and RAPD, do not provide information on the expression of the "target" genes, while the technologies for the study of gene expression (like microarrays) require prior knowledge of the genomic sequence of the species and do not provide information on DNA polymorphisms in different genotypes. Moreover, these technologies result very costly in terms of time and money and do not allow high-throughput analysis. This is especially true for food matrixes and samples whose genomic and transcriptomic information are constantly increasing, but have not yet reached an established standard, as it had happened for higher level organisms.

On the contrary, cDNA sequencing with new ultra-massive sequencers allows the obtainment of *de novo* sequence information (and therefore of panels of DNA polymorphisms estimated in thousands of SNPs per genome). At the same time, it is possible to obtain gene expression profiles at whole genome level and, therefore, information on how genes are modulated (e.g., in different tissues or at different stages of the plant or of the fruit development) at extremely low costs and in few hours.

The availability of new-generation, ultra-massive sequencers allows an extreme increase in the yield in terms of base pairs sequenced in a single experiment, the reduction of the sequencing costs, and the time required. 454-based transcriptome sequencing was employed for the high-throughput acquisition of gene-associated SNPs (Barbazuk et al. 2007), where a first-generation massive pyrosequencing technology was used to sequence the transcriptomes of isolates from two inbred lines of maize. The validation rate on a subgroup of these SNPs (85%) led to the identification of at least 4900 valid SNPs within more than 2400 maize genes. More recently, the combined use of next-generation sequencing and high-throughput genotyping allowed to obtain a higher resolution genetic map in the anchoring and orienting of most of the soybean sequence that was not completed (~34%) in Soybean Consensus Map 4.0 project (Hyten et al. 2010). Illumina Genome Analyzer reads were mapped on the existing reference scaffold assembly for the discovery of putative SNPs. The procedure added reliable genetic markers to 335 scaffolds, 23 of which were previously unmapped in the preliminary scaffold assembly.

The improvements achieved in both technologies in recent years promise to increase the knowledge in the field by multiplying the amount of information gathered from a single experiment of orders of magnitude respect to traditional techniques and also to first-generation instruments. In 2010, the 454 Titanium protocol generated 500 Mb sequence in a single run, with an average reads length of 400 bp; on the other hand, Illumina technology greatly increased the sequencing yield, generating 40 Gb sequence, but produced shorter reads (average length 100 bp). The integration of these two platforms seems to be really promising in particular in the field of new molecular markers discovery for varietal genotyping and food quality assessment.

### 2.5.3 NEW HIGH-THROUGHPUT MICROARRAY METHODS FOR PHENOTYPIC CHARACTERIZATION IN LIVESTOCK

One of the "grand challenges" in modern biology is to understand the genetic basis of phenotypic diversity within and among species. Thousands of years of selective breeding of domestic animals has created a diversity of phenotypes among breeds that is only matched by that observed among species in nature. Livestock, therefore, constitutes a unique resource for understanding the genetic basis of phenotypic variation and, when its genome sequences become available, the identification of the mutations that underlie the transformation from a wild to a domestic species will be a realistic and important target (Andersson and Georges 2004). The advances in genomics technology provided by high-throughput array have created the opportunity to greatly expand our ability to study the genetics of the organisms in the world around us. The rationale would be to genotype a collection of SNPs that occur at regular intervals and cover the whole genome to detect genomic regions in which the frequencies of the SNP allele differ between experimental populations. Affymetrix released a commercial bovine chip (25.000 SNPs) and Illumina offers a bovine chip for 50.000 SNPs and a new pig 60k SNPs chip. These methodologies empower applications such as genome-wide-enabled selection, identification of QTL, evaluation of genetic merit of individuals, and comparative genetic studies. For example, the International Bovine HapMap project (Gibbs et al. 2009) used the bovine SNP50 Genotyping BeadChip (Illumina, San Diego, CA) for characterizing the genome in dairy and beef cattle breeds. Comparisons between breed groups have the potential to identify genomic regions influencing complex traits with no need for complex equipment and the collection of extensive phenotypic records and can contribute to the identification of candidate genes and to the understanding of the biological mechanisms controlling complex traits.

## 2.6 CONCLUSIONS

As more pathogen genomes and targeted genes are sequenced, costs associated with microarray-based technologies will probably decrease in the near future. Thus, both diagnostic and quality-related applications of microarray-based analyses will continue to expand. At the same time, the advent of new sequencing methods and instruments will suggest new targets, techniques, and field of application. In food safety, this means the possibility to more precisely identify genomic regions unique to the target bacteria with no interaction with the foreign matrix environment and the increase in the information about emerging pathogens or bacteria recently discovered to be potentially dangerous to human health. Moreover, the genomics revolution is allowing the scientific community to increase the understanding of how selection has created genetic differences between subspecies populations, both in agriculture and livestock. Thanks to these advancements, our comprehension of the mechanisms underlying the development of complex traits is also increasing.

The main issues related to the extensive use of advanced technologies in food industry are that new materials and methods used are very often not yet assessed as new chemicals and, currently, the industries have to follow established guidelines. The small number of commercial assays already present in the market (i.e., Eppendorf DualChip and Promega Biosmart Allin 1.0 for GMO detection and Clondiag ArrayTubes for antibiotic resistance) confirms that some difficulties still remain before an advanced technology-based assay can be routinely used in food industry.

Acquiring evidence in this area is fundamental for the development of new kits and methods to be introduced on the market. Significant modifications should also be made in associated legislation to make microarray-, or, in general, DNA-based methods the standard for assessing safety and quality in food and all related products.

## REFERENCES

Aarts, H. J., J. P. van Rie, and E. J. Kok. 2002. Traceability of genetically modified organisms. *Expert Rev Mol Diagn* 2:69–76.

Abee, T., W. van Schaik, and R. J. Siezen. 2004. Impact of genomics on microbial food safety. *Trends Biotechnol* 22:653–660.

Ahn, S. and D. R. Walt. 2005. Detection of *Salmonella* spp. using microsphere-based, fiber-optic DNA microarrays. *Anal Chem* 77:5041–5047.

Altschul, S. F., W. Gish, W. Miller, E. W. Myers, and D. J. Lipman. 1990. Basic local alignment search tool. *J Mol Biol* 215:403–410.

Andersson, L. 2001. Genetic dissection of phenotypic diversity in farm animals. *Nat Rev Genet* 2:130–138.

Andersson, L. and M. Georges. 2004. Domestic-animal genomics: Deciphering the genetics of complex traits. *Nat Rev Genet* 5:202–212.

Baeumner, A. J. 2003. Biosensors for environmental pollutants and food contaminants. *Anal Bioanal Chem* 377:434–445.

Balaban, N. and A. Rasooly. 2000. *Staphylococcal* enterotoxins. *Int J Food Microbiol* 61:1–10.

Barbazuk, W. B., S. J. Emrich, H. D. Chen, L. Li, and P. S. Schnable. 2007. SNP discovery via 454 transcriptome sequencing. *Plant J* 51:910–918.

Bergonier, D., X. Berthelot, M. Romeo et al. 1999. Fréquence des différents germes responsables de mammites cliniques et subcliniques chez les petits ruminants laitiers. In *Milking and Milk Production of Dairy Sheep and Goats*, eds. F. Barillet and N. P. Zervas, pp. 130–136.Wageningen, the Netherlands.

Birch, L., C. L. Archard, H. C. Parkes, and D. G. McDowell. 2001. Evaluation of LabChip™ technology for GMO analysis in food. *Food Control* 12:535–540.

Boettcher, P. J., A. Caroli, A. Stella et al. 2004. Effects of casein haplotypes on milk production traits in Italian Holstein and Brown Swiss cattle. *J Dairy Sci* 87:4311–4317.

Bottero, M. T., A. Dalmasso, D. Soglia et al. 2004. Development of a multiplex PCR assay for the identification of pathogenic genes of *Escherichia coli* in milk and milk products. *Mol Cell Probes* 18:283–288.

Braunschweig, M., C. Hagger, G. Stranzinger, and Z. Puhan. 2000. Associations between casein haplotypes and milk production traits of Swiss Brown cattle. *J Dairy Sci* 83:1387–1395.

Bresee, J. S., M. A. Widdowson, S. S. Monroe, and R. I. Glass. 2002. Foodborne viral gastroenteritis: Challenges and opportunities. *Clin Infect Dis* 35:748–753.

Breton, C., D. Claux, I. Metton, G. Skorski, and A. Berville. 2004. Comparative study of methods for DNA preparation from olive oil samples to identify cultivar SSR alleles in commercial oil samples: Possible forensic applications. *J Agric Food Chem* 52:531–537.

Brookes, A. J. 1999. The essence of SNPs. *Gene* 234:177–186.

Busconi, M. F. C., M. Corradi, C. Bongiorni, F. Cattapan, and C. Fogher. 2003. DNA extraction from olive oil and its use in the identification of the production cultivar. *Food Chem* 83:127–139.

Cankar, K., D. Stebih, T. Dreo, J. Zel, and K. Gruden. 2006. Critical points of DNA quantification by real-time PCR—Effects of DNA extraction method and sample matrix on quantification of genetically modified organisms. *BMC Biotechnol* 6:37.

Chen, J., M. A. Iannone, M. S. Li et al. 2000. A microsphere-based assay for multiplexed single nucleotide polymorphism analysis using single base chain extension. *Genome Res* 10:549–557.

Chessa, S., F. Chiatti, G. Ceriotti et al. 2007. Development of a single nucleotide polymorphism genotyping microarray platform for the identification of bovine milk protein genetic polymorphisms. *J Dairy Sci* 90:451–464.

Chiang, Y. C., C. Y. Yang, C. Li et al. 2006. Identification of *Bacillus* spp., *Escherichia coli*, *Salmonella* spp., *Staphylococcus* spp. and *Vibrio* spp. with 16S ribosomal DNA-based oligonucleotide array hybridization. *Int J Food Microbiol* 107:131–137.

Chizhikov, V., A. Rasooly, K. Chumakov, and D. D. Levy. 2001. Microarray analysis of microbial virulence factors. *Appl Environ Microbiol* 67:3258–3263.

Chou, C. C., C. H. Chen, T. T. Lee, and K. Peck. 2004. Optimization of probe length and the number of probes per gene for optimal microarray analysis of gene expression. *Nucleic Acids Res* 32:e99.

Claros, M. G., R. Crespillo, M. L. Aguilar, and F. M. Canovas. 2000. DNA fingerprint and classification of geographically related genotypes of olive-tree (*Olea europaea* L.). *Euphytica* 116:131–142.

Consolandi, C., L. Palmieri, S. Doveri et al. 2007. Olive variety identification by ligation detection reaction in a universal array format. *J Biotechnol* 129:565–574.

Consolandi, C., L. Palmieri, M. Severgnini, E. Maestri, N. Marmiroli, C. Agrimonti, L. Baldoni, P. Donini, G. De Bellis, and B. Castiglioni. 2008. A procedure for olive oil traceability and authenticity: DNA extraction, multiplex PCR and LDR–universal array analysis. *Eur Food Res Technol* 227:1429–1438.

Cremonesi, P., G. Pisoni, M. Severgnini et al. 2009. Pathogen detection in milk samples by ligation detection reaction-mediated universal array method. *J Dairy Sci* 92:3027–3039.

Damiani, G., S. Florio, E. Budelli, P. Bolla, and A. Caroli. 2000. Single nucleotide polymorphisms (SNPs) within Bov-A2 SINE in the second intron of bovine and buffalo κ-casein (CSN3) gene. *Anim Genet* 31:277–279.

De Buyser, M. L., B. Dufour, M. Maire, and V. Lafarge. 2001. Implication of milk and milk products in food-borne diseases in France and in different industrialised countries. *Int J Food Microbiol* 67:1–17.

Dekkers, J. C. and F. Hospital. 2002. The use of molecular genetics in the improvement of agricultural populations. *Nat Rev Genet* 3:22–32.

Di Stasio, L. and P. Mariani. 2000. The role of protein polymorphism in the genetic improvement of milk production. *Zootec Nutr Anim* 26:69–90.

Doveri, S., D. M. O'Sullivan, and D. Lee. 2006. Non-concordance between genetic profiles of olive oil and fruit: A cautionary note to the use of DNA markers for provenance testing. *J Agric Food Chem* 54:9221–9226.

Edelstein, R. L., C. R. Tamanaha, P. E. Sheehan et al. 2000. The BARC biosensor applied to the detection of biological warfare agents. *Biosens Bioelectron* 14:05–13.

Eom, H. S., B. H. Hwang, D. H. Kim et al. 2007. Multiple detection of food-borne pathogenic bacteria using a novel 16S rDNA-based oligonucleotide signature chip. *Biosens Bioelectron* 22:845–853.

Farrell, H. M., R. Jimenez-Flores, Jr., G. T. Bleck et al. 2004. Nomenclature of the proteins of cows' milk—Sixth revision. *J Dairy Sci* 87:1641–1674.

Favis, R., J. P. Day, N. P. Gerry et al. 2000. Universal DNA array detection of small insertions and deletions in BRCA1 and BRCA2. *Nat Biotechnol* 18:561–564.

Ferretti, L., P. Leone, and V. Sgaramella. 1990. Long range restriction analysis of the bovine casein genes. *Nucleic Acids Res* 18:6829–6833.

Fox, L. K., J. H. Kirk, and A. Britten. 2005. *Mycoplasma* mastitis: A review of transmission and control. *J Vet Med B Infect Dis Vet Public Health* 52:153–160.

Frahm, E., I. Heiber, S. Hoffmann et al. 1998. Application of 23S rDNA-targeted oligonucleotide probes specific for enterococci to water hygiene control. *Syst Appl Microbiol* 21:450–453.

Gemas, V. J. V., M. C. Almadanim, R. Tenreiro, A. Martins, and P. Fevereiro. 2004. Genetic diversity in the olive tree (*Olea europaea* L. subsp. europaea) cultivated in Portugal revealed by RAPD and ISSR markers. *Genet Resour Crop Evol* 51:501–511.

Germini, A., A. Mezzelani, F. Lesignoli et al. 2004. Detection of genetically modified soybean using peptide nucleic acids (PNAs) and microarray technology. *J Agric Food Chem* 52:4535–4540.

Germini, A., S. Rossi, A. Zanetti et al. 2005. Development of a peptide nucleic acid array platform for the detection of genetically modified organisms in food. *J Agric Food Chem* 53:3958–3962.

Gerry, N. P., N. E. Witowski, J. Day et al. 1999. Universal DNA microarray method for multiplex detection of low abundance point mutations. *J Mol Biol* 292:251–262.

Giannino, M. L., M. Aliprandi, M. Feligini et al. 2009. A DNA array based assay for the characterization of microbial community in raw milk. *J Microbiol Meth* 78:181–188.

Gibbs, R. A., J. F. Taylor, C. P. Van Tassell et al. 2009. Genome-wide survey of SNP variation uncovers the genetic structure of cattle breeds. *Science* 324:528–532.

Gilmour, M. W., M. Graham, G. Van Domselaar et al. 2010. High-throughput genome sequencing of two *Listeria monocytogenes* clinical isolates during a large foodborne outbreak. *BMC Genomics* 11:120.

Gu, X. X., R. Rossau, G. Jannes et al. 1998. The rrs (16S)-rrl (23S) ribosomal intergenic spacer region as a target for the detection of *Haemophilus ducreyi* by a heminested-PCR assay. *Microbiology* 144:1013–1019.

Hacia, J. G. 1999. Resequencing and mutational analysis using oligonucleotide microarrays. *Nat Genet* 21:42–47.

Hamid, M. E., A. Roth, O. Landt et al. 2002. Differentiation between *Mycobacterium farcinogenes* and *Mycobacterium senegalense* strains based on 16S–23S ribosomal DNA internal transcribed spacer sequences. *J Clin Microbiol* 40:707–711.

Hassan, A. A., O. Akineden, and E. Usleber. 2005. Identification of *Streptococcus canis* isolated from milk of dairy cows with subclinical mastitis. *J Clin Microbiol* 43:1234–1238.

Hayes, H., E. Petit, C. Bouniol, and P. Popescu. 1993. Localization of the alpha-S2-casein gene (CASAS2) to the homoeologous cattle, sheep, and goat chromosomes 4 by in situ hybridization. *Cytogenet Cell Genet* 64:281–285.

Helps, C. R., D. A. Harbour, and J. E. Corry. 1999. PCR-based 16S ribosomal DNA detection technique for *Clostridium esthertheticum* causing spoilage in vacuum-packed chill-stored beef. *Int J Food Microbiol* 52:57–65.

Hemmer, W. 1997. Foods derived from genetically modified organisms and detection methods. BATS-Report 2/1997. Agency for Biosafety Research and Assessment of Technology Impacts of the Swiss Priority Programme Biotechnology of the Swiss National Science Foundation. Basel, Switzerland.

Hernandez, M., M. Pla, T. Esteve et al. 2003a. A specific real-time quantitative PCR detection system for event MON810 in maize YieldGard based on the 3'-transgene integration sequence. *Transgenic Res* 12:179–189.

Hernandez, M., D. Rodriguez-Lazaro, T. Esteve, S. Prat, and M. Pla. 2003b. Development of melting temperature-based SYBR Green I polymerase chain reaction methods for multiplex genetically modified organism detection. *Anal Biochem* 323:164–170.

Holst-Jensen, A., S. B. Ronning, A. Lovseth, and K. G. Berdal. 2003. PCR technology for screening and quantification of genetically modified organisms (GMOs). *Anal Bioanal Chem* 375:985–993.

Hong, B. X., L. F. Jiang, Y. S. Hu, D. Y. Fang, and H. Y. Guo. 2004. Application of oligonucleotide array technology for the rapid detection of pathogenic bacteria of foodborne infections. *J Microbiol Meth* 58:403–411.

Huang, H. Y. and T. M. Pan. 2004. Detection of genetically modified maize MON810 and NK603 by multiplex and real-time polymerase chain reaction methods. *J Agric Food Chem* 52:3264–3268.

Hyten, D. L., S. B. Cannon, Q. Song et al. 2010. High-throughput SNP discovery through deep resequencing of a reduced representation library to anchor and orient scaffolds in the soybean whole genome sequence. *BMC Genomics* 11:38.

Ikonen, T., H. Bovenhuis, M. Ojala, O. Ruottinen, and M. Georges. 2001. Associations between casein haplotypes and first lactation milk production traits in Finnish Ayrshire cows. *J Dairy Sci* 84:507–514.

International Olive Council. 2006. *Trade Standard Applying to Olive Oils and Olive-Pomace Oils*. http:// www.internationaloliveoil.org/downloads/NORMAEN1.pdf (accessed date: June 26, 2006).

Ivnitski, D., D. J. O'Neil, A. Gattuso et al. 2003. Nucleic acid approaches for detection and identification of biological warfare and infectious disease agents. *Biotechniques* 35:862–869.

James, D., A. M. Schmidt, E. Wall, M. Green, and S. Masri. 2003. Reliable detection and identification of genetically modified maize, soybean, and canola by multiplex PCR analysis. *J Agric Food Chem* 51:5829–5834.

Jayarao, B. M., B. E. Gillespie, M. J. Lewis, H. H. Dowlen, and S. P. Oliver. 1999. Epidemiology of *Streptococcus uberis* intramammary infections in a dairy herd. *Zentrolbl Veterinarimed B* 46:433–442.

Kaminski, S., A. Ahman, A. Rusc, E. Wojcik, and T. Malewski. 2005. MilkProtChip—A microarray of SNPs in candidate genes associated with milk protein biosynthesis—Development and validation. *J Appl Genet* 46:45–58.

Kaminski, S., P. Brym, A. Rusc et al. 2006. Associations between milk performance traits in Holstein cows and 16 candidate SNPs identified by arrayed primer extension (APEX) microarray. *Anim Biotechnol* 17:1–11.

Kaminski, S., H. Help, P. Brym, A. Rusc, and E. Wojcik. 2008. SNiPORK—A microarray of SNPs in candidate genes potentially associated with pork yield and quality—Development and validation in commercial breeds. *Anim Biotechnol* 19:43–69.

Kim, H. J., S. H. Park, T. H. Lee et al. 2008. Microarray detection of food-borne pathogens using specific probes prepared by comparative genomics. *Biosens Bioelectron* 24:238–246.

Kurg, A., N. Tonisson, I. Georgiou et al. 2000. Arrayed primer extension: Solid-phase four-color DNA resequencing and mutation detection technology. *Genet Test* 4:1–7.

Leimanis, S., M. Hernandez, S. Fernandez et al. 2006. A microarray-based detection system for genetically modified (GM) food ingredients. *Plant Mol Biol* 61:123–139.

Li, Y., D. Liu, B. Cao et al. 2006. Development of a serotype-specific DNA microarray for identification of some *Shigella* and pathogenic *Escherichia coli* strains. *J Clin Microbiol* 44:4376–4383.

Madico, G., T. C. Quinn, J. Boman, and C. A. Gaydos. 2000. Touchdown enzyme time release-PCR for detection and identification of *Chlamydia trachomatis*, *C. pneumoniae*, and *C. psittaci* using the 16S and 16S–23S spacer rRNA genes. *J Clin Microbiol* 38:1085–1093.

Margulies, M., M. Egholm, W. E. Altman et al. 2005. Genome sequencing in microfabricated high-density picolitre reactors. *Nature* 437:376–380.

Marmiroli, N., C. Peano, and E. Maestri. 2003. Advanced PCR techniques in identifying food components. In *Food Authenticity and Traceability*, ed. M. Lees, pp. 3–33. Cambridge, U.K.: CRC Press.

Martin, P., M. Szymanowska, L. Zwierzchowski, and C. Leroux. 2002. The impact of genetic polymorphisms on the protein composition of ruminant milks. *Reprod Nutr Dev* 42:433–459.

Martins-Lopes, P., S. Gomes, E. Santos, and H. Guedes-Pinto. 2008. DNA markers for Portuguese olive oil fingerprinting. *J Agric Food Chem* 56:11786–11791.

Matar, G. M., J. E. Koehler, G. Malcolm et al. 1999. Identification of *Bartonella* species directly in clinical specimens by PCR-restriction fragment length polymorphism analysis of a 16S rRNA gene fragment. *J Clin Microbiol* 37:4045–4047.

Matsuoka, T., H. Kuribara, H. Akiyama et al. 2001. A multiplex PCR method of detecting recombinant DNAs from five lines of genetically modified maize. *Shokuhin Eiseigaku Zasshi* 42:24–32.

Miraglia, M., K. G. Berdal, C. Brera et al. 2004. Detection and traceability of genetically modified organisms in the food production chain. *Food Chem Toxicol* 42:1157–1180.

Montemurro, C., A. Pasqualone, R. Simeone, W. Sabetta, and A. Blanco. 2008. AFLP molecular markers to identify virgin olive oils from a single Italian cultivars. *Eur Food Res Technol* 226:1439–1444.

Murray, M. G. and W. F. Thompson. 1980. Rapid isolation of high molecular weight plant DNA. *Nucleic Acids Res* 8:4321–4325.

Muzzalupo, I., M. Pellegrino, and E. Perri. 2007. Detection of DNA in virgin olive oils extracted from destoned fruits. *Eur Food Res Technol* 224:469–475.

Nolan, J. P. and L. A. Sklar. 2002. Suspension array technology: Evolution of the flat-array paradigm. *Trends Biotechnol* 20:9–12.

Pafundo, S., C. Agrimonti, E. Maestri, and N. Marmiroli. 2007. Applicability of SCAR markers to food genomics: Olive oil traceability. *J Agric Food Chem* 55:6052–6059.

Pafundo, S., C. Agrimonti, and N. Marmiroli. 2005. Traceability of plant contribution in olive oil by amplified fragment length polymorphisms. *J Agric Food Chem* 53:6995–7002.

Panicker, G., D. R. Call, M. J. Krug, and A. K. Bej. 2004. Detection of pathogenic *Vibrio* spp. in shellfish by using multiplex PCR and DNA microarrays. *Appl Environ Microbiol* 70:7436–7444.

Pasqualone, A., C. Montemurro, C. Summo et al. 2007. Effectiveness of microsatellite DNA markers in checking the identity of protected designation of origin extra virgin olive oil. *J Agric Food Chem* 55:3857–3862.

Pastinen, T., M. Raitio, K. Lindroos et al. 2000. A system for specific, high-throughput genotyping by allele-specific primer extension on microarrays. *Genome Res* 10:1031–1042.

Peano, C., R. Bordoni, M. Gulli et al. 2005a. Multiplex polymerase chain reaction and ligation detection reaction/universal array technology for the traceability of genetically modified organisms in foods. *Anal Biochem* 346:90–100.

Peano, C., F. Lesignoli, M. Gulli et al. 2005b. Development of a peptide nucleic acid polymerase chain reaction clamping assay for semiquantitative evaluation of genetically modified organism content in food. *Anal Biochem* 344:174–182.

Peano, C., M. C. Samson, L. Palmieri, M. Gulli, and N. Marmiroli. 2004. Qualitative and quantitative evaluation of the genomic DNA extracted from GMO and non-GMO foodstuffs with four different extraction methods. *J Agric Food Chem* 52:6962–6968.

Perreten, V., L. Vorlet-Fawer, P. Slickers et al. 2005. Microarray-based detection of 90 antibiotic resistance genes of gram-positive bacteria. *J Clin Microbiol* 43:2291–2302.

Popescu, C. P., S. Long, P. Riggs et al. 1996. Standardization of cattle karyotype nomenclature: Report of the committee for the standardization of the cattle karyotype. *Cytogenet Cell Genet* 74:259–261.

Prinzenberg, E. M., C. Weimann, H. Brandt et al. 2003. Polymorphism of the bovine CSN1S1 promoter: Linkage mapping, intragenic haplotypes, and effects on milk production traits. *J Dairy Sci* 86:2696–2705.

Ramsay, G. 1998. DNA chips: State-of-the art. *Nat Biotechnol* 16:40–44.

Raspor, P. 2005. Bio-markers: Traceability in food safety issues. *Acta Biochim Pol* 52:659–664.

Relogio, A., C. Schwager, A. Richter, W. Ansorge, and J. Valcarcel. 2002. Optimization of oligonucleotide-based DNA microarrays. *Nucleic Acids Res* 30:e51.

Rudi, K., I. Rud, and A. Holck. 2003. A novel multiplex quantitative DNA array based PCR (MQDA-PCR) for quantification of transgenic maize in food and feed. *Nucleic Acids Res* 31:e62.

Sanz-Cortes, F., D. E. Parfitt, C. Romero, D. Struss, G. Llacer, and M. L. Badenes. 2003. Intraspecific olive diversity assessed with AFLP. *Plant Breed* 122:173–177.

Sasaki, Y., K. Yamamoto, K. Amimoto et al. 2001. Amplification of the 16S–23S rDNA spacer region for rapid detection of *Clostridium chauvoei* and *Clostridium septicum*. *Res Vet Sci* 71:227–229.

Schwerin, M. 2001. Structural and functional genomics in domestic animals: The way to understand the phenotype. *J Appl Genet* 42:293–308.

Sergeev, N., M. Distler, M. Vargas et al. 2006. Microarray analysis of *Bacillus cereus* group virulence factors. *J Microbiol Meth* 65:488–502.

Severgnini, M., P. Cremonesi, C. Consolandi et al. 2009. ORMA: A tool for identification of species-specific variations in 16S rRNA gene and oligonucleotides design. *Nucleic Acids Res* 37:e109.

Siqueira, J. F., Jr., I. N. Rocas, A. Favieri, and K. R. Santos. 2000. Detection of *Treponema denticola* in endodontic infections by 16S rRNA gene-directed polymerase chain reaction. *Oral Microbiol Immunol* 15:335–337.

Smith, J. G., L. Kong, G. K. Abruzzo et al. 1996. PCR detection of colonization by *Helicobacter pylori* in conventional, euthymic mice based on the 16S ribosomal gene sequence. *Clin Diagn Lab Immunol* 3:66–72.

Song, J. Y., H. G. Park, S. O. Jung, and J. Park. 2005. Diagnosis of HNF-1alpha mutations on a PNA zip-code microarray by single base extension. *Nucleic Acids Res* 33:e19.

Stenberg, J., M. Nilsson, and U. Landegren. 2005. ProbeMaker: An extensible framework for design of sets of oligonucleotide probes. *BMC Bioinformatics* 6:229.

Straub, J. A., C. Hertel, and W. P. Hammes. 1999. A 23S rDNA-targeted polymerase chain reaction-based system for detection of *Staphylococcus aureus* in meat starter cultures and dairy products. *J Food Prot* 62:1150–1156.

Suo, B., Y. He, G. Paoli et al. 2010. Development of an oligonucleotide-based microarray to detect multiple foodborne pathogens. *Mol Cell Probes* 24:77–86.

Taverniers, I., E. Van Bockstaele, and M. De Loose. 2001. Use of cloned DNA fragments as reference materials for event specific quantification of genetically modified organisms (GMOs). *Meded Rijksuniv Gent Fak Landbouwkd Toegep Biol Wet* 66:469–472.

Tengs, T., A. B. Kristoffersen, K. G. Berdal et al. 2007. Microarray-based method for detection of unknown genetic modifications. *BMC Biotechnol* 7:91.

Tesfaye, M. and F. B. Holl. 1998. Group-specific differentiation of *Rhizobium* from clover species by PCR amplification of 23S rDNA sequences. *Can J Microbiol* 44:1102–1105.

Thiyagarajan, S., M. Karhanek, M. Akhras, R. W. Davis, and N. Pourmand. 2006. PathogenMIPer: A tool for the design of molecular inversion probes to detect multiple pathogens. *BMC Bioinformatics* 7:500.

Threadgill, D. W. and J. E. Womack. 1990. Genomic analysis of the major bovine milk protein genes. *Nucleic Acids Res* 18:6935–6942.

Urbanczyk-Wochniak, E., A. Luedemann, J. Kopka et al. 2003. Parallel analysis of transcript and metabolic profiles: A new approach in systems biology. *EMBO Rep* 4:989–993.

Vijaya Satya, R., N. Zavaljevski, K. Kumar, and J. Reifman. 2008. A high-throughput pipeline for designing microarray-based pathogen diagnostic assays. *BMC Bioinformatics* 9:185.

Volokhov, D., V. Chizhikov, K. Chumakov, and A. Rasooly. 2003. Microarray-based identification of thermophilic *Campylobacter jejuni*, *C. coli*, *C. lari*, and *C. upsaliensis*. *J Clin Microbiol* 41:4071–4080.

Wang, R. F., M. L. Beggs, L. H. Robertson, and C. E. Cerniglia. 2002a. Design and evaluation of oligonucleotide-microarray method for the detection of human intestinal bacteria in fecal samples. *FEMS Microbiol Lett* 213:175–182.

Wang, R. F., S. J. Kim, L. H. Robertson, and C. E. Cerniglia. 2002b. Development of a membrane-array method for the detection of human intestinal bacteria in fecal samples. *Mol Cell Probes* 16:341–350.

Wang, X. W., L. Zhang, L. Q. Jin et al. 2007. Development and application of an oligonucleotide microarray for the detection of foodborne bacterial pathogens. *Appl Microbiol Biotech* 76:225–233.

Weiler, J., H. Gausepohl, N. Hauser, O. N. Jensen, and J. D. Hoheisel. 1997. Hybridisation based DNA screening on peptide nucleic acid (PNA) oligomer arrays. *Nucleic Acids Res* 25:2792–2799.

Whitesides, G. M. 2006. The origins and the future of microfluidics. *Nature* 442:368–373.

Wilson, K. H., W. J. Wilson, J. L. Radosevich et al. 2002. High-density microarray of small-subunit ribosomal DNA probes. *Appl Environ Microbiol* 68:2535–2541.

Windels, P., S. De Buck, E. Van Bockstaele, M. De Loose, and A. Depicker. 2003. T-DNA integration in Arabidopsis chromosomes. Presence and origin of filler DNA sequences. *Plant Physiol* 133:2061–2068.

Wong, H. C., Y. L. Chen, and C. L. F. Chen. 1988. Growth, germination and toxigenic activity of *Bacillus cereus* in milk products. *J Food Prot* 51:707–710.

Wong, H. C., S. H. Liu, L. W. Ku et al. 2000. Characterization of *Vibrio parahaemolyticus* isolates obtained from foodborne illness outbreaks during 1992 through 1995 in Taiwan. *J Food Prot* 63:900–906.

Woolfe, M. and S. Primrose. 2004. Food forensics: Using DNA technology to combat misdescription and fraud. *Trends Biotechnol* 22:222–226.

Xu, X., Y. Li, H. Zhao et al. 2005. Rapid and reliable detection and identification of GM events using multiplex PCR coupled with oligonucleotide microarray. *J Agric Food Chem* 53:3789–3794.

Xu, J., H. Miao, H. Wu et al. 2006. Screening genetically modified organisms using multiplex-PCR coupled with oligonucleotide microarray. *Biosens Bioelectron* 22:1–7.

Xu, J., S. Zhu, H. Miao et al. 2007. Event-specific detection of seven genetically modified soybean and maizes using multiplex-PCR coupled with oligonucleotide microarray. *J Agric Food Chem* 55:5575–5579.

Yang, L., J. Guo, A. Pan et al. 2007. Event-specific quantitative detection of nine genetically modified maizes using one novel standard reference molecule. *J Agric Food Chem* 55:15–24.

Yang, L., A. Pan, H. Zhang et al. 2006. Event-specific qualitative and quantitative polymerase chain reaction analysis for genetically modified canola T45. *J Agric Food Chem* 54:9735–9740.

# 3 Metabolomics and Food Science

## Concepts and Serviceability in Plant Foods and Nutrition

*Noureddine Benkeblia*

## CONTENTS

## 3.1 INTRODUCTION

Metabolomics (or metabonomics) is considered one of the recent "omics," joining genomics, transcriptomics, and proteomics as a science employed toward the understanding of systems biology (Schmidt 2004). Although there is some overlap in terminology with metabolomics and metabonomics, for simplicity, the term metabolomics is preferred and is defined as a "measurement of time-related multiparametric metabolic responses of biological systems to a physiological or environmental stimulus or genetic modification" (Nicholson et al. 1999).

The term metabolomics has its root from metabolites, which result from the interaction of the system's genome with its environment. They are not merely the end product of gene expression but also form a part of the regulatory system in an integrated manner. The field of metabolomics entails the study of global metabolite profiles in a system (organelle, cell, tissue, or organism) under a given set of conditions (Goodacre et al. 2004).

The challenge is to analyze the complete range of primary and secondary metabolites that are present within a biological system or excreted from this system. The analysis shall reflect the exact biological face of this system at a defined developmental stage or under specific environmental factors or stresses. The metabolomics experiment ranges from sampling and sample preparation through analytical strategies to raw data processing and data analysis (Brown et al. 2005). Due to this complex route, no single analytical technology can detect all metabolites present, and currently several promising comprehensive technologies, such as chromatographic techniques coupled to mass spectrometry, are employed to study these wide arrays of metabolites (Dunn and Ellis 2005).

Metabolomics potential is significant, and because it is considered as an emerging idea so far, it has the potential to revolutionize an entire field of scientific endeavor. It is now imperative for us to detect subtle perturbations within the phenomenally complex biochemical matrix of living organisms (Mitchell et al. 2002). This discipline is promising an all-encompassing approach to understanding comprehensive, yet fundamental changes occurring in living organisms (Fell and Wagner 2002, Glassbrook et al. 2000, Mitchell et al. 2002).

From its first description in the literature of the 1950s, metabolomics developed slowly during the following four decades. However, during the last 10 years and with the development of new analytical technologies and "omics," metabolomics has become an area of major research interest. To illustrate this recent

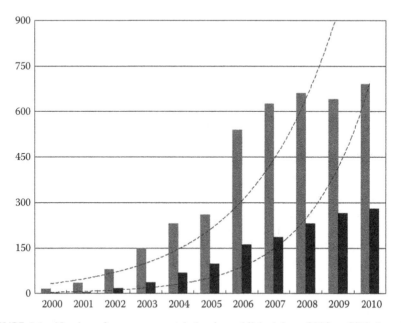

**FIGURE 3.1**  Number of papers on metabolomics published from 2000 to 2010 (last date estimation). Database searched: ASFA, Biological abstracts, CAB Direct, CiNii, Current Contents, Highwire, ISI, Medline, ProQuest, Publimed, and Science Direct. Search term used: metabolomics and nutrigenomics.

development, the number of publications in the last 5 years (January 2005 through December 2010) increased logarithmically and is more than double of the total number in regard to this topic that have been published in the last 20 years combined (Figure 3.1).

From early life, plants provide the major part of human food intake, and cereals and other starchy plants have been our major source of energy. Over the past century, to support the growing human population, much of the systematic effort in plant breeding has focused on increasing the yield per hectare and in protecting crops from pests, diseases, and other attacks, which cause losses during cultivation, harvesting, handling, transportation, and storage. Research regarding the quality of horticultural crops, in particular cereals, fruits, and vegetables, was primarily designed to improve their utility for processing, for example, baking or brewing, rather than to improve their nutritional values. With the development of new analytical techniques and technologies, these approaches began to change in the early 1960s with the discovery of new varieties (Mertz et al. 1964, Rochfort 2005).

For most common disorders and diseases that afflict man, including obesity, diabetes, CVD, and many cancers, diets that are rich in plant foods, fruits and vegetables, are associated with lower risk (World Health Organization/Food and Agriculture Organization [WHO/FAO] 2003).

## 3.2 ROLE OF FOODS IN HUMAN HEALTH

Now that scientific knowledge of the nutrients that are the basis of nutrient deficiency and diseases is established, determining the role of foods and nutrients in metabolic regulation has become a key scientific objective of nutrition research. The importance of diet has become even more obvious with the realization that many of life's modern diseases are the result of subtle but chronic metabolic imbalances related in great part (>35%) to diet. Although many of the diseases that medicine has dealt with successfully over the past century have been those caused by exogenous toxins or pathogenic organisms, the metabolic diseases including atherosclerosis, obesity, hypertension, diabetes, osteoporosis, and various inflammatory diseases are caused by chronic imbalances of normal metabolic pathways (Barsh and Schwartz 2002, Seeman 2002, Tabas 2002). These diseases thus pose a great challenge for all aspects of traditional public health intervention, including nutrition.

Foods are a part of the problem, and nutrition should play a vital role in metabolic disease prevention. Metabolic balance is responsive to the presence of essential nutrients at the limits of their adequacy, as well as to the proportion of essential nutrients and to the abundance of nonessential components in the diet. As dietary strategies seek to modify metabolism for health benefits, the importance of understanding precisely how much of each nutrient is optimal leads to the necessity to redefine safety of nutrients consumed in amounts beyond those necessary for adequacy. New strategies, technologies, and knowledge must be established to evaluate both the efficacy and the safety of diets designed specifically to influence metabolism on a continuous basis.

## 3.3  "OMICS" AND FOOD AND NUTRITION SCIENCES

Investigators of food and nutrition sciences, as well as medical fields, are developing novel approaches and furthering existing methods to study metabolites and to detect and prevent metabolic disorders and imbalances (Ravussin and Bouchard 2000). New tools in the scientific field to support these approaches are emerging from "omics" and related global technologies, including gene expression, transcription, and metabolism (Scalbert et al. 2009, Watkins et al. 2001). In addition, "omics" has propelled a change in the perspective of biological scientists to "the systems approach." In the recent past, rigorous studies of biological signals, structures, reactions, and catalysts were largely simplistic. Researchers reduced their focus to increasingly narrow spheres to understand molecular mechanisms of genes and their expression. On the other hand, nutritionists also focused attention on molecular details to understand how nutrients could exert in the diet their biological effects. However, although these approaches allowed understanding of specific mechanisms, the ability to examine the larger behavior of entire biological systems or organisms was lost (Rist et al. 2006).

Later, genomics and proteomics technologies changed the strategy of food and nutrition researchers. Presently, it is possible to measure simultaneously thousands of biological events in molecular detail (Roberts et al. 2001). With these principles in place, researchers extended the analysis of not only genes and their expression, but also went to another global perspective to examine the biological system and its organization. This led to the study of the proteins and metabolites, which were studied separately under the field of proteomics and metabolomics, respectively (German et al. 2002).

Furthermore, the expansion of data management through the use of bioinformatics has made it possible to see a new future for food and nutrition sciences intervention. Scientists from different biological disciplines are embracing bioinformatics as the ultimate key to understanding biodiversity and its evolution (Mendes 2002, Noordewier and Brown 2002, Servant et al. 2002, Wickware 2000). Interestingly, the field of food science is moving toward the complex issue of biodiversity and the variation between individuals (Shastry 2002). Thus, "omics" will not be the only, and probably not the most important, platform for food sciences. However, food technologists and scientists of other related disciplines will use the downstream products of "omics" from genomics to proteomics and metabolomics.

## 3.4  ANALYTICAL TECHNIQUES

After the first publications dealt with the metabolites of specific compounds, studies soon expanded to include multiple classes of compounds and more recently full or partial metabolomic analysis has been exploited (Dunn and Ellis 2005, Weichert et al. 2002). Recent work has focused on the improvement of analytical techniques and data management systems. Although nuclear magnetic resonance (NMR), Fourier transform infrared (FTIR), and high-performance liquid chromatography (HPLC-UV) techniques are used, mass spectrometry (MS) currently is the most frequently used analytical tool for metabolomics in plants. Recent advances include localization of metabolite profiles within tissues, cells, and organelles in real time as well (Gidman et al. 2003, Johnson et al. 2003). During the last few years, gas chromatography, as well as liquid chromatography, coupled with mass spectrometry (GC-MS and LC-MS) have been useful analytical techniques for metabolomic analysis and spatially metabolite profiling of plants. Several MS techniques have been used in these approaches and applied in several studies (Kopka 2006, Taylor et al. 2002). With the development of MS technologies, strategies in metabolomic profiling by HPLC-MS are of interest for future developments.

Combinations of techniques have also been expected for metabolome analysis (Castrillo et al. 2003), such as electrospray ionization time-of-flight mass spectrometry (ESI-TOF-MS) used in plant analysis (Goodacre et al. 2004) and electrospray ionization mass spectrometry (ESI-MS) used to detect oligosaccharides, glycosides, amino sugars, amino acids, and sugar nucleotides in plant tissue (Tolstikov and Fiehn 2002). On the other hand, deconvolution and peak identification tools such as the automated mass spectral deconvolution and identification system (AMDIS, http://www.amdis.net) and National Institute of Standards and Technology (NIST, http://nist.gov) database are useful for specific compound identification in GC-MS. Useful bioinformatics programs such as MSFACTS and MET-IDEA (Broeckling et al. 2006, Duran et al. 2003) have been developed by the scientists of the Samuel Roberts Noble Foundation (Ardmore, Oklahoma), which can import and reformat large data sets to easily handled Excel sheets, and these programs have been demonstrated using GC-MS data generated from different tissues in a legume (Duran et al. 2003). Other researchers have also been active, and a new visualization tool named COMPSARI has been recently released, which facilitates the identification of small differences in MS data (Katz et al. 2004).

Nevertheless, measurement of metabolites is not easy, because (a) the dynamic of metabolites makes problematic the harvesting protocols and experimental design and (b) their chemistry, which makes their identification more complex than it seems (Kell 2004).

In metabolomics studies, quenching of metabolism is an important first step, due to the swift turnover of many metabolites in the cell, which vary rapidly (e.g., ATP has a biological half-life ($t_{1/2}$) of less than 0.1 s) (Walsh and Koshland 1984). Thus, the metabolism of cells should be stopped instantaneously by using liquid nitrogen. Moreover, as enzyme activities are only affected by the metabolite concentrations in their direct environment, it is more appropriate to analyze metabolites in the different compartments of the cell separately (e.g., cytoplasm, mitochondria, extracellular matrix, and cell wall). After quenching, metabolites are extracted from the different compartments and their concentrations are determined. This is accomplished by a nonaqueous fractionation (NAQF) procedure to separate subcellular compartments under enzymatically inactive conditions (Gerhardt and Heldt 1984, Stitt et al. 1989).

## 3.5 METABOLOMICS AND PLANT FOOD SCIENCE

From the practical point of view, food sciences and nutrition are not well prepared for applying and exploiting "omics" technologies; however, research in these fields is moving the genome into the center of all the processes that essentially determine human metabolism and health (Muller and Kersten 2003). Despite the fact that metabolomics has been applied to identify biological markers of diseases (Griffin et al. 2001, Wang et al. 2004), the plant research community has also been active in the development of metabolomics, as well as other "omics." From the fundamental point of view, plants accumulate thousands of metabolites with important functions in their ecology, physiology, and stresses responses. Presently, metabolomics, because it is highly sensitive, allows scientists to resolve small differences between wild-type and transgenic plants and offers subtle tools and new technologies to analyze the complex interaction occurring in plants (Fiehn 2002, Rochfort 2005).

However, because of the diversity of eating behaviors and the wide range of consumed plant foods, the intra- and interindividual heterogeneity of consumption make the characterization and quantification of dietary exposure more complex than it seems (Mathers 2006). This complexity is worsened in cases of specific foods because of changes that occur in plant foods during storage and processing and also the lack of information regarding the digestion, absorption, and metabolic transformation of most food constituents, especially nonnutrient food constituents.

Presently, metabolomics-based protocols have the capacity to characterize dietary exposure to plant foods and to focus on (a) the large number of plant metabolites (plant metabolome), (b) the metabolomic profiling of processed foods (food metabolome), and (c) the nutritional evolution (digestion and absorption) of plant-derived metabolites (absorbed metabolome), and these processes offer the potential to develop novel approaches to track nutritional exposure to plants and plant-derived foods over prolonged time periods (Mathers 2004a).

## 3.6 METABOLOMICS AND NATURAL BIOLOGICALLY ACTIVE COMPOUNDS

The genome in every cell is continually exposed to both exogenous and endogenous factors, which cause damage to nucleic acids, and cells have evolved a range of DNA repair mechanisms that sense and repair different kinds of damage. The major types of DNA repair in mammalian cells include one-step repair, base excision repair, nucleotide excision repair, DNA mismatch repair, and recombinational repair. Recent research suggests that dietary antioxidants may protect the cell through upregulating DNA repair (Brash and Havre 2002). Importantly, there is now evidence from a human intervention trial that improved nutrition may enhance DNA repair in human subjects *in vivo*. Because genomic damage is the primary step in the development of some pathologies, plant-derived bioactive food components could have a protective effect against such pathologies by intervening in the pathways regulating gene expression (Bovy et al. 2007, Milner 2004). Cells have evolved numerous mechanisms that minimize such damage, including inhibition of oxidative reactions by free radical scavenging, detoxification of potential mutagens, repairing the damage, and removing severely damaged cells by shunting them into apoptosis (Mathers 2004b). Thus, understanding the interrelationships between genes and diets is fundamental for nutritional strategies, and this concept is the root of a new approach namely "nutrigenomics." Nutrigenomics is a science that considers the interaction of specific genes and food components, including bioactive compounds. This information could be a key to a personalized guide to nutrition (Trujillo et al. 2006).

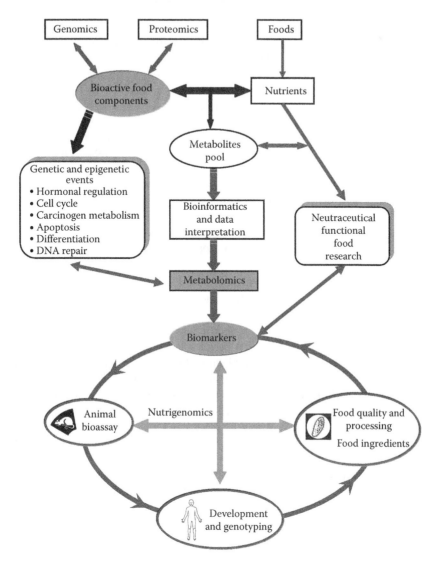

**FIGURE 3.2** Metabolomic approach and its integration in food and nutrition sciences: nutrigenomics.

The dual application of metabolomics, with nutrigenomics, has been of great help in the discovery of the mode of action (MOA) of natural biological compounds, as well as in functional food analyses (Figure 3.2). The use of metabolomic approaches and appropriate statistical analyses has the potential to allow rapid analysis of the complex data obtained from these analyses. For example, NMR technique has been used to cluster the spectra of crude plant extracts to determine the biochemical MOA of a medicinal extract of *Anoectochilus formosanus* (an herb), and its activity was compared using metabolomics and transcriptomics analyses (Yang et al. 2004).

However, these MOA are potentially modifiable by active components in foods, such as phenolics and carotenoids, and also by nutritional status of the organisms (Steele 2003). This fact may help explain why diets rich in plant foods, particularly fruits and vegetables, which are the main source of these biological molecules, appear to be protective against a wide range of common diseases (WHO/FAO 2003).

To highlight this example, during the past decade, there has been vast expansion in the research of fructooligosaccharides (FOS), including their chemistry, biochemistry, and enzymology in living organisms, as well as nutritional and health benefits (Benkeblia and Shiomi 2006, Cherbut 2002, Cummings et al. 1997, Flamm et al. 2001). FOS fit well within the current concept of the class of dietary material and are even labeled as "functional foods" since their vast health benefits are continuously reported (Roberfroid 2002). Likely due to their specific properties, FOS affect several functions and contribute to reduce the risk of many diseases. Thus, they may contribute in a significant way to a well-being by their specific effects on several physiological functions (Cummings et al. 2001, Roberfroid 2000, Roberfroid and Salvin 2000, Weaver 2005).

However, in spite of these considerable advances in FOS science, many other aspects of the mechanisms of FOS behind their involvement in well-being have not been fully understood.

Bearing in mind their functional properties, such as the bioavailability of minerals, prebiotic effects and modulation of colonic microflora, improvement of the gastrointestinal physiology, the metabolism of lipids, or prevention of some cancers, further basic researches on their metabolism are needed. Thus, metabolomic approaches could be considered as a "key" tool to investigate and profile the metabolomes to help answer the questions about their proven and/or putative roles in human health.

Furthermore, much of the work in the area of natural biological compounds has focused on plant secondary metabolites and micronutrients, such as flavonoids, quercetins, vitamins A, C, and E, and trace minerals including Zn, Se, and Mn that are believed to prevent oxidative damage (Ames and Wakimoto 2002, Collins et al. 2003, Wei et al. 2003).

## 3.7 METABOLOMICS AND FOOD NUTRIENTS ASSESSMENT

As in the expression: "the dose makes the poison," the nutrition and health fields are expanding their influences beyond considering only acute toxicity to address chronic metabolic imbalance. Undoubtedly, toxicity has become associated either with damaging molecules or with molecules and foods that generate metabolic disorders, causing sustained imbalances. On the other hand, when disorders occur, dosage is of high importance although essential nutrients are required up to certain levels, these same nutrients, in overabundance, can alter the metabolism in a destructive fashion. However, the changes induced in metabolic biomarkers by food ingredients are very small compared to those induced by drugs, and nutritionists are attempting to resolve these problems with increasingly accurate and reproducible techniques (Goodacre 2007). Alternatively, the application of metabolomics will allow us to screen and identify a broad range of metabolic determinants of health, rather than to focus on a few surrogate biomarkers (Gibney et al. 2005, Wishart 2008). For example, at the intracellular level, each amino acid is influenced by several biochemical reactions that occur either between amino acids or between amino acids and nonamino acid metabolites produced by other nutrients such as sugar and lipid, or by nucleotide metabolism. The regulation of biochemical reaction occurs at multiple levels of the organism; therefore, it could be expected that some information related to the relationships among various metabolites would be lost by traditional approaches, while it would be detected by metabolomics (Oresic 2009).

From this assumption, one of the approaches to metabolomics research in nutrition is to identify the maximum number of metabolites, build an appropriate model of a metabolic network, and elucidate their relationships (Hall et al. 2008, Manach et al. 2009), if any. From this stage, useful information may be gained by the metabolomic profiling of amino acids to detect potential changes in the relationships of these metabolites (Noguchi et al. 2003). For example, the amino acid metabolome seemed to be especially relevant in studying the effects of excessive intake of protein and amino acids and was a convenient model to focus on in order to analyze metabolomic data. The change in plasma amino acid concentrations over time, after the ingestion of a meal, has been well studied (Hegarty et al. 1982, Moundras et al. 1993).

Measuring the consequences of polyunsaturated fatty acids (PUFAs) in the diet on gene expression using metabolomics has also yielded interesting results (German et al. 2003, Oresic 2009). Effects of 18 carbon PUFAs on the transcriptional responses in the liver and hippocampus were compared in animals to determine whether varying amounts and compositions of fatty acids have an influence on any aspect of metabolism and genetic regulation (Berger et al. 2002). The number of genes that were differentially expressed in the livers and brains of these animals due the consumption of different dietary PUFAs was determined. The results have shown that from the 12,000 discrete genetic elements of the murine genome whose abundance is measurable on gene arrays, over 300 genes in both liver and hippocampus differed.

Metabolomics could also be a useful tool to determine the quality and authenticity of foods by analyzing the complete metabolome of these foods or food ingredients (Burdock et al. 2006, Vogels et al. 1993, 1996). For example, using the quality attributes of wheat, it is possible to predict the quality of bread produced from the flour of this wheat. Also, biomolecules or their specific ratios in the raw material can be identified by spacially metabolomic profiling (van der Werf et al. 2001). Moreover, human responses to diet are different and are not the consequence of genetic variation, but life stage, lifestyle, and personal environment also influence the human organism, and metabolomic analyses would help in designing a personalized diet rather than waiting for a predictive knowledge of genetic variation (Fay and German 2008). On the other hand, the quality attributes and safety of fresh and processed food crops have become topics of considerable interest during the last decade, and much attention is being paid on how to satisfy consumers' needs. Thus, metabolomics, as well as other "omic" technologies, could be considered as an interesting new road to the detailed knowledge of the composition and the variation of the biochemical of fresh and processed food crops and how they change during the postharvest handling and processing (Capanoglu et al. 2010, Stewart et al. 2011).

## 3.8   METABOLOMICS, FOOD MICROBIOLOGY, AND FERMENTATION TECHNOLOGY

Currently, microorganisms are used in the preparation and processing of foods and beverages in the human diet, and microbial fermentations is perhaps the oldest technique known for the preservation of foods. Fermented foods and beverages now represent a significant portion of the food processing industry (Campbell-Platt 1994, McKay and Baldwin 1990). Microorganisms are directly involved in the success of food manufacturing processes such as alcoholic fermentations, baking, sausage manufacture, vegetable fermentations, production of food ingredients (e.g., industrial enzymes, nutritive additives, flavor components, sweeteners, and stabilizers) as well as dairy products and numerous other traditional or local fermented foods (DellaPenna 1999). Lactic acid bacteria (LAB) play an essential role in these food and beverage fermentation processes, and many of these fermentations depend on LAB strains for manufacturing and production. LAB have also been considered beneficial to human health (Fleet 1999, Tannock 1999), and, currently, LAB are employed in numerous probiotic products considered as "functional foods," or foods that provide a health benefit aside from satisfying nutritional needs (Sanders 1998). During the last decade, this segment of the food industry experienced a vast expansion due to an increasing public awareness of the role of nutrition in maintaining health and well-being (Hilliam 1998). Recent investigations have linked probiotic LAB to a large assortment of health benefits, including resistance to pathogens, immune system modulation, cancer prevention, and reduction of cardiovascular diseases (Sanders and Int'l Veld, 1999).

Thus, sequence annotation of LAB and metabolomic approaches, in addition to transcriptomics and proteomics, are of great help to define the molecular nature of metabolic networks within these utile microorganisms. Moreover, one of the most difficult issues of metabolic engineering is to decide whether it is necessary to change the metabolic pathway or not, and if the answer is yes, then where to change it in order to more efficiently produce desired molecules or to divert the fermentation process toward a desired pathway. This scientific knowledge, aided by the development of new technological, genetic, and molecular tools, will enable the selection and/or tailoring of strains for various fermentation or probiotic rationales (Breidt 2004, Mills 2004). Understanding of microbial ecology of fermented foods and its metabolic pathways will also help to reduce the amount of salts used in vegetable fermentations and may also help the use of starter cultures, because most vegetable fermentations are carried out without the use of starter cultures (Breidt 2004, Lee et al. 2009).

## 3.9   METABOLOMICS AND GM FOOD CROPS

Understanding the biology of food crops and developing crops with improved qualities are the main objectives of the research community in agricultural science (Gibbon and Larkins 2005). Herbicide-resistant varieties of soybean (Padgette et al. 1995) and resistance-enhanced maize strains (Koziel et al. 1993) are among the first generation of engineered GM food crops. However, it is important to assess the safety of GM food crops for human consumption. A multicompositional analysis, using metabolomic profiling, of biologically active compounds in plants could indicate if potentially unintended effects have taken place as a result of genetic modification (Kuiper et al. 2002, Schilter and Constable 2002). Metabolomic approaches based on targeted compositional analyses have shown efficacy in describing intended or unintended effects (Barros et al. 2010). Moreover and from the purely biological point of view, the following questions would be answered: (1) Would a transgene that has been inserted into the novel crop survive within the human intestine, (2) Would it be taken up by the gut microflora and incorporated into the bacterial genome, and (3) Is there horizontal gene transfer to enterocytes or other human cells? Many studies have been conducted regarding these hypotheses (Martin-Orúe et al. 2002, Mazza et al. 2005, Netherwood et al. 2004, Nielsen and Townsend 2004, Rossi et al. 2005), leading the authors to conclude that it is unlikely that the occurrence of genetic transfer associated with GM plants is higher than that from conventional plants.

## 3.10  METABOLOMICS AND SUSTAINABLE AGRICULTURE

Products obtainable through genomics and modern biotechnology are of crucial importance within the context of sustainable development of the world economy, particularly, to developing and poor countries. The greatest ultimate impact will be on agricultural genomics, especially for marker-assisted selection and breeding programs in crop and animal agriculture, for crop genetic engineering to overcome abiotic and biotic stresses, and for the improvement of the nutritional quality of major foods (Figure 3.3). It is imperative that sustainable agriculture becomes a "key target" in the "gene revolution" because the cost of "damage reparation" of these stresses may be higher than the cost of developing new concepts (Benkeblia 2011).

Presently, there is no distinctive line between basic and applied "omics" research, since most basic research often has direct bearing on applied sciences. For example, basic biochemical studies of oil, protein, starch, cellulose synthesis, and secondary metabolism, or research concerning fruits and vegetables, metabolism, soil fertility, seed development, and growth characteristics have obvious applications in agriculture at the farm field and postharvest storage levels (Somerville and Somerville 1999). In addition, "omics" technologies, which will confer the agronomic traits to crop and plant foods, and engineering of novel traits could be considered the foundation of sustainable agriculture and environment care (Campbell et al. 2003, Mazur et al. 1999, Somerville and Somerville 1999, Walbot 1999). The metabolomic approaches will allow unraveling of biochemical pathways and identification and characterization of genes encoding biosynthetic enzymes, which produce secondary and intermediary metabolites in crop plants (Fridman and Pichersky 2005, Gianchandani et al. 2006, Girke et al. 2003, Stitt and Fernie 2003, Sweetlove et al. 2003, Weckwerth and Fiehn 2002).

Typically, target points of sustainable agriculture fall into three classes: (a) agronomic, (b) nutritional quality, and (c) physical trait. An agronomic point can be biotic (e.g., resistance to diseases, parasites, insects, and weeds) or abiotic (e.g., better adaptation to heat, drought, salinity, acidity, heavy metals, water logging, and nutrient [especially nitrogen and phosphorus] availability). A nutritional point includes content and quality of starch, protein, oil, or nutritional elements (Mazur et al. 1999),

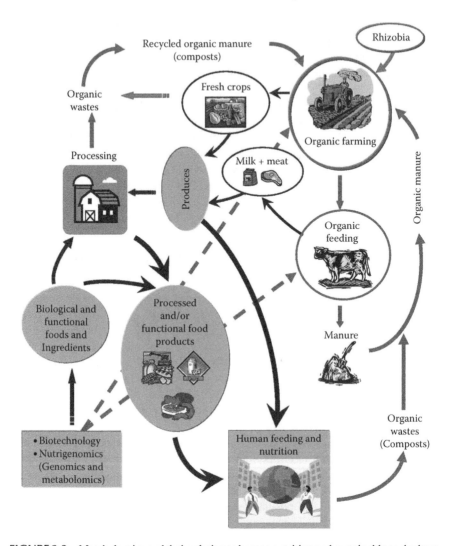

**FIGURE 3.3** Metabolomics and their relation to human nutrition and sustainable agriculture.

while a physical point includes plant architecture and shelf life (Ait-Ali et al. 2003). Directly or indirectly, plants provide a major part of humanity's food, most of which comes from cereals such as wheat, rice, and maize. During the majority of agricultural history, the focus has been on an agronomic point such as yield, productivity, and pest resistance, while nutritional quality has been ignored, with the result that most plant foods have limited nutritional qualities. To alleviate this problem, research has been conducted to enhance levels of essential and nonessential micronutrients and macronutrients, such as vitamins (e.g., A, C, E, and folate), minerals (e.g., iron and zinc), and proteins (Beyer and Potrykus 2001, Beyer et al. 2002, Klöti and Potrykus 1999, Potrykus 2001, Wu et al. 2003, Ye et al. 2000). For example, many genes have been cloned for vitamin pathways and for the synthesis of many other "nonessential" compounds and macronutrients (DellaPenna 1999, 2001). In the near future, it will probably be possible to manipulate the content and composition of many nutrients in food crops. Other benefits will include reducing the levels of antinutritional factors (e.g., phytates), toxins (e.g., cyanide in cassava), and allergens in seeds, food grains, leaves, and tubers (Graham et al. 2001, Tada et al. 1996).

## 3.11 CONCLUDING COMMENTS

Undoubtedly, synergistic evolvement of "omics" and associated modern technologies will provide a greater understanding of plant foods and the environmental factors that influence their biological systems. They can also contribute to designing new foods with specific health protective properties. The use of such approaches may surely allow for prevention measures to block or suppress the initiation, promotion, or progression of pathways that lead to metabolic disorders, nutritional deficiencies, and thereby decrease risk of diseases.

It should be admitted that there is no way to identify or to design a single "miracle" compound, given the complexity of foods. To this end, the potential usefulness of metabolomics, of course with other technologies such as genomics and proteomics, in modern plant breeding should be further explored and given priority. The strategic vision is to improve the safe exploitation of plants to "produce better quality and healthy plant foods offering consumers real options to improve their 'quality of life'." One of the potential benefits of application of metabolomic approaches in plant science is the design of novel food crops with enhanced health benefits and to reduce the risk of food-related diseases. The aim includes creating foods to help maintain the health of people specially the third age. Finally, success depends upon the ability to identify and validate bioactive compounds, to determine their role in health promotion, and to help define the efficacious range of intake of macro- and micronutrients. It will be necessary to develop effective collaborative research programs between plant scientists and others, because it is unlikely that single individuals and/or institutions have sufficient capabilities to encompass all desired issues. Aside that, creation of multidisciplinary teams and development of scientific exchange on metabolomics would likely be a creative solution to many problems related to foods and human health and answer at least some of our questions.

## ACKNOWLEDGMENTS

Part of this work was supported by a New Initiative Research Grant from the Office of Graduate Studies and Research, The University of the West Indies, Mona.

## REFERENCES

Ait-Ali, T., C. Rands, and N. P. Harberd. 2003. Flexible control of plant architecture and yield via switchable expression of *Arabidopsis gai*. *Plant Biotechnol J* 1:337–342.

Ames, B. N. and P. Wakimoto. 2002. Are vitamin and mineral deficiencies a major cancer risk? *Nat Rev Cancer* 2:694–704.

Barros, E., S. Lezar, M. J. Anttonen et al. 2010. Comparison of two GM maize varieties with a near-isogenic non-GM variety using transcriptomics, proteomics and metabolomics. *Plant Biotechnol J* 8:436–451.

Barsh, G. S. and M. W. Schwartz. 2002. Genetic approaches to studying energy balance: Perception and integration. *Nat Rev Genet* 3:589–600.

Benkeblia, N. 2011. *Sustainable Agriculture and New Biotechnologies*. Boca Raton, FL: CRC Press.

Benkeblia, N. and N. Shiomi. 2006. Fructooligosaccharides in edibles Allium: Occurrence, chemistry and health benefits. *Curr Nutr Food Sci* 2:181–191.

Berger, A., D. M. Mutch, J. B. German, and M. A. Roberts. 2002. Dietary effects of arachidonate-rich fungal oil and fish oil on murine hepatic and hippocampal gene expression. *Lipids Health Dis* 1:1–23.

Beyer, P. and I. Potrykus. 2001. Golden Rice: Proof of concept and beyond. http://www. agbioworld.org (accessed November 18, 2010).

Beyer, J. A., A. Salim, Y. Xudong, P. Lucca, P. Schaub, R. Welsch, and I. Potrykus. 2002. "Golden Rice": Introducing the β-carotene biosynthetic pathway into rice endosperm by genetic engineering to defeat vitamin A-deficiency. *J Nutr* 132:S506–S510.

Bovy, A., E. Schijlen, and R. D. Hall. 2007. Metabolic engineering of flavonoids in tomato (*Solanum lycopersicum*): The potential for metabolomics. *Metabolomics* 3:399–412.

Brash, D. E. and P. A. Havre. 2002. New careers for antioxidants. *Proc Natl Acad Sci USA* 99:13969–13971.

Breidt, Jr. E. 2004. A genetic study of the molecular ecology of sauerkraut fermentations. *J Food Sci* 69:30–32.

Broeckling, C. D., I. R. Reddy, A. L. Duran, X. Zhao, and L. W. Sumner. 2006. MET-IDEA: A data extraction tool for mass spectrometry-based metabolomics. *Anal Chem* 78:4334–4341.

Brown, M., W. B. Dunn, D. I. Ellis et al. 2005. A metabolome pipeline: From concept to data to knowledge. *Metabolomics* 1:39–41.

Burdock, G. A., I. G. Carabin, and J. C. Griffiths. 2006. The importance of GRAS to the functional food and nutraceutical industries. *Toxicology* 221:17–27.

Campbell, M. M., A. M. Brunner, H. M. Jones, and S. H. Strauss. 2003. Forestry's fertile crescent: The application of biotechnology to forest trees. *Plant Biotechnol J* 1:141–154.

Campbell-Platt, G. 1994. Fermented foods: A world perspective. *Food Res Int* 27:253–257.

Capanoglu, E., J. Beekwilder, D. Boyacioglu, R. C. H. De Vosb, and R. D. Hall. 2010. The effect of industrial food processing on potentially health-beneficial tomato antioxidants. *Crit Rev Food Sci* 50:919–930.

Castrillo, J. I., A. Hayes, S. Mohammed, S. J. Gaskell, and S. G. Oliver. 2003. An optimized protocol for metabolome analysis in yeast using direct infusion electrospray mass spectrometry. *Phytochemistry* 62:929–937.

Cherbut, C. 2002. Inulin and oligofructose in the dietary fiber concept. *Br J Nutr* 87 (Suppl. 2): S159–S162.

Collins, A. R., V. Harrington, J. Drew, and R. Melvin. 2003. Nutritional modulation of DNA repair in a human intervention study. *Carcinogenesis* 24:511–515.

Cummings, J. H., G. T. Macfarlane, and H. N. Englyst. 2001. Prebiotic digestion and fermentation. *Am J Clin Nutr* 73 (Suppl.):S415–S420.

Cummings, J. H., M. B. Roberfroid, H. Andersson et al. 1997. A new look at dietary carbohydrate: Chemistry, physiology and health. *Eur J Clin Nutr* 51:417–423.

DellaPenna, D. 1999. Nutritional genomics: Manipulating plant micronutrients to improve human health. *Science* 285:375–379.

DellaPenna, D. 2001. Plant metabolic engineering. *Plant Physiol* 125:160–163.

Dunn, W. B. and D. I. Ellis. 2005. Metabolomics, current analytical platforms and methodologies. *Trends Anal Chem* 24:285–294.

Duran, A. L., J. Yang, L. Wang, and L. W. Sumner. 2003. Metabolomics spectral formatting, alignment and conversion tools (MSFACTs). *Bioinformatics* 19:2283–2293.

Fay, L. B. and J. B. German. 2008. Personalizing foods: Is genotype necessary? *Curr Opin Biotechnol* 19:121–128.

Fell, D. A. and A. Wagner. 2002. The small world of metabolism. *Nature* 18:1121–1122.

Fiehn, O. 2002. Metabolomics—The link between genotypes and phenotypes. *Plant Mol Biol* 48:155–171.

Flamm, G., W. Glinsman, D. Kritchevsky, L. Prosky, and M. Roberfroid. 2001. Inulin and oligofructose as dietary fiber: A review of the evidence. *Crit Rev Food Sci Nutr* 41:353–362.

Fleet, G. H. 1999. Microorganisms in food ecosystems. *Int J Food Microbiol* 50:101–117.

Fridman, E. and E. Pichersky. 2005. Metabolomics, genomics, proteomics, and the identification of enzymes and their substrates and products. *Curr Opin Plant Biol* 8:242–248.

Gerhardt, R. and H. W. Heldt. 1984. Measurement of subcellular metabolite levels in leaves by fractionation of freeze-stopped material in nonaqueous media. *Plant Physiol* 75:542–547.

German, J. B., M. A. Roberts, L. Fay, and S. M. Watkins. 2002. Metabolomics and individual metabolic assessment: The next great challenge for nutrition. *J Nutr* 132:2486–2487.

German, J. B., M. A. Roberts, and S. M. Watkins. 2003. Genomics and metabolomics as markers for the interaction of diet and health: Lessons from lipids. *J Nutr* 133:S2078–S2083.

Gianchandani, E. P., D. L. Brautigan, and J. A. Papin. 2006. Systems analyses characterize integrated functions of biochemical networks. *Trends Biochem Sci* 5:284–291.

Gibbon, B. C. and B. A. Larkins. 2005. Molecular genetic approaches to developing quality protein maize. *Trends Genet* 21:227–233.

Gibney, M. J., M. Walsh, L. Brennan, H. M. Roche, B. German, and B. van Ommen. 2005. Metabolomics in human nutrition: Opportunities and challenges. *Am J Clin Nutr* 82:497–503.

Gidman, E., R. Goodacre, B. Emmett, A. R. Smith, and D. Gwynn-Jones. 2003. Investigating plant–plant interference by metabolic fingerprinting. *Phytochemistry* 63:705–710.

Girke, T., M. Ozkan, D. Carter, and N. V. Raikhel. 2003. Towards a modeling infrastructure for studying plant cells. *Plant Physiol* 132:410–414.

Glassbrook, N., C. Beecher, and J. Ryals. 2000. Metabolic profiling on the right path. *Nat Biotechnol* 18:1157–1161.

Goodacre, R. 2007. Metabolomics of a superorganism. *J Nutr* 137:S259–S266.

Goodacre, R., S. Vaidyanathan, W. B. Dunn, G. G. Harrigan, and D. B. Kell. 2004. Metabolomics by numbers: Acquiring and understanding global metabolite data. *Trends Biotechnol* 22:245–252.

Graham, R. D., R. M. Welch, and H. E. Bouis. 2001. Addressing micronutrient malnutrition through enhancing the nutritional quality of staple foods: Perspectives and knowledge gaps. *Adv Agron* 70:77–142.

Griffin, J. L., H. J. Williams, E. Sang, K. Clarke, C. Rae, and J. K. Nicholson. 2001. Metabolic profiling of genetic disorders: A multitissue [1]H nuclear magnetic resonance spectroscopic and pattern recognition study into dystrophic tissue. *Anal Biochem* 293:16–21.

Hall, R. D., I. D. Brouwer, and M. A. Fitzgerald. 2008. Plant metabolomics and its potential application for human nutrition. *Physiol Plant* 132:162–175.

Hegarty, J. E., P. D. Fairclough, K. J. Moriarty, M. L. Clark, M. J. Kelly, and A. M. Dawson. 1982. Comparison of plasma and intraluminal amino acid profiles in man after meals containing a protein hydrolysate and equivalent amino acid mixture. *Gut* 23:670–674.

Hilliam, M. 1998. The market for functional foods. *Int Dairy J* 8:349–353.

Johnson, H. E., D. Broadhurst, R. Goodacre, and A. R. Smith. 2003. Metabolic fingerprinting of salt-stressed tomatoes. *Phytochemistry* 62:919–928.

Katz, J. E., D. S. Dumlao, S. Clarke, and J. Hau. 2004. A new technique (COMSPARI) to facilitate the identification of minor compounds in complex mixtures by GC/MS and LC/MS: Tools for the visualization of matched datasets. *J Am Soc Mass Spectrom* 15:580–584.

Kell, D. B. 2004. Metabolomics and systems biology: Making sense to the soup. *Curr Opin Microbiol* 7:296–307.

Klöti, A. and I. Potrykus. 1999. Rice improvement by genetic transformation. In *Molecular Biology of Rice*, ed. K. Shimamoto, pp. 283–301. Tokyo, Japan: Springer-Verlag.

Kopka, J. 2006. Current challenges and development in GC-MS based metabolite profiling technology. *J Biotechnol* 124:312–322.

Koziel, M. G., G. L. Beland, C. Bowman, N. B. Carozzi, and R. Crenshaw. 1993. Field performance of elite transgenic maize plants expressing an insecticidal protein derived from *Bacillus thuringiensis. Biotechnology* 11:194–200.

Kuiper, H. A., H. P. J. M. Noteborn, E. J. Kok, and G. A. Kleter. 2002. Safety aspects of novel foods. *Food Res Int* 35:267–271.

Lee, J. E., G.-S. Hwang, C.-H. Lee, and Y.-S. Hong. 2009. Metabolomics reveals alterations in both primary and secondary metabolites by wine bacteria. *J Agric Food Chem* 57:10772–10783.

Manach, C., J. Hubert, R. Llorach, and A. Scalbert. 2009. The complex links between dietary phytochemicals and human health deciphered by metabolomics. *Mol Nutr Food Res* 53:1303–1315.

Martin-Orúe, S. M., A. G. O'Donnell, J. Ariño, T. Netherwood, H. J. Gilbert, and J. C. Mathers. 2002. Degradation of transgenic DNA from genetically modified soya and maize in human intestinal simulations. *Br J Nutr* 87:533–542.

Mathers, J. C. 2004a. What can we expect to learn from genomics? *Proc Nutr Soc* 63:1–4.

Mathers, J. C. 2004b. The biological revolution—Towards a mechanistic understanding of the impact of diet on cancer risk. *Mutat Res* 551:43–49.

Mathers, J. C. 2006. Plant foods for human health: Research challenges. *Proc Nutr Soc* 65:198–203.

Mazur, B., E. Krebbers, and S. Tingey. 1999. Gene discovery and product development for grain quality traits. *Science* 285:372–375.

Mazza, R., M. Soave, M. Morlacchini, G. Piva, and A. Marocco. 2005. Assessing the transfer of genetically modified DNA from feed to animal tissues. *Transgen Res* 14:775–784.

McKay, L. L. and K. A. Baldwin. 1990. Applications for biotechnology: Present and future improvements in lactic acid bacteria. *FEMS Microbiol Rev* 7:3–14.

Mendes, P. 2002. Emerging bioinformatics for the metabolome. *Brief Bioinform* 3:134–145.

Mertz, E. T., L. S. Bates, and O. E. Nelson. 1964. Mutant maize that changes the protein composition and increases the lysine content of maize endosperm. *Science* 145:279–280.

Mills, D. A. 2004. Fermentation technology. The lactic acid bacteria project. *J Food Sci* 69:28–30.

Milner, J. A. 2004. Molecular targets for bioactive food components. *J Nutr* 134:S2492–S2498.

Mitchell, S., E. Holmes, and P. Carmichael. 2002. Metabonic and medicine: The biochemical oracle. *Biologist (London)* 49:217–221.

Moundras, C., C. Remesy, and C. Demigne. 1993. Dietary protein paradox: Decrease of amino acid availability induced by high-protein diets. *Am J Physiol* 264:G1057–G1065.

Muller, M. and S. Kersten. 2003. Nutrigenomics goals and strategies. *Nat Rev Genet* 4:315–322.

Netherwood, T., S. M. Martin-Orúe, A. G. O'Donnell et al. 2004. Assessing the survival of transgenic plant DNA in the human gastrointestinal tract. *Nat Biotechnol* 22:204–209.

Nicholson, J. K., J. C. Lindon, and E. Holmes. 1999. 'Metabonomics': Understanding the metabolic responses of living systems to pathophysiological stimuli via multivariate statistical analysis of biological NMR spectroscopic data. *Xenobiotica* 29:1181–1189.

Nielsen, K. M. and J. P. Townsend. 2004. Monitoring and modeling horizontal gene transfer. *Nat Biotechnol* 22:1110–1114.

Noguchi, Y., R. Sakai, and T. Kimura. 2003. Metabolomics and its potential for assessment of adequacy and safety amino acid intake. *J Nutr* 133:S2097–S2100.

Noordewier, M. and J. Brown. 2002. Unfolding the secrets of the *Salmonella* genome to aid drug development. *Trends Pharmacol Sci* 23:397–399.

Oresic, M. 2009. Metabolomics, a novel tool for studies of nutrition, metabolism and lipid dysfunction. *Nutr Metab Cardiovasc Dis* 19:816–824.

Padgette, S. R., K. H. Kolacz, X. Delannay et al. 1995. Development, identification, and characterization of a glyphosate-tolerant soybean line. *Crop Sci* 35:1451–1461.

Potrykus, I. 2001. Golden rice and beyond. *Plant Physiol* 125:1157–1161.

Ravussin, E. and C. Bouchard. 2000. Human genomics and obesity: Finding appropriate drug targets. *Eur J Pharmacol* 410:131–145.

Rist, M. J., U. Wenzel, and H. Daniel. 2006. Nutrition and food science go genomic. *Trends Biotechnol* 24:172–178.

Roberfroid, M. B. 2000. Fructo-oligosaccharides: Benefit for gastrointestinal functions. *Curr Opin Gastroenterol* 16:173–177.

Roberfroid, M. B. 2002. Functional foods: Concepts and application to inulin and oligofructose. *Br J Nutr* 87 (Suppl. 2):S139–S143.

Roberfroid, M. and J. Slavin. 2000. Nondigestible oligosaccharides. *Crit Rev Food Sci Nutr* 40:461–480.

Roberts, M. A., D. Mutch, and J. B. German. 2001. Genomics in food and nutrition. *Curr Opin Biotechnol* 12:516–522.

Rochfort, S. 2005. Metabolomics reviewed: A new "omics" platform technology for systems biology and implications for natural products research. *J Nat Prod* 68:1813–1820.

Rossi, F., M. Morlacchini, G. Fusconi, A. Pietri, R. Mazza, and G. Piva. 2005. Effect of Bt corn on broiler growth performance and fate of feed-derived DNA in the digestive tract. *Poult Sci* 84:1022–1030.

Sanders, M. E. 1998. Overview of functional foods: Emphasis on probiotic bacteria. *Int Dairy J* 8:341–347.

Sanders, M. E. and J. H. Int'l Veld. 1999. Bringing a probiotic-containing functional food to the market: Microbiological, product, regulatory and labeling issues. *Ant van Leeuwenhoek* 76:293–315.

Scalbert, A., L. Brennan, O. Fiehn et al. 2009. Mass-spectrometry-based metabolomics: Limitations and recommendations for future progress with particular focus on nutrition research. *Metabolomics* 5:435–458.

Schilter, B. and A. Constable. 2002. Regulatory control of genetically modified (GM) foods: Likely developments. *Toxicol Lett* 127:341–349.

Schmidt, C. 2004. Metabolomics takes its place as latest up-and-coming "omic" science. *J Natl Cancer I* 96:732–734.

Seeman, E. 2002. Pathogenesis of bone fragility in women and men. *Lancet* 359:1841–1850

Servant, A., S. Laperche, F. Lallemand et al. 2002. Genetic diversity within human erythroviruses: Identification of three genotypes. *J Virol* 76:9124–9134.

Shastry, B. S. 2002. SNP alleles in human disease and evolution. *J Hum Genet* 47:561–566.

Somerville, C. and S. Somerville. 1999. Plant functional genomics. *Science* 285:380–383.

Steele, V. E. 2003. Current mechanistic approaches to chemoprevention of cancer. *J Biochem Mol Biol* 36:78–81.

Stewart, D., L. V. T. Shepherd, R. D. Hall, and P. D. Fraser. 2011. Crops and tasty, nutritious food—How can metabolomics help? In *Biology of Plant Metabolomics*, Annual Plant Reviews Vol. 43, ed. R. D. Hall, doi: 10.1002/9781444339956.ch7. Oxford, U.K.: Wiley-Blackwell.

Stitt, M. and A. R. Fernie. 2003. From measurements of metabolites to metabolomics: An 'on the fly' perspective illustrated by recent studies of carbon–nitrogen interactions. *Curr Opin Biotechnol* 14:136–144.

Stitt, M., R. McC Lilley, R. Gerhardt, and H. Heldt. 1989. Metabolite level in specific cells and subcellular compartments of plant leaves. *Methods Enzymol* 174:518–552.

Sweetlove, L. J., R. L. Last, and A. R. Fernie. 2003. Predictive metabolic engineering: A goal for systems biology. *Plant Physiol* 132:420–425.

Tabas, I. 2002. Cholesterol in health and disease. *J Clin Invest* 110:583–590.

Tada, Y., M. Nakase, T. Adachi et al. 1996. Reduction of 14–16kDa allergenic proteins in transgenic rice plants by antisense gene. *FEBS Lett* 391:341–345.

Tannock, G. W. 1999. *Probiotics: A Critical Review*. Norfolk, VA: Horizon Scientific Press.

Taylor, J., R. D. King, T. Altmann, and O. Fiehn. 2002. Application of metabolomics to plant genotype discrimination using statistics and machine learning. *Bioinformatics* 18 (Suppl. 2):S241–S248.

Tolstikov, V. V. and O. Fiehn. 2002. Analysis of highly polar compounds of plant origin: Combination of hydrophilic interaction chromatography and electrospray ion trap mass spectrometry. *Anal Biochem* 301:298–307.

Trujillo, E., C. Davis, and J. Milner. 2006. Nutrigenomics, proteomics, metabolomics, and the practice of dietetics. *J Am Diet Assoc* 106:403–413.

van der Werf, M. J., E. H. J. Schuren, S. Bijlsma, A. C. Tas, and B. van Ommen. 2001. Nutrigenomics: Application of genomics technologies in nutritional sciences and food technology. *J Food Sci* 66:773–779.

Vogels, J. W. T. E., A. C. Tas, F. van den Berg, and J. van der Greef. 1993. A new method for classification of wines based on proton and C-13 NMR spectroscopy in combination with pattern recognition techniques. *Chemom Intell Lab Syst* 21:249–258.

Vogels, J. W. T. E., L. Terwel, A. C. Tas, F. van den Berg, F. Dukel, and van J. der Greef. 1996. Detection of adulteration in orange juices by a new screening method using proton NMR spectroscopy in combination with pattern recognition techniques. *J Agric Food Chem* 44:175–180.

Walbot, V. 1999. Genes, genomes, genomics. What can plant biologists expect from the 1998 national science foundation plant genome research program? *Plant Physiol* 119:1151–1155.

Walsh, K. and D. E. Koshland. 1984. Determination of flux through the branch point of two metabolic cycles. The tricarboxylic acid cycle and the glyoxylate shunt. *J Biol Chem* 259:9646–9654.

Wang, Y. L., E. Holmes, J. K. Nicholson et al. 2004. Metabonomic investigations in mice infected with *Schistosoma mansoni*: An approach for biomarker identification. *Proc Natl Acad Sci USA* 101:12676–12681.

Watkins, S. M., B. D. Hammock, J. W. Newman, and J. B. German. 2001. Individual metabolism should guide agriculture toward foods for improved health and nutrition. *Am J Clin Nutr* 74:283–286.

Weaver, C. M. 2005. Inulin, oligofructose and bone health: Experimental approaches and mechanisms. *Brit J Nutr* 93 (Suppl. 1):S99–S103.

Weckwerth, W. and O. Fiehn. 2002. Can we discover novel pathways using metabolomic analysis? *Curr Opin Biotechnol* 13:156–160.

Wei, Q., H. Shen, L. E. Wang et al. 2003. Association between low dietary folate intake and suboptimal cellular DNA repair capacity. *Cancer Epidemiol Biomarkers Prev* 12:963–969.

Weichert, H., A. Kolbe, A. Kraus, C. Wasternack, and I. Feussner. 2002. Metabolic profiling of oxylipins in germinating cucumber seedlings—Lipoxygenase-dependent degradation of triacylglycerols and biosynthesis of volatile aldehydes. *Planta* 215:612–619.

Wickware, P. 2000. Next-generation biologists must straddle computation and biology. *Nature* 404:683–684.

Wishart, D. S. 2008. Metabolomics: Applications to food science and nutrition research. *Trends Food Sci Tech* 19:482–493.

World Health Organization/Food and Agriculture Organization (WHO/FAO). 2003. Diet, Nutrition and the Prevention of Chronic Diseases. WHO Technical Report Series, No. 916.

Wu, X. R., Z. H. Chen, and W. R. Folk. 2003. Enrichment of cereal protein lysine content by altered tDNA[lys] coding during protein synthesis. *Plant Biotechnol J* 1:187–194.

Yang, N. S., L. F. Shyur, C. H. Chen, S. Y. Wang, and C. M. Tzeng. 2004. Medicinal herb extract and a single-compound drug confer similar complex pharmacogenomic activities in MCF-7 cells. *J Biomed Sci* 11:418–422.

Ye, X., S. Al Babili, A. Klöti et al. 2000. Engineering the provitamin A (β-carotene) biosynthetic pathway into (carotenoid-free) rice endosperm. *Science* 287:303–305.

# 4 Foodomics
## *A New Omics for a New Food Era*

*Virginia Garcia-Cañas, Carolina Simó,
Miguel Herrero, Elena Ibañez,
and Alejandro Cifuentes*

## CONTENTS

## 4.1 INTRODUCTION TO FOODOMICS

Nowadays, boundaries among the different research disciplines are becoming diffuse giving rise to impressive possibilities in the emerging interdisciplinary areas. In food science and nutrition, this trend has given rise to the development of new methodologies in which advanced analytical methodologies, mainly "omics" and bioinformatics—frequently together with *in vitro*, *in vivo*, and/or clinical assays—are applied to investigate topics considered unapproachable few years ago. As a result, researchers in food science and nutrition are being pushed to move from classical methodologies to more advanced strategies usually borrowing methods well established in medical, pharmacological, and/or biotechnological research.

One of the main goals in modern food science and nutrition is to improve our limited understanding of the roles of nutritional compounds at the molecular level (i.e., their interaction with genes and their subsequent effect on proteins and metabolites) for the rational design of strategies to manipulate cell functions through diet, which is expected to have an extraordinary impact on our health. The problem to solve is huge, and it includes the study of the individual variations in gene sequences, particularly in single nucleotide polymorphisms (SNPs), and their expected different answers to nutrients. Moreover, nutrients can be considered as signaling molecules that are recognized by specific cellular-sensing mechanisms. However, unlike pharmaceuticals, the simultaneous presence of a variety of nutrients, with diverse chemical structures and concentrations, having numerous targets with different affinities and specificities, increases enormously the complexity of the problem. It is therefore a necessity to look at hundreds of test compounds simultaneously and observe the diverse temporal and spatial responses.

Another good example of the application of advanced approaches in food science is the development of new transgenic (also called genetically modified, GM) foods in which molecular biology, chemistry, agriculture, and food science are put together in order to adequately develop these new foods. Moreover, monitoring the composition, traceability, and quality of these GM foods (e.g., for discarding the existence of unintended modifications or for labeling issues) has been recommended using advanced analytical techniques (EFSA 2006) including omics techniques that are able to provide a broad profile of these GM foods (Garcia-Villaba et al. 2008, Levandi et al. 2008, Simó et al. 2010).

This trend has generated the emergence of new areas of research, which usually try to dissect the research problem into smaller and more feasible challenges, and with them, a completely new terminology. Thus, terms such as nutrigenomics, nutrigenetics, nutritional genomics, transgenics, functional foods, nutraceuticals, GM foods, nutritranscriptomics, nutriproteomics, nutrimetabolomics, systems biology, etc., are nowadays frequently used in food science (Powell 2007, Rezzi et al. 2007a,b, Rist et al. 2006, Subbiah 2006, Trujillo et al. 2006). Interestingly, in practically all these new areas, it is observed that the number of works dealing with opinions, comments, and revisions is much higher than the expected number of works showing real experimental data, indicating the interest on these hot topics, but demonstrating the complexity of these approaches and the long way to go.

The number of opportunities (e.g., new methodologies, new generated knowledge, new products, etc.) derived from these multidisciplinary approaches is, therefore, impressive, and it includes the possibility to account for food products tailored to promote the health and well-being of groups of population identified on the basis of their individual genomes. However, to achieve these goals researchers involved in modern food science need to rely on an adequate background of several advanced tools (genomics, transcriptomics, proteomics, metabolomics, bioinformatics, etc.) and multiple disciplines (chemistry, microbiology, biotechnology, nutrition, medicine, etc.) in order to extract all the potential from these new technologies. In this way, researchers will be able to adequately understand and put together all the information and data that can be generated by these approaches. Usually, a *sine qua non* condition is to work within multidisciplinary teams in order to be able to face the huge complexity of the problem and to handle the generated results in a rational way.

In this context, we have recently defined for the first time *foodomics* as a new discipline that studies the food and nutrition domains through the application of advanced omics technologies (Cifuentes 2009, Herrero et al. 2010). Thus, foodomics is intended to be not only a useful concept able to cover in a simple and straightforward way all the aforementioned new terminologies, but also, more importantly, it is intended to be a global discipline that includes all the emerging working areas in which food (including nutrition), advanced analytical techniques (mainly omics tools),

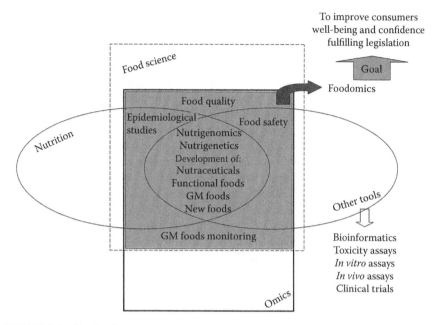

**FIGURE 4.1** Foodomics: covered areas, subdisciplines, tools, and goals.

and bioinformatics are put together. A representation of the areas covered by foodo-mics and its main goal (i.e., to improve consumers' well-being and confidence and fulfilling legislation) can be seen in Figure 4.1. For instance, foodomics would cover, for example, the development of new transgenic foods using molecular tools, the genomic/transcriptomic/proteomic and/or metabolomic study of foods for com-pound profiling/authenticity and/or biomarker analysis related to food quality, new investigations on food bioactivity and its effect on human health following nutrig-enomics and/or nutrigenetics approaches, development of global omics strategies to explore food safety issues, etc. Moreover, the interest in foodomics coincides with a clear shift in medicine and biosciences toward prevention of future diseases through adequate food intake, improving well-being and confidence of consumers while ful-filling the legislation.

In the following sections, we will provide a description of the fundamentals of foodomics, including the main tools that are used, the subdisciplines that foodomics integrate, some representative applications, and its direct interaction with systems biology. The chapter concludes by discussing the future challenges and foreseen developments of this emerging discipline in the new food era.

## 4.2 FOODOMICS TOOLS

Foodomics involves the use of multiple tools to deal with its different subdisci-plines and applications. Thus, the use of omics tools such as genomics, transcrip-tomics, proteomics, and metabolomics is a must in this new discipline. Although a detailed description on these tools is out of the scope of this chapter (readers inter-ested in these topics can find useful information elsewhere [Dettmer et al. 2007,

Garcia-Cañas et al. 2010, Griffiths and Wang 2009, Raqib and Cravioto 2009] including other chapters in this book), some fundamentals about these techniques are provided in the following.

Regarding genomics and transcriptomics, for years, the expression of individual genes has been determined by quantification of mRNA with northern blotting. This classical technique has gradually been replaced by more sensitive techniques such as real-time PCR. It has to be considered that both techniques can only analyze gene expression for a limited number of genes at a time. This can be very useful to monitor the up- or downregulation of a given gene for a specific problem. However, it is an important limitation for many foodomics applications since it only provides the analysis of a reduced number of genes, while the global analysis of gene expression may offer better opportunities in foodomics (e.g., for the identification of the effect of bioactive food constituents on homeostatic regulation and how this regulation is potentially altered in the development of certain chronic diseases [Hu and Kong 2004]). Two conceptually different analytical approaches have emerged to allow quantitative and comprehensive analysis of changes in mRNA expression levels of hundreds or thousands of genes. One approach is based on microarray technology, and the other group of techniques is based on DNA sequencing (Morozova and Marra 2008).

In proteomics, the huge dynamic concentration range of proteins in biological samples causes many detection difficulties due to many proteins that are below the level of sensitivity of the most advanced instruments. For this reason, fractionation and subsequent concentration of the proteome are often needed (Fang and Zhang 2008, Pernemalm et al. 2008). Besides, the use and development of high-resolving separation techniques as well as highly accurate mass spectrometers are nowadays essential to solve the proteome complexity (Chen 2008, Han et al. 2008). Currently, more than a single electrophoretic or chromatographic step is used to separate the thousands of proteins found in a biological sample. This separation step is followed by analysis of the isolated proteins (or peptides) by mass spectrometry (MS) via the so-called soft ionization techniques, such as electrospray ionization (ESI) and matrix-assisted laser desorption/ionization (MALDI), combined with the everyday more powerful mass spectrometers. Two fundamental analytical strategies can be employed: the *bottom-up* and the *top-down* approach. Both methodologies differ on the separation requirements and the type of MS instrumentation (Bogdanov and Smith 2005, Motoyama and Yates 2008, Wiesner et al. 2008). New proteomic approaches based on array technology are also being employed. Protein microarrays can be composed by recombinant protein molecules or antibodies immobilized in a high-density format on the surface of a substrate material. There are two major classes of protein micro(or nano-)arrays: analytical and functional protein microarrays, the antibody-based microarray being the most common platform in proteomic studies (Borrebaeck and Wingren 2007).

Regarding metabolomics, there are three basic approaches that can be used here: target analysis, metabolic profiling, and metabolic fingerprinting. Target analysis aims the quantitative measurement of selected analytes, such as specific biomarkers or reaction products. Metabolic profiling is a nontargeted strategy that focuses on the study of a group of related metabolites or a specific metabolic pathway. It is one of the basic approaches to phenotyping, because the study of metabolic profiles of a cell gives a more accurate description of a phenotype (Lee and Go 2005). Meanwhile, metabolic fingerprinting does not aim to identify all metabolites, but to compare patterns of metabolites that change in response to the cellular environment (Fiehn 2002). Unlike nucleic acid- or protein-based omics techniques, which intend to determine a single chemical class of compounds, metabolomics has to deal with very different compounds of very diverse chemical and physical properties. Moreover, the relative concentration of metabolites in the biological fluids can vary from millimolar level (or higher) to picomolar, making it easy to exceed the linear range of the analytical techniques employed. As no single technique can be expected to meet all these requirements, many metabolomics approaches can employ several analytical tools (Koulman and Volmer 2008), being nuclear magnetic resonance (NMR) and MS (usually combined with a separation technique) the two most common techniques used so far in metabolomics. The large amount of metabolomic data is normally studied using principal component analysis (PCA) or other related techniques. PCA is a tool for exploratory data analysis that determines correlation differences among sample sets, which can be caused by either a biological difference or a methodological bias. It is usually used as a first step to obtain information about the quality of the data. After data reduction, a multivariate analysis is usually performed. The most common is partial least square discriminant analysis (PLS-DA). The aim of PLS-DA is to discriminate the complete data list and reduce it with the most relevant ones (Koulman and Volmer 2008).

The development of genomics, transcriptomics, proteomics, and metabolomics (Ferguson et al. 2007) has given rise to extraordinary opportunities for increasing our understanding about different issues that can be addressed by foodomics. This includes (a) to understand the biochemical, molecular, and cellular mechanisms that underlie the beneficial or adverse effects of certain bioactive food components; (b) to know the identity of genes that are involved in the previous stage to the onset of the disease, and therefore, possible molecular biomarkers (Greenspan 2001); (c) to determine the effect of bioactive food constituents on crucial molecular pathways (Müller and Kersten 2003); (d) to carry out investigation on unintended effects in GM crops (García-Villalba et al. 2008, Levandi et al. 2008, Simó et al. 2010).

Due to the huge amount of data usually obtained from omics studies, it has been necessary to develop strategies to convert the complex raw data obtained into useful information. Thus, bioinformatics has also become a crucial tool in foodomics. Over the last few years, the use of biological knowledge accumulated in public databases by means of bioinformatics allows to systematically analyze large data lists in an attempt to assemble a summary of the most significant biological aspects (Waagmeester et al. 2008). Also, statistical tools are usually applied, for example, for exploratory data analysis to determine correlations among samples (which can be caused by either a biological difference or a methodological bias), for discriminating the complete data list and reducing it with the most relevant ones for biomarker discovery, etc.

Moreover, the use of other more classical approaches in foodomics, such as toxicity studies, *in vitro* or *in vivo* assays, and/or clinical trials, can provide an important added value to the results achieved by this new discipline. Some examples and applications of these combinations will be discussed in Section 4.4.

## 4.3  FOODOMICS AND SYSTEMS BIOLOGY

Foodomics has to face important difficulties derived, among others, from food complexity, the huge natural variability, the large number of different nutrients and bioactive food compounds, their very different concentrations and the numerous targets with different affinities and specificities that they may have. As described earlier and in other chapters of this book, transcriptomics, proteomics, and metabolomics represent powerful analytical platforms developed for the analysis of genes, proteins, and metabolites. However, "omics" platforms need to be integrated in order to understand the biological meaning of the results on the investigated system (e.g., cell, tissue, and organ), giving rise to the growing of a new discipline called systems biology (Hood et al. 2004). Systems biology can be defined as an integrated approach for studying biological systems at the level of cells, organs, or organisms by measuring and integrating genomic, proteomic, and metabolic data (Panagiotou and Nielsen 2009). Thus, systems biology approaches may encompass molecules, cells, organs, individuals, or even ecosystems, and it is regarded as an integrative approach to all the information at the different levels of genomic expression (mRNA, protein, and metabolite).

However, in foodomics studies, biologic responses may be subtle, and, therefore, careful attention needs to be given to the methodologies used to identify these responses. Unlike any reductionist approach that would take these techniques individually, systems biology exploits global data sets to derive useful information (Feng et al. 2008). Each large data set contains sufficient noise to preclude the identification of multiple minor, but relevant changes could be unnoticed without adequate statistical tools since the researcher is focused on the changes that are really significant within the whole data set. Systems biology, however, by confining the information, can provide a filter for "distracting" noise generated in each individual platform and minimize the data to be interpreted by focusing on only those end points common between the various experimental platforms (Mutch et al. 2005). To achieve this, appropriate statistical models have to be used in order to filter through the large data sets and highlight only those important changes. Although systems biology has been scarcely applied in foodomics studies, its potential is underlined by its adoption by other disciplines. For instance, a systems biology approach has been applied to investigate carbohydrate metabolism in yeast (Weston and Hood 2004). In a recent work, Kohanski et al. (2008) used the context likelihood of relatedness (CLR) algorithm (gene network analysis) in combination with gene expression microarrays and gene ontology-based enrichment analysis to construct and filter gene connectivity maps of bacteria under antibiotic treatment (Kohanski et al. 2008). The gene networks were further enriched with data derived from antibiotic growth high-throughput screening to provide insight into the pathway, whereby the antibiotic under study triggers its bactericide action.

## 4.4  APPLICATIONS OF FOODOMICS

The use of omics technologies in food science and/or nutrition research has given rise to the emergence of several specialities within the area covered by foodomics as shown in Figure 4.1. This is the case of nutritional genomics that includes

(a) nutrigenetics, whose main goal is to understand the gene-based differences in response to a specific dietary pattern, a functional food, or a supplement for a specific health outcome and (b) nutrigenomics, which deals with the interactions between dietary components and the genome as well as the resulting changes in proteins and other metabolites (Cortesy-Theulaz et al. 2005). Foodomics intends to enable the identification of biomarkers that can guide the assessment of the health status of humans and/or provide quantitative measures for diet-derived effects on human health (Hood et al. 2004, Kaput 2008). Within nutrigenomics, the fields of nutri-transcriptomics, nutriproteomics, and nutrimetabolomics study—using the respective transcriptomics, proteomics, and metabolomics tools—the dependence of gene transcription, protein expression, and metabolite generation, respectively, on dietary changes. As a result, the number of successful examples of transcriptome, proteome, and metabolome profiling, as stand-alone tools for capturing the cellular responses to nutrients and identifying their molecular targets, has grown significantly. Some examples are listed in Table 4.1. The ultimate goal of these high-throughput studies is to enable scientists to make recommendations for personalized health maintenance based on molecular signatures of food-derived nutrients and nonnutrients that lead to a specific phenotype and subsequently to prevent the onset and progression of disease (Fay and German 2008, Kaput 2008).

In the last few years, interesting examples of gene expression microarray applications in foodomics have been reported for transcriptome analysis. Early applications of microarray to this new field were related to the effects of caloric restriction on aging (Kayo et al. 2001, Lee et al. 1999). Soon, the technology was extended to study other interesting aspects in foodomics including the effects of dietary protein in the gene expression of cells (Kato and Kimura 2003), the mechanisms of dietary long-chain polyunsaturated fatty acids in the molecular functions of cancer and normal cells (Narayanan et al. 2003), and the effects on transcriptome of a high- or low-carbohydrate intake (van Erk et al. 2006). The molecular mechanisms of certain bioactive food constituents have also been investigated by microarray technology. More specifically, research has been focused on the study of the expression of lipid or energy metabolism-related genes by anthocyanins (Tsuda et al. 2006), the induction of changes in the expression of estrogen-responsive genes by genistein (Niculescu et al. 2007), the modulating action on the expression of genes involved in cell-cycle arrest and apoptosis of cultured colon cancer cells by quercetin (Murtaza et al. 2006), the anticancer and chemopreventive molecular mechanisms induced by epicatechin and epigallocatechin-3-gallate in human colon carcinoma and bronchial epithelial cells (see Figure 4.2) (McLoughlin et al. 2004, Vittal et al. 2004, Wang and Mukhar 2002), the chemopreventive action by sulforaphane in model animals (Thimmulappa et al. 2002), and the effect on the expression of diabetes-related genes by the natural carotenoid astaxanthin (Naito et al. 2006).

The number of studies on the effect of specific natural compounds, nutrients, or diets on the proteome is also continuously increasing. Most of them are based on the *bottom-up* approach, more precisely in classical combination of 2DE and MS, although LC-MS also has been applied with this purpose. As an example, the potential beneficial effect (atherosclerosis prevention, vascular protection) of isoflavones from different food matrices has been studied by using several differential proteomic

**TABLE 4.1**
**Some Foodomics Applications Related to Nutrigenomics**

| Bioactive Compound | Food/ Beverage | Studied Model | Issue | "Omic" Approach | Analytical Tool | Reference |
|---|---|---|---|---|---|---|
| Sulforaphane | Cruciferous vegetables | Mice | Chemopreventive agent in cancer | Transcriptomics | DNA microarray | Thimmulappa et al. (2002) |
| Omega-3 fatty acid | Fish oil | Human colon adenocarcinoma Caco-2 cells | Chemopreventive agent in cancer | Transcriptomics | DNA microarray | Narayanan et al. (2003) |
| Quercetin | Fruits and vegetables | CO115 colon-adenocarcinoma cells | Chemopreventive agent in cancer | Transcriptomics | DNA microarray | Murtaza et al. (2006) |
| Genistein | Soybean | Postmenopausal women (peripheral lymphocytes) | Regulation cAMP signaling and cell differentiation | Transcriptomics | DNA microarray | Niculescu et al. (2007) |
| Isoflavones | Cereal bars | Human peripheral blood mononuclear cells | Atherosclerosis-preventive activities | Proteomics | 2DE, MALDI-TOF MS | Fuchs et al. (2007) |
| Isoflavones | Soya foods | Human serum | Vascular protection | Proteomics | DIGE, LC-MS/MS | Wong et al. (2008) |
| Polyphenols | Green tea | Human lung adenocarcinoma A549 cells | Anticancer activity | Proteomics | 2DE, nLC-ESI-Q-TOF MS/MS | Lu et al. (2007) |
| Quercetin | — | Human SW480 colon carcinoma cells | Colorectal cancer prevention | Proteomics | 2DE, MALDI-TOF MS | Mouat et al. (2005) |
| Flavonoids/ phenolic compounds | Red wine/red grape juice/tea | Human urine, plasma, and feces | Cardiovascular disease prevention | Metabolomics | GC-TOF-MS | Grün et al. (2008) |
| Polyphenols | Wine/grape juice | Human feces | Inflammatory bowel prevention | Metabolomics | $^1$H-NMR | Jacobs et al. (2008) |
| Isoflavones | Soy | Human urine | Improvement in kidney function | Metabolomics | $^1$H-NMR | Solanky et al. (2005) |

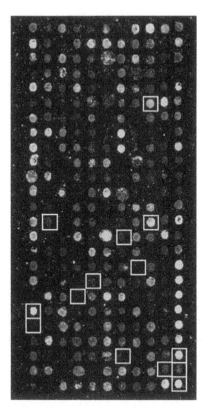

**FIGURE 4.2** Scanned image of a microarray composed of a total of 250 kinases and phosphatases, showing the expression profile obtained from human prostate carcinoma LNCaP cells treated with 12 mM EGCG or water only for 12 h. (From Wang, S.I. and Mukhar, H., *Cancer Lett.*, 182, 43, 2002. With permission.)

approaches (Fuchs et al. 2007, Wong et al. 2008). However, most of the research in this field is carried out on the activity of food ingredients using *in vitro* and *in vivo* tumor models for a deeper knowledge of their mechanisms on disease prevention. Some examples (Lu et al. 2007, Mouat et al. 2005) are given in Table 4.1.

One of the objectives of metabolomics within the frame of foodomics is to investigate the metabolic alterations produced by the effect of nutrients or bioactive food constituents on different metabolic pathways. Its importance lays not only on the information obtained on the molecular events involved and how the body adapts the metabolic pathways to different nutrient fluxes, but also on the identification of certain metabolites as biomarkers for health or disease status (Kussman et al. 2008). Many applications of metabolomics in this area focus on the study on the potential health benefits derived from the ingestion of functional compounds or foods, such as flavonoids (Grün et al. 2008), polyphenols (Jacobs et al. 2008), and isoflavones (Solanky et al. 2005).

Regarding the possibilities of other more global foodomics approaches, they have still a long way to go. The combination of systems biology with a subdiscipline as nutrigenomics should provide a holistic view of the molecular mechanisms underlying the beneficial or adverse effects of certain bioactive food components. Also, it should help in other foodomics subdiscipline such as nutrigenetics in the discovery of key genes and proteins that function to regulate metabolic pathways and whose expression is affected by specific bioactive food compounds. This will aid in rapidly identifying new biomarkers for nutritional status and disease progression and designing a novel concept for dietary prevention and intervention of disease (van Ommen and Stierum 2002).

As mentioned earlier, foodomics tools offer enormous potential to study the molecular basis of biological processes with agronomic interest and economic relevance, such as the interaction between crops and its pathogens, as well as physicochemical changes that take place during fruit ripening. In this line, successful examples of transcriptome analysis are based on recently developed microarray chips covering the genome of important crop species such as watermelon (Wechter et al. 2008), citrus (Martinez-Godoy et al. 2008), melon (Mascarell-Creus et al. 2009), and canola (Xiang et al. 2008).

Also, proteomics and metabolomics represent powerful analytical platforms to acquire more detailed and complete information on food composition even beyond the traditional food component analysis. This comprehensive knowledge of biochemical composition of foods will provide a better understanding of metabolic networks allowing food research community for a better insight of the molecular basis of important food characteristics such as flavor, color, texture, aroma, added-value nutrition, as well as the discovery of novel bioactive compounds in foods. As an example, rice is an important food crop plant that has been extensively studied using multiple proteomic approaches and also used in many cases as an excellent model plant in cereal crop research (Agrawal et al. 2009). In a recent work, Shu et al. (2008) used GC-MS to analyze a broad spectrum of low molecular weight rice constituents for the investigation of time-dependent metabolic changes in the course of the germination of rice, establishing the basis of the research of the potential advantageous nutritional properties of germinated rice.

The ability of different transcriptomic, proteomic, and metabolomic approaches may also be important to assess food safety and quality at every stage of production to ensure food safety for human consumption. It is also a valuable tool to distinguish between similar food products and to detect food frauds (adulteration, origin, authenticity, etc.), food-borne pathogens, toxic species, food allergens, etc.

In the context of food safety, several DNA microarray chips have been developed for the detection of food-borne pathogens (Kim et al. 2008, Wang et al. 2007) and toxigenic microorganisms (Liu et al. 2007). Also, DNA microarray technology has found many practical applications in genetically modified organism (GMO) analysis. In spite of the controversy of whether GMOs are beneficial or harmful for humans, animals, and environment, there is an increasing number of GMOs developed every year. Many countries have already established regulations regarding their development, authorization, as well as the labeling and traceability of the authorized GMOs in food. To date, DNA microarray technology has demonstrated to have impressive multiplexing capabilities for GMO analysis, and many examples can be found in the literature (Hammels et al. 2009, Tengs et al. 2007, von Götz 2010, Zhou et al. 2008).

In addition to the aforementioned applications, DNA microarrays for gene expression analysis have also demonstrated to be helpful on detecting mycotoxins in foods. This approach offers new possibilities to study the influence of environmental and technological parameters like pH, temperature, and water activity on the activation of mycotoxin biosynthesis (Schmidt-Heydt and Geisen 2007). The effect of the consumption of hypoallergenic wheat flour on the expression of a wide spectrum of genes is another example on the use of gene expression microarray technology in food safety. This technique can be applied in animal and cellular models demonstrating to be an efficient strategy for evaluating different aspects concerning food safety (Narasaka et al. 2006).

A particular case on the application of "omics" approaches to guarantee food safety is the biomarker discovery in body fluids and tissues regarding prion diseases (Huzarewich et al. 2010). In this sense, big effort is being carried out by the scientific community to achieve early detection of prion diseases in animals, which have not only a known risk of transmission to humans but also an economic impact on animal production.

Proteomic and metabolic changes also occur during crop growing conditions, food processing/preparation (fermentation, baking, boiling, etc.), and food conservation/storage (freezing, smoking, drying, etc.). These tools are, therefore, very useful for getting a deeper understanding of molecular details of foods and food-related matrices. Thus, it has been demonstrated the utility of metabolomic studies to improve quality control of beverage production. In this sense, NMR was successfully employed for the detection of adulteration of orange juices by the addition of lower cost grapefruit juices (Cuny et al. 2008) and for monitoring beer production, studying the effect on beer metabolic composition of site- and time-related variables during brewing process (Almeida et al. 2006). In a recent work, microbial spoilage of beef was studied by analyzing the release of volatile organic compounds by GC-MS (Ercolini et al. 2009).

The usefulness of foodomics for achieving a complete characterization of GMO has also been mentioned (Herrero et al. 2010), following the corresponding European regulations on GMO labeling and traceability in food and feed. A scheme of this approach can be seen in Figure 4.3.

For instance, gene expression microarray has shown to be a valuable profiling method to assess possible unintended effects of genetic transformation in plants. With this technology, detailed information has also been obtained on nontargeted effects of transgenes in several plant species including potato, rice, wheat, and maize. In these cases, the genetic modification did not considerably alter overall gene expression that falls within the range of natural variation of landraces and varieties (Baudo et al. 2006, Coll et al. 2009, Dubouzet et al. 2007, Gregersen et al. 2005), supporting the possibility of producing transgenic plants that are substantially equivalent to nontransformed plants at the transcriptomic level.

Also, MS-based technologies have wide possibilities to evaluate GM crops based on their proteomic and metabolic profiles, as demonstrated through the large number of applications that use GC-MS, LC-MS, CE-MS, or MS as a stand-alone technique. Thus, proteomics can be applied to study potential alterations in the GM crop proteome. For this purpose, comparative proteomics strategy is mainly used. Representative examples to the study of substantial equivalence of GM are given in Table 4.2.

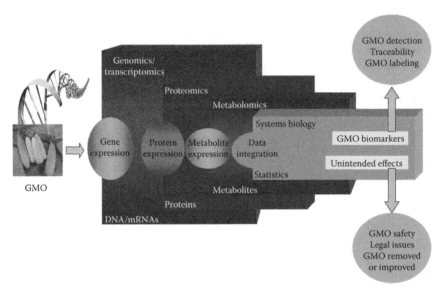

**FIGURE 4.3**　Ideal foodomics platform to analyze genetically modified foods. GMO, genetically modified organism.

## TABLE 4.2
## Some Foodomics Applications Related to Food Safety and Quality

| Issue | Food/Beverage | "Omic" Approach | Analytical Tool | Reference |
|---|---|---|---|---|
| Crop improvement | Melon | Transcriptomics | Gene expression microarray | Mascarell-Creus et al. (2009) |
| Monitoring mycotoxin production | Wheat | Transcriptomics | Gene expression microarray | Schmidt-Heydt and Geisen (2007) |
| Study of substantial equivalence | Maize | Transcriptomics | Gene expression microarray | Coll et al. (2009) |
| GMO detection | Maize | Genomics | DNA microarray | Hammels et al. (2009) |
| Food research | Rice | Proteomics | Review | Agrawal et al. (2009) |
| Prion disease discovery | Meat | Proteomics | Review | Huzarewich et al. (2010) |
| Food research | Rice | Metabolomics | GC-MS | Shu et al. (2008) |
| Beverage authenticity | Fruit juice | Metabolomics | $^1$H-NMR | Cuny et al. (2008) |
| Production monitoring | Beer | Metabolomics | $^1$H NMR | Almeida et al. (2006) |
| Microbial spoilage detection | Meat | Metabolomics | GC-MS | Ercolini et al. (2009) |

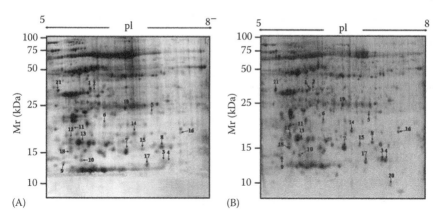

**FIGURE 4.4**   2DE proteomic maps of tobacco (*N. tabacum*) leaves from (A) untransformed tobacco plants (NN) and (B) transgenic tobacco plants overexpressing tomato prosystemin gene (MZ119). (From Rocco, M., *J. Proteomics*, 71, 176, 2008. With permission.)

For instance, the expression of recombinant antibodies in two transgenic crops (tomato and tobacco), as a strategy to confer self-protection against virus attack, did not significantly alter the leaf-proteome profile (Di Carli et al. 2009). However, Rocco et al. (2008) observed that a tobacco transformed with the tomato prosystemin gene affected the expression of a number of proteins involved in protection from pathogens and oxidative stress and in carbon/energy metabolism (Figure 4.4). Zhou et al. (2009) reported the combined use of GC-FID and GC-MS to investigate possible unintended effects on the metabolome of a transgenic line of rice that expressed two genes that confer distinct insect resistance. In addition to GC-MS, LC-MS has been demonstrated as a useful methodology for the metabolomic analysis of GM crops, enabling the separation and detection of polar/nonvolatile, large, and/or thermolabile compounds, without the need of chemical derivatization. Tesniere et al. (2006) provided complementary and interesting data in the investigation of metabolism alterations in transgenic grapevine by LC-MS. Systems biology can be applied to deeply analyze GMOs in order to exclude any unintended effect by monitoring possible translocation in the foreign genes inserted in the GMO, possible proteins generated as response to this modification and the possible metabolites pathways that can be influenced by the activity of the new synthesized proteins. The application of foodomics following a systems biology approach should allow to detect and to identify these unintended modifications, providing in this way more sounded data on the equivalent nature of GMOs compared to their natural counterparts.

Functional wine-omics has also been defined and involves research partners in viticulture, oenology, food science, and chemistry (Moore et al. 2008). This functional wine-omics would use a systems biology scheme to wine-related organisms. Data generated within the program is proposed to be integrated with other data sets from viticulture, oenology, analytical chemistry, and the sensory sciences through chemometrics and other statistical tools. The aim of the program is to model aspects of the wine-making process, from the vineyard to the finished product.

## 4.5  FOODOMICS: FUTURE CHALLENGES AND DEVELOPMENTS

There are a large number of challenges in food science and nutrition to be faced in the near future. These include (a) the production of new functional foods with scientifically proved claims; (b) the assessment of food safety, quality, and traceability as a whole using omics approaches; (c) the development, production, and monitoring of new transgenics foods (including the so-called second-generation GM crops); (d) the understanding of the effects of gene–food interaction on human health (nutrigenomics); and (e) the explanation of the different answers from individuals to food, including the long-distance achievement of recommending personalized diet (nutrigenetics). A detailed discussion on these topics is provided hereafter.

Foodomics approaches can help to overcome the important limitations detected by several regulatory institutions, including the European Food Safety Authority (EFSA), related to the controversial demonstration about the health claims on different foods and food ingredients. Thus, as discussed in a recent article (Daniells 2010), the announcement by the Panel on Dietetic Products, Nutrition and Allergies (NDA) at the EFSA (2010) indicates that no evidence has been provided to establish that a food ingredient having antioxidant activity/content and/or antioxidant properties can have a beneficial physiological effect on human health. This decision will not only have an important economical impact on the antioxidant market that is calculated to move billions of euros per year but also have a negative influence on the consumers' confidence about the possibility to promote health through foods. Therefore, more sophisticated approaches than the ones used so far will be required to demonstrate with strong scientific evidences the positive health effect derived from the intake of determined foods and food ingredients. In this regard, foodomics applied to study the *in vitro* and *in vivo* mechanisms of these compounds (including, if required, foodomics of biological samples from randomized clinical trials) is the right way to prove that antioxidant activity is indeed associated with a beneficial physiological effect. Moreover, this approach can be extended to better prove (or not) the health claims linking health benefits to many other different compounds, most of them rejected by EFSA so far. Just to describe a few, melatonin does not benefit sleep; xanthan gum does not boost satiety; green and black tea extracts do not protect DNA, proteins, and lipids from oxidative damage; C12-peptide does not help to maintain normal blood pressure; *Lactobacillus plantarum* BFE 1685 does not decrease potentially pathogenic intestinal microorganisms; *Lactobacillus rhamnosus* LB21 NCIMB 40564 does not decrease potentially pathogenic intestinal microorganisms; *L. plantarum* 299v (DSM 9843) does not support the immune system (insufficiently defined effect); linoleic acid does not maintain normal neurological function; vitamin D does not benefit cardiovascular health; etc. (EFSA 2010, Starling 2010).

In this regard, it has been mentioned that it is probably too early to conclude on the value of many substances for health, and the same can apply to other health relationships that are still in the process. Thus, foodomics could help to overcome the main limitations detected by EFSA to reject these proposals, namely, lack of information to identify the substance on which the claim is based, lack of evidence that the claimed effect is indeed beneficial to the maintenance or improvement of the functions of the body, and lack of human studies with reliable measures of the claimed health benefit. However, it is also interesting to mention that the traditional medical world has often noted that although many of the omics tools and foodomics approaches provide academically interesting research (Breikers et al. 2006, Fardet et al. 2007, Griffiths and Grant 2006, Narasaka et al. 2006, Rezzi et al. 2007a,b, Smolenski et al. 2007), they have not been translated to methods or approaches with medicinal impact and value, because the data integration when dealing with such complex systems is not straightforward. Definitely, one of the major challenges in the analysis and interpretation of these omic data from foodomics will be to deliver models of causation from correlations (Hirai et al. 2004, Schnackenberg et al. 2006).

In the near future, nutritional genomics may be the answer to a personalized nutrition, but (a) it will be necessary to carry out more studies in terms of, for example, discovering more polymorphisms of one nucleotide, identifying genes related to complex disorders, and demonstrating a higher degree of evidence through epidemiological studies based in foodomics that can lead to public recommendations and (b) it will be mandatory to support a better nutritional education and to extend the research on new food products. As a long-term result, a personalized diet depending on a particular genetic profile will become possible.

Therefore, it is necessary to better analyze the interrelationship among genetic variants, nutrients, and environmental factors. This knowledge can only be generated using multidisciplinary approaches, considering international consortia and working on foodomics based on extensive populations. Foodomics can also be important in terms of public health considering two different approaches: at short term, involving the clinical application to treat metabolic alterations such as diabetes, etc., and at long term, more related to the public primary prevention, that is, inhibiting the development of disease before it occurs.

Regarding the omics tools used in foodomics, they will also have to overcome important limitations for optimal implementation in the nondistant future. Thus, limitations of DNA microarrays associated with the high background noise that specially hinders the detection of low signals (i.e., low-signal-to-noise ratios) and the efficiency and specificity of the hybridization probes have to be addressed. Novel approaches focused on the use of electrochemical transducers in combination with enzymatic, redox-active indicators, or nanoparticle labels, as well as with label-free hybridization strategies, are being investigated as cheaper and sensitive alternatives to current optical detection systems (Privett et al. 2008). Also, some interesting alternatives to typical linear probes have been proposed such as molecular beacon probes and peptide nucleic acids (Sassolas et al. 2008). These probes offer high specificity and appear as good candidates for mismatch discrimination. Next-generation methods in transcriptomics will undoubtedly continue to technically improve in several ways within the next few years. New improvements will probably include the establishment of routine data analysis methods and increase in the numbers and lengths of sequence reads as well (Maricic and Paabo 2009, Quail et al. 2008). It is also expected that the cost of these analyses will continue decreasing in the near future, allowing new applications and extensive use of these technologies in foodomics research.

In proteomics, MS alone or combined with two-dimensional electrophoresis (2DE), liquid chromatography, and capillary electrophoresis has become the most used methodology. There is an evident need of developing improved or alternative technologies (e.g., protein microarrays) to bring into a reality the routine analysis for proteome research, including improvements in the resolution of peptides to provide increased protein coverage. Apart of the everyday more sophisticated sample treatments and separation techniques, MS will keep essential for the systematic investigation in proteomics. In this sense, conventional mass spectrometers are giving way to the more sophisticated and compact mass spectrometers, most of them hybrid instruments in a combination of two or more analyzers. As can be deduced from the low number of proteomic applications in foodomics studies, it is expected that new innovations in proteomic technology will help proteomic profiling to also become a standard practice in foodomics.

A great advance in metabolomics is expected with the incorporation of new MS interfaces for which nearly no sample preparation is needed (Chen et al. 2006, Feng et al. 2008, Huang et al. 2007). Comprehensive multidimensional techniques, such as GC × GC or LC × LC, are also a revolutionary improvement in separation techniques that will be implemented in metabolomics studies in the near future. They not only provide enhanced resolution and a huge increase in the peak number but also an increase in selectivity and sensitivity in comparison with conventional separation techniques. As an example, comprehensive GC × GC coupled to TOF-MS has demonstrated to be a promising tool for metabolic profiling (Pasikanti et al. 2008).

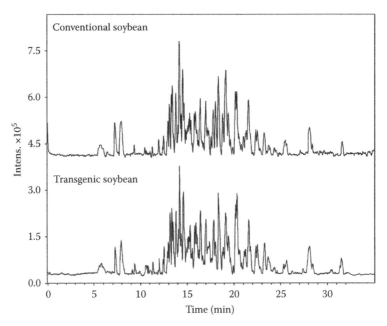

**FIGURE 4.5**   CE-TOF MS base peak electropherogram of the digested protein extract from conventional and transgenic soybean. CE-TOF MS analysis conditions: bare silica capillary (50 μm id, 90 cm); BGE: 0.5 M formic acid; injection time: 20 s at 0.5 psi (34.5 mbar); separation voltage: 25 kV; sheath liquid: isopropanol–water (50:50, v/v) at a 3 μL/min flow rate; nebulizer gas: 0.4 bar; drying gas: 4 L/min $N_2$ at 200°C; MS is used in positive ion mode; scan: 50–3000 m/z. (Redrawn from Simó, C. et al., *Electrophoresis*, 31, 1175, 2010.)

Also, capillary electrokinetic techniques and their coupling to mass spectrometry (CE and CE-MS) are ideal tools for metabolomics, as they do not require extensive sample preparation and due to their wide range of applications, great efficiency and resolution, and low sample consumption. Although CE and CE-MS have not been widely used in foodomics (Herrero et al. 2010), they have already been identified as a very promising tool for metabolomic studies (García-Villalba et al. 2008, Levandi et al. 2008, Oh et al. 2010). Interesting examples on the use of CE-MS in foodomics can be found in very recent works, such as the study of substantial equivalence of transgenic and conventional soybean from their peptidic profiles using a shot-gun approach (see Figure 4.5) (Simó et al. 2010).

The challenge in the combination of foodomics and systems biology is not only at the technological level, where, as mentioned earlier, great improvements are being made and expected in the "omics" technologies, but also on the bioinformatics side (data processing, clustering, dynamics, integration of the various "omics" levels, etc.) that will have to progress for systems biology to demonstrate all its potential in the new foodomics discipline (Gehlenborg et al. 2010).

## ACKNOWLEDGMENT

This work was supported by projects AGL2008-05108-C03-01 and CONSOLIDER INGENIO 2010 CSD2007-00063 FUN-C-FOOD (Ministerio de Educación y Ciencia).

## REFERENCES

Agrawal, G. K., N. S. Jwa, and R. Rakwal. 2009. Rice proteomics: Ending phase I and the beginning of phase II. *Proteomics* 9:935–963.

Almeida, C., I. F. Duarte, A. Barros, J. Rodrigues, M. Spraul, and A. A. Gil. 2006. Composition of beer by $^1$H NMR spectroscopy: Effects of brewing site and date of production. *J Agric Food Chem* 54:700–706.

Baudo, M. M., R. Lyons, S. Powers et al. 2006. Transgenesis has less impact on the transcriptome of wheat grain than conventional breeding. *Plant Biotechnol J* 4:369–380.

Bogdanov, B. and R. D. Smith. 2005. Proteomics by FTICR mass spectrometry: Top down and bottom up. *Mass Spectrom Rev* 24:168–200.

Borrebaeck, C. A. K. and C. Wingren. 2007. High-throughput proteomics using antibody microarrays: An update. *Expert Rev Mol Diagn* 7:673–686.

Breikers, G., S. G. J. van Breda, F. G. Bouwman et al. 2006. Potential protein markers for nutritional health effects on colorectal cancer in the mouse as revealed by proteomics analysis. *Proteomics* 6:2844–2852

Chen, C. H. 2008. Review of a current role of mass spectrometry for proteome research. *Anal Chim Acta* 624:16–36.

Chen, H., Z. Pan, N. Talaty, D. Raftery, and R. G. Cooks. 2006. Combining desorption electrospray ionization mass spectrometry and nuclear magnetic resonance for differential metabolomics without sample preparation. *Rapid Comm Mass Spectrom* 20:1577–1584.

Cifuentes, A. 2009. Food analysis and foodomics. *J Chromatogr A* 1216:7109–7110.

Coll, A., A. Nadal, R. Collado et al. 2009. Gene expression profiles of MON810 and comparable non-GM maize varieties cultured in the field are more similar than are those of conventional lines. *Transgenic Res* 18:801–808.

Cortesy-Theulaz, I., J. T. den Dunnen, P. Ferre et al. 2005. Nutrigenomics: The impact of biomics technology on nutrition research. *Ann Nutr Metab* 49:355–365.

Cuny, M., E. Vigneau, G. Le Gall, I. Colquhoun, M. Lees, and D. N. Rutledge. 2008. Fruit juice authentication by ¹H NMR spectroscopy in combination with different chemometrics tools. *Anal Bioanal Chem* 390:419–427.

Daniells, S. 2010. *EFSA's Antioxidant Rejections could be Blessing in Disguise.* http://www.foodqualitynews.com/Legislation/EFSA-s-antioxidant-rejections-could-be-blessing-in-disguise (accessed April 7, 2010).

Dettmer, K., P. A. Aronov, and B. D. Hammock. 2007. Mass spectrometry based metabolomics. *Mass Spectrom Rev* 26:51–78.

Di Carli, M., M. E. Villani, G. Renzone et al. 2009. Leaf proteome analysis of transgenic plants expressing antiviral antibodies. *J Proteome Res* 8:838–848.

Dubouzet, J. G., A. Ishihara, F. Matsuda, H. Miyagawa, H. Iwata, and K. Wakasa. 2007. Integrated metabolomic and transcriptomic analyses of high-tryptophan rice expressing a mutant anthranilate synthase alpha subunit. *J Exp Bot* 58:3309–3321.

EFSA. 2006. (European Food Safety Agency. 2006). *Guidance Document of the Scientific Panel on Genetically Modified Organisms for the Risk Assessment of Genetically Modified Plants and Derived Food and Feed.* Parma, Italy: EFSA Communications Department.

EFSA. 2010. Opinions of the NDA Panel Published on 2009 and 2010. http://www.efsa.europa.eu/cs/Satellite (accessed on April 7, 2010).

Ercolini, D., F. Russo, A. Nasi, P. Ferranti, and F. Villani. 2009. Mesophilic and psychrotrophic bacteria from meat and their spoilage potential in vitro and in beef. *Appl Environ Microbiol* 75:1990–2001.

Fang, X. and W. W. Zhang. 2008. Affinity separation and enrichment methods in proteomic analysis. *J Proteomics* 71:284–303.

Fardet, A., C. Canlet, G. Gottardi et al. 2007. Whole-grain and refined wheat flours show distinct metabolic profiles in rats as assessed by a H-1 NMR-based metabonomic approach. *J Nutr* 137:923–929.

Fay, L. B. and J. B. German. 2008. Personalizing foods: Is genotype necessary? *Curr Opin Biotechnol* 19:121–128.

Feng, X., X. Liu, Q. Luo, and B. F. Liu. 2008. Mass spectrometry in systems biology: An overview. *Mass Spectrom Rev* 27:635–660.

Ferguson, L. R., M. Philpott, and P. Dryland. 2007. Nutrigenomics in the whole-genome scanning era: Crohn's disease as example. *Cell Mol Life Sci* 64:3105–3118.

Fiehn, O. 2002. Metabolomics—The link between genotype and phenotype. *Plant Mol Biol* 48:155–171.

Fuchs, D., K. Vafeiadou, W. L. Hall et al. 2007. Health benefits of isoflavones in functional foods? Proteomic and metabonomic advances. *Am J Clin Nutr* 86:1369–1375.

Garcia-Cañas, V., C. Simó, C. Leon, and A. Cifuentes. 2010. Advances in nutrigenomics research: Novel and future analytical approaches to investigate the biological activity of natural compounds and food functions. *J Pharm Biomed Anal* 51:290–304.

García-Villalba, R., C. León, G. Dinelli A. Segura-Carretero, R. Fernández-Gutiérrez, V. Garcia-Cañas, A. Cifuentes. 2008. Transgenic vs. conventional soybean: A comparative metabolomic study using capillary electrophoresis-time of flight-mass spectrometry. *J Chromatogr A* 1195:164–173.

Gehlenborg, N., S. L. O'Donoghue, N. S. Baliga et al. 2010. Visualization of omics data for systems biology. *Nat Methods* 7:S56–S68

Greenspan, R. J. 2001. The flexible genome. *Nat Rev Gen* 2:383–387.

Gregersen, P. L., H. Brinch-Pedersen, and P. B. Holm. 2005. A microarray-based comparative analysis of gene expression profiles during grain development in transgenic and wild type wheat. *Transgenic Res* 14:887–905.

Griffiths, H. R. and M. M. Grant. 2006. The use of proteomic techniques to explore the holistic effects of nutrients in vivo. *Nutr Res Rev* 19:284–293.

Griffiths, W. J. and Y. Q. Wang. 2009. Mass spectrometry: From proteomics to metabolomics and lipidomics. *Chem Soc Rev* 38:1882–1896.

Grün, C. H., F. A. van Dorsten, D. M. Jacobs et al. 2008. GC–MS methods for metabolic profiling of microbial fermentation products of dietary polyphenols in human and in vitro intervention studies. *J Chromatogr B* 871:212–219.

Hammels, S., T. Glouden, K. Gillard et al. 2009. A PCR-microarray method for the screening of genetically modified organisms. *Eur Food Res Technol* 228:531–541.

Han, X., A. Aslanian, and J. R. Yates III. 2008. Mass spectrometry for proteomics. *Curr Opin Chem Biol* 12:483–490.

Herrero, M., V. García-Cañas, C. Simo, and A. Cifuentes. 2010. Recent advances in the application of CE methods for food analysis and foodomics. *Electrophoresis* 31:205–228.

Hirai, M. Y., M. Yano, D. B. Goodenowe et al. 2004. Integration of transcriptomics and metabolomics for understanding of global responses to nutritional stress in *Arabidopsis thaliana*. *PNAS* 101:10205–10210.

Hood, L., J. R. Health, M. E. Phelps, and B. Lin. 2004. Systems biology and new technologies enable predictive and preventative medicine. *Science* 306:640–643.

Hu, R. and A. T. Kong. 2004. Activation of MAP kinases, apoptosis and nutrigenomics of gene expression elicited by dietary cancer-prevention compounds. *Nutrition* 20:83–88.

Huang, J. T., F. M. Leweke, T. M. Tsang et al. 2007. CSF metabolic and proteomic profiles in patients prodromal for psychosis. *PLoS ONE* 2:e756.

Huzarewich, R. L., C. G. Siemens, and S. A. Booth. 2010. Application of "omics" to prion biomarker discovery. *J Biomed Biotechnol* 2010:613504.

Jacobs, D. M., N. Deltimple, E. van Velzen et al. 2008. $^1$H NMR metabolite profiling of feces as a tool to assess the impact of nutrition on the human microbiome. *NMR Biomed* 21:615–626.

Kaput, J. 2008. Nutrigenomics research for personalized nutrition and medicine. *Curr Opin Biotechnol* 19:110–120.

Kato, H. and T. Kimura. 2003. Evaluation of the effects of the dietary intake of proteins and amino acids by DNA microarray technology. *J Nutr* 133:2073S–2077S.

Kayo, T., D. B. Allison, R. Weindruch, and T. A. Prolla. 2001. Influences of aging and caloric restriction on the transcriptional profile of skeletal muscle from rhesus monkeys. *PNAS* 98:5093–5098.

Kim, H. J., S. H. Park, T. H. Lee, B. H. Hanm, R. Kim, and H. Y. Kim. 2008. Microarray detection of food-borne pathogens using specific probes prepared by comparative genomic. *Biosens Bioelectron* 24:238–246.

Kohanski, M. A., D. J. Dwyer, J. Wierzbowski, G. Cottarel, and J. J. Collins. 2008. Mistranslation of membrane proteins and two-component system activation trigger antibiotic-mediated cell death. *Cell* 135:679–690.

Koulman, A. and D. A. Volmer. 2008. Perspectives for metabolomics in human nutrition: An overview. *Nutr Bull* 33:324–330.

Kussman, M., S. Rezzi, and H. Danelore. 2008. Profiling techniques in nutrition and health research. *Curr Opin Biotechnol* 19:83–99.

Lee, W. N. P. and V. L. Go. 2005. Nutrient–gene interaction: Tracer-based metabolomics. *J Nutr* 135:3027S–3032S.

Lee, C. K., R. G. Klopp, R. Weindruch, and A. Prolla. 1999. Gene expression profile of aging and its retardation by caloric restriction. *Science* 285:1390–1393.

Levandi, T., C. Leon, M. Kaljurand, V. Garcia-Cañas, and A. Cifuentes. 2008. Capillary electrophoresis-time of flight-mass spectrometry for comparative metabolomics of transgenic vs. conventional maize. *Anal Chem* 80:6329–6335.

Liu, Y., B. Elsholz, S. O. Enfors, and M. Gabig-Ciminska. 2007. Confirmative electric DNA array-based test for food poisoning Bacillus cereus. *J Microbiol Methods* 70:55–64.

Lu, Q. Y., Y. S. Jin, Z. F. Zhang et al. 2007. Green tea induces annexin-I expression in human lung adenocarcinoma A549 cells: Involvement of annexin-I in actin remodeling. *Lab Invest* 87:456–465.

Maricic, T. and S. Paabo. 2009. Optimization of 454 sequencing library preparation from small amounts of DNA permits sequence determination of both DNA strands. *Biotechnology* 46:51–57.

Martinez-Godoy, M. A., N. Mauri, J. Juarez et al. 2008. A genome-wide 20 K citrus microarray for gene expression analysis. *BMC Genomics* 9:318–324.

Mascarell-Creus, A., J. Cañizares, J. Vilarrasa-Blasi et al. 2009. An oligo-based microarray offers novel transcriptomic approaches for the analysis of pathogen resistance and fruit quality traits in melon (*Cucumis melo* L.). *BMC Genomics* 10:467–482.

McLoughlin, P., M. Roengvoraphoj, C. Gissel, J. Hescheler, U. Certa, and A. Sachinidis. 2004. Transcriptional responses to epigallocatechin-3 gallate in HT 29 colon carcinoma spheroids. *Genes Cells* 9:661–669.

Moore, J. P., B. Divol, P. R. Young et al. 2008. Wine biotechnology in South Africa: Towards a systems approach to wine science. *Biotechnol J* 3:1355–1367.

Morozova, O. and M. A. Marra. 2008. Applications of next-generation sequencing technologies in functional genomics. *Genomics* 92:255–264.

Motoyama, A. and J. R. Yates III. 2008. Multidimensional LC separations in shotgun proteomics. *Anal Chem* 80:7187–7193.

Mouat, M. F., K. Kolli, R. Orlando, J. L. Hargrove, and A. Grider. 2005. The effects of quercetin on SW480 human colon carcinoma cells: A proteomic study. *Nutr J* 4:1–7.

Müller, M. and S. Kersten. 2003. Nutrigenomics: Goals and strategies. *Nat Rev Gen* 4:315–322.

Murtaza, L., G. Marra, R. Schlapbach, A. Patrignani, M. Kunzli, and U. Wagner. 2006. A preliminary investigation demonstrating the effect of quercetin on the expression of genes related to cell-cycle arrest, apoptosis and xenobiotic metabolism in human CO115 colonadenocarcinoma cells using DNA microarray. *Biotechnol Appl Biochem* 45:29–36.

Mutch, D. M., W. Wahli, and G. Williamson. 2005. Nutrigenomics and nutrigenetics: The emerging faces of nutrition. *FASEB J* 19:1602–1616.

Naito, Y., K. Uchiyama, K. Mizushima et al. 2006. Microarray profiling of gene expression patterns in glomerular cells of astaxanthin-treated diabetic mice: A nutrigenomic approach. *Int J Mol Med* 18:685–695.

Narasaka, S., Y. Endo, Z. W. Fu et al. 2006. Safety evaluation of hypoallergenic wheat flour by using a DNA microarray. *Biosci Biotechnol Biochem* 70:1464–1470.

Narayanan, B. A., N. K. Narayanan, B. Simi, B. S. Reddy. 2003. Modulation of inducible nitric oxide synthase and related proinflammatory genes by the omega-3 fatty acid docosahexaenoic acid in human colon cancer cells. *Cancer Res* 62:972–979.

Niculescu, M. D., E. A. Pop, L. M. Fischer, and S. H. Zeisel. 2007. Dietary isoflavones differentially induce gene expression changes in lymphocytes from postmenopausal women who form equol as compared with those who do not. *J Nutr Biochem* 18:380–390.

Oh, E., M. N. Hasan, M. Jamshed et al. 2010. Growing trend of CE at the omics level: The frontier of systems biology. *Electrophoresis* 31:74–92.

Panagiotou, G. and J. Nielsen. 2009. Nutritional systems biology: Definitions and approaches. *Ann Rev Nutr* 29:329–339.

Pasikanti, K. K., P. C. Ho, and E. C. Chan. 2008. Gas chromatography/mass spectrometry in metabolic profiling of biological fluids. *J Chromatogr B* 871:202–211.

Pernemalm, M., L. M. Orre, J. Lengqvist, P. Wikström, R. Lewensohn, and J. Lehtiö. 2008. Evaluation of three principally different intact protein prefractionation methods for plasma biomarker discovery. *J Proteome Res* 7:2712–2722.

Powell, K. 2007. Functional foods from biotech—An unappetizing prospect? *Nature* 25:525–531.

Privett, B. J., J. H. Shin, and M. H. Schoenfisch. 2008. Electrochemical sensors. *Anal Chem* 80:4499–4517.

Quail, M. A., I. Kozarewa, F. Smith et al. 2008. A large genome center's improvements to the Illumina sequencing system. *Nat Methods* 5:1005–1010.

Raqib, R. and A. Cravioto. 2009. Nutrition, immunology, and genetics: Future perspectives. *Nutr Rev* 67:S227–S236.

Rezzi, S., Z. Ramadan, L. B. Fay, and S. Kochhar. 2007a. Nutritional metabonomics: Applications and perspectives. *J Proteome Res* 6:513–525.

Rezzi, S., Z. Ramadan, F. P. Martin et al. 2007b. Human metabolic phenotypes link directly to specific dietary preferences in healthy individuals. *J Proteome Res* 6:4469–4477.

Rist, M. J., U. Wenzel, and H. Daniel. 2006. Nutrition and food science go genomic. *Trends Biotechnol* 24:1–7.

Rocco, M., G. Corrado, S. Arena et al. 2008. The expression of tomato prosystemin gene in tobacco plants highly affects host proteomic repertoire. *J Proteomics* 71:176–185.

Sassolas, A., B. D. Leca-Bouvier, and L. J. Blum. 2008. DNA biosensors and microarrays. *Chem Rev* 108:109–139.

Schmidt-Heydt, M. and R. Geisen. 2007. A microarray for monitoring the production of mycotoxins in food. *Int J Food Microbiol* 117:131–140.

Schnackenberg, L. K., R. C. Jones, S. Thyparambil et al. 2006. An integrated study of acute effects of valproic acid in the liver using metabonomics, proteomics, and transcriptomics platforms. *OMICS* 10:1–13.

Shu, X. L., T. Frank, Q. Y. Shu, and K. H. Engel. 2008. Metabolite profiling of germinating rice seeds. *J Agric Food Chem* 6:11612–11620.

Simó, C., E. Domínguez-Vega, M. L. Marina, M. C. García, G. Dinelli, and A. Cifuentes. 2010. CE-TOF MS analysis of complex protein hydrolyzates from genetically modified soybeans. A tool for foodomics. *Electrophoresis* 31:1175–1183.

Smolenski, G., S. Haines, F. Y. S. Kwan et al. 2007. Characterization of host defense proteins in milk using a proteomic approach. *J Proteome Res* 6:207–215.

Solanky, K. S., N. J. Bailey, B. M. Beckwith-Hall et al. 2005. Biofluid $^1$H NMR-based metabonomic techniques in nutrition research—Metabolic effects of dietary isoflavones in humans. *J Nutr Biochem* 16:236–244.

Starling, S. 2010. EFSA Mass Rejects Probiotics and Antioxidants as Article 13.1 Batch Two Published. http://www.beveragedaily.com/Product-Categories/Ingredients-and-additives/EFSA-mass-rejects-probiotics-and-antioxidants-as-article-13.1-batch-two-published (accessed on April 7, 2010).

Subbiah, M. T. R. 2006. Nutrigenetics and nutraceuticals: The next wave riding on personalized medicine. *Transl Res* 149:55–61.

Tengs, T., A. B. Kristoffersen, K. G. Berdal et al. 2007. Microarray-based method for detection of unknown genetic modifications. *BMC Biotechnol* 7:91–98.

Tesniere, C., L. Torregrosa, M. Pradal et al. 2006. Effects of genetic manipulation of alcohol dehydrogenase levels on the response to stress and the synthesis of secondary metabolites in grapevine leaves. *J Exp Bot* 57:91–99.

Thimmulappa, R. K., K. H. Mai, S. Srisuma, T. W. Kensler, M. Yamamoto, and S. Biswal. 2002. Identification of nrf2-regulated genes induced by the chemopreventive agent sulforaphane by oligonucleotide microarray. *Cancer Res* 62:5196–5203.

Trujillo, E., C. Davis, and J. Milner. 2006. Nutrigenomics, proteomics, metabolomics and the practice of diets. *J Am Diet Assoc* 106:403–414.

Tsuda, T., Y. Ueno, T. Yoshikawa, H. Kojo, and T. Osawa. 2006. Microarray profiling of gene expression in human adipocytes in response to anthocyanins. *Biochem Pharm* 71:1184–1197.

van Erk, M. J., W. A. Blom, V. Van Ommen, and H. F. Hendriks. 2006. High-protein and high-carbohydrate breakfasts differentially change the transcriptome of human blood cells. *Am J Clin Nutr* 84:1233–1241.

van Ommen, B. and R. Stierum. 2002. Nutrigenomics: Exploiting systems biology in the nutrition and health arena. *Curr Opin Biotechnol* 13:517–521.

Vittal, R., Z. E. Selvanayagam, Y. Sun et al. 2004. Gene expression changes induced by green tea polyphenol (–)-epigallocatechin-3-gallate in human bronchial epithelial 21BES cells analyzed by DNA microarray. *Mol Cancer Ther* 3:1091–1099.

von Götz, F. 2010. See what you eat-broad GMO screening with microarrays. *Anal Bioanal Chem* 393:1961–1967.

Waagmeester, A. S., T. Kelder, and C. T. A. Evelo. 2008. The role of bioinformatics in pathway curation. *Genes Nutr* 3:139–142.

Wang, S. I. and H. Mukhar. 2002. Gene expression profile in human prostate LNCaP cancer cells by (–) epigallocatechin-3-gallate. *Cancer Lett* 182:43–51.

Wang, X. W., L. Zhang, L. Q. Jin et al. 2007. Development and application of an oligonucleotide microarray for the detection of food-borne bacterial pathogens. *Appl Microbiol Biotechnol* 76:225–233.

Wechter, W. P., A. Levi, K. R. Harris et al. 2008. Gene expression in developing watermelon fruit. *BMC Genomics* 9:275–280.

Weston, A. D. and L. Hood. 2004. Systems biology, proteomics, and the future of health care: Toward predictive, preventative, and personalized medicine. *J Proteome Res* 3:179–196.

Wiesner, J., T. Premsler, and A. Sickmann. 2008. Application of electron transfer dissociation (ETD) for the analysis of posttranslational modifications. *Proteomics* 8:4466–4483.

Wong, M. C. Y., P. W. Emery, V. R. Preedy, and H. Wiseman. 2008. Health benefits of isoflavones in functional foods? Proteomic and metabonomic advances. *Inflammopharmacology* 16:235–239.

Xiang, D., R. Datla, F. Li et al. 2008. Development of a Brassica seed cDNA microarray. *Genome* 51:236–242.

Zhou, J., C. Ma, H. Xu et al. 2009. Metabolic profiling of transgenic rice with cryIAc and sck genes: An evaluation of unintended effects at metabolic level by using GC-FID and GC–MS. *J Chromatogr B* 877:725–732.

Zhou, P. P., J. A. Zhang, Y. H. You, and Y. N. Wu. 2008. Detection of genetically modified crops by combination of multiplex PCR and low-density DNA microarray. *Biomed Environ Sci* 21:53–62.

# 5 Proteomics in Food Biotechnology

*Gu Chen and Xuewu Zhang*

## CONTENTS

## 5.1 INTRODUCTION

Human food is a very complex biological mixture. Food quality and safety are issues of high concern for the food industry worldwide as they are directly linked to public health and welfare. Increasingly, high-throughput techniques are developed and applied to monitor and evaluate food quality and safety. Proteomics is one of the choices. Proteomics is the global study of the whole set of proteins encoded by a genome under certain conditions and at a certain time. Based on the high-performance separation techniques and high-resolution mass spectrometry, proteomics can monitor the protein compositions of foods and their fluctuation during processing to evaluate the food quality and safety related to protein efficiently. In this chapter, we outline the state of the art of proteomic techniques and review their application in the control of food quality and evaluation of food safety.

## 5.2 PROTEOMIC PLATFORM—STATE OF THE ART

Typical proteomic workflows encompass protein extraction, protein separation and quantification, protein identification, and data analysis and interpretation.

Protein extraction itself can be a difficult task given the diversity of food and their raw material. Generally, each technique focuses on a particular set of proteins due to the complex chemical nature and broad dynamic range of proteins. Carpentier et al. listed a detailed protocol of protein extraction for a series of plants (banana, pear, apple, potato, and maize) (Carpentier et al. 2008). Prefractionation techniques such as organelle fractionation using differential density ultracentrifugation can help to enrich target proteins (Ho et al. 2006).

### 5.2.1 Protein Separation

Nowadays proteins are separated using either gel-based or gel-free approaches.

#### 5.2.1.1 Gel-Based Protein Separation

The gel-based proteomic approach starts from two-dimensional electrophoresis (2-DE) separation of proteins, which is based on two distinct features of proteins: isoelectric point (pI) and molecular weight. O'Farrell introduced this technique in the 1970s (Ofarrell et al. 1977). First, in isoelectric focusing (IEF) proteins are separated according to their pI on a pH gradient created in the gel or strip. Proteins then migrate toward cathode or anode according to their total charge up to the point where the gel pH equals their pI. Then a common electrophoresis on a polyacrylamide gel (SDS-PAGE) is run perpendicularly to the original orientation of electrodes. Before this second dimension SDS-PAGE, focused proteins need to be equilibrated in an excess of SDS to eliminate the intrinsic charges as well as the secondary and tertiary structures so that proteins migrate in the second direction solely dependent on their molecular weight. Once proteins are separated, they were visualized and quantified with staining strategies such as colloidal coomassie blue, silver, radiolabeling, and fluorescence (reviewed by Miller et al. 2006). The resulting "maps" of proteins can be compared to identify differentially expressed proteins. The identity of proteins is verified after "cutting out" the area of the gel with the given difference and subsequent analysis using mass spectrometry. One of the pitfalls of comparative 2-DE is the high gel-to-gel variation that makes it difficult to distinguish biological variation from technical variation. To overcome this issue, two-dimensional in-gel electrophoresis (DIGE) was developed in 1997 (Unlu et al. 1997). In DIGE, samples were first labeled with different dyes (Cy2, Cy3, and Cy5) and mixed together to be resolved on the same 2-DE gel. An internal standard (representing average of all samples) can be included to normalize protein abundance across multiple gels, thus improving the confidence of inter-gel spot matching and quantification.

Gel-based proteomics is the choice to study isoforms and posttranslational modifications of proteins and is powerful for non-model organisms (Carpentier et al. 2008), but it still has disadvantages such as the low resolving power of low-abundant proteins, hydrophobic or very acidic proteins, comigration of proteins with similar pI and molecular weight, and the difficulty for automation.

### 5.2.1.2 Gel-Free Protein Separation

Gel-free approaches are successful for relatively simple protein mixtures from sequenced organisms. Here proteins are first proteolyzed and the resulting mixture of peptides is separated through reverse-phase chromatography based on hydrophobicity. The subsequently eluted peptides are detected by mass spectrometer. All the tandem mass spectra are used to search databases and reconstruct the original proteins (Roe and Griffin 2006). Multidimensional protein identification technology (MudPit) aided to resolve proteins from complex samples (Roe and Griffin 2006, Washburn et al. 2001) and stable isotope labeling and dilution strategies are introduced for relative quantification of proteins through gel-free approaches (Gygi et al. 1999, Ong et al. 2002, Roe and Griffin 2006, Ross et al. 2004). Gel-free approaches have some pitfalls such as the lack of qualitative and quantitative information on protein isoforms and posttranslational modifications and the difficulty in cross-species identification of poorly sequenced genomes (Carpentier et al. 2008).

### 5.2.2 Protein Identification—Mass Spectrometry

Proteins need to be digested by trypsin or other proteolytic enzyme to smaller peptides before being introduced into a mass spectrometer. A mass spectrometer consists of an ion source to produce ions from sample, mass analyzer to separate the ions according to their mass to charge ratio (m/z), a detector to record the number of ions from the analyzer, and a computer to process data and provide mass spectra (Lane 2005).

Two "soft" ionization techniques of mass spectrometry, matrix-assisted laser desorption ionization (MALDI) (Karas and Hillenkamp 1988) and electrospray ionization (ESI) (Fenn et al. 1989) enabled the high-throughput identification of proteins and revolutionized the proteomic platform. Different mass analyzers, such as time of flight (TOF), quadrupole (Q), and ion traps, have their strengths and weaknesses, respectively. The mass spectra measured from samples are then compared with theoretical spectra that are calculated from protein sequences in available databases (using bioinformatics tools). Genomics data provided the groundwork for proteomics in many model organisms, which have been sequenced, but also provided groundwork for other related species in which sequences have not been revealed completely. To get a significant hit, only a subset of all peptides from the protein digest need to be matched in fully sequenced organisms. For proteins from non-model organisms with a poorly characterized genome, cross-species identification is performed by comparing proteins of interest to orthologous proteins from species that are well characterized (Pedreschi et al. 2010). Tandem mass spectrometry couples two stages of MS and enables de novo peptide sequencing. In tandem MS, a particular peptide is isolated and fragmentized typically down the peptide bond by collision with inert gas. From the mass spectrum of the resulting fragments, sequence information of the peptide is obtained. Aided by various algorithms such as MASCOT, SEQUEST, X Tandem, and PHENYX, this de novo peptide sequencing by MS/MS provides great opportunities in non-model organisms (e.g., most animal- and plant-based food) (Pedreschi et al. 2010).

Apart from protein identification, MS is also a powerful tool for protein post-translational modification analysis, for example, carbonylation of milk proteins (Fenaille et al. 2005), deamidation within peptides (Schmid et al. 2001), determination of disulfide linkages (Wu et al. 2009a), and N-glycosylation and O-glycosylation (Bykova et al. 2006, Holland et al. 2005).

### 5.2.3 DATA ANALYSIS AND INTERPRETATION

Proteomics generates tremendous amount of data from which high-quality data should be filtered. Both gel-based and gel-free approaches require proper data analysis and interpretation, but first of all a good experimental design should be emphasized (Pedreschi et al. 2010). Sources of variability and appropriate replication should be considered in experimental design to characterize technical and biological differences (Chich et al. 2007, Horgan 2007). The missing values and multiple testing problems in gel-based approaches must be addressed (Albrecht et al. 2010). Appropriate statistical tests should be used depending on the questions asked. Univariate statistical tests (e.g., t-test, ANOVA, Kolmogorov–Smirnov, and Kruskall–Wallis test) account for changes in abundance for each individual protein. Multivariate statistical tests (e.g., principal component analysis, partial least squares discriminant analysis, and clustering) consider the multivariate context of proteins. The combination of both statistical approaches (univariate and multivariate) is powerful and has been performed in several reports (Kjaersgard et al. 2006, Pedreschi et al. 2007, 2008b).

## 5.3 PROTEOMICS IN FOOD BIOTECHNOLOGY

### 5.3.1 PROTEOMICS IN FOOD QUALITY

#### 5.3.1.1 Animal-Based Food

##### 5.3.1.1.1 Meat

Protein is largely responsible for the characteristics of many meat products during manufacturing process and storage. Proteomics offers a powerful tool to identify the specific proteins that may be indicative of alterations in meat quality. Meat quality is a complex trait influenced by genetic components and environmental factors, such as the handling of animals and the slaughter process. Early proteomic analysis characterized postmortem changes in porcine muscle (Lametsch and Bendixen 2001, Lametsch et al. 2002). Several specific peptides resulting from proteolytic activity in meat can serve as good candidates for meat quality markers and further studies of these specific fragments will lead to a better understanding of the proteolytic activities involved in the postmortem conversion of muscle to meat. The influence of postmortem storage time and preslaughter conditions (transport the day before slaughter or immediately before slaughter) on proteome changes of pork meat was also investigated (Morzel et al. 2004).

2-DE maps of tissues from many meat-producing animals have been published, for example, porcine muscles (Lametsch and Bendixen 2001, Lametsch et al. 2002), bovine semitendinosus muscle (Bouley et al. 2004), and layer chicken pectoralis muscle (Doherty et al. 2004). These maps help identify markers for meat quality traits and quality control during meat processing.

Inconsistent tenderness is one of the most detrimental factors of meat quality. 2-DE was used to compare Longissimus sarcoplasmic protein abundance between two groups (tough meat and tender meat) in cooked pork (Laville et al. 2007). Fourteen protein spots differing in quantity ($P < 0.05$) between the two groups were identified, which suggest that the lower post-cooking shear force could at least in part be related to muscle adipogenetic and/or myogenetic status. Functional proteomic analysis was used to predict beef tenderness and its differential (Zapata et al. 2009). Zapata et al. associated electrophoretic bands from the myofibrillar muscle fraction with meat tenderness to explore the mechanisms controlling tenderness. The proteins identified in these bands encompass a wide array of cellular pathways related to structural, metabolic, chaperone, and developmental functions, which may help lead to the establishment of a coherent mechanism accounting for meat tenderness.

Next to tenderness, color development is another organoleptic characteristic responsible for meat quality. 2-DE was used to investigate sarcoplasmic protein expression in pig semimembranosus muscles between 2 groups (light and dark) of 12 pigs (Sayd et al. 2006); 22 proteins or fragments ($P < 0.05$) were differentially expressed. Muscles leading to darker meat had a more oxidative metabolism, indicated by more abundant mitochondrial enzymes of the respiratory chain, hemoglobin, and chaperone or regulator proteins. Conversely, enzymes of glycolysis were overexpressed in the lighter group. This protein pattern is likely to have severe implications on postmortem metabolism, namely, acceleration of ATP depletion and pH fall and subsequent enhanced protein denaturation, well known to induce discoloration.

### 5.3.1.1.2  Seafood

The early application included proteomic analysis of seafood quality (reviewed by Pineiro et al. 2003). Proteomics with multivariate data analysis was applied to analyze protein changes in cod muscle proteins during different storage conditions (Kjaersgard et al. 2006). MALDI-TOF peptide mass fingerprint from arginine kinase tryptic digests was used for the identification of seven commercial, closely related species of Decapoda shrimps (Ortea et al. 2009). It was suggested that MS characterization of species-specific peptides is a good tool for rapid and effective identification and authentication of food, providing and guaranteeing the quality and safety of the foodstuffs to consumers.

*5.3.1.1.3 Milk*

Caseins and whey protein are the major proteins in milk and milk products (Fong et al. 2008). Proteomics has been applied to describe the minor proteins in bovine milk and human colostrum to elucidate their biological role and implications for animal and human health (Palmer et al. 2006, Reinhardt and Lippolis 2006, 2008, Smolenski et al. 2007). Proteomic approaches have also been applied to analyze milk of other species such as donkey, horse, and marsupials (D'Auria et al. 2005, Miranda et al. 2004).

*5.3.1.1.4 Others*

Comparative proteomic analyses of livers were conducted from two different *Bos taurus* breeds: "Chianina and Holstein Friesian" (Timperio et al. 2009). MS identified 39 differentially expressed proteins in 2-DE. Combined with transcriptomics analyses and pathway analysis, it was revealed that Chianina (beef cattle) expressed proteins that focused on metabolic and anabolic pathways, while Holstein Friesian (dairy cattle) increased milk productions at the expenses of thermoregulatory capacity.

Avian eggs are nutritious food and also major sources of biologically active compounds. Proteomics and transcriptomics have been applied to identify and functionally characterize new egg proteins, which may be a source of useful active compounds beneficial for human and animal health (Gautron et al. 2010). These newly identified proteins could be used in marker-assisted genetic selection and breeding.

An exclusive food for the queen honey bee, royal jelly is also widely used in medical products, in cosmetics, and as health food. Comprehensive proteomic analysis of royal jelly reveals novel royal jelly proteins and potential phospho/glycoproteins (Furusawa et al. 2008). Proteomic analysis of major royal jelly protein changes under different storage conditions suggested that MRJP5 protein is a reliable freshness marker and that the best way to maintain quality of royal jelly is under freezing conditions (Li et al. 2008).

### 5.3.1.2 Plant-Based Food

*5.3.1.2.1 Cereals*

Proteomics was widely applied in cereal science. As the main staple food for more than half of the world's population, rice is considered as a model cereal for genetics and molecular studies. Rice anthers proteins at the young microspore stage were identified early by proteome (Imin et al. 2001). Systematic and comparative proteomic analysis of rice leaf, root, and seed tissue revealed ubiquitous proteins and tissue-specific proteins involved in metabolic pathways, indicating the presence of distinct regulatory mechanisms in different tissues (Koller et al. 2002). As the "cornerstone" of cereal proteomes, numerous proteomic studies in rice have been performed during growth and development and against a wide variety of environmental factors, which have been reviewed by Agrawal et al. (2009).

Protein composition and functionality are tightly related with the quality of products derived from wheat. Application of proteome analysis in wheat grain included protein profile of grain and kernels (Amiour et al. 2002, Rathmell et al. 2000), flour quality control (Skylas et al. 2000, Yahata et al. 2005), characterization of heat-responsive proteins (Majoul et al. 2003, 2004) and abiotic stress responsive proteins (Kamal et al. 2010), characterization of gliadin proteins for varietal polymorphisms (Mamone et al. 2005), identification of proteins in aleurone layer (Laubin et al. 2008), and distinguishing durum wheat cultivars for pasta making (De Angelis et al. 2008). Foam-forming soluble proteins from wheat dough were also identified through proteomic methods (Salt et al. 2005). They may play important roles in stabilizing gas bubbles in dough, and thus influence structure of bread.

Barley is a major cereal crop grown mainly for feed and malting. Proteomic analysis in barley have revealed water-soluble seed and malt protein patters (Bak-Jensen et al. 2004) and identified heat-stable proteins possibly involved in the texture of head foams (Perrocheau et al. 2005). Proteomics of barley seed was reviewed recently (Finnie and Svensson 2009).

### 5.3.1.2.2 Fruit and Vegetable

Proteomic studies focusing on understanding the fruit-ripening process have been reported in tomato (Faurobert et al. 2007, Rocco et al. 2006), grape berry (Giribaldi et al. 2007), and some stone fruits (Abdi et al. 2002). Differentially expressed proteomic analysis in placental tissues from nonpungent and pungent peppers during fruit development revealed protein markers related to pungency (Lee et al. 2006). These proteins are involved in a complex biosynthesis network of capsaicinoids in pepper cells. Proteomic approaches enhanced the understanding of phytopathological disorder in fruits. Studies focused on understanding the physiological disorders in tomato fruit affected with blossom-end rot (Casado-Vela et al. 2005), tomato fruit infected with tobacco mosaic virus (Casado-Vela et al. 2006), and peach fruit influenced with antagonist yeast *Pichia membranifaciens* and salicylic acid (Chan et al. 2007). Other studies focused on understanding the physiological changes during the postharvest process in order to further improve the storage processes. Pedreschi and coworkers elucidated the mechanisms of core breakdown disorder in Conference pears by proteomics (Pedreschi et al. 2007, 2008a), and they also assessed the effect of extreme gas conditions (anoxia and air) on pear slices with DIGE (Pedreschi et al. 2009). Lliso et al. studied major protein changes in the albedo of the citrus fruit peel during postharvest ageing through 2-DE. This proteomic survey in matured-on-tree fruits and in fruits stored in nonstressing, cold, and drought conditions indicates that major protein changes in the postharvest stored citrus fruits are apparently related to the activation of programmed cell death (Lliso et al. 2007).

### 5.3.1.2.3 Wine and Beer

In the wine industry, proteomic approaches have been applied to understand grape berry development under different environmental conditions (Giribaldi et al. 2007, Sarry et al. 2004) and to track Champagne wine quality (Cilindre et al. 2008). Metabolite profiles, especially the volatile organic compounds, determine the quality and authenticity of wine (Lund and Bohlmann 2006). However, with the published grape genome (Travis 2008), proteomics provides useful tool for linking wine proteome (grape and yeast derived) with the sensory features of wine to improve wine processing.

The beer proteome has been evaluated recently by different groups to reveal barley proteins and yeast proteins (Fasoli et al. 2010, Iimure et al. 2010). Beer proteome provides a platform for the detection and potential manipulation of beer-quality-related proteins to enrich flavor and texture.

### 5.3.1.2.4 *Organically versus Nonorganically Grown Plants*

Organic crops can be expected to contain fewer agrochemical residues than nonorganically grown alternatives, but whether or not organically grown products are healthier and safer is a matter of debate (Magkos et al. 2006). The increased disease pressure in organically grown plants due to no pesticides can increase the level of antioxidant compounds but also the protective allergenic proteins (Asami et al. 2003, Carbonaro et al. 2002, Vian et al. 2006, Young et al. 2005). Proteomic approach was used to quantify the effects of different farming systems on the protein profiles of potato tubers (Lehesranta et al. 2007). Principal component analysis showed that only fertilization practices (organic matter versus mineral fertilizer based) had a significant effect on protein composition and suggested that organic fertilization leads to an increased stress response in potato tubers.

### 5.3.1.3 Microorganism-Based Food

#### 5.3.1.3.1 *Fermentation*

Proteome and metabolome of cultures in fermentation processes (beer, cheese, sausage, etc.) can be used to predict the quality of the fermented end product. In the fermentation industry, proteomics was combined with enzyme activity assays to analyze metabolic pathway of glycerol fermentation by *Klebsiella pneumoniae* (Wang et al. 2003). Proteomics of milk and bacteria used in fermented dairy products has been reviewed recently (Gagnaire et al. 2009). Based on the reference proteome map of lactic acid bacteria, proteomics can detect the strain-to-strain variations and elucidate the mechanisms of bacterial adaptation to environment *in vitro* and *in vivo* (Gagnaire et al. 2009). Proteomic analysis of bacteria entrapped in cheese revealed the predominant metabolic pathways (Gagnaire et al. 2007, 2009).

#### 5.3.1.3.2 *Probiotics*

Some bacteria colonizing the human gastrointestinal tract have health-promoting properties and can be used as food additives (Salminen and Gueimonde 2004). *Bifidobacteria* and *lactobacilli* are the most popular probiotics added as live bacteria to food. After the proteome maps were obtained in *Bifidobacterium infantis* (Vitali et al. 2005) and *Bifidobacterium longum* NCC2705 (Yuan et al. 2006), investigation was continued to explore the host-inducing proteome changes in *B. longum* NCC2705 grown *in vivo* (Yuan et al. 2008) and stress response in Bifidobacterium (Sanchez et al. 2008). Quantitative proteomics was reported on two *B. longum* strains that differ in heat shock resistance (Guillaume et al. 2009). Proteomic analysis was recently reported on *Lactobacillus casei Zhang*, a new probiotic bacterium isolated from traditional homemade koumiss in Inner Mongolia, China (Wu et al. 2009b).

#### 5.3.1.4 Fungus-Based Food

Mushroom can be defined as a macrofungus with a distinctive fruiting body. Proteomics of two cultivated mushrooms *Sparassis crispa* and *Hericium erinaceum* provides insight into their numerous functional protein components and diversity (Horie et al. 2008).

### 5.3.2 PROTEOMICS IN FOOD SAFETY

The public are more and more aware of and concerned about food safety. Proteomics provides new tools for monitoring food safety related to proteins.

#### 5.3.2.1 Microorganism Contamination

Pathogenic microorganisms and microbial toxins remain a threat to human beings and their monitoring during food manufacturing process is an essential issue. For the most common food poisoning bacteria, like *Staphylococcus aureus*, *Campylobacter jejuni*, some *Salmonella* and *Staphylococcus* spp., some *Bacillus* strains and *Escherichia coli* O157:H7 strain, well-established detection methods are available, mostly immunochemical methods. However, proteomics provides more sensitive and specific methods for the characterization of microbial contaminants and relative toxins (Scott and Cordwell 2009). Applications include MS identification of enterohemorrhagic *E. coli* O157:H7 from ground beef (Ochoa and Harrington 2005); detection, confirmation, and quantification of staphylococcal enterotoxin B in food matrixes using liquid chromatography–mass spectrometry (Callahan et al. 2006); detection and discrimination of *Salmonella* associated with food (Levin 2009). Staphylococcal enterotoxins are major causing agents of food-borne diseases. The combination of immunocapture and protein standard absolute quantification, which uses isotope-labeled enterotoxins as internal standards for MS-based analysis, is powerful in specifically identifying and quantifying these contaminating agents in food matrices. This approach is believed to significantly improve the elucidation of staphylococcal food-poisoning outbreaks (Dupuis et al. 2008). *C. jejuni* is the leading cause of food- and water-borne illness worldwide. Proteomics helps to identify membrane-associated proteins from *C. jejuni* strains (Cordwell et al. 2008), and novel surface polypeptides of *C. jejuni* were discovered by proteomics as traveler's diarrhea vaccine candidates (Prokhorova et al. 2006). Guidelines, challenges, and future perspectives of Campylobacter proteomics were reviewed recently (Scott and Cordwell 2009).

Bacterial communities that are attached to a surface are called biofilms. Their inherent resistances to antimicrobial agents are a cause of many persistent and chronic bacterial infections. In the food industry, the biofilm-forming bacteria can survive on stainless steel surface and resist sanitation cleaning or survive food processing. Recent comparative proteomic studies between biofilm and planktonic mode have identified many proteins differentially expressed during biofilm formation. For example, studies in *Bacillus cereus* (Oosthuizen et al. 2002, Vilain and Brozel 2006), *Listeria monocytogenes* (Tremoulet et al. 2002b), and *E. coli* O157:H7 NCTC 12900 (Tremoulet et al. 2002a) reveal the complexity of this developmental process.

*Staphylococcus xylosus* is a gram-positive bacterium found on the skin of mammals and frequently isolated from food plants and fermented cheese or meat. A comparative proteomic analysis between planktonic and sessile cells revealed novel proteins that could be involved in the exopolysaccharide biosynthetic pathway in biofilms as well as in several enzymes related to polyketide biosynthesis (Planchon et al. 2009).

As the most important target of high hydrostatic pressure (HHP) treatment, proteins of *B. cereus* were analyzed by proteomic analysis through 2D-DIGE (Martnez-Gomariz et al. 2009). Flagellin was the protein that decreased the most. The differential expression of some proteins after HHP may suggest a reduction of virulence and protective response against oxidative stress in flagellated Bacillus.

In summary, in addition to other analyses, proteomic analyses of food-related pathogenic microorganisms give valuable information about their behavior during food processing and help detect and eliminate contamination by these bacteria.

### 5.3.2.2 Prion

Prion diseases are characterized by the infection of an abnormal conformation (PrP[Sc]) of normal cellular protein (PrP[C]) in neural tissues of humans and animals. They cause scrapie in sheep and goats, and bovine spongiform encephalopathy (BSE). Humans get infectious Creutzfeldt–Jakob disease (CJD) after consumption of prion-infected meat or meat products (Knight 2001). The outbreaks of infectious prion diseases have prompted the need for detection and elimination of prion infections as part of the safety control for meat and meat products. Immunoaffinity reactors are suggested for prion protein qualitative analysis (Bilkova et al. 2005). And prion protein binding proteins (Petrakis and Sklaviadis 2006, Strom et al. 2006) and biomarkers for prion infection were identified with the help of proteomics (Giorgi et al. 2009, Steinacker et al. 2010). Proteomic profiling of cerebrospinal fluid (CSF) was developed for the multiple marker diagnostics of prion disease (Herbst et al. 2009). Though extensive studies have been performed, reliable biomarkers for prion infection are still rather limited, and true positive rate was low. Autoantibody to glial fibrillary acidic protein was identified in the sera of cattle with BSE, which might be useful in understanding the pathogenesis and in developing a serological diagnosis of BSE in live cattle (Nomura et al. 2009). Fast and reliable screening methods of prion infection in animals and meat are expected to prevent these kinds of food-borne diseases.

### 5.3.2.3 Allergens

The application of proteomics to study allergenic proteins is referred to as "allerge-nomics" (Monaci and Visconti 2009, Yagami et al. 2004). It is important to detect and monitor allergenic proteins, given that proteins are not only major constituents of foods but also used as food additives. Combining immunoblot of IgE on 2-DE with mass spectrometry, allergenic proteins (IgE-binding antigens) were successfully detected in food of plant origin, such as wheat flour (Akagawa et al. 2007), wheat (Sotkovsky et al. 2008), peanut (Chassaigne et al. 2007, 2009, Piersma et al. 2005, Schmidt et al. 2009, Stevenson et al. 2009), tomato seed (Bassler et al. 2009), maize kernels (Fasoli et al. 2009), and ryegrass pollen (De Canio et al. 2009). Food of animal origin, especially seafood and milk products, can also cause allergies (Lehrer et al. 2003). Allergenic proteins were characterized by mass spectrometry from frog (Taka et al. 2000) and shrimp (Shiomi et al. 2008, Yu et al. 2003). Oxidative modifications of milk protein, for example, carbonylation of beta-lactoglobulin during industrial treatments, tend to increase the natural allergenicity of milk proteins. Immunoblot and tandem mass spectrometry were used to monitor the allergenicity in milk powder (Fenaille et al. 2005). Proteomics also revealed that postharvest storage, like the controlled atmosphere, can alter the amounts of allergenic proteins in apples and pears (Pedreschi et al. 2007, Sancho et al. 2006).

### 5.3.2.4   Genetically Modified Food

Safety of genetically modified organisms (GMO) is one of the concerns of food safety. For GMOs and food derived from GMOs, safety assessment is to determine the intended and unintended effects of transgenes and whether GMOs are substantially equivalent to existing food with long history of safe use. Other than compositional analysis of major nutrients and toxicants, proteomics provide complementary tools to address these questions.

In proteomic comparison of virus-resistant (genetically modified, GM) tomato and its counterpart seedlings, no significant differences, either qualitative or quantitative, were detected, indicating that the expression of major proteins was unmodified by the genetic manipulation (Corpillo et al. 2004). Proteomics was used to compare proteins from conventional and transgenic maize (Erny et al. 2007, Zolla et al. 2008). Recently, proteomic analysis was reported of two GM maize varieties with a near-isogenic non-GM variety in three different locations over three growing seasons (Barros et al. 2010). Together with data from transcriptomics and metabolomics, the authors concluded that environmental factors caused more variation in the different transcript/protein/metabolite profiles than the different genotypes (Barros et al. 2010). Similar conclusion was obtained in transgenic *Arabidopsis* that the transgenic events had a weaker impact on the plants than the environmental stresses (Ren et al. 2009). But comparative proteomics of transgenic and nontransgenic soybean seeds suggested that potential allergen exists in transgenic lines (Brandao et al. 2010).

### 5.3.2.5   Toxin and Plant Lectin

Botulinum neurotoxin (BoNT) causes the disease botulism, which can be lethal if untreated. Rapid determination of exposure to BoNT is an important public health goal. Detection of botulinum neurotoxin A in a spiked milk sample with subtype identification was reported through toxin proteomics (Kalb et al. 2005). Proteomic identification of azaspiracid toxin biomarkers was reported in blue mussels, *Mytilus edulis* (Nzoughet et al. 2009). Four proteins were characterized to be present only in the hepatopancreas of toxin-contaminated mussels, and they share their identity or homology with cathepsin D, superoxide dismutase, glutathione S-transferase Pi, and a bacterial flagellar protein (Nzoughet et al. 2009).

Plant lectins, mostly secretory proteins, for example, Ricin and legume seeds lectins, can cause food poisoning, and consumption of raw or incorrectly processed beans has been shown to cause outbreaks of gastroenteritis, nausea, and diarrhea.

Proteomic approaches were used to study structure, functions, and toxicity of legume seed lectins in either raw or processed foods and have been reviewed recently (Nasi et al. 2009).

### 5.3.2.6 Others

Illicit treatment of livestock with growth-promoting agents, like anabolic steroids, can increase muscle accretion and reduce fat deposition, but they pose great threat on the health of consumers. These chemical agents are difficult to detect by conventional analytical approaches due to the use of synergistic formulations at very low dosage and the use of uncharacterized novel compounds. However, illicit treatment of steroids in cattle can be detected by metabonomics (Dumas et al. 2005) and proteomics (Gardini et al. 2006). Differential expression of adenosine kinase and reticulocalbin in the liver of calves treated with anabolic compound was found (Gardini et al. 2006). Recently a low-mass-range proteomic platform has been developed to detect illicit treatments in bovine serum samples and a polypeptide fragment from beta2-glycoprotein-I was found strongly associated (Della Donna et al. 2009).

Long-time and low-dose administration of antibiotics, mainly tetracycline, has been used as growth promoter in livestock. But systematic use of antibiotic promotes the generation of resistant bacterial population and is banned in the European Union. Effects of tetracycline administration on the proteomic profile of pig muscle samples were demonstrated by proteomics (Gratacos-Cubarsi et al. 2008). They found that although tetracyclines are rapidly eliminated, differentially expressed proteins were detected in tetracycline-treated pigs, which may be used as biomarkers to detect illegal administration of tetracyclines.

## 5.4 CONCLUSION AND PERSPECTIVE

At a time when consumers are demanding healthier and safer foods, proteomics offers us the scientific approach to monitor the quality and safety of food at the protein level. As a powerful tool that can simultaneously analyze several hundred proteins in complex mixtures, proteomics has largely expanded our knowledge of food components and compositions and has been widely applied for quality control and safety assessment in food biotechnology.

Beginning with the identification of protein, proteomics stepped into quantitative analysis (Domon and Aebersold 2010, Elliott et al. 2009), and now it also deals with assessment of modification, three-dimensional structure of proteins, and their interactions (Ebina et al. 2009). Apart from characterizing proteins in the food matrix, proteomics can be applied to study protein–protein interactions in raw and processed foods and also the interactions between proteins and other food components.

So far, genomes of only a few food-related organisms have been completed. Thus, some proteomic approaches have been restricted by the uncertain cross-species protein identifications. The ongoing sequencing projects of a lot of food-related organisms and the rapidly developing sequencing platforms are expected to overcome this obstacle in the near future.

In conclusion, proteomics provides great opportunities for the food industry in quality control, traceability, process optimization, food safety, and nutritional assessment (Pedreschi et al. 2010). Moreover, when proteomics is combined with other OMICS platforms, such as genomics, bioinformatics, transcriptomics, and metabonomics, surely more comprehensive information will be provided. It can be expected that other than helping provide nutrient and safe food, proteomics will help us design better food to enhance human health.

## ACKNOWLEDGMENT

The authors acknowledge the support of the National Natural Science Foundation of China (30800609) and the Fundamental Research Funds for the Central Universities (SCUT 2009ZM0006).

## REFERENCES

Abdi, N., P. Holford, and B. McGlasson. 2002. Application of two-dimensional gel electrophoresis to detect proteins associated with harvest maturity in stonefruit. *Postharvest Biol Technol* 26:1–13.

Agrawal, G. K., N. S. Jwa, and R. Rakwal. 2009. Rice proteomics: Ending phase I and the beginning of phase II. *Proteomics* 9:935–963.

Akagawa, M., T. Handoyo, T. Ishii, S. Kumazawa, N. Morita, and K. Suyama. 2007. Proteomic analysis of wheat flour allergens. *J Agric Food Chem* 55:6863–6870.

Albrecht, D., O. Kniemeyer, A. A. Brakhage, and R. Guthke. 2010. Missing values in gel-based proteomics. *Proteomics* 10:1202–1211.

Amiour, N., M. Merlino, P. Leroy, and G. Branlard. 2002. Proteomic analysis of amphiphilic proteins of hexaploid wheat kernels. *Proteomics* 2:632–641.

Asami, D. K., Y. J. Hong, D. M. Barrett, and A. E. Mitchell. 2003. Comparison of the total phenolic and ascorbic acid content of freeze-dried and air-dried marionberry, strawberry, and corn grown using conventional, organic, and sustainable agricultural practices. *J Agric Food Chem* 51:1237–1241.

Bak-Jensen, K. S., S. Laugesen, P. Roepstorff, and B. Svensson. 2004. Two-dimensional gel electrophoresis pattern (pH 6–11) and identification of water-soluble barley seed and malt proteins by mass spectrometry. *Proteomics* 4:728–742.

Barros, E., S. Lezar, M. J. Anttonen et al. 2010. Comparison of two GM maize varieties with a near-isogenic non-GM variety using transcriptomics, proteomics and metabolomics. *Plant Biotechnol J* 8:436–451.

Bassler, O. Y., J. Weiss, S. Wienkoop et al. 2009. Evidence for novel tomato seed allergens: IgE-reactive legumin and vicilin proteins identified by multidimensional protein fractionation-mass spectrometry and in silico epitope modeling. *J Proteome Res* 8:1111–1122.

Bilkova, Z., A. Castagna, G. Zanusso et al. 2005. Immunoaffinity reactors for prion protein qualitative analysis. *Proteomics* 5:639–647.

Bouley, J., C. Chambon, and B. Picard. 2004. Mapping of bovine skeletal muscle proteins using two-dimensional gel electrophoresis and mass spectrometry. *Proteomics* 4:1811–1814.

Brandao, A. R., H. S. Barbosa, and M. A. Z. Arruda. 2010. Image analysis of two-dimensional gel electrophoresis for comparative proteomics of transgenic and non-transgenic soybean seeds. *J Proteomics* 73:1433–1440.

Bykova, N. V., C. Rampitsch, O. Krokhin, K. G. Standing, and W. Ens. 2006. Determination and characterization of site-specific N-glycosylation using MALDI-Qq-TOF tandem mass spectrometry: Case study with a plant protease. *Anal Chem* 78:1093–1103.

Callahan, J. H., K. J. Shefcheck, T. L. Williams, and S. M. Musser. 2006. Detection, confirmation, and quantification of staphylococcal enterotoxin B in food matrixes using liquid chromatography-mass spectrometry. *Anal Chem* 78:1789–1800.

Carbonaro, M., M. Mattera, S. Nicoli, P. Bergamo, and M. Cappelloni. 2002. Modulation of antioxidant compounds in organic vs conventional fruit (peach, *Prunus persica* L., and pear, *Pyrus communis* L.). *J Agric Food Chem* 50:5458–5462.

Carpentier, S. C., B. Panis, A. Vertommen et al. 2008. Proteome analysis of non-model plants: A challenging but powerful approach. *Mass Spectrom Rev* 27:354–377.

Casado-Vela, J., S. Selles, and R. B. Martinez. 2005. Proteomic approach to blossom-end rot in tomato fruits (*Lycopersicon esculentum* M.): Antioxidant enzymes and the pentose phosphate pathway. *Proteomics* 5:2488–2496.

Casado-Vela, J., S. Selles, and R. B. Martinez. 2006. Proteomic analysis of tobacco mosaic virus-infected tomato (*Lycopersicon esculentum* M.) fruits and detection of viral coat protein. *Proteomics* 1(Suppl. 6):S196–S206.

Chan, Z. L., G. Z. Qin, X. B. Xu, B. Q. Li, and S. P. Tian. 2007. Proteome approach to characterize proteins induced by antagonist yeast and salicylic acid in peach fruit. *J Proteome Res* 6:1677–1688.

Chassaigne, H., J. V. Norgaard, and A. J. van Hengel. 2007. Proteomics-based approach to detect and identify major allergens in processed peanuts by capillary LC-Q-TOF (MS/MS). *J Agric Food Chem* 55:4461–4473.

Chassaigne, H., V. Tregoat, J. V. Norgaard, S. J. Maleki, and A. J. van Hengel. 2009. Resolution and identification of major peanut allergens using a combination of fluorescence two-dimensional differential gel electrophoresis, Western blotting and Q-TOF mass spectrometry. *J Proteomics* 72:511–526.

Chich, J. F., O. David, F. Villers, B. Schaeffer, D. Lutomski, and S. Huet. 2007. Statistics for proteomics: Experimental design and 2-DE differential analysis. *J Chromatogr B* 849:261–272.

Cilindre, C., S. Jegou, A. Hovasse et al. 2008. Proteomic approach to identify champagne wine proteins as modified by *Botrytis cinerea* infection. *J Proteome Res* 7:1199–1208.

Cordwell, S. J., C. L. L. Alice, R. G. Touma et al. 2008. Identification of membrane-associated proteins from *Campylobacter jejuni* strains using complementary proteomics technologies. *Proteomics* 8:122–139.

Corpillo, D., G. Gardini, A. M. Vaira et al. 2004. Proteomics as a tool to improve investigation of substantial equivalence in genetically modified organisms: The case of a virus-resistant tomato. *Proteomics* 4:193–200.

D'Auria, E., C. Agostoni, M. Giovannini et al. 2005. Proteomic evaluation of milk from different mammalian species as a substitute for breast milk. *Acta Paediatr* 94:1708–1713.

De Angelis, M., F. Minervini, L. Caputo et al. 2008. Proteomic analysis by two-dimensional gel electrophoresis and starch characterization of *Triticum turgidum* L. var. durum cultivars for pasta making. *J Agric Food Chem* 56:8619–8628.

De Canio, M., S. D'Aguanno, C. Sacchetti et al. 2009. Novel IgE recognized components of lolium perenne pollen extract: Comparative proteomics evaluation of allergic patients sensitization profiles. *J Proteome Res* 8:4383–4391.

Della Donna, L., M. Ronci, P. Sacchetta et al. 2009. A food safety control low mass-range proteomics platform for the detection of illicit treatments in veal calves by MALDI-TOF-MS serum profiling. *Biotechnol J* 4:1596–1609.

Doherty, M. K., L. McLean, J. R. Hayter et al. 2004. The proteome of chicken skeletal muscle: Changes in soluble protein expression during growth in a layer strain. *Proteomics* 4:2082–2093.

Domon, B. and R. Aebersold. 2010. Options and considerations when selecting a quantitative proteomics strategy. *Nat Biotechnol* 28:710–721.

Dumas, M. E., C. Canlet, J. Vercauteren, F. Andre, and A. Paris. 2005. Homeostatic signature of anabolic steroids in cattle using H-1-C-13 HMBC NMR metabonomics. *J Proteome Res* 4:1493–1502.

Dupuis, A., J. A. Hennekinne, J. Garin, and V. Brun. 2008. Protein standard absolute quantification (PSAQ) for improved investigation of staphylococcal food poisoning outbreaks. *Proteomics* 8:4633–4636.

Ebina, T., H. Toh, and Y. Kuroda. 2009. Loop-length-dependent SVM prediction of domain linkers for high-throughput structural proteomics. *Biopolymers* 92:1–8.

Elliott, M. H., D. S. Smith, C. E. Parker, and C. Borchers. 2009. Current trends in quantitative proteomics. *J Mass Spectrom* 44:1637–1660.

Erny, G. L., M. L. Marina, and A. Cifuentes. 2007. CE-MS of zein proteins from conventional and transgenic maize. *Electrophoresis* 28:4192–4201.

Fasoli, E., G. Aldini, L. Regazzoni, A. V. Kravchuk, A. Citterio, and P. G. Righetti. 2010. Les Maitres de l'Orge: The proteome content of your beer mug. *J Proteome Res* 9:5262–5269.

Fasoli, E., E. A. Pastorello, L. Farioli et al. 2009. Searching for allergens in maize kernels via proteomic tools. *J Proteomics* 72:501–510.

Faurobert, M., C. Mihr, N. Bertin et al. 2007. Major proteome variations associated with cherry tomato pericarp development and ripening. *Plant Physiol* 143:1327–1346.

Fenaille, F., V. Parisod, J. C. Tabet, and P. A. Guy. 2005. Carbonylation of milk powder proteins as a consequence of processing conditions. *Proteomics* 5:3097–3104.

Fenn, J. B., M. Mann, C. K. Meng, S. F. Wong, and C. M. Whitehouse. 1989. Electrospray ionization for mass-spectrometry of large biomolecules. *Science* 246:64–71.

Finnie, C. and B. Svensson. 2009. Barley seed proteomics from spots to structures. *J Proteomics* 72:315–324.

Fong, B. Y., C. S. Norris, and K. P. Palmano. 2008. Fractionation of bovine whey proteins and characterisation by proteomic techniques. *Int Dairy J* 18:23–46.

Furusawa, T., R. Rakwal, H. W. Nam et al. 2008. Comprehensive royal jelly (RJ) proteomics using one- and two-dimensional proteomics platforms reveals novel RJ proteins and potential phospho/glycoproteins. *J Proteome Res* 7:3194–3229.

Gagnaire, V., J. Jardin, G. Jan, and S. Lortal. 2009. Invited review: Proteomics of milk and bacteria used in fermented dairy products: From qualitative to quantitative advances. *J Dairy Sci* 92:811–825.

Gagnaire, V., D. Molle, J. Jardin, and S. Lortal. 2007. Quantitative proteomic analysis of bacterial enzymes released in cheese during ripening. *J Dairy Sci* 90:630–640.

Gardini, G., P. Del Boccio, S. Colombatto et al. 2006. Proteomic investigation in the detection of the illicit treatment of calves with growth-promoting agents. *Proteomics* 6:2813–2822.

Gautron, J., S. Rehault-Godbert, V. Jonchere, V. Herve-Grepinet, K. Mann, and Y. Nys. 2010. High-throughput technology (proteomics and transcriptomics) to identify and functionally characterise new egg proteins. *Prod Anim* 23:133–141.

Giorgi, A., L. Di Francesco, S. Principe et al. 2009. Proteomic profiling of PrP27–30-enriched preparations extracted from the brain of hamsters with experimental scrapie. *Proteomics* 9:3802–3814.

Giribaldi, M., L. Perugini, F. X. Sauvage, and A. Schubert. 2007. Analysis of protein changes during grape berry ripening by 2-DE and MALDI-TOF. *Proteomics* 7:3154–3170.

Gratacos-Cubarsi, M., M. Castellari, M. Hortos, J. A. Garcia-Regueiro, R. Lametsch, and F. Jessen. 2008. Effects of tetracycline administration on the proteomic profile of pig muscle samples (L. *dorsi*). *J Agric Food Chem* 56:9312–9316.

Guillaume, E., B. Berger, M. Affolter, and M. Kussmann. 2009. Label-free quantitative proteomics of two *Bifidobacterium longum* strains. *J Proteomics* 72:771–784.

Gygi, S. P., B. Rist, S. A. Gerber, F. Turecek, M. H. Gelb, and R. Aebersold. 1999. Quantitative analysis of complex protein mixtures using isotope-coded affinity tags. *Nat Biotechnol* 17:994–999.

Herbst, A., S. McIlwain, J. J. Schmidt, J. M. Aiken, C. D. Page, and L. J. Li. 2009. Prion disease diagnosis by proteomic profiling. *J Proteome Res* 8:1030–1036.

Ho, E., A. Hayen, and M. R. Wilkins. 2006. Characterisation of organellar proteornes: A guide to subcellular proteomic fractionation and analysis. *Proteomics* 6:5746–5757.

Holland, J. W., H. C. Deeth, and P. F. Alewood. 2005. Analysis of O-glycosylation site occupancy in bovine kappa-casein glycoforms separated by two-dimensional gel electrophoresis. *Proteomics* 5:990–1002.

Horgan, G. W. 2007. Sample size and replication in 2D gel electrophoresis studies. *J Proteome Res* 6:2884–2887.

Horie, K., R. Rakwal, M. Hirano et al. 2008. Proteomics of two cultivated mushrooms *Sparassis crispa* and *Hericium erinaceum* provides insight into their numerous functional protein components and diversity. *J Proteome Res* 7:1819–1835.

Iimure, T., N. Nankaku, N. Hirota et al. 2010. Construction of a novel beer proteome map and its use in beer quality control. *Food Chem* 118:566–574.

Imin, N., T. Kerim, J. J. Weinman, and B. G. Rolfe. 2001. Characterisation of rice anther proteins expressed at the young microspore stage. *Proteomics* 1:1149–1161.

Kalb, S. R., M. C. Goodnough, C. J. Malizio, J. L. Pirkle, and J. R. Barr. 2005. Detection of botulinum neurotoxin A in a spiked milk sample with subtype identification through toxin proteomics. *Anal Chem* 77:6140–6146.

Kamal, A. H. M., K. H. Kim, K. H. Shin et al. 2010. Abiotic stress responsive proteins of wheat grain determined using proteomics technique. *Aust J Crop Sci* 4:196–208.

Karas, M. and F. Hillenkamp. 1988. Laser desorption ionization of proteins with molecular masses exceeding 10000 Daltons. *Anal Chem* 60:2299–2301.

Kjaersgard, I. V. H., M. R. Norrelykke, and F. Jessen. 2006. Changes in cod muscle proteins during frozen storage revealed by proteome analysis and multivariate data analysis. *Proteomics* 6:1606–1618.

Knight, R. 2001. Creutzfeldt-Jakob disease: A protein disease. *Proteomics* 1:763–766.

Koller, A., M. P. Washburn, B. M. Lange et al. 2002. Proteomic survey of metabolic pathways in rice. *Proc Natl Acad Sci USA* 99:11969–11974.

Lametsch, R. and E. Bendixen. 2001. Proteome analysis applied to meat science: Characterizing post mortem changes in porcine muscle. *J Agric Food Chem* 49:4531–4537.

Lametsch, R., P. Roepstorff, and E. Bendixen. 2002. Identification of protein degradation during post-mortem storage of pig meat. *J Agric Food Chem* 50:5508–5512.

Lane, C. S. 2005. Mass spectrometry-based proteomics in the life sciences. *Cell Mol Life Sci* 62:848–869.

Laubin, B., V. Lullien-Pellerin, I. Nadaud, B. Gaillard-Martinie, C. Chambon, and G. Branlard. 2008. Isolation of the wheat aleurone layer for 2D electrophoresis and proteomics analysis. *J Cereal Sci* 48:709–714.

Laville, E., T. Sayd, C. Terlouw et al. 2007. Comparison of sarcoplasmic proteomes between two groups of pig muscles selected for shear force of cooked meat. *J Agric Food Chem* 55:5834–5841.

Lee, J. M., S. Kim, J. Y. Lee et al. 2006. A differentially expressed proteomic analysis in placental tissues in relation to pungency during the pepper fruit development. *Proteomics* 6:5248–5259.

Lehesranta, S. J., K. M. Koistinen, N. Massat et al. 2007. Effects of agricultural production systems and their components on protein profiles of potato tubers. *Proteomics* 7:597–604.

Lehrer, S. B., R. Ayuso, and G. Reese. 2003. Seafood allergy and allergens: A review. *Mar Biotechnol* 5:339–348.

Levin, R. E. 2009. The use of molecular methods for detecting and discriminating salmonella associated with foods—A review. *Food Biotechnol* 23:313–367.

Li, J. K., M. Feng, L. Zhang, Z. H. Zhang, and Y. H. Pan. 2008. Proteomics analysis of major royal jelly protein changes under different storage conditions. *J Proteome Res* 7:3339–3353.

Lliso, I., F. R. Tadeo, B. S. Phinney, C. G. Wilkerson, and M. Talon. 2007. Protein changes in the albedo of citrus fruits on postharvesting storage. *J Agric Food Chem* 55:9047–9053.

Lund, S. T. and J. Bohlmann. 2006. The molecular basis for wine grape quality—A volatile subject. *Science* 311:804–805.

Magkos, F., F. Arvaniti, and A. Zampelas. 2006. Organic food: Buying more safety or just peace of mind? A critical review of the literature. *Crit Rev Food Sci* 46:23–56.

Majoul, T., E. Bancel, E. Triboi, J. Ben Hamida, and G. Branlard. 2003. Proteomic analysis of the effect of heat stress on hexaploid wheat grain: Characterization of heat-responsive proteins from total endosperm. *Proteomics* 3:175–183.

Majoul, T., E. Bancel, E. Triboi, J. Ben Hamida, and G. Branlard. 2004. Proteomic analysis of the effect of heat stress on hexaploid wheat grain: Characterization of heat-responsive proteins from non-prolamins fraction. *Proteomics* 4:505–513.

Mamone, G., F. Addeo, L. Chianese et al. 2005. Characterization of wheat gliadin proteins by combined two-dimensional gel electrophoresis and tandem mass spectrometry. *Proteomics* 5:2859–2865.

Martnez-Gomariz, M., M. L. Hernaez, D. Gutierrez, P. Ximenez-Embun, and G. Prestamo. 2009. Proteomic analysis by two-dimensional differential gel electrophoresis (2D DIGE) of a high-pressure effect in *Bacillus cereus*. *J Agric Food Chem* 57:3543–3549.

Miller, I., J. Crawford, and E. Gianazza. 2006. Protein stains for proteornic applications: Which, when, why? *Proteomics* 6:5385–5408.

Miranda, G., M. F. Mahe, C. Leroux, and P. Martin. 2004. Proteomic tools to characterize the protein fraction of Equidae milk. *Proteomics* 4:2496–2509.

Monaci, L. and A. Visconti. 2009. Mass spectrometry-based proteomics methods for analysis of food allergens. *Trac-Trends Anal Chem* 28:581–591.

Morzel, M., C. Chambon, M. Hamelin, V. Sante-Lhoutellier, T. Sayd, and G. Monin. 2004. Proteome changes during pork meat ageing following use of two different pre-slaughter handling procedures. *Meat Sci* 67:689–696.

Nasi, A., G. Picariello, and P. Ferranti. 2009. Proteomic approaches to study structure, functions and toxicity of legume seeds lectins. Perspectives for the assessment of food quality and safety. *J Proteomics* 72:527–538.

Nomura, S., T. Miyasho, N. Maeda, K. Doh-ura, and H. Yokota. 2009. Autoantibody to glial fibrillary acidic protein in the sera of cattle with bovine spongiform encephalopathy. *Proteomics* 9:4029–4035.

Nzoughet, J. K., J. T. G. Hamilton, C. H. Botting et al. 2009. Proteomics identification of azaspiracid toxin biomarkers in blue mussels, *Mytilus edulis*. *Mol Cell Proteomics* 8:1811–1822.

Ochoa, M. L. and P. B. Harrington. 2005. Immunomagnetic isolation of enterohemorrhagic *Escherichia coli* O157: H7 from ground beef and identification by matrix-assisted laser desorption/ionization time-of-flight mass spectrometry and database searches. *Anal Chem* 77:5258–5267.

Ofarrell, P. Z., H. M. Goodman, and P. H. Ofarrell. 1977. High-resolution 2-dimensional electrophoresis of basic as well as acidic proteins. *Cell* 12:1133–1141.

Ong, S. E., B. Blagoev, I. Kratchmarova et al. 2002. Stable isotope labeling by amino acids in cell culture, SILAC, as a simple and accurate approach to expression proteomics. *Mol Cell Proteomics* 1:376–386.

Oosthuizen, M. C., B. Steyn, J. Theron et al. 2002. Proteomic analysis reveals differential protein expression by *Bacillus cereus* during biofilm formation. *Appl Environ Microb* 68:2770–2780.

Ortea, I., B. Canas, and J. M. Gallardo. 2009. Mass spectrometry characterization of species-specific peptides from arginine kinase for the identification of commercially relevant shrimp species. *J Proteome Res* 8:5356–5362.

Palmer, D. J., V. C. Kelly, A. M. Smit, S. Kuy, C. G. Knight, and G. J. Cooper. 2006. Human colostrum: Identification of minor proteins in the aqueous phase by proteomics. *Proteomics* 6:2208–2216.

Pedreschi, R., M. L. A. T. M. Hertog, S. C. Carpentier et al. 2008b. Treatment of missing values for multivariate statistical analysis of gel-based proteomics data. *Proteomics* 8:1371–1383.

Pedreschi, R., M. Hertog, K. S. Lilley, and B. Nicolai. 2010. Proteomics for the food industry: Opportunities and challenges. *Crit Rev Food Sci* 50:680–692.

Pedreschi, R., M. Hertog, J. Robben et al. 2009. Gel-based proteomics approach to the study of metabolic changes in pear tissue during storage. *J Agric Food Chem* 57:6997–7004.

Pedreschi, R., M. Hertog, J. Robben, J. P. Noben, and B. Nicolai. 2008a. Physiological implications of controlled atmosphere storage of 'Conference' pears (*Pyrus communis* L.): A proteomic approach. *Postharvest Biol Technol* 50:110–116.

Pedreschi, R., E. Vanstreels, S. Carpentier et al. 2007. Proteomic analysis of core breakdown disorder in Conference pears (*Pyrus communis* L.). *Proteomics* 7:2083–2099.

Perrocheau, L., H. Rogniaux, P. Boivin, and D. Marion. 2005. Probing heat-stable water-soluble proteins from barley to malt and beer. *Proteomics* 5:2849–2858.

Petrakis, S. and T. Sklaviadis. 2006. Identification of proteins with high affinity for refolded and native PrPC. *Proteomics* 6:6476–6484.

Piersma, S. R., M. Gaspari, S. L. Hefle, and S. J. Koppelman. 2005. Proteolytic processing of the peanut allergen Ara h 3. *Mol Nutr Food Res* 49:744–755.

Pineiro, C., J. Barros-Velazquez, J. Vazquez, A. Figueras, and J. M. Gallardo. 2003. Proteomics as a tool for the investigation of seafood and other marine products. *J Proteome Res* 2:127–135.

Planchon, S., M. Desvaux, I. Chafsey et al. 2009. Comparative subproteome analyses of planktonic and sessile *Staphylococcus xylosus* C2a: New insight in cell physiology of a coagulase-negative *Staphylococcus* in biofilm. *J Proteome Res* 8:1797–1809.

Prokhorova, T. A., P. N. Nielsen, J. Petersen et al. 2006. Novel surface polypeptides of *Campylobacter jejuni* as traveller's diarrhoea vaccine candidates discovered by proteomics. *Vaccine* 24:6446–6455.

Rathmell, W. G., D. J. Skylas, F. Bekes, and C. W. Wrigley. 2000. Wheat-grain proteomics: The full compliment of proteins in developing and mature grain. *R Soc Chem* 548:117–121.

Reinhardt, T. A. and J. D. Lippolis. 2006. Bovine milk fat globule membrane proteome. *J Dairy Res* 73:406–416.

Reinhardt, T. A. and J. D. Lippolis. 2008. Developmental changes in the milk fat globule membrane proteome during the transition from colostrum to milk. *J Dairy Sci* 91:2307–2318.

Ren, Y. F., J. Lv, H. Wang, L. C. Li, Y. F. Peng, and L. J. Qu. 2009. A comparative proteomics approach to detect unintended effects in transgenic *Arabidopsis*. *J Genet Genomics* 36:629–639.

Rocco, M., C. D'Ambrosio, S. Arena, M. Faurobert, A. Scaloni, and M. Marra. 2006. Proteomic analysis of tomato fruits from two ecotypes during ripening. *Proteomics* 6:3781–3791.

Roe, M. R. and T. J. Griffin. 2006. Gel-free mass spectrometry-based high throughput proteomics: Tools for studying biological response of proteins and proteomes. *Proteomics* 6:4678–4687.

Ross, P. L., Y. L. N. Huang, J. N. Marchese et al. 2004. Multiplexed protein quantitation in *Saccharomyces cerevisiae* using amine-reactive isobaric tagging reagents. *Mol Cell Proteomics* 3:1154–1169.

Salminen, S. and M. Gueimonde. 2004. Human studies on probiotics: What is scientifically proven. *J Food Sci* 69:M137–M140.

Salt, L. J., J. A. Robertson, J. A. Jenkins, F. Mulholland, and E. N. C. Mills. 2005. The identification of foam-forming soluble proteins from wheat (*Triticum aestivum*) dough. *Proteomics* 5:1612–1623.

Sanchez, B., L. Ruiz, C. G. de los Reyes-Gavilan, and A. Margolles. 2008. Proteomics of stress response in Bifidobacterium. *Front Biosci* 13:6905–6919.

Sancho, A. I., R. Foxall, T. Browne et al. 2006. Effect of postharvest storage on the expression of the apple allergen Mal d 1. *J Agric Food Chem* 54:5917–5923.

Sarry, J. E., N. Sommerer, F. X. Sauvage et al. 2004. Grape berry biochemistry revisited upon proteomic analysis of the mesocarp. *Proteomics* 4:201–215.

Sayd, T., M. Morzel, C. Chambon et al. 2006. Proteome analysis of the sarcoplasmic fraction of pig semimembranosus muscle: Implications on meat color development. *J Agric Food Chem* 54:2732–2737.

Schmid, D. G., F. von der Mulbe, B. Fleckenstein, T. Weinschenk, and G. Jung. 2001. Broadband detection electrospray ionization Fourier transform ion cyclotron resonance mass spectrometry to reveal enzymatically and chemically induced deamidation reactions within peptides. *Anal Chem* 73:6008–6013.

Schmidt, H., C. Gelhaus, T. Latendorf et al. 2009. 2-D DIGE analysis of the proteome of extracts from peanut variants reveals striking differences in major allergen contents. *Proteomics* 9:3507–3521.

Scott, N. E. and S. J. Cordwell. 2009. Campylobacter proteomics: Guidelines, challenges and future perspectives. *Expert Rev Proteomic* 6:61–74.

Shiomi, K., Y. Sato, S. Hamamoto, H. Mita, and K. Shimakura. 2008. Sarcoplasmic calcium-binding protein: Identification as a new allergen of the black tiger shrimp *Penaeus monodon*. *Int Arch Allergy Immunol* 146:91–98.

Skylas, D. J., J. A. Mackintosh, S. J. Cordwell et al. 2000. Proteome approach to the characterisation of protein composition in the developing and mature wheat-grain endosperm. *J Cereal Sci* 32:169–188.

Smolenski, G., S. Haines, F. Y. S. Kwan et al. 2007. Characterisation of host defence proteins in milk using a proteomic approach. *J Proteome Res* 6:207–215.

Sotkovsky, P., M. Hubalek, L. Hernychova et al. 2008. Proteomic analysis of wheat proteins recognized by IgE antibodies of allergic patients. *Proteomics* 8:1677–1691.

Steinacker, P., W. Rist, M. Swiatek-de-Lange et al. 2010. Ubiquitin as potential cerebrospinal fluid marker of Creutzfeldt-Jakob disease. *Proteomics* 10:81–89.

Stevenson, S. E., Y. Chu, P. Ozias-Akins, and J. J. Thelen. 2009. Validation of gel-free, label-free quantitative proteomics approaches: Applications for seed allergen profiling. *J Proteomics* 72:555–566.

Strom, A., S. Diecke, G. Hunsmann, and A. W. Stuke. 2006. Identification of prion protein binding proteins by combined use of far-Western immunoblotting, two dimensional gel electrophoresis and mass spectrometry. *Proteomics* 6:26–34.

Taka, H., N. Kaga, T. Fujimura et al. 2000. Rapid determination of parvalbumin amino acid sequence from Rana catesbeiana (pI 4.78) by combination of ESI mass spectrometry, protein sequencing, and amino acid analysis. *J Biochem-Tokyo* 127:723–729.

Timperio, A. M., A. D'Alessandro, L. Pariset, G. M. D'Amici, A. Valentini, and L. Zolla. 2009. Comparative proteomics and transcriptomics analyses of livers from two different *Bos taurus* breeds: "Chianina and Holstein Friesian". *J Proteomics* 73:309–322.

Travis, J. 2008. Uncorking the grape genome. *Science* 320:475–477.

Tremoulet, F., O. Duche, A. Namane et al. 2002b. Comparison of protein patterns of listeria monocytogenes grown in biofilm or in planktonic mode by proteomic analysis. *Fems Microbiol Lett* 210:25–31.

Tremoulet, F., O. Duche, A. Namane, B. Martinie, and J. C. Labadie. 2002a. A proteomic study of *Escherichia coli* O157: H7 NCTC 12900 cultivated in biofilm or in planktonic growth mode. *Fems Microbiol Lett* 215:7–14.

Unlu, M., M. E. Morgan, and J. S. Minden. 1997. Difference gel electrophoresis: A single gel method for detecting changes in protein extracts. *Electrophoresis* 18:2071–2077.

Vian, M. A., V. Tomao, P. O. Coulomb, J. M. Lacombe, and O. Dangles. 2006. Comparison of the anthocyanin composition during ripening of Syrah grapes grown using organic or conventional agricultural practices. *J Agric Food Chem* 54:5230–5235.

Vilain, S. and V. S. Brozel. 2006. Multivariate approach to comparing whole-cell proteomes of *Bacillus cereus* indicates a biofilm-specific proteome. *J Proteome Res* 5:1924–1930.

Vitali, B., V. Wasinger, P. Brigidi, and M. Guilhaus. 2005. A proteomic view of *Bifidobacterium infantis* generated by multi-dimensional chromatography coupled with tandem mass spectrometry. *Proteomics* 5:1859–1867.

Wang, W., J. B. Sun, M. Hartlep, W. D. Deckwer, and A. P. Zeng. 2003. Combined use of proteomic analysis and enzyme activity assays for metabolic pathway analysis of glycerol fermentation by *Klebsiella pneumoniae*. *Biotechnol Bioeng* 83:525–536.

Washburn, M. P., D. Wolters, and J. R. Yates. 2001. Large-scale analysis of the yeast proteome by multidimensional protein identification technology. *Nat Biotechnol* 19:242–247.

Wu, S. L., H. T. Jiang, Q. Z. Lu, S. J. Dai, W. S. Hancock, and B. L. Karger. 2009a. Mass spectrometric determination of disulfide linkages in recombinant therapeutic proteins using online LC-MS with electron-transfer dissociation. *Anal Chem* 81:112–122.

Wu, R., W. Wang, D. Yu et al. 2009b. Proteomics analysis of *Lactobacillus casei* Zhang, a new probiotic bacterium isolated from traditional home-made koumiss in inner Mongolia of China. *Mol Cell Proteomics* 8:2321–2338.

Yagami, T., Y. Haishima, T. Tsuchiya, A. Tomitaka-Yagami, H. Kano, and K. Matsunaga. 2004. Proteomic analysis of putative latex allergens. *Int Arch Allergy Immunol* 135:3–11.

Yahata, E., W. Maruyama-Funatsuki, Z. Nishio et al. 2005. Wheat cultivar-specific proteins in grain revealed by 2-DE and their application to cultivar identification of flour. *Proteomics* 5:3942–3953.

Young, J. E., X. Zhao, E. E. Carey, R. Welti, S. S. Yang, and W. Q. Wang. 2005. Phytochemical phenolics in organically grown vegetables. *Mol Nutr Food Res* 49:1136–1142.

Yu, C. J., Y. F. Lin, B. L. Chiang, and L. P. Chow. 2003. Proteomics and immunological analysis of a novel shrimp allergen, Pen m 2. *J Immunol* 170:445–453.

Yuan, J., B. Wang, Z. K. Sun et al. 2008. Analysis of host-inducing proteome changes in *Bifidobacterium longum* NCC2705 grown in vivo. *J Proteome Res* 7:375–385.

Yuan, J., L. Zhu, X. K. Liu et al. 2006. A proteome reference map and proteomic analysis of *Bifidobacterium longum* NCC2705. *Mol Cell Proteomics* 5:1105–1118.

Zapata, I., H. N. Zerby, and M. Wick. 2009. Functional proteomic analysis predicts beef tenderness and the tenderness differential. *J Agric Food Chem* 57:4956–4963.

Zolla, L., S. Rinalducci, P. Antonioli, and P. G. Righetti. 2008. Proteomics as a complementary tool for identifying unintended side effects occurring in transgenic maize seeds as a result of genetic modifications. *J Proteome Res* 7:1850–1861.

# 6 Challenges in Feasible Problem Construction in Nutritional Genomics
## An Empirical Study*

*Bart Penders, Klasien Horstman, and Rein Vos*

## CONTENTS

## 6.1 INTRODUCTION

Scientists need to know what lunch consists of, what *defines* a lunch […]. Some of us are exploring the intricacies of lunch, reducing it to our intellectually preferred level of understanding. The physical biochemistry of toasting […]; the physiology of water homeostasis in lettuce, and how to keep it from wilting; the molecular biology of casein digestion by bacteria […]; and innumerable studies on pastrami and its relatives. This is, in short, why science is so hard. We ask so many hard questions, at so many different levels. [Now] look how many people have contributed to our study of lunch, and none of them comes up on a PubMed search for "lunch" (Mole 2004).

---

* This chapter is a reworked and extended version of Penders et al. (2009a). Elements from the original publication are reproduced with permission by *Interdisciplinary Science Reviews* and Maney Publishing (see http://www.maney.co.uk/journals/isr).

Whether it is food or "lunch," global warming, cancer, and sustainable energy, the majority of societal problems of today are studied by very diverse groups of scientists. Scientists of diverse plumage work together in large organizations or consortia of scientists, policymakers, industry representatives, and sometimes even ethicists and social scientists to prioritize and address research questions. This trend toward large-scale cooperation in science has been addressed in the literature dealing with the "New Production of Knowledge" and in the literature dealing with the "Triple Helix of Science-Government-Industry," for instance (see, e.g., Etzkowitz and Leydesdorff 1998, Gibbons et al. 1994, Hessels and van Lente 2008, Nowotny et al. 2001, 2003). The large-scale cooperation between different scientists is stimulated because of the idea that it contributes to the solving of complex research problems and therefore to various identified normative goals of science—be it a cure against a disease or the construction of a desired tool or technology to solve a social problem. However, Science and Technology Studies have taught that problem solving as well as cooperation is very hard and takes a lot of work (Latour 1987, Latour and Woolgar 1986). Therefore, solving a problem together can surely be considered an immense task. In this chapter, we will explore the idea that large-scale, multisited, interdisciplinary scientific cooperation helps to achieve a certain goal, in this case the promotion of population health. This exploration will lead us to a counter-intuitive conclusion, namely, that this cooperative work leads to different practices of establishing health. To that purpose we will present the field of nutrigenomics as an empirical example.

The work scientists do, whether in solitude or in cooperative initiatives, and the knowledge they construct, is riddled with norms or standards. This work is about establishing technical norms, such as threshold values in measurements or statistics, but also about setting moral norms on what constitutes "proper" scientific practice, "proper" content, or "proper" scientific behavior. Scientists use these norms, but they also set them, by means of new technical standards or new machines in which norms are embedded. In nutrition science, and in particular nutrigenomics, the combination of nutrition science with genetics, multiple norms can be identified. We will focus on the two most prominent ones: *health* and *personalization*. In the case of nutrition science, these norms are clearly visible in the stated goals of the field: *normative goals*. Namely, nutrition scientists work together to solve health problems both on a personal and a population level (Kaput 2008, Müller and Kersten 2003). Personal health and population health are related, since each individual's personal health contributes to population health and vice versa. Nutrigenomics is, as most practices, a heterogeneous practice. The balance between personal and public health approaches may vary from program to program and from lab to lab. It must be noted though, that overall, public health, that is, the improvement of population health, is identified as the major political goal in societal contextualization of the research programs (e.g., NuGO 2003), as well as articles by nutrigenomicists (Lampe 2006), and those who have commented upon the practice (Bergmann et al. 2008). Making populations healthier with the help of nutrigenomics is about understanding how diet influences widespread, complex, and chronic conditions, including but not restricted to Alzheimer's, diabetes, metabolic syndrome, and for instance, Crohn's disease. Nevertheless, excursions toward personal diets are occasionally undertaken and we will not ignore them in this chapter.

We will demonstrate how a normative goal, such as health in the case of nutrigenomics, is subject to change as the research process proceeds. As argued earlier, norms are set by scientists while they do research. When research goals contain such norms, they too are subject to change. We will show how this change arises as a result of solving research problems in terms of "making research problems doable." To this end, our chapter will consist of three sections. First, we will start developing a conceptual framework to deal with large-scale problem solving in research practices. We will use the notion of "doability," introduced by Joan Fujimura as a conceptual tool to understand problem solving strategies in science (Fujimura 1987, 1992, 1996). We will amend this notion in four specific ways in order to facilitate the analysis of contemporary large-scale, multisited, and interdisciplinary ways of science. Second, we will demonstrate the merits of this conceptual framework by providing an empirical account of problem solving in the large-scale, multisited, and interdisciplinary research practice of nutrigenomics. What exactly nutrigenomics entails, will be introduced in more detail at the beginning of this section of the chapter. Third, and finally, we will discuss the normative effects of this way of problem solving: what kinds of norms regarding health are produced while making research problems doable and how do these changing norms affect the goal of nutrigenomics, which is to improve population health.

## 6.2    FROM DOABLE TASKS TO DOABLE NETWORKS

In her widely acknowledged study on how the protooncogene theory became a widely accepted research problem, Joan Fujimura developed the concept of "doability" (Fujimura 1987) to grasp the particular quality assigned to research problems by scientists. She developed doability into a theoretical frame for explaining and understanding decisions on all levels of scientific practice. Fujimura's concept encompasses the levels of experiment and bench work, all the way to acquiring funds and societal support. Scientists can only spend resources, personal, intellectual, and tangible, on problems that are perceived to be doable or that have the potential of becoming doable. This approach can be considered the scientific parallel to the strategic rule of engagement Sun Tzu left us in "The Art of War": "Thus it is in war the victorious strategist only seeks battle after the victory has been won," which can be rephrased into: "Thus it is in science the successful researcher only engages a problem after it is considered doable" (Giles 1910 [2005]).

Fujimura uses a scheme in her 1987 paper to explain how she conceptualizes doability. She distinguishes three levels of "work" to be done by scientists: work on the experimental level, the laboratory level, and the social world level. In order for a research problem to be doable, all three levels need to be aligned so that tasks belonging to each of them can relate to one another (Figure 6.1)

Although understanding laboratory practices in terms of doability has motivated many studies (Eriksson and Webster 2008, Palmer 2006), Fujimura has been criticized of not living up to the promise she made in developing the model mentioned earlier (Löwy 1998, Palladino 1998). The critique says that she focused on the laboratory at the expense of other sites of scientific practice and trimmed the notion of doability of much of its value for the analysis of contemporary scientific practice. We will nonetheless show that the groundwork Fujimura has invested in "doability" can be taken beyond a single laboratory up to a level of large-scale research work, incorporating

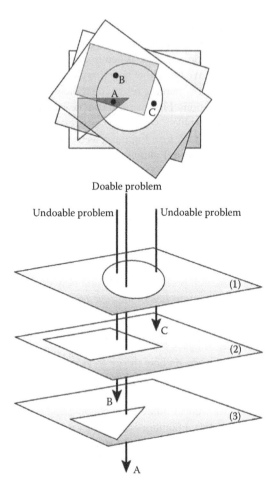

**FIGURE 6.1** Doability as alignment. Doability is the situation in which all the actors and elements in the research situation are aligned. The act of pursuing doability and rearticulating the elements in the research situation to reach alignment can be conceptualized as shuffling and manipulating three layers filled with tasks, until tasks on every level exist in vertical alignment and the doable problem, visualized as an arrow, can traverse all layers. The arrow representing the doable research problem is able to traverse tasks on all three layers of organization, whereas arrow representing the "undoable" problem cannot. The three layers are distinct from one another, but their vertical organization has no direct hierarchical meaning. (1) Social world, (2) laboratory, and (3) experiment; A–C: research problems. Bottom: side view; top: vertical view. (Redrawn from Fujimura, J.H., *Soc. Stud. Sci.*, 17, 257, 1987.)

various laboratories in many disciplines, as well as multiple sites of scientific practice such as conference and meeting rooms, committee meetings, expert panels, lecture halls, and desks. Therefore, we will introduce four additions to the work of Fujimura. First, we will extend the notion of research tasks to include all elements in the research situation, a Latourian twist to Fujimura's model, shifting from tasks to networks containing a heterogeneous composition of elements—ranging from computers and apparatus to cell lines and secretaries. The second addition is a shift from a single laboratory to multiple laboratories, enabling the large-scale character of contemporary science to be taken into account. The third addition is to pay attention to the existence of laboratories in different social words. That is, the various styles of science enable us to cope with the different disciplinary characters of these laboratories. Finally, the fourth addition aims to include other research sites than laboratories, since conferences, meetings, lectures, special issues, etc., are equally part of a research practice.

### 6.2.1 Toward a Network of Local Doabilities

To shift from tasks to networks, means aligning next to tasks also actors and artifacts such as chemicals, reagents, apparatus, and protocols. For instance, performing a PCR reaction (a task) now needs to be complemented by the availability of the DNA fragment to be amplified, free nucleotides, *taq* or *pfu* polymerase, the right buffer, Eppendorf tubes, a PCR machine, and the technician performing the experiment. At the laboratory level, a building is required; as is power from the sockets; the technician needs a contract, a job description, and a boss. By directly incorporating all elements in the alignment, the diagram shifts from reflecting a doable problem as solely doable in terms of work, toward a socially and materially doable research practice.

Secondly, large-scale research dealing with problems such as cancer or global warming, cannot easily be reduced to a single social world, a single laboratory, or a single experiment—such problems are too big and too complex. Consortia or organizations dealing with such problems, attempt to divide the main problem into smaller bits, which are handed to specific laboratories based upon the material configuration in that laboratory, such as the availability of specific machines or tools or the presence of specific expertise. Each laboratory, each research site deals with a module of the overall research problem. The number of modules can range from just a handful up to several hundreds. All of these laboratories or research sites can be considered modules in a network with respect to the research problem. Each one of these labs is trying to get the answer to its module of the research question, getting its bit "to work." As a result, the modular configuration of the overall research problem is accompanied by a modular configuration of laboratories simultaneously pursuing a doable problem at their local site. These "quests for doability" are not the same, since each site for research deals with its own unique problem module and each research site has its own unique combination of elements in its particular research situation. Just as the problem modules relate to the overall problem, the modular doabilities relate to the doability of the overall problem. Between the labs and the modules, several ties can exist, that is "intermodular" ties, such as shared methodologies, shared materials, or shared funding. Thus, the visualization of doability as shown in Figure 6.1 is valid for one research site only: it is a "local doability."

This implies that the "overall doability" of the "overall problem" cannot be visualized as a single three-level alignment. The doability of large-scale research problems is much more of a network, an intricate web of interconnections, all requiring some version of alignment but also operating in smaller subunits. After all, no lab is an island. Scientists act inside a module, managing the doability of "their" problem module. However, because of the connections between the modules, shared materials, notions, fundings, methods, and their actions, aimed at achieving or maintaining doability, echo into the adjacent modules. As a result, the overall goal may be subject to different processes of doability construction and may be subjected to a number of simultaneous articulations.

### 6.2.2 TOWARD DIFFERENT STYLES AND DIFFERENT ALIGNMENTS

Thirdly, it is necessary to pay attention to the existence of laboratories in different social words, in other words, to take into account the interdisciplinary character of today's science. Science can be considered an intricate epistemological topography, a world map if you will, which is filled with boundaries of various types. The boundaries between disciplines, which are often troublesome, can nevertheless be overcome from time to time. Adjacent disciplines share a lot of materials and expertise. For instance, a PCR machine can be found in almost all the biology departments, as well as in various chemistry and (neuro-)psychology departments. Such machines, or other shared elements in research practices, can act as a common ground between diverse research sites, as boundary objects (Star and Griesemer 1989). Besides boundaries between disciplines, there is, however, another boundary that traverses the topography of science, which can be considered to create more of a challenge to the notion of boundary-crossing ability. The large consortia, studying the "big problems," are not confined to a single style of scientific reasoning (Crombie 1994, Davidson 1999, Hacking 1992a–c). In the biomedical field, the large-scale scientific champions of our day, currently laboratory initiatives are combined with information technology and bioinformatics, in a single consortium.

While the difference between laboratory science and informatics is based upon the object of study, this is not its sole basis. Sites at which "lab science" is performed differ from sites at which "information science" is performed, not solely because of the different problem module they address, but also because of the way of approaching and dealing with this problem. Methods, elements, conventions, rules, and truths that are commonplace within a certain style of science, may be considered irrelevant within another one. At all three levels of the alignment shown in Figure 6.3, the "rules of engagement" can be considered different. Thus, it is a matter of object of study, as well as method of study. As a result, in a network of local doabilities, not only do these local doabilities differ from one another because of a number of contingencies or a difference in the object of enquiry (the problem module), but the method of enquiry also results in different "styles of alignment" and different flavors of doability. The boundary between two different styles may be an epistemological minefield, but we have previously demonstrated that it is not impenetrable (Penders et al. 2007a,b, 2008). As a result of hard work, boundaries can be overcome by the material and social characteristics of specific boundary objects, which enable cooperation across styles. Nevertheless, the ways of constructing doability, as well as the articulation of work taking place, differ between styles. Again, this may result in a diversification of doability.

### 6.2.3 TOWARD INCOMPLETE ALIGNMENTS

Our fourth and final expansion of Fujimura's model takes it beyond the lab to include other sites such as conferences, meetings, lectures, books, articles, or television. All of those sites have something in common, when compared to a laboratory: experiments are not the scientific purpose of these venues. At each of these sites, tasks are performed and elements are present that are of key importance that contribute to the doability of the research problem. Social support, public acceptance, and understanding and valorization efforts are as important to "overall doability" as getting the experiments to work.

Nevertheless, it may seem a bit odd to talk about "local doabilities" in terms of the three-level alignment depicted in Figure 6.1 when there is no lab and there is no experiment. What would a three-level alignment look in such a situation? Although the experiments are not conducted at such sites, the experiments can be represented by other elements, such as laboratory notebooks, graphs, tables or articles, or even technicians who are present. Often, the elements that are present at a certain site do not equally represent every layer of organization. Consider for instance a programmatic journal publication; such publications are meant to clear the way for a certain research problem, display its social significance or show other interesting research niches currently unaddressed. Such publications (or lectures that serve similar goals) often precede the conducting of actual experiments or even the selection of laboratories that are to be part of a research consortium. At every site in the knowledge production process, the collection of elements present is different. Since elements correspond to a particular layer in the organization of scientific practice (Figure 6.1), within every one of these collections one or more layers may be more (or less) prominently present. At the sites mentioned earlier, the social world layer can be said to be overrepresented with respect to elements present and tasks performed, as compared to the laboratory level and the experiment level.

When certain tasks or elements are over- or underrepresented from a research site, they are also over- or underrepresented in the local alignment pertaining to that site. For instance, to "abstract from practical requirement of the laboratory" is regularly noticed in expectations uttered in, for instance, conference lectures or programmatic publications. This is only possible in a situation where the laboratory is underrepresented in the alignment of elements.

In Figure 6.2, such a "modified" alignment is shown. Because of a relative underrepresentation of some layers compared to others, more research problems are doable at this site of practice. It is important to consider that Figure 6.2 may be put upside down. To a laboratory technician, public acceptance and understanding of the overall research problem may appear just as absent from the experiment he or she is conducting as the specific experiments may be absent to a research institute director being interviewed on TV.

The modules of a research problem differ from one another. A particular problem module may be doable at a certain site because of a relative over or underrepresentation of particular elements in the research situation. Since, as a mirror to the overrepresentation of the social world level at a conference, an overrepresentation of the experiment level exists at the bench, in the network of local doabilities that together form the overall doability of the research problem, these asymmetries even out. This implies that the doability of a large-scale research problem cannot easily be determined, since its local equivalents may differ in their degree of doability. For more thorough evaluation, multiple sites of scientific practice have to be visited. This is why scientists attend meetings and conferences and this is why science and technology studies (STS) researchers should not (and generally do not) settle for a single observation at a single site.

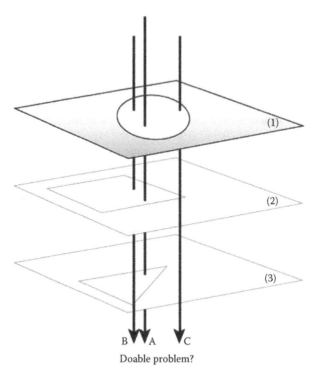

Doable problem?

**FIGURE 6.2** Incomplete alignment. When elements or tasks from the laboratory or the experimental world are absent or underrepresented at a site of nutrigenomic practice, they are also absent or underrepresented in the alignment. The possible restrictions or limitations they pose can be ignored and a larger subset of problems can be considered doable (as is represented by arrows B and C ignoring one or two absent tasks or elements, respectively). (1) Social world, (2) laboratory, (3) and experiment.

The doability of a research problem in a single lab is part of a network of multiple local doabilities, each contingent upon the availability of tasks and elements at this particular site, together forming an interconnected web: *a network of doabilities*. The complete network forms the "overall doability" of the large-scale research problem. The process of constructing, creating, and maintaining all these coinciding doabilities and the creation and maintenance of the ties between is immensely complex. The four additions we have made to Fujimura's conceptualization of doable problems enable us to analyze how in a large-scale, multisited, multidisciplinary science program, research problems are addressed and dealt with.

## 6.3　MAKING DOABLE EQUALS DIVERSIFICATION?

We will now turn to an empirical demonstration of how the expanded notion of doability helps us to study and understand a large-scale research practice. To this end, we have visited numerous sites in the research practice of nutrigenomics. We have studied nutrigenomics research practice for over 4 years, from 2003 to 2007. Observations were conducted in laboratories, three of which were as participant observation for over a month each, supplemented with observations at conferences and meetings in many places, for example, the Netherlands, Spain, Italy, Poland, Australia, and New Zealand. Next to these observations, the nutrigenomic literature was analyzed and in-depth interviews (n = 38) were conducted with scientists (both in academia and in industry), administrators, and other nutrigenomic professionals up to saturation level, when no apparent new issues or insights came to the fore. Excerpts from interviews, notes, and lectures have—where relevant—been translated from Dutch and German into English by B.P. Respecting the privacy of the scientists who have cooperated, their names have been replaced by codes if requested and the names of scientists willing to be identified have been left unaltered.

Nutrigenomics is the study of the interaction between genes, proteins, and metabolites of the (human) body, with the nutrients the body ingests and the effects of health. The main research problem of nutrigenomics, the "overall problem," is how to understand these relationships so that they can be mobilized for the benefit of public health, through stimulating population health, or via promoting individual health for the benefit of population health (Kaput 2005, Kaput and Rodriguez 2004, Müller and Kersten 2003, van Ommen 2004). It should be noted that the latter trajectory is less prominent in nutrigenomic research practices.

The main research program we studied is called "An integrated genomics approach towards gut health and nutrition." It is a Dutch program in which eight labs from four universities cooperate. This name is considered too lengthy for day-to-day communication and generally is abbreviated to the "*Gut Health*" *program* by scientists and administrators alike. Because of its close ties to the European Nutrigenomics Organization (NuGO), which range from shared goals and equipment up to individual memberships, empirical detours have been made into this European research program as well.

### 6.3.1   NETWORK OF LOCAL DOABILITIES

Let us first look into how multiple laboratories studying a common problem, can be accounted for. The goal of the Gut Health program is to provide insight and understanding in gut function and gut health, given that the gut is the main site for interaction between body and nutrients. The eight laboratories that participate in the program were each assigned a module of the problem based upon existing expertise in the labs, as well as the research infrastructure of the institutes these labs are part of. The problem modules were formulated based upon two main sets of variables. The first was the exemplar nutrient that was going to be used in the experimental strategies. The second was the type of molecular effect of the nutrient to be studied, coupled to an experimental platform. Combined, these lead to a modular problem topography as shown in Figure 6.3, in which each lab is assigned both a nutrient and an experimental platform.

In this topography, every scientist conducts his experiments in his lab, in his discipline, attempting to address his problem module. *Together*, all the scientists in the Gut Health program work on "gut health and function," but individually none of them do. Dealing with a particular problem module is difficult enough, pushing the overall problem to the background. Similar to the motto at the top of this chapter,

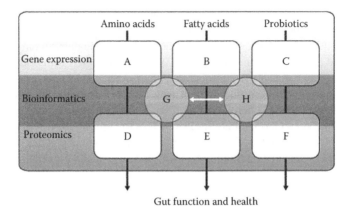

Gut function and health

**FIGURE 6.3** Division of work in Gut Health. This (topo)graphical representation of the division of work in the project is redrawn from the final project proposal for Gut Health. Divisions were made in two dimensions, one distinguishing between the compounds under investigation—amino acids, fatty acids, and bacteria—and the other distinguishing the entities to be measured: genes or proteins. Bioinformatics "hovers" above all six quadrants laden with the task of integration. The codes in each quadrant refer to the laboratory in which most of the particular subproject research was conducted.

the word "health" will not, or rarely, pop(s) up in a PubMed search. Their own problem module has their primary interest:

> I think that everybody does his own thing, eventually [...]. I cannot say that people who work in a different group add something to my subject. Everybody does one's own thing. I am together with [Z003 and Z002] and others have teamed up in other groups.

**Interview Scientist W006, 20050919.**

The primary efforts of the scientists working in a single laboratory are concentrated onto devising an experimental strategy, making an experiment work, assembling and creating the tools to do so, and finally publishing a research paper. Combined, they all add up to a doable problem module. All the labs are simultaneously constructing doable problem modules, it is their core business, and scientists excel at it. Constructing a problem module into a doable problem module carries consequences for adjacent modules, as some elements in the research situation are shared between them. Let us provide an example that very clearly describes how through the creation of local doability, the doability of other problem modules, as well as the "overall doability" of the gut health and function problem, was influenced.

Doing genomic research entails the measurements of thousands of variables simultaneously. The laboratories measuring gene expressions (see Figure 6.3), use a certain tool to do so: the microarray, also called the Gene Chip, a small device able to simultaneously register the activity of tens of thousands of genes. Since laboratories A, B, and C all study gene expression profiles, they share the experimental machinery that enables them to do so, establishing an important tie between the modules. Such microarrays are, however, extremely expensive. That is why they are often not bought by single labs but in bulk by institutes or universities, which can obtain a significant discount. Labs A, B, and C, however, are part of different universities, which made deals with different commercial producers of microarrays. Every lab did get access to the technology—at a discount—which enabled them to perform the desired experiments. However, because of different microarray platforms being part of the experimental strategies of the program, the experiments from the individual labs could no longer be compared to one another, or be integrated into the overall research problem:

> A central database was envisioned, in which all data would be saved so that everybody in the programme would be able to have access to it. Subsequently, the analysis would be performed altogether. But this has not happened. Everybody started using their own […] platforms […]. Both cannot be compared amongst each other. That database would, if it would come have into being, not have worked.

**Interview Scientist E001, 20050308.**

The bioinformatics labs in the program were supposed to perform overall analysis, integration, and comparison of the experiments in the individual labs, in order to address the overall problem of gut health and function. By buying different arrays at minimal costs, most of the laboratories made sure their local problem module became doable, but at the same time they decreased the local doability of the bioinformatics modules as well as the overall doability of the gut health and function research question.

Now that we have established the modular character of research problems and research programs and possible implications for problem-solving strategies, we can turn to a second type of consequence. For example, the data derived from the measurements of gene and protein expressions have been used to construct claims about nutrients and health. These claims can be quite modest, referring to small sets or single experiments: "The level of the project at this time is 'what does glutamine do in a cell?'" (Observation Scientist W002, 20050301). But such claims can also be more far reaching, such as specific claims about health that are constructed out of measurements on a molecular level. Information about the concentration of RNA molecules or specific proteins is translated into potential health information. Food industry representatives, for instance, talk about health effects that are based upon "genes that are to be up or down regulated" (Observation Industry Representative I001, 20050301) or based upon "molecular markers with a clinical relevance" (Observation Industry Representative I003, 20040524). Nutrigenomic research in general, and the Gut Health program or NuGO in particular, are research initiatives in which health is the main normative goal while methodology and level of enquiry are restricted to the molecular. Rose has argued that such a combination, especially in large-scale research, will result in the "molecularization of health" (Rose 2001, 2007). In the Gut Health program, this molecularization of health can be understood as the aforementioned quotes by two representatives from the food industry illustrate.

It is important to consider the dynamics of doable problem construction in more detail. Laboratories pursue doable problem modules and buying microarrays is one of the actions performed to enable this. As a result, only molecules can be measured and since it is health that is the ultimate goal, health is articulated into an entity that exists (mainly) out of an array of molecular concentrations. Interestingly, the experiments performed with different microarrays cannot be compared, since the measurements and corresponding outcomes are different. Consequently, the claims on which genes are proper markers for (gut) health are equally difficult to compare. Different genes or proteins, different cut-off values, and different technical norms coexist as an effect of the different doable problem modules. Thus, while a trend toward molecularization can be identified, different molecularized healths are produced corresponding to diverse sets of norms.

### 6.3.2 DIFFERENT STYLES AND DIFFERENT ALIGNMENTS

Having accounted for the effects of multiple laboratories cooperating on a common problem, now we shall turn our attention to the multidisciplinarity of these various laboratories. Differences between modules of a research program can be understood in many ways. There are geographical, cultural, organizational, and material differences, all of which add to different decisions made to enhance local doability. In this section, we would like to present a specific difference between problem modules: a difference in *style of science*. We have discerned two specific styles of science in large-scale nutrigenomic research in general and in the Gut Health and NuGO programs in particular, namely, a "wet" and a "dry" style of the science. The first corresponds to the "laboratory style," to the laboratory work bench or laboratory work, and the second to the "statistical style," referring to desktop or in silico work, both previously described by Hacking (1992a–c). In Figure 6.3, laboratories G and H can be identified as acting in a "dry" style, whereas the other labs largely act in a "wet" style. Cooperation between the two sets of labs can be quite difficult, as their different styles are accompanied by different criteria for significance or importance, methods of identifying these and different claims or truth sentences (Hacking 1992c). Scientist W008 shares the frustration that arises out of such cooperation:

> Initially, in the very beginning [...] I got some data back from [lab H]. They struck out all high gene expressions, because they did not fit in a linear gradient for the dye. To us, those are the most important ones and they just strike them out. Not that they ask us, or even tell us. I just got the data back and then I saw it. I thought 'hey, how is that possible?'. I checked it, and then I asked them. Then they told me what was going on. When I saw that, and when I heard [the explanation] I thought I was going to quit. I was that angry. I simply just do not understand it [...]. I know quite a bit about statistics. I want to understand and I tried, but it simply doesn't work.

**Observation Scientist W008, 20040416.**

Labs G and H are just as keen on constructing doable problems as labs A–F but the problem module that is their responsibility differs greatly from the problem modules the other labs deal with. Performing a microarray experiment or performing an in silico dimensional reduction of millions of measurements into a graph displaying similarities, are very different things. Nevertheless, between "wet" and "dry" modules of the Gut Health program, ties do exist, for example, shared notions of gene expression or the actual gene expression measurement values that are emailed from one lab to another. For instance, the "shared data" in the aforementioned quote is such a tie. Nevertheless, these ties are not necessarily identified as "shared" because of the epistemological differences in criteria for significance or importance, methodology and different truth claims.

Labs working in different styles of research conduct different types of experiments, use different materials and concepts, and end up with different alignments to construct doable problems. In the previous sections, we have seen that "wet" laboratories construct doable problems by articulating health as a molecular entity, "dry" laboratories act differently. "Dry" labs are scattered with computers, algorithms, databases, and datasets, and instead of performing experiments, computations, calculations and data analyses are performed, all within a strict set of methodological rules. Bioinformaticians working in the dry labs, attempt to "read" a health status out of the data sets. This requires a large number of very complex calculations using huge numbers of numbers. While these numbers represent the molecules measured by the "wet" colleagues, these numbers are "treated" in ways that do not necessarily correspond to the "wet" world, as scientist W008 found out.

In the process of assembling clusters of genes that respond in similar ways to nutrient exposure and the calculations of relative and absolute changes in gene expression values, "dry" scientists are also constructing their doable problem module and by doing so actively articulate the elements inside, one of these elements being health:

> 800 Genes can be a marker, if clustered right. Can we say, based upon 800 genes that the gut is healthier?

**Scientist M004, 20050301.**

"Dry" scientists talk of health and markers, and, as in the aforementioned quote, of large numbers of clustered genes as a single marker. Similarly, Müller and Kersten (2003) argue that "patterns of gene expression, protein expression and metabolite production in response to particular nutrients or nutritional regimes can be viewed as dietary signatures." In such statements, the interaction between health and nutrition is framed in terms of molecular information or signals. Such information and signals can be quantified and used for statistical analyses, for instance, a method called "principal component analysis" (PCA) through the use of which a *normal* metabolic profile can be mapped into three-dimensional space, a "cloud" (Ebbels et al. 2003) that occupies *the normal space* or *the space of normality*. If one moves further away from this space, ones health risk rises accordingly.

The observations that revealed this conceptualization of health were conducted at a NuGO Workshop in Krakow, Poland, at which both "wet" and "dry" scientists sat together to determine standards and norms for health ("Defining markers of health," March 25–26). Here, a number of healths "collided" and the often subtle differences between the various heaths came to the fore.

Where "wet" health was articulated as a molecular entity, a "dry" health is articulated as an entity that is comprised out of risks or risk profiles. In the different "dry" labs, problem modules also differ, alignments differ, and thus articulations differ, just as they do in "wet" labs, resulting in various technical norms for these risk profiles and thus several coexisting "dry" health standards.

### 6.3.3  INCOMPLETE ALIGNMENTS

Science and research practices are not solely about laboratories. Other sites where science is performed should be included in our analysis as well. Scientists venture beyond the lab, quite regularly, and visit scientific conferences, attend local and global meetings, and workshops. The tasks performed at such sites, including lecturing, presenting, publishing, and discussing, are just as much part of science as is experimenting. Here we will focus on a selection of such different sites, specifically directed at agenda-setting activities: programmatic publications and lectures at conferences. To demonstrate and understand the differences between various sites of scientific activities, we have chosen a highly debated "part" of nutrigenomics: the personalized diet. What does personalized diet look like, what is it all about? Personalized nutrition is very much a line of research in which a lot of promises, imaginaries, and expectations are uttered, while simultaneously people are working in laboratories who disagree with these expectations. We will focus on the interplay between expectations and laboratories, promises and practice, rhetoric and doability (Douglas 2005, van Lente 1993, 2000). Please note that the explicit focus on the individual in the rhetoric surrounding the personalized diet does not debunk the goal of public health. It presents an alternative trajectory that has its own set of consequences for scientific inquiry, as much as a set of societal and ethical consequences.

In 1937, Schwartz Rose wrote that "all men [of] all races of men have the same nutrition needs" (1937, p. 259). Now, 70 years later, that statement is being contested. Currently, phrases such as the "basis of differences among individuals that relate diet and health" and "distinguishing individual differences" are used to carefully construct personalization in terms of individuals. Talk of genetic or nongenetic individuality is not new, but it is being discussed more prominently in the last few years. Older references are rare (Williams 1956, Young and Scrimshaw 1979), but in the last few years, a large number of papers have been published focusing on genetic or biochemical individuality (Arai 2005, German et al. 2003, Kaput 2004, Kaput et al. 1994, Klaus and Keijer 2004, Watkins et al. 2001). Scientist M001 is convinced that the future will enable the personalized diet:

> I still am convinced that we will, in the end reach a personalised dietary advice, based upon nutrigenomics. Because I remain to be convinced that the effects of nutrition are immensely different between people and that can only be, based upon differences in genes and constitutions [...]. It might be very complicated, but in the end one must be able to find the right combinations that can predict why one's cholesterol rises and the other's doesn't. And [...] with the calculation power and the immense acceleration at which several things are being analysed [...] that sort of information becomes available faster [...].

**Interview Scientist M001, 20050316.**

In their expectations, scientists present a picture of what the personalized diet is about. They are sure that it is indeed the future and that it is going to be tailored to the unique needs of every individual, whether based upon "difference in genes and constitutions" as scientist M001 stated earlier, or based upon "nutritional status, lifestyle, disease-risk and genetic-makeup," according to Hoolihan and Harlander (2004).

Such expectations have the luxury of being abstracted from certain practical requirements that actually doing the experiments in a laboratory may introduce. Many of the practical requirements disappear by expecting or assuming technological advancements. For instance, scientist M001 dismisses practical requirements and limitations when he refers to the "immense acceleration at which several things are being analysed," or sometimes are simply ignored. Practical requirements exist out of elements that can be found in laboratories and in experiments: materials, expertises, samples, and much more. But at the programmatic conferences and in the agenda-setting publications, laboratories are absent, as are experiments. Scientists who are embedded in the research practice, in their labs, designing or performing experiments, argue that monitoring and charting all the differences between individuals is both impossible (1) and unnecessary (2):

(1) The number of combinations and permutations of genes and environmental factors are so huge that one will never be able to evaluate all such interactions.

**Observation Larry Parnell, 20050910.**

(2) If you reason the other way around, there are a number of pathological deviations known from differences in genotype. There are lethal mutations and there are a number of mutations that make people truly obese, pathologically obese. But there are only six of them. If you go to the more subtle deviations ... at a certain moment the relevance of the difference between the trees in the forest disappears. The art is not to wander to deep into the forest but still notice the use of your work. [...] It matters that one is capable of separating sense from nonsense and useful from the useless and find out for which nutritional parameter it is useful to keep looking for differences.

**Interview Ben van Ommen, 20060115.**

Nutrigenomicists Parnell and Van Ommen do not contest the idea that people are different. They argue that a number of practical and material limitations need to be taken into account to reach a dietary stratification that can be considered doable. This does not mean that scientist M001, Hoolihan or Harlander are intentionally deceiving us by expecting personalization as individualization. At the sites where they uttered their expectations, various elements belonging to the social world layer of scientific organization (see Figure 6.1) were overrepresented. In other words, at sites such as conferences or programmatic papers, research agenda's, issues of public–private research relationships and funding priorities outweighed test tubes, lab benches, and tacit experimental expertises. Thus, in the process of aligning the social world, laboratory, and experiment, the latter two were locally underrepresented and personalization as individualization was locally doable.

Van Ommen and Parnell are also seeking doability and position themselves in a research situation that involves both labs and experiments. In order to reach doability, they are aligning all three levels of scientific organization and by doing so, they are actively articulating the notion of the "personalized" to facilitate alignment. To them, personalization is not about genetically unique individuals, but about groups of people sharing a number of traits that are relevant to dietary advice (Penders 2010, Penders et al. 2007a,b), thus effectively shifting *personalization as individualization* toward *personalization as categorization*. As a result, the ideal of individual health has become group health or category health. How these categories will exactly be defined currently is at the heart of nutrigenomic research.

## 6.4  NORMATIVE EFFECTS OF LARGE-SCALE DOABILITY IN NUTRITION SCIENCE

In nutrigenomics, the overall goal is to understand (gut) health and function, and to use these insights to improve and promote human health. To craft doable research problems, scientists have engaged in huge amounts of articulation work, as we have seen earlier. Here, we have focused on health and the personal as key elements subject to active articulation and change, because of the central position of these norms in nutrigenomics. Norms matter, for in the midst of all of this cooperation and problem solving, realignment and integration, the notion of health acts as a compass, providing direction to nearly all such shifts. The existence of norms for what health or healthy is, subtly provides direction for an entire research practice.

A large part of the dynamics of articulating research problems is a result of the interplay between the diverse problem modules among one another, versus the overall problem. In other words, the dynamics of local doability construction need not correspond to the dynamics of overall doability construction. Thus, the dynamics of doable problem construction does not necessary coincide with the goal of promoting public health. Because of this, scientist N002 concludes that:

> [T]he deliverable 'we will make people healthy and prevent all disease' is stupid. However, eventually we will need to take this path because politics opens the doors to funding only there [...].

**Interview Scientist N002, 20051211.**

Scientist X003 even argues that health "is a very dangerous concept" (Interview Scientist X003, 20060505). We would not go that far. Recalling the goal of nutrigenomics, namely to understand the relationship between diet and nutrition and subsequently mobilize this understanding for the benefit of human health, this turned out to be very hard indeed: something that was expected by almost all participants. Scientist X003 states that "health means different things and it is different in every experimental context and I am convinced that we know [this]" (Interview Scientist X003, 20060505).

What are the consequences of having large-scale science deal with a normative goal, such as health? Well, the goal did not necessarily come any closer. In its attempt to construct a doable problem, the goal the research problem was a part of, changed. In this chapter, we demonstrated that as a result of the interplay doable problem construction and the interconnected problem modules several rearticulations have taken place in the nutrigenomic research situation. In summary these are (1) the articulation of health as a molecular entity, (2) the articulation of health as a risk-based entity, and (3) the articulation of the personal as category based. Furthermore, it is worth noting that especially with respect to the first two articulation processes, these are not singular articulations. Multiple molecularized (wet) healths coexist in the research situation as do multiple computation-based (dry) healths (Penders et al. 2009a,b). Phrased differently, where a unified definition of health was sought, many situated norms for health were found (Figure 6.4). In the case of the personalized diet, *personalization as individualization* was articulated as *personalization as categorization*, resulting in a situation in which the goal of a particular diet is not uniform as the notion of health may vary between groups, as opposed to a uniform ideal of public health. The standard of health shifted from a singular toward a plural, while the plurality of the ideal healthy diet was constrained. The large-scale, interdisciplinary approach of Gut Health implied that a lot of smaller research problems have been made doable. However, at the same time, and as an effect of the fragmentation of the research problem, the overall global goal of gut health has not. Paradoxically, the quest for health has made that goal harder to reach.

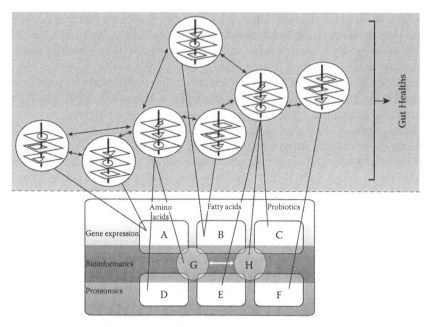

**FIGURE 6.4** A network of doabilities. The lower image, based upon Figure 6.3, represents the Gut Health organization. As every laboratory deals with a small subset of problems, all of which have to be constructed into doable problems, a variety of interacting, doable subproblems emerge (schematically represented in the gray area). A complex mixture of doable problems results in a mixture of health.

The merit of using a framework enabling one to track a doable problem construction is that it enables the observer to perceive the normative differences produced in the research practice, as we have seen earlier, as well as provides the first clues toward possible political effects that may arise out of such normative articulations. What can be considered "health" or "healthy" is by no means static. Shifts in what is considered healthy, are not new. For instance, Steven Shapin shows how, already 500 years ago, an orientation toward health transformed into an orientation toward disease:

> [Initially] (1470–1530), the doctors' presumption was that you were basically healthy, occasionally needing medical expertise to maintain you in that state of health, but [afterwards] (1530–70) the experts were trying to convince their readers that they were basically ill, requiring constant dietetic monitoring to prevent sickness from becoming disabling or even fatal (Shapin 2002).

Such shifts are not the result of the doctors' humor or even their cash purses. Around the 1530s, the concept of health changed in interaction with changes in the field of medicine and people's daily lives.

Over time, categories such as health and disease or notions of normal and pathological, have not been stable. Changes occur in the ways in which health is understood or materialized in biomedical technology and technical norms or protocols. In literature from social theory, a prominent trend is suggested, namely that health may *molecularize* (Rose 2007). Rose argues that the process of molecularization is a "reorganisation of the gaze of the life sciences, their institutions, procedures, instruments, spaces of operation and forms of capitalization" (Rose 2001, 2007, Shostak 2005). In our study of nutrigenomic research practice, we have observed that out of the vast array of potential healths existing next to one another, some can indeed be conceptualized in terms of molecularization. The mobilization of such norms for health can be described in terms of molecular politics (Rose 2001, 2007). Yet molecular politics alone cannot account for the shifts we have observed.

Many papers dealing with normative effects of biomedical science in terms of molecularization focus on rather monolithic, top-down alterations in the conceptualization of health and very few studies show empirical examples of "biopolitics bottom-up" (Lemke 2007, p. 127). We, however, have shown that subtle, situated processes such as experiments, the management of single programs, and the construction of a network of situated doabilities, are perfectly capable of influencing contemporary norms of health bottom-up.

The aforementioned analysis demonstrates a vast complexity for nutrition science, but it also shows that nutrition scientists are able to deal with this complexity and manage to craft doable problems out of it. Normative effects of the process of creating doable problems are the creation of several healths, where only one was sought. The outcome of large-scale nutrition research may be very surprising; because of the dynamics of doability being pursued at many sites simultaneously, each rearticulating multiple elements in the research situation. In the case described earlier, it is a surprise with far reaching political and practical effects. For the pursuit of doable problems cannot be separated from the active construction and reconstruction of norms, a process of coevolution that nutrition science would be wise to continuously monitor.

It is because of this, the importance of large-scale science in our world and for our world, that it needs to be studied thoroughly and continuously. Take, for instance, the sequencing of individual genomes, which is just starting to take off by the release of the genomes of James Watson and the publication of that of J. Craig Venter (Check 2007, Gross 2007, Ledford 2007, Levy et al. 2007, Marshall 2007), or the relatively new field of epigenomics, researching how traits acquired during life are stored and passed on to the next generations (Davis and Milner 2004, Gosden and Feinberg 2007, Liu 2007), or existing trends toward individualization and a focus on risk. Contemporary nutrition science will have to come to terms with these and other movements or trends, and "contemporary norms of selfhood" (Novas and Rose 2000, Rose 2007) will coevolve with the sciences and be incorporated into them. The better we learn to understand large science, the better we learn to understand what it does to us. For instance, does super sizing science help (Vermeulen 2009)? It most certainly does not make the practice of performing science easier, that much has been demonstrated earlier. Nonetheless, if it *works* by enabling to unlock additional research problems, it may be worth the effort. However, given the situated nature of scientific practice, the local character of doable problems, it may very well be the case that, sometimes (or often), scaling down science may be a more prudent strategy.

## ACKNOWLEDGMENTS

We acknowledge support from the Societal Component of Genomics Research Programme (MCG) of the Netherlands Organisation for Scientific Research (NWO) to B.P. (Project no. 050-32-011; "Nutrigenomics and society in the making") and would like to thank all the nutrition scientists for their participation and cooperation. B.P. is currently being supported by the Netherlands Genomics Initiative (NGI). Furthermore, we are grateful to Dr. I. Van Hoyweghen, Dr. E. Aarden, and Dr. M.-H. Derksen for valuable discussions and suggestions and three anonymous reviewers for their constructive comments. We gratefully acknowledge the permission granted by Maney Publishing to expand upon the text previously published in *Interdisciplinary Science Reviews*.

## REFERENCES

Arai, S. 2005. Functional food science. *J Sci Food Agric* 85:1603–1605.
Bergmann, M. M., U. Görman, and J. C. Mathers. 2008. Bioethical considerations for human nutrigenomics. *Annu Rev Nutr* 28:447–467.
Check, E. 2007. Celebrity genomes alarm researchers. *Nature* 447:358–359.
Crombie, A. C. 1994. *Styles of Scientific Thinking in the European Tradition: The History of Argument and Explanation in the Mathematical and Biomedical Sciences and Arts.* 3 Volumes. London, U.K.: Duckworth.
Davidson, A. I. 1999. Styles of reasoning, conceptual history and the emergence of psychiatry. In *The Science Studies Reader*, ed. M. Biagioli, pp. 124–136. New York: Routledge.
Davis, C. D. and J. Milner. 2004. Frontiers in nutrigenomics, proteomics, metabolomics and cancer prevention. *Mutat Res* 551:51–64.
Douglas, C. M. W. 2005. Managing HuGE expectations: Rhetorical strategies in human genome epidemiology. *Sci Stud* 18:26–45.

Ebbels, T., H. Keun, O. Beckonert, H. Antti, M. Bollard, E. Holmes, and J. C. Lindon. 2003. Toxicity classification from metabonomic data using a density superposition approach: 'CLOUDS'. *Anal Chim Acta* 490:109–122.

Eriksson, L. and A. Webster. 2008. Standardizing the unknown: Practicable pluripotency as doable futures. *Sci Cult* 17:57–69.

Etzkowitz, H. and L. Leydesdorff. 1998. Triple helix of innovation. *Sci Public Policy* 25:358–364.

Fujimura, J. H. 1987. Constructing 'do-able' problems in cancer research: Articulating alignment. *Soc Stud Sci* 17:257–293.

Fujimura, J. H. 1992. Crafting science: Standardized packages, boundary objects and translation. In *Science as Practice and Culture*, ed. A. Pickering, pp. 168–214. Chicago, IL: University of Chicago Press.

Fujimura, J. H. 1996. *Crafting Science: A Sociohistory of the Quest for the Genetics of Cancer.* Cambridge, MA: Harvard University Press.

German, J. B., M.-A. Roberts, and S. M. Watkins. 2003. Personal metabolomics as a next generation nutritional assessment. *J Nutr* 133:4260–4266.

Gibbons, M., C. Limoges, H. Nowotny, S. Schwartzman, P. Scott, and M. Trow. 1994. *The New Production of Knowledge: The Dynamics of Science and Research in Contemporary Societies.* London, U.K.: Sage.

Giles, L. 2005. *Sun Tzu on the Art of War. The Oldest Military Treatise in the World.* 1910 http://www.chinapage.com/sunzi-e.html (accessed September 27, 2005).

Gosden, R. G. and A. P. Feinberg. 2007. Genetics and epigenetics—Nature's pen-and-pencil set. *New Engl J Med* 356:731.

Gross, L. 2007. A new human genome sequence paves the way for individualized genomics. *PLoS Biol* 5:e266.

Hacking, I. 1992a. The self-vindication of the laboratory sciences. In *Science as Practice and Culture*, ed. A. Pickering, pp. 29–64. Chicago, IL: University of Chicago Press.

Hacking, I. 1992b. Statistical language, statistical truth and statistical reason: The self-authentication of a style of scientific reasoning. In *The Social Dimensions of Science*, ed. E. McMullin. Notre Dame, IN: University of Notre Dame Press.

Hacking, I. 1992c. 'Style' for historians and philosophers. *Stud Hist Philos Sci* 23:1–20.

Hessels, L. and H. van Lente. 2008. Re-thinking new knowledge production: A literature review and a research agenda. *Res Pol* 37:740–760.

Hoolihan, L. and S. Harlander. 2004. Individualization of nutritional recommendations and food choices. *Compr Rev Food Sci F* 3:140–141.

Kaput, J. 2004. Diet–disease gene interactions. *Nutrition* 20:26–31.

Kaput, J. 2005. Decoding the pyramid: A systems-biological approach to nutrigenomics. *Ann NY Acad Sci* 1055:64–79.

Kaput, J. 2008. Nutrigenomics research for personalized nutrition and medicine. *Curr Opin Biotech* 19:110–120.

Kaput, J. and R. L. Rodriguez. 2004. Nutritional genomics: The next frontier in the postgenomic era. *Physiol Genomics* 16:166–177.

Kaput, J., D. Swartz, E. Paisley, H. Mangian, W. L. Daniel, and W. J. Visek. 1994. Diet–disease interactions at the molecular level: An experimental paradigm. *J Nutr* 124:1296S–1305S.

Klaus, S. and J. Keijer. 2004. Gene expression profiling of adipose tissue: Individual, depot-dependent, and sex-dependent variabilities. *Nutrition* 20:115–120.

Lampe, J. W. 2006. For debate: Investment in nutrigenomics will advance the role of nutrition in public health. *Cancer Epidemiol Biomark* 15:2329–2330.

Latour, B. 1987. *Science in Action: How to Follow Scientists and Engineers through Society?* Cambridge, MA: Harvard University Press.

Latour, B. and S. Woolgar. 1986. *Laboratory Life: The Construction of Scientific Facts.* Princeton, NJ: Princeton University Press.

Ledford, H. 2007. All about Craig: The first "full" genome sequence. *Nature* 449:6–7.

Lemke, T. 2007. *Biopolitik zur Einführung*. Hamburg, Germany: Junius Verlag.

Levy, S., G. Sutton, P. C. Ng et al. 2007. The diploid genome sequence of an individual human. *PLoS Biol* 5:e254.

Liu, Y. 2007. Like father like son. A fresh review of the inheritance of acquired characteristics. *EMBO Rep* 8:798–803.

Löwy, I. 1998. Book review: Joan H Fujimura, Crafting science: A sociohistory of the quest for the genetics of cancer. *Med Hist* 42:252–253.

Marshall, E. 2007. Sequencers of a famous genome confront privacy issues. *Science* 315:1780.

Mole, 2004. No free lunches. *J Cell Sci* 117(5):653–654.

Müller, M. and S. Kersten. 2003. Nutrigenomics: Goals and strategies. *Nat Rev Genet* 4:315–322.

Novas, C. and N. Rose. 2000. Genetic risk and the birth of the somatic individual. *Econ Soc* 29:485–513.

Nowotny, H., P. Scott, and M. Gibbons. 2001. *Re-Thinking Science. Knowledge and the Public in an Age of Uncertainty*. Oxford, U.K.: Blackwell.

Nowotny, H., P. Scott, and M. Gibbons. 2003. 'Mode 2' revisited: The new production of knowledge. *Minerva* 41(3):179–194.

NuGO. 2003. European Nutrigenomics Organisation: Linking genomics, nutrition and health research. In *Network of Excellence Proposal*. Brussels, Belgium: EU.

Palladino, P. 1998. Book review: Joan H Fujimura, Crafting science: A sociohistory of the quest for the genetics of cancer. *Br J Hist Sci* 31:373–375.

Palmer, C. L. 2006. Weak information work and doable problems in interdisciplinary science. *P Am Soc Inform Sci Tech* 43:108.

Penders, B. 2010. *The Diversification of Health. Politics of Large-Scale Cooperation in Nutrition Science*. Bielefeld (D), Germany: Transcript Verlag.

Penders, B., K. Horstman, W. H. M. Saris, and R. Vos. 2007a. From individuals to groups: A review of the meaning of 'personalized' in nutrigenomics. *Trends Food Sci Tech* 18:333–338.

Penders, B., K. Horstman, and R. Vos. 2007b. Proper science in moist biology. *EMBO Rep* 8:613.

Penders, B., K. Horstman, and R. Vos. 2008. Walking the line between lab and computation: The 'moist' zone. *BioScience* 58(8):747–755.

Penders, B., K. Horstman, and R. Vos. 2009a. Large-scale research and the goal of health: An analysis of doable problem construction in 'new' nutrition science. *Interdiscip Sci Rev* 34:332–349.

Penders, B., R. Vos, and K. Horstman. 2009b. Side effects of problem-solving strategies in large-scale nutrition science: Towards a diversification of health. *Br J Nutr* 102:1400–1403.

Rose, N. 2001. The politics of life itself. *Theory Cult Soc* 18:1–30.

Rose, N. 2007. *The Politics of Life Itself. Biomedicine, Power and Subjectivity in the Twenty-First Century*. ed by P. Rabinow. In *Formation*. Princeton, NJ & Woodstock, U.K.: Princeton University Press.

Schwartz Rose, M. 1937. Racial food habits in relation to health. *Sci Mon* 44:257–267.

Shapin, S. 2002. Barbecue of the vanities: A short history of diet books. *Lond Rev Books* 16:21–23.

Shostak, S. 2005. The emergence of toxicogenomics: A case study of molecularization. *Soc Stud Sci* 35:367–403.

Star, S. L. and J. R. Griesemer. 1989. Institutional ecology, "translations", and boundary objects. Amateurs and professionals in Berkeley's museum of vertebrate zoology, 1907–1939. *Soc Stud Sci* 19:387–420.

van Lente, H. 1993. *Promising Technology. The Dynamics of Expectations in Technological Developments*. Delft, the Netherlands: Eburon.

van Lente, H. 2000. Forceful futures: From promise to requirement. In *Contested Futures. A Sociology of Prospective Techno-Science*, eds. N. Brown, B. Rappert, and A. Webster. London, U.K.: Ashgate.

van Ommen, B. 2004. Nutrigenomics: Exploiting systems biology in the nutrition and health arena. *Nutrition* 20:4–8.

Vermeulen, N. 2009. *Supersizing Science: On Building Large-Scale Research Projects in Biology*. Maastricht, the Netherlands: Maastricht University Press.

Watkins, S. M., B. D. Hammock, J. W. Newman, and J. B. German. 2001. Individual metabolism should guide agriculture toward foods for improved health and nutrition. *Am J Clin Nutr* 74:283–286.

Williams, R. J. 1956. *Biochemical Individuality: The Basis for the Genetotrophic Concept.* New York: John Wiley & Sons.

Young, V. R. and N. S. Scrimshaw. 1979. Genetic and biological variability in human nutrient requirements. *Am J Clin Nutr* 32:486–500.

# 7 Genomics and Breeding in Food Crops

*Allan Brown, Andrew H. Paterson, and Li Li*

## CONTENTS

## 7.1 INTRODUCTION

Plant biology is in the midst of a revolution, based on a dramatic increase in the number of crops and noncrop models for which reference genome sequences are available, with a growing subset of these also enjoying sequence data for multiple genotypes that permits massively parallel identification of informative DNA markers useful in breeding and genetics. Several surprising fundamental messages have been revealed by the first 10 sequences that shed new light on the "prehistory" of crop evolution, and the genome sequences empower new approaches to crop improvement. The generation of tremendous volumes of sequence information introduces new technical challenges into plant biology and agriculture—the relatively new field of bioinformatics addresses these challenges by utilizing efficient data management strategies, generating and maintaining web-based interfaces to access and submit information, and developing the algorithms necessary to compare multiple sequences and identify homology or conserved motifs in a reliable manner.

Among the many new opportunities created by increased genomic data, of singular importance for crop improvement is the possibility of genotyping thousands of genes in a single pass, already a reality in some crops. One can envision the ability to routinely query entire transcriptomes or even genomes to identify variants that are of potential phenotypic importance—the limiting factor thus becoming the acquisition of ample high-quality phenotypic data. In crops or noncrop plants where structural and functional information is limited, data from related or model crops can often be utilized.

The extensive gene discovery resulting from "omics" technology, in addition to the development of ever more efficient gene transfer technologies, permits acceleration of crop improvement through biotechnological approaches. We review some of the best known cases of using genetic engineering techniques to breed biotech crops with value-added traits beyond those that improve plant performance in the field. Increased understanding of plant metabolic pathways permits the generation of biotech food crops with improved nutritional value and premium quality, complementing conventional and marker-aided approaches to provide plant breeders with unprecedented scope for crop improvements.

## 7.2   GENOMIC SEQUENCING

The release of the first plant genomic sequence, *Arabidopsis thaliana* (a distant relative of cruciferous crops), a decade ago foreshadowed a new era in plant improvement (Initiative 2000). As of this writing, subsequent drafts of 10 angiosperm genome sequences have been published, including *Populus trichocarpa* (poplar or black cottonwood), *Vitis vinifera* (grapevine), *Carica papaya* (papaya), *Cucumis sativus* (cucumber), *Glycine max* (soya), and the monocots *Oryza sativa* (rice, including each of two subspecies), *Sorghum bicolor* (sorghum), *Zea mays* (maize), and *Brachypodium distachyon* (Goff et al. 2002, Huang et al. 2009a,b, International Rice Genome Sequencing 2005, Jaillon et al. 2007, Ming et al. 2008, Paterson et al. 2009, Schmutz et al. 2010, Schnable et al. 2009, Tuskan et al. 2006, Yu et al. 2002, 2005b). Sequencing is in progress for many more. As recently as 2006, one of the authors projected that "the sequencing of 200 domesticated plants would take a relatively short 14 years" (Paterson 2006). At the time considered audacious, this projection now looks conservative.

Two factors are largely responsible for the rapid acceleration in crop genome sequencing. First, there is increasing understanding of how whole-genome shotgun (WGS) approaches might be integrated into existing information networks including genetic and physical maps to yield high-quality draft genome sequences.

Arguments against the WGS approaches in many crop plants have generally focused on the generally higher content and more recent origin of repetitive DNA than in animal or microbe genomes (where WGS methods were developed). However, traditionally inclusive definitions of repetitive DNA, for example, as collections of elements that comprise a family based on 70%–80% matches along a predetermined length of DNA sequence, fail to reflect the power of modern DNA sequencing to distinguish among the vast majority of members of such heterogeneous families. In humans, sequencing error rates have recently been estimated to be 1%–5% of the average polymorphism rate of about 0.1% between alleles (Collins et al. 2004). A level of sequence divergence of 0.1% reflects about 100,000 years of neutral evolution, suggesting that all but the most recent sequence duplications may be resolved even in genome-wide comparisons. The use of paired end-sequences from several size classes of subclones in virtually all WGS efforts often permits circumscription of the size of intervals that contain elements too similar to distinguish by other means, thus offering contiguity approaching that of clone-based efforts. Second, the reduction to practice of sequencing methodologies able to provide deep coverage of angiosperm-sized genomes in single experiments costing tens of thousands of dollars or less has substantially reduced the "heavy lifting" needed to obtain a useful genome sequence.

Several surprising fundamental messages have been revealed by the first 10 sequences that shed new light on the "prehistory" of crop evolution. First and foremost, all crop genomes studied to date (and very probably all that exist) have experienced polyploidy in their evolutionary history, with a genome triplication that affected most if not all dicots (Jaillon et al. 2007, Tang et al. 2008a), at least two genome duplications that affected all Poaceae monocots (with the earlier one probably affecting additional taxa for which sequences are not yet available) (Paterson et al. 2004, Tang et al. 2010), and additional lineage-specific duplications superimposed on these in many lineages. In most lineages, however, gene and chromosome numbers have been restored to a relatively narrow range following these events, by loss of many of the resulting duplicated genes and chromosome mergers. The vast majority of gene functional groups show postduplication gene preservation/loss rates in angiosperms that are indistinguishable from the genome-wide average. Such "neutral" loss of duplicated genes presumably involves inactivating mutations opposed by very weak selection (Haldane 1933). However, genes in a few specific functional categories duplicate and reduplicate in successive genome duplications (Blanc and Wolfe 2004, Chapman et al. 2006, Maere et al. 2005, Paterson et al. 2006, Seoighe and Gehring 2004, Tang et al. 2008b, Thomas et al. 2006), and their fates may be integrally intertwined with the evolution of morphological complexity (Freeling and Thomas 2006).

Second, different genomes evolve at remarkably different speeds—rates of nucleotide substitution per synonymous site (Ks) between corresponding genes remaining from the paleo-triplication range from 1.27 in *Vitis* to 1.83 in *Carica*, with *Populus* being intermediate (1.51), all highly significant differences. Since all these species share the same triplication, if they evolved at comparable rates then the respective sets of paleologs should show similar Ks values. *Arabidopsis* has a still faster molecular clock—genes remaining after a lineage-specific duplication after their divergence with *Carica* have median Ks values of ~1.8, near that of the much older gamma-duplicates in the other dicots. Indeed, the many merits of *A. thaliana* as a botanical model notwithstanding, it is something of an outlier among angiosperm genomes in being very rapidly evolving, having experienced at least one triplication and two duplications in its evolutionary history (Bowers et al. 2003), and having undergone 30% genome size reduction and at least nine rearrangements in the short time since its divergence from *A. lyrata* (Hansson et al. 2006, Kawabe et al. 2006, Koch and Kiefer 2005, Kuittinen et al. 2004). It is important that our understanding of angiosperm evolution grows to reflect the histories of more plants.

Third, most angiosperm genomes include two highly differentiated "components" within each chromosome. An early observation about eukaryotic genome organization was that some regions of a genome showed differential staining with DNA-detecting dyes (Stack et al. 1974). It has long been recognized that "heterochromatic" genomic domains such as the pericentromeric space are generally repeat rich. Careful comparison of the rice and sorghum genomes showed euchromatic and heterochromatic regions, as defined cytologically (Cheng et al. 2001, Kim et al. 2005), to represent evolutionarily distinct components of genomes that can be independently detected by several comparative or in silico approaches (Bowers et al. 2005). Nearly all genetic recombinations are confined to the euchromatin. Greater microcolinearity in recombinogenic (euchromatic) than nonrecombinogenic (heterochromatic) regions is consistent with the hypothesis that genomic rearrangements are usually deleterious, thus more likely to persist in nonrecombinogenic regions by virtue of "Muller's ratchet." Single-copy genes in a genome are largely found in euchromatin, while even small multigene families show enrichment in heterochromatin. Modern cereal chromosomes that result from a genome duplication thought to have occurred about 70 million years ago (Paterson et al. 2009) continue to show very close correlation in the abundance of genes and repetitive DNA despite nearly complete turnover of specific repetitive DNA elements, suggesting that the euchromatic and heterochromatic states, respectively, have persisted for at least 70 million years. This general pattern of genome organization appears to hold true in additional angiosperms (Schmutz et al. 2010).

The genome sequences empower new approaches to crop improvement. Access to a virtually unlimited set of prospective DNA markers mitigates the need for marker discovery by costly and tedious genetic mapping. Indeed, access to the entire set of genes opens the door to genetic analysis approaches that focus on the genes directly rather than relying on diagnostic DNA markers. Combined with new "resequencing" approaches, "genotyping by sequencing" may become the most cost-effective means to characterize individual segregants in plant populations. Likewise, massively parallel sequencing may soon (if not already) be the most cost-effective means to study gene expression patterns in specific organs, developmental stages, or in response to exogenous treatments.

Particularly exciting is the opportunity to greatly accelerate the characterization of "gene banks" for most of the world's leading crops. A reference sequence provides a static picture of a genome, while the reality is that genomes are dynamically changing. The ability to obtain substantial sequence information for "core collections" sampled from much larger collections of germplasm provides insight into the levels and patterns of contemporaneous evolution that are occurring in a gene pool and has also proven to be a powerful means to identify high-probability candidate genes likely to be responsible for some traits (Harjes et al. 2008, Thornsberry et al. 2001, Weber et al. 2008, Yu et al. 2008, 2005a). Much as mammalian geneticists are now working to characterize the entire spectrum of allelic variants in human, the ability to resequence the contents of the world's plant gene banks (numbering more than 1 million accessions in the CGIAR and USDA germplasm collections alone) would provide a resource of unprecedented power for use in deterministic plant breeding approaches.

While it is now feasible to sequence many crop genomes, several challenges remain to be overcome. In particular, we do not yet have a high-quality reference sequence for any autopolyploid, thus excluding a host of important crops particularly among forages and biomass crops. In principle, the challenge of being able to identify four, six, or more alleles that might segregate among the members of a homologous series of chromosomes in an autopolyploid is manageable—high depth of sequence coverage permits the distinction of alleles from errors by virtue of redundant sampling (Dehal et al. 2002). However, assembly of such genomes into their linear arrangement, in a manner that permits us to visualize the arrangement of allelic variation along each member of a homologous series of chromosomes, is extremely challenging, requiring high-quality sequencing reads that are sufficiently long to cover multiple single-nucleotide polymorphisms (SNPs) that distinguish among allelic variants. No doubt this will come, but it is not in place yet. An interim step for such genomes may be to "revert" to a bacterial artificial chromosome (BAC)-based approach, revealing the basic gene set by sequencing a tiling path of clones that cover the basic chromosomal complement and setting aside the task of detecting allelic variation until sequencing is cheaper or alternative approaches emerge.

## 7.3  BIOINFORMATICS

The generation of tremendous volumes of sequence information would be of limited value without the concurrent development of the resources and tools necessary to store, distribute, analyze, and annotate information in a timely fashion. The relatively new field of bioinformatics addresses these challenges by utilizing efficient data management strategies, generating and maintaining web-based interfaces to access and submit information, and developing the algorithms necessary to compare multiple sequences and identify homology or conserved motifs in a reliable manner. Bioinformatics is a rapidly evolving field and it is likely by the time this chapter is in press, that much of the information contained here will be supplemented or replaced. The journal *Nucleic Acids Research* publishes a database issue each January to introduce new resources and provide updates on existing ones. The most current version included 58 new data resources and updates to 73 previously published data resources (Cochrane and Galperin 2010). The online database collection currently holds 1230 data resources (http://www.oxfordjournals.org/nar/database/a/). The objective here is not to provide a comprehensive overview, but to discuss how available resources are being utilized by those working on improvement of food crops. Recently, we have seen the development of bioinformatic tools that are tailored to breeders, yet also provide the opportunity to view selection and improvement from a broader biological interpretation; one that is consistent with the integration of multiple "omic" disciplines in plant science toward a single systems biology approach.

Simply put, the purpose of a database is to store information and to allow for efficient submissions and timely retrieval. As mundane as this might appear at first glance, databases and the information they contain are of limited value if they cannot be accessed and utilized readily by biologists who may have only rudimentary knowledge of informatics. Today's databases serves as functional interfaces between informatics and research applications, and have greatly benefited from the concurrent spread of the world wide web and the increase in computational power and speed of modern personal computers. Great strides have occurred since Genbank, developed by the National Center for Biotechnology Information (NCBI) originated in the early 1980s with a skeleton crew manually keying in sequences from published papers (Sayers et al. 2009). Through query interfaces and appropriate cross-links, searches through hundreds of millions of sequences can be accomplished both rapidly and reliably, and even novice users can obtain useful information with little prior training.

Databases are classified as primary or secondary sites depending on how broad or focused their scope and objectives are. Primary databases serve as initial sites for the collection and distribution of nucleotide or protein sequence information for multiple organisms. In addition to Genbank, the most familiar of these include the European Molecular Biology Laboratory Nucleotide Sequence Database (EMBL) and the DNA database of Japan (DDBJ) (Stoesser et al. 1997). Along with Genbank, these databases are partner organizations in the International Nucleotide Sequence Database Collaboration (INSDC), which provides for exchanges of information and uniformity of content among the sites (Benson et al. 2010). In addition to the sequence information and appropriate references, each record in a primary database can also provide available passport information such as the scientific name and taxonomy of the source organism, annotations, and areas of biological significance (coding regions and their protein translations, transcription units, repeat regions, and sites of mutations or modifications). Cross-references are provided to protein sequence databases and to Pubmed (if literature references for the sequence are available).

Analogous primary databases for proteins include the Universal Protein Resource (UniProt) that consists of two parts: UniProtKB/Swissprot developed by the Swiss Institute of Bioinformatics (SIB) and UniProtKB/TrEMBL(Translated EMBL). Swissprot provides manual annotation of each submission and is considered the gold standard of protein databases (Bairoch and Apweiler 2008, UniProt Consortium 2010). TrEMBL includes automated translation of DNA submissions to EMBL and other primary DNA sequence databases. Manual annotation of both protein and nucleotide sequences remains the greatest challenge facing database curators as it consumes considerable time and financial resources to conduct critical reviews of available literature and to examine in-depth the experimental or computer-generated data associated with each submission. Curators must examine evidence from expressed sequence tags (ESTs), full length cDNAs, and known proteins in addition to available evidences from direct assays, genetic interactions, and mutant phenotype studies before assigning a function to a given sequence. The need for high value, actively curated databases has increased dramatically over the past decade and calls for community annotation and creative strategies such as "annotation jamborees" have done little to solve the backlogs of sequence information awaiting manual annotation in most crop species (Ohyanagi et al. 2006).

Several ab initio or automated gene finding programs such as GlimmerM or GeneMark (based on standard or modified Hidden Markov Model algorithms) have been developed in recent years to provide initial annotation to the enormous amount of sequencing data produced by de novo sequencing projects but even the best of these programs requires manual curation to remove discrepancies and refine predictions (Baldi et al. 1994, Lomsadze et al. 2005, Pertea and Salzberg 2002). These programs predict putative genes within the sequence by identifying features such as transcription initiation and stop sites, splice sites, and polyadenylated tails. The programs either utilize training sets of known full length cDNAs or can be completely ab initio.

Secondary databases cater to specific niches such as individual plant species or clades, specific gene families or to specialized genomic features. Examples include the Arabidopsis Information Resource (TAIR), Genome database for Rosaceae (GDR), and SOL-Solanaceus Genomics Network (SGN) (Jung et al. 2008, Mueller et al. 2005, Swarbreck et al. 2008). Secondary databases can be as simple as a resource for a single research lab to multi-institutional resource providing information to hundreds of labs around the world. What these databases lack in computational power or available resources is made up for in flexibility and in providing expertise to address specific needs of their respective communities. Gramene (http://www.gramene.org), for example, serves a resource for comparative grass genomics (Liang et al. 2008). The focus on comparative genomics and the transfer of information from model crops such as rice and sorghum to complex polyploids such as wheat, allows it to tailor and prioritize their efforts to study micro- and macrosynteny across grass species.

Bioinformatic tools, either stand-alone programs or those imbedded within databases, allow users to perform searches based on homology or ontological features; to align multiple sequences; to visualize sequences in relation to other genomic features; and to identify conserved features such as open reading frames, coding regions, SNPs, or tandem repeats. A list of some of the more common tools is provided in Table 7.1. Basic local alignment search tool (Blast) has become such a standardized tool for identifying homologous sequences that the program name is often used to describe its function (Altschul et al. 1990). NCBI-Blast is arguably the most commonly used bioinformatic tool and contains multiple algorithms for searching protein and nucleotide databases. BlastN and BlastP allow for searches of nucleotide and protein databases, respectively, using similar queries. Tblastn allows users to query a nucleotide database with a protein sequence by translating all nucleotide sequences into six theoretically protein sequences based on all possible reading frames. Results of such searches generally produce identity scores (a ratio of identical nucleotides to total nucleotides) and similarity scores (a measure of how likely one sequence is related to another over evolutionary time).

One of the most significant breakthroughs in bioinformatics has been the standardized usage of terms associated with assignment of genes into functional classes. Gene Ontology (GO) established by the GO consortium allows for the classification of genes based on s categories: biological process, molecular function, and the cellular localization (Harris et al. 2004). Blast2Go incorporates initial blast search results from NCBI with ontology results from the GO database to provide an annotation of unknown sequences that can be weighted by the user (Götz et al. 2008).

ClustalW and a host of similar programs allow for the alignment of multiple DNA and protein sequences (Chenna et al. 2003). Most programs generally allow for adjustable gap penalties based on position, content, and the length of the sequence for insertions or deletions that might occur between distantly related sequences. Multiple alignment programs have become particularly important in identifying

**TABLE 7.1**

**List of Useful Bioinformatic Resources**

| Resource | URL | Description |
|---|---|---|
| NCBI | http://www.ncbi.nih.gov/ | Database and tools available through NCBI (Blast, Pubmed) |
| SwissProt | http://us.expasy.org/sprot/ | Primary protein database |
| TAIR database | http://www.arabidopsis.org/ | *Arabidopsis* database |
| SOL database | http://solgenomics.net/ | Solanaceae crops |
| Gramene | http://www.gramene.org/ | Comparative genome analysis of grasses |
| GDR | http://www.rosaceae.org/ | Rosaceae genomics |
| ClustalW | http://www.clustal.org/ | Multiple sequence alignment |
| Gbrowse | http://webgbrowse.cgb.indiana.edu/ | Web version of generic genome browser |
| Apollo | http://www.gmod.org/wiki/Main_Page | Genome browser with editing function |
| Artemis | http://www.sanger.ac.uk/resources/software/artemis | Genome browser with editing function |
| Cmap | http://www.gmod.org/wiki/Main_Page | Comparison of genetic, physical, and sequence maps |
| Primer3 | http://www-genome.wi.mit.edu/genome_software/other/primer3.html | Design of PCR primers |
| Gmap | http://research-pub.gene.com/gmap/ | Mapping and aligning cDNA sequences to a genome |
| repeatmasker | http://www.repeatmasker.org | Screens DNA sequences for interspersed repeats and low complexity DNA sequences |
| Blast2GO | http://www.blast2go.org | Functional annotation of novel sequences and analysis of annotation data |
| GO Database | http://www.geneontology.org/ | Contains ontology, gene product, sequence, and manual annotation data |
| GlimmerM | http://www.cbcb.umd.edu/software/glimmerm/index.shtml | A gene finder developed specifically for eukaryotes |
| GeneMark | http://exon.gatech.edu/ | Gene prediction in eukaryotes |
| KEGG | http://www.genome.ad.jp/kegg/ | Pathway maps for metabolism and other cellular processes |
| MISA | http://pgrc.ipk-gatersleben.de/misa/ | Identification and localization microsatellites |
| SeqMap | http://www.stanford.edu/group/wonglab/jiangh/seqmap/ | Mapping short sequence reads to reference genome |
| Mosaik | http://bioinformatics.bc.edu/marthlab/Mosaik | SNP and INDEL discovery from short reads |

relationships among related individuals and among members of gene families. A particularly important use of these tools has been in identifying polymorphisms that can be used to design molecular markers from accessions in databases, from collections of ESTs, or from database entries, amplicon resequencing, and directed next-generation genomic sequencing efforts.

Genomic browsers provide graphical interfaces of sequence information in relation to other genomic features. These browsers provide visualization that ranges from megabases of sequence information to the level of individual nucleotides and offers a way to visually inspect the available evidence from gene prediction programs, cDNAs, and protein sequences to determine the appropriate modeling of a specific gene and to infer the presence of alternative splicing within a given coding region. Linking genomic sequencing data with molecular markers and genetic linkage maps through programs such as CMap provides a mechanism for identifying putative markers close to the gene of interest, and in the case of quantitative trait loci (QTLs) also allows for the identification of putative candidate genes within the confidence intervals. CMap, originally written for the Gramene project, and now available through Generic model organism database (GMOD) is also an important tool for comparative analysis across closely related organisms (Youens-Clark et al. 2009). NCBI's embedded map viewer allows for cross links to all of the tools and sequence information available in NCBI's associated databases, but it suffers from not allowing third party data to be utilized (Wheeler et al. 2009). GBrowse (The Generic Genome Browser) allows third party data and has gained considerable favor by utilizing flexible plug-ins to allow customization by the numerous projects that have adopted it as their default viewer. A web-based accessible version is currently available (Podicheti et al. 2009). One of the few drawbacks associated with GBrowse has been the lack of an editing function. Even the earliest sequenced plant genomes continue to undergo refinement as new experimental data is evaluated. Plant genomic sequences should be seen as dynamic and not fixed and will continue to require input from the community (with appropriate curation) to refine and improve the working draft. Apollo and Artemis are examples of stand-alone genomic browsers that allow editing function and contain many of the same features associated with GBrowse (Lewis et al. 2002, Rutherford et al. 2000). Apollo and Gbrowse, and several other useful open source programs are available through the GMOD, a consortium of intuitions that provides links and downloads for several useful programs (http://gmod.org).

Of particular interest to breeders are algorithms that identify potential molecular markers from databases, ESTs libraries, or from genomic sequencing data. Arguably, the two most commonly used molecular markers are microsatellites or Simple Sequence Repeats (SSRs) and SNPs. SSRs are tandem di-, tri-, and tetranucleotide repeats found within coding regions of genes and throughout the intergenic regions of plant genomes. Perfect SSRs are stretches of repeats without interruption, while imperfect SSRs are disrupted by nonrepeating nucleotides. Complex SSRs are made up of one or more simple SSRs adjacent to each other. A number of algorithms have developed to identify SSRs but they differ primarily in their speed and ability to recognize imperfect and complex SSRs (Leclercq et al. 2007). MIcroSAtellite (Misa), simple sequence repeat identification tool (SSRIT), and RepeatFinder are some of the more commonly used programs available (Agarwal et al. 2007, Temnykh et al. 2001,

Volfovsky et al. 2001). An additional benefit of some programs such as Misa is that they allow for the installation of the primer design software primer3, which simplifies the primer design (Rozen and Skaletsky 2000).

Traditionally, identifying SNPs has been accomplished through data mining of redundant EST accessions or through sequencing of selected amplicons using panels of divergent genotypes. A number of programs such as Polybayes and SNPDetector are available to identify polymorphisms from chromatography trace files (Marth et al. 1999, Zhang et al. 2005). The drawback of these approaches is that they are limited to utilizing only what sequence information has been previously generated and is dependent on the quality of the data itself: data mining requires the generation of well-annotated, high-quality ESTs, while sequencing amplicon is dependent on having primer information. Amplicon sequencing can also be a time consuming effort. When a draft genomic sequence is available, identifying large numbers of SNPs through resequencing with next-generation sequencing (NGS) platforms has been accomplished. In *Arabidopsis*, >15X resequencing of two ecotypes followed by alignment to Col-0 led to the identification of 823,325 SNPs and ~80,000 1–3 bp insertion/deletions (Ossowski et al. 2008). Numerous programs to align short NGS reads have been developed including Mosaik, SeqMap, and SOAP (Jiang and Wong 2008, Li et al. 2008).

## 7.4  MOLECULAR MARKERS AND IMPROVEMENT OF FOOD PLANTS

Molecular markers are the most common way genomic information is utilized in plant improvement. Markers represent visualized polymorphisms in the DNA sequence and function as "fingerprints" at specific locations on the chromosome and provide a method of indirect selection for traits that are difficult to score due to cost or to incomplete expression of traits at a particular developmental stage or environment. Early selection using markers, particularly for woody perennials like grape or blueberry, saves considerable time and expense over conventional selection strategies.

The first markers described were phenotypic in nature and represented highly heritable traits such as seed or flower color. Sax (1923) described a statistical relationship between seed color (a physical marker) and seed weight (a quantitative trait) and is often credited with the first description of a QTL. Often, phenotypic markers were due to deleterious recessive mutations that limited their use, as did the difficulty of assembling significant numbers of these mutants in a single selection population. Restriction fragment length polymorphisms (RFLPs) began a new era in QTL detection as these markers were plentiful, but they required the use of radioactive probes and were labor intensive. RFLPs were largely replaced by PCR-based marker systems in the late 1990s. Many of the earliest PCR markers systems such as random amplified polymorphic DNAs (RAPDs) and amplified fragment length polymorphisms (AFLPs) were highly informative but suffered from a lack of reproducibility. These early systems were themselves largely replaced by SSRs and SNPs that are much more amendable to automation and high-throughput genotyping.

Early DNA markers were generally random in nature due to a lack of available genomic information. Identifying associations between markers and genes of interest depended on having evenly spaced informative markers across a well-defined genetic linkage map. Moving from the marker to the actual gene or genes that produced the desired effect was itself a challenge as the distance of a few centimorgans along a chromosome might well represent several hundred putative genes.

With the advent of high-throughput transcriptome and genomic sequencing, the availability of bioinformatic tools to assign putative function to the sequences, and the adaptation of microarray technology, the possibility of genotyping thousands of genes in a single pass has become a reality in some crops, and commercial genotyping arrays have become available for a number of crops (Jeremy et al. 2008, Winzeler et al. 1998). Currently, Illumina GoldenGate assays are able to genotype up to 1,536 polymorphic sites in 384 individuals in a single reaction and custom-designed Affymetrix arrays can genotype 44,100 SNPs (Oliphant et al. 2002, Tung et al. 2010). Recently, whole genome resequencing has also been demonstrated to be a viable alternative to array genotyping and may ultimately become the method of choice as the cost of short read sequencing becomes more affordable and the higher error of these techniques is accounted for (Huang et al. 2009a,b).

On the subject of molecular markers, the fields of breeding and molecular genetics are sometimes at odds with each other. Breeders look to manipulate naturally occurring variation to pursue a specific applied end (e.g., electing plants that are higher yielding or better suited to meet challenges in a specific environment). Geneticists seek to understand the variation in terms of specific features (e.g., coding region polymorphisms, variation in gene copy number, or noncoding factors that affect gene expression). While these pursuits are not mutually exclusive, they sometimes result in different experimental approaches. As Bernardo (2008) points out: "they require different emphases on gene discovery versus selection, require different levels of stringency for declaring the presence of a QTL, require different levels of resolution for pinpointing QTL location, and usually require different types of germplasm."

The candidate gene identification (CGI) is generally favored by geneticists and utilizes markers based on known gene sequences to validate their involvement in the trait of interest (Pflieger et al. 2001). The benefit of this approach is that the marker and the gene are in near or complete linkage disequilibrium that reduces the potential of linkage drag and increases the statistical power to estimate the effect. An additional benefit to the geneticists is that the polymorphism that produces the marker is also potentially the causative factor of the observed phenotype. The success of this strategy depends on the a priori knowledge about the physiological, biochemical, or functional aspects of the possible candidates (Zhu and Zhao 2007). The absence of such knowledge in regard to complex and quantitative traits limits the usage of CGI but it has been effective, particularly, in regard to gene–disease research of humans and animals (Tabor et al. 2002).

In crops where structural and functional information is limited, research from related or model crops can be utilized. *Arabidopsis*, a relative of the economically important oilseed, vegetable and condiments in the Brassicaceae family has provided considerable candidate gene information to their improvement. Alignment of common markers between *Arabidopsis* and the *Brassicas* has demonstrated considerable localized synteny and colinearity (Lagercrantz et al. 1996). Consensus primers derived from conserved regions of *Arabidopsis* have been useful in amplifying partial sequences of *B. napus* genes impacting fatty-acid synthesis, disease resistance, and flowering time (Fourmann et al. 2002). Recently, consensus primer sequences from conserved regions of *Arabidopsis* γ-tocopherol methyltransferase were used to develop markers associated with modified vitamin E content in oilseed rape (Endrigkeit et al. 2009). The FLOWERING LOCUS C (FLC) originally cloned in *Arabidopsis* plays an important role in flowering and response to vernalization. Markers based on this sequence have cosegregated with QTLs in several *Brassica* crops (Lou et al. 2007, Okazaki et al. 2007, Osborn et al. 1997, Schranz et al. 2002, Tadege et al. 2001, Teutonico and Osborn 1995).

While CGI has worked well with simply inherited traits, the complex and polygenic nature of many economic traits and the difficulty involved in selecting or introgressing these multiple genes (or QTLs) into elite breeding material has limited its use. In all fairness, it should be noted that these difficulties are not limited to CGI, and, in general, the utilization of QTLs has lagged significantly behind our ability to identify them (Bernardo 2008). In the 30 years since our coauthor first described some of the first principles of QTL analysis, we have witnessed the development of increasingly more sophisticated algorithms for detecting QTL position, effect, and interactions.

## 7.5 RECOMBINANT TECHNIQUES IN CROP IMPROVEMENT

The advance of "omics" research also facilitates novel gene discovery. The extensive gene discovery in addition to the development of gene transfer technologies accelerates crop improvement through biotechnological approach. Plant biotechnology has become an import adjunct to traditional plant breeding (Shewry et al. 2008). While traditional plant breeding involves selective breeding to produce desired traits by crossing of a thousand genes, plant biotechnology allows plant breeders to develop crops with specific traits by using one or a few genes. The common recombinant techniques used in generating biotech crops are described in the following.

### 7.5.1 MANIPULATION OF GENE EXPRESSION

The first crucial step in the production of biotech crops is to construct suitable chimeric DNA transformation constructs that contain "genes of interest" driven by specific promoters. Diverse DNA sources from different species can be used. Manipulation of transgene expression is achieved by using specific promoters. The cauliflower mosaic virus 35S gene promoter, maize polyubiquitin, and rice *actin* promoter are commonly used in plants for constitutive expression of "genes of interest." In many cases, the desire to target transgene products in agriculturally important tissues and organs makes the tissue-specific or inducible promoters of particular interest. A number of tissue-specific promoters have been identified and used. These include globulin (*glb*) and glutelin (*glu*) promoter that produces endosperm-specific gene expression in rice and maize, and starch granular bound starch synthase (GBSS) and patatin promoters that drive tuber-specific expression in potato tubers.

## 7.5.2 GENE STACKING

The simultaneous transfer of multiple genes into plants is rapidly gaining popularity in biotech crop production to stack different genes and traits (Halpin 2005). Various techniques and strategies have been developed (Naqvi et al. 2010). The conventional stacking methods include crossing transgenic lines or sequential transformation, but suffer from a long and labor-intensive development process. Cotransformation is one of the most promising approaches for simultaneous introduction of multiple transgenes into crops (Halpin 2005, Naqvi et al. 2010). In this method, multiple genes are constructed either within a single transferred DNA (T-DNA) or on different T-DNA. Cotransformation strategy has been successfully used for the production of Golden Rice (Ye et al. 2000) and multivitamin corn (Naqvi et al. 2009). A more recent development of gene stacking technology is the use of engineered minichromosome to transfer and express multiple sets of genes into crops (Houben and Schubert 2007).

## 7.5.3 RNA INTERFERENCE

While many plant biotechnology applications aim at producing more specifically desired compounds in food crops through enhancing expression of genes of interest, genetic engineering of food crops that contain reduced levels of unwanted compounds is achieved by downregulating the endogenous gene expression using a targeted gene silencing approach such as RNA interference (RNAi). RNAi that refers to several different types of RNA-mediated gene silencing is an effective and highly specific knockdown technology (Chen 2010). This technology involves the use of double-stranded RNA (dsRNA) as a trigger to degrade a targeted gene or its promoter region in a homology dependent manner, leading to posttranscriptional or transcriptional targeted gene silencing (McGinnis 2010). The use of DNA constructs that generate hairpin dsRNA greatly improves the efficiency of targeted gene silencing (Waterhouse et al. 1998). The transgene construct can be designed to simultaneously silence multiple, closely related target genes. In comparison with dsRNA, artificial microRNA (miRNA) technology offers more specificity that permits more controlled silencing of specific genes (Schwab et al. 2006). Because of the effectiveness and specificity at silencing one or more genes in a wide range of plant species, transgene-induced RNAi techniques have potential for broad applications such as a powerful functional genomics tool. RNAi has become the technology of choice preferred over earlier approaches of using antisense or cosuppression, although the commercial biotech crops, such as ringspot-resistant papaya, were originally developed using antisense technology.

## 7.5.4 GENE TRANSFER TECHNIQUES

A prerequisite for crop genetic engineering is the ability to transfer genes of interest into plant cells. During the past decades, a number of plant transformation techniques have been developed (Rao et al. 2009). *Agrobacterium*-mediated transformation and particle bombardment represent the two major methods that are used extensively in crop species.

The soil-born *Agrobacterium tumefaciens* is well known to cause the crown-gall disease of plants. The tumor-inducing (Ti) plasmid was found to carry a piece of DNA, T-DNA, which is inserted into the plant genome during infection (Chilton et al. 1977). This exciting discovery led to the use of the Ti plasmid of *Agrobacterium* as vectors for plant transformation (Hernalsteens et al. 1980). Binary vectors that contain T-DNA borders, selectable marker genes, and replicate origins for both *Escherichia coli* and *A. tumefaciens* were developed in 1984 (Bevan 1984), which form the basis of plant transformation vectors commonly used today. T-DNA transfer also requires the virulence genes. The development of T-DNA binary systems that contain binary vectors and disarmed Ti plasmids opens up the era of plant genetic engineering for crop improvement. Both binary vectors and the *Agrobacterium* strains containing disarmed Ti plasmids have been improved during the past decades to meet the specific needs of plant transformation (Lee and Gelvin 2008).

Particle bombardment or biolistic transformation is a direct gene transfer technology. It involves the coating of naked DNA with micron-sized metal particles and the high-velocity bombardment to deliver DNA into intact recipient plant cells (Sanford 2000). This technology was developed in the 1980s and has been widely adopted since early 1990s. Particle bombardment is relatively genotype independent and can be used for a broad range of plant species. Many important transgenic crop species were first generated by using this technology.

The ability to regenerate plants following gene transfer in plant cells is another key step for crop genetic engineering. In many cases, production of transgenic crops requires tissue culture phase. Advances in developing a large number of reliable regeneration protocols for different plant species facilitate the progress in genetic engineering of food crops.

### 7.5.5 SELECTABLE MARKER REMOVAL

Selectable marker genes in the transformation constructs allow the selection of transformed individuals. Some commonly used selectable marker genes are *nptII*, *hpt*, and *bar* whose products resist to kanamycin, hygromycin, and BASTA/Biolophos, respectively. Because of the public concerns for the presence of antibiotic marker genes in genetically engineered crops, several techniques are developed to remove marker genes after selection to produce "marker-free" biotech crops. These approaches include the use of homologous recombination to excise the marker genes, different transformation constructs followed by genetic segregation of the markers from traits of interest, and transposon-mediated marker gene elimination (Gidoni et al. 2008). The use of site-specific recombination technique, however, becomes a popular approach for marker removal. The most commonly used site-specific recombination systems are *Cre/lox* and flippase recognition target/*flippase recombination enzyme* (*FLP/FRT*) that involve the interaction of a single recombinase of *Cre* or *FLP* with a pair of identical recognition target sites of *lox* or *FRT* (Broach 1982, Sternberg and Hamilton 1981). The selectable marker genes are flanked between directly oriented recombination sites in the DNA transformation constructs. Following the selection, a *Cre* or *FLP* gene encoding the recombinase is stably or transiently expressed to excise away the flanked marker gene (Srivastava and Gidoni 2010). This technology has been successfully implemented for the generation of the first U.S. regulatory approval marker-free high-lysine transgenic maize, LY038 (Ow 2007). Less controversial types of selectable marker systems such as phosphomannose isomerase (PMI) avoid the use of antibiotic marker genes (Bojsen et al. 1999).

## 7.6   BIOTECH CROPS WITH VALUE-ADDED TRAITS

Biotech crops were first commercially grown in 1994. Since the large-scale cultivation of major commodity crops in 1996, biotech crops have obtained wide adoption with over 330 million acres (134 million hectares) in 25 countries in 2009 (James 2009). While the first generation of biotech crops focuses on traits that improve crop performance in the field, biotech crops with value-added traits that benefit consumers are on the way for commercial production.

### 7.6.1   GOLDEN RICE

Worldwide, some 250 million preschool children are vitamin A deficient (World Health Organization), which is caused primarily by simple diets of staple foods with low levels of provitamin A carotenoids. Golden Rice is a rice variety engineered to produce beta-carotene provitamin A carotenoid in seed endosperm. It was developed to fortify food to help combat global vitamin A deficiency. Golden Rice represents the most well-publicized case for genetically engineered crops with nutritional enhancement.

*Agrobacterium*-mediated transformation was used to simultaneously transfer multiple genes encoding enzymes for the entire beta-carotene biosynthetic pathway in two vectors into rice endosperm (Beyer et al. 2002, Ye et al. 2000). Daffodil phytoene synthase and a bacterial phytoene desaturase under control of the endosperm-specific glutelin and CaMV35S promoter, respectively, were placed in one vector. Daffodil lycopene beta cyclase under control of the rice glutelin promoter was constructed in another vector with *hpt* as selectable marker. Cotransformation of these two vectors results in the production of Golden Rice containing 1.6 µg/g carotenoids in the endosperm (Ye et al. 2000). Subsequently, Golden Rice 2 with more intensely colored seeds was generated by Syngenta using maize phytoene synthase with nonantibiotic PMI marker gene as selectable marker. The Golden Rice 2 contains up to 31 µg/g total beta-carotene, a level adequate for the potential to reduce vitamin A malnutrition in small children (Paine et al. 2005). Following the regulatory approval for field trials, Golden Rice has been integrated with local rice cultivars in a number of countries (http://www.goldenrice.org/). Since no rice germplasms produce beta-carotene in the endosperm, genetic engineering represents the only way to introduce beta-carotene trait in the crop.

### 7.6.2   HIGH-OLEIC-ACID SOYBEAN

Soybeans provide approximately 70%–80% of total fat and oil consumption in the United States (http:/www/soystats.com). Soybean oil contains over 50% polyunsaturated fatty acids (linoleic 18:2 and linolenic 18:3). The usual hydrogenation process increases oil stability but also causes the formation of trans fatty acids, which are associated with increased risk of cardiovascular diseases (Remig et al. 2010).

High-oleic-acid (18:1) oil represents a healthy product that contains zero trans fatty acids along with significantly increased oil stability (Damude and Kinney 2008).

A high-oleic-acid biotech soybean developed by Pioneer Hi-Bred, a Dupont company, has been recently approved by USDA for commercial production in the United States (DuPont News Release). It will be the first biotech crop with improved oil trait to be on market. The high-oleic-acid soybean was produced by using particle bombardment technology to transform embryos with a construct containing two cassettes. One cassette has a fragment of soybean *fad2-1* under control of soybean seed-preferred kunitz trysin inhibitor gene promoter and the other one contains soybean acetolactate synthase gene regulated by S-adenosyl-L-methionine synthetase promoter as selectable marker (GM Crop Database: http://www.cera-gmc.org/). The use of antisense *fad2-1* causes tissue-specific silencing of the expression of the endogenous omega-6 desaturase gene, resulting in blocking the synthesis of downstream products and accumulating over 75% oleic acid in seeds. High-oleic-acid biotech soybean, marketed as Plenish™ by DuPont, is anticipated to be on the U.S. market in 2012 (DuPont News Release).

### 7.6.3 FOLATE BIOFORTIFIED RICE

Folates are B vitamins. Folate deficiency is a global health problem, affecting not only many people in developing countries, but also a surprisingly large population in developed countries (Bekaert et al. 2008). Recent research has established that it is possible to biofortify rice by engineering folate biosynthetic pathway to satisfy the daily folate requirement for an average adult person (Storozhenko et al. 2007).

Folates are synthesized from pteridine, p-aminobenzoate (PABA), and glutamate precursor. *Agrobacterium*-mediated transformation technology was used to introduce rice with a T-DNA construct stacking with guanosine-5′-triphosphate (GTP) cyclohydrolase I (*GCHI*) and aminodeoxychorismate synthase (*ADCS*) genes, which encode the first enzyme for pteridin and PABA synthesis, respectively. The transgenic lines expressing *GCHI* and *ADCS* under control of either the rice endosperm-specific globulin (*glb-1*) or the glutelin B1 promoter accumulate folates to 1723 µg/100 g fresh weight rice seeds (Storozhenko et al. 2007), a level that is adequate for a micronutrient daily requirement.

The aforementioned examples represent some best known cases of using genetic engineering techniques to broad biotech crops with value-added traits beyond those that improve plant performance in the field. The fast development of "omics" technology and an increased understanding of plant metabolic pathways permit the generation of biotech food crops with improved nutritional value and premium quality. Plant biotechnology in the "omics" era provides plant breeders an unprecedented opportunity for crop improvement.

## 7.7  CONCLUSIONS

We are entering an exciting and challenging time in the course of crop improvement. The past decade has seen the release of 10 genomic draft sequences of various plant species, and more are currently being generated with NGS platforms. Concurrently, we have seen the development of high-throughput genotyping and expression arrays, the availability of bioinformatic tools and resources, and ever more efficient ways of introducing novel genes into elite breeding material through the use of molecular markers and recombinant techniques. Equally exciting is the prospect of multiple "omics" disciplines converging into an integrated plant systems approach that provides not only additional tools, but also opportunities to examine in greater detail the biological and physiological processes that currently limit the improvement of food crops. Metabolomics, for example, with the promise of accurately identifying and quantifying thousands of small molecular weight compounds with tandem liquid chromatography and mass spec, could revolutionize breeding for human nutrition and health.

These advancements could not come at a more opportune time. Breeders have made impressive gains throughout the years in developing higher yielding plants that are better adapted to environmental challenges, but the combined pressures of population growth, limited production areas, and dwindling genetic resources make it even more imperative that we continue to stay ahead of the curve in producing high-quality productive crops for the twenty-first century.

## REFERENCES

Agarwal, R. K., P. S. Hendre, R. K. Varshney, P. R. Bhat, V. Krishnakumar, and L. Singh. 2007. Identification characterization and utilization of EST-derived genic microsatellite markers for genome analysis of coffee and related species. *Theor Appl Genet* 114:359–372.

Altschul, S. F., W. Gish, W. Miller, E. W. Myers, and D. J. Lipman. 1990. Basic local alignment search tool. *J Mol Biol* 215:403–410.

Bairoch, A. and R. Apweiler. 2008. The SWISS-PROT protein sequence database and its supplement TrEMBL in 2000. *Nucleic Acids Res* 28:45–48.

Baldi, P., Y. Chauvin, T. Hunkapiller, and M. A. McClure. 1994. Hidden Markov models of biological primary sequence information. *Proc Natl Acad Sci USA* 91:1059–1063.

Bekaert, S., S. Storozhenko, P. Mehrshahi et al. 2008. Folate biofortification in food plants. *Trends Plant Sci* 13:28–35.

Benson, D. A., I. Karsch-Mizrachi, D. J. Lipman, J. Ostell, and E. W. Sayers. 2010. GenBank. *Nucleic Acids Res* 38:46–51.

Bernardo, R. 2008. Molecular markers and selection for complex traits in plants: Learning from the last 20 years. *Crop Sci* 48:1649–1664.

Bevan, M. 1984. Binary agrobacterium vectors for plant transformation. *Nucleic Acids Res* 12:8711–8721.

Beyer, P., S. Al Babili, X. Ye et al. 2002. Golden Rice: Introducing the beta-carotene biosynthesis pathway into rice endosperm by genetic engineering to defeat vitamin A deficiency. *J Nutr* 132:506S–510S.

Blanc, G. S. and K. H. Wolfe. 2004. Widespread paleopolyploidy in model plant species inferred from age distributions of duplicate genes. *Plant Cell* 16:1667–1678.

Bojsen, K., I. Donaldson, A. Haldrup et al. 1999. Positive selection. United States Patent, No. 5, 994, 629.

Bowers, J. E., M. A. Arias, R. Asher et al. 2005. Comparative physical mapping links conservation of microsynteny to chromosome structure and recombination in grasses. *Proc Natl Acad Sci USA* 102:13206–13211.

Bowers, J. E., B. A. Chapman, J. Rong, and A. H. Paterson. 2003. Unravelling angiosperm genome evolution by phylogenetic analysis of chromosomal duplication events. *Nature* 422:433–438.

Broach, J. R. 1982. The yeast plasmid 2 mu circle. *Cell* 28:203–204.

Chapman, B. A., J. E. Bowers, F. A. Feltus, and A. H. Paterson. 2006. Buffering crucial functions by paleologous duplicated genes may impart cyclicality to angiosperm genome duplication. *Proc Natl Acad Sci USA* 103:2730–2735.

Chen, X. 2010. Small RNAs—Secrets and surprises of the genome. *Plant J* 61:941–958.

Cheng, Z. K., C. R. Buell, R. A. Wing, M. H. Gu, and J. M. Jiang. 2001. Towards a cytological characterization of the rice genome. *Genome Res* 11:2133–2141.

Chenna, R., H. Sugawara, T. Koike et al. 2003. Multiple sequence alignment with the Clustal series of program. *Nucleic Acids Res* 31:3497–3500.

Chilton, M. D., M. H. Drummond, D. J. Merio et al. 1977. Stable incorporation of plasmid DNA into higher plant cells: The molecular basis of crown gall tumorigenesis. *Cell* 11:263–271.

Cochrane, G. R. and M. Y. Galperin. 2010. The 2010 Nucleic Acids Research Database Issue and online database collection: A community of data resources. *Nucleic Acids Res* 38:1–4.

Collins, F. S., E. S. Lander, J. Rogers, and R. H. Waterston. 2004. Finishing the euchromatic sequence of the human genome. *Nature* 431:931–945.

Damude, H. G. and A. J. Kinney. 2008. Enhancing plant seed oils for human nutrition. *Plant Physiol* 147:962–968.

Dehal, P., Y. Satou, R. K. Campbell et al. 2002. The draft genome of *Ciona intestinalis*: Insights into chordate and vertebrate origins. *Science* 298:2157–2167.

Endrigkeit, J., X. Wang, D. Cai et al. 2009. Genetic mapping, cloning, and functional characterization of the BnaX.VTE4 gene encoding a gamma-tocopherol methyltransferase from oilseed rape. *Theor Appl Genet* 119:567–575.

Fourmann, M., P. Barret, N. Froger et al. 2002. From *Arabidopsis thaliana* to *Brassica napus*: Development of amplified consensus genetic markers (ACGM) for construction of a gene map. *Theor Appl Genet* 105:1196–1206.

Freeling, M. and B. C. Thomas. 2006. Gene-balanced duplications, like tetraploidy, provide predictable drive to increase morphological complexity. *Genome Res* 16:805–814.

Gidoni, D., V. Srivastava, and N. Carmi. 2008. Site-specific excisional recombination strategies for elimination of undesirable transgenes from crop plants. *In Vitro Cell Dev Biol-Plant* 44:457–467.

Goff, S. A., D. Ricke, T. H. Lan et al. 2002. A draft sequence of the rice genome (*Oryza sativa* L. spp *japonica*). *Science* 296:92–100.

Götz, S., J. M. García-Gómez, J. Terol et al. 2008. High-throughput functional annotation and data mining with the Blast2GO suite. *Nucleic Acids Res* 36:3420–3435.

Haldane, J. B. S. 1933. The part played by recurrent mutation in evolution. *Am Nat* 67:5–19.

Halpin, C. 2005. Gene stacking in transgenic plants—The challenge for 21st century plant biotechnology. *Plant Biotech J* 3:141–155.

Hansson, B., A. Kawabe, S. Preuss, H. Kuittinen, and D. Charlesworth. 2006. Comparative gene mapping in *Arabidopsis lyrata* chromosomes 1 and 2 and the corresponding *A. thaliana* chromosome 1: Recombination rates, rearrangements and centromere location. *Genet Res* 87:75–85.

Harjes, C. E., T. R. Rocheford, L. Bai et al. 2008. Natural genetic variation in lycopene epsilon cyclase tapped for maize biofortification. *Science* 319:330–333.

Harris, M. A., J. Clark, A. Ireland et al. 2004. The Gene Ontology (GO) database and informatics resource. *Nucleic Acids Res* 32:258–261.

Hernalsteens, J. P., F. V. Vliet, M. D. Beuckeleer et al. 1980. The *Agrobacterium tumefaciens* Ti plasmid as a host vector system for introducing foreign DNA in plant cells. *Nature* 287:654–656.

Houben, A. and I. Schubert. 2007. Engineered plant minichromosomes: A resurrection of B chromosomes? *Plant Cell* 19:2323–2327.

Huang, X., Q. Feng, Q. Qian et al. 2009b. High-throughput genotyping by whole-genome resequencing. *Genome Res* 19:1068–1076.

Huang, S., R. Li, Z. Zhang et al. 2009a. The genome of the cucumber, *Cucumis sativus* L. *Nat Genet* 41:1275–1281.

Initiative, T. A. G. 2000. Analysis of the genome sequence of the flowering plant *Arabidopsis thaliana. Nature* 408:796–815.

International Rice Genome Sequencing. 2005. The map-based sequence of the rice genome. *Nature* 436:793–800.

Jaillon, O., J. M. Aury, B. Noel et al. 2007. The grapevine genome sequence suggests ancestral hexaploidization in major angiosperm phyla. *Nature* 449:463–467.

James, C. 2009. Global status of commercialized biotech/GM crops: 2009. *ISAAA Brief* No. 41. ISAAA: Ithaca, NY.

Jeremy, E., J. Jaroslav, S. Megan et al. 2008. Development and evaluation of a high-throughput, low-cost genotyping platform based on oligonucleotide microarrays in rice. *Plant Methods* 4:13.

Jiang, H. and W. H. Wong. 2008. SeqMap: Mapping massive amount of oligonucleotides to the genome. *Bioinformatics* 24:2395–2396.

Jung, S., M. Staton, T. Lee et al. 2008. GDR (Genome Database for Rosaceae): Integrated web-database for rosaceae genomics and genetics data. *Nucleic Acids Res* 36:1034–1040.

Kawabe, A., B. Hansson, J. Hagenblad, A. Forrest, and D. Charlesworth. 2006. Centromere locations and associated chromosome rearrangements in *Arabidopsis lyrata* and *A. thaliana. Genetics* 173:1613–1619.

Kim, J. S., M. N. Islam-Faridi, P. E. Klein et al. 2005. Comprehensive molecular cyto-genetic analysis of sorghum genome architecture: Distribution of euchromatin, heterochromatin, genes and recombination in comparison to rice. *Genetics* 171:1963–1976.

Koch, M. A. and M. Kiefer. 2005. Genome evolution among cruciferous plants: A lecture from the comparison of the genetic maps of three diploid species—*Capsella rubella, Arabidopsis lyrata* subsp *Petraea*, and *A. thaliana. Am J Bot* 92:761–767.

Kuittinen, H., A. A. de Haan, C. Vogl et al. 2004. Comparing the linkage maps of the close relatives *Arabidopsis lyrata* and *A. thaliana. Genetics* 168:1575–1584.

Lagercrantz, U., J. Putterill, G. Coupland, and D. Lydiate. 1996. Comparative mapping in *Arabidopsis* and *Brassica*, Wine scale genome collinearity and congruence of genes controlling flowering time. *Plant J* 9:13–20.

Leclercq, S., E. Rivals, and P. Jarne. 2007. Detecting microsatellites within genomes: Significant variation among algorithms. *BMC Bioinform* 8:125–143.

Lee, L. Y. and S. B. Gelvin. 2008. T-DNA binary vectors and systems. *Plant Physiol* 146:325–332.

Lewis, S. E., S. M. Searle, N. Harris et al. 2002. Apollo: A sequence annotation editor. *Genome Bio* 3:1–14.

Li, R., Y. Li, K. Kristiansen, and J. Wang. 2008. SOAP: Short oligonucleotide alignment program. *Bioinformatics* 24: 713–714.

Liang, C., P. Jaiswal, C. Hebbard et al. 2008. Gramene: A growing plant comparative genomics resource. *Nucleic Acids Res* 36:D947–D953.

Lomsadze, A., V. Ter-Hovhannisyan, Y. Chernoff, and M. Borodovsky. 2005. Gene identification in novel eukaryotic genomes by self-training algorithm. *Nucleic Acids Res* 33:6494–6506.

Lou, P., J. J. Zhao, J. S. Kim et al. 2007. Quantitative trait loci for flowering time and morphological traits in multiple populations of *Brassica rapa. J Exp Bot* 58:4005–4016.

Maere, S., S. De Bodt, J. Raes et al. 2005. Modeling gene and genome duplications in eukaryotes. *Proc Natl Acad Sci USA* 102:5454–5459.

Marth, G., M. D. Yandell, I. Korf et al. 1999. A general approach to single-nucleotide polymorphism discovery. *Nat Genet* 23:452–456.

McGinnis, K. M. 2010. RNAi for functional genomics in plants. *Brief Funct Genomics* 9:111–117.

Ming, R., S. Hou, Y. Feng et al. 2008. The draft genome of the transgenic tropical fruit tree papaya (*Carica papaya* L.). *Nature* 452:991–997.

Mueller, L. A., T. H. Solow, N. Taylor et al. 2005. The SOL genomics network: A comparative resource for Solanaceae biology and beyond. *Plant Physiol* 138:1310–1317.

Naqvi, S., G. Farre, G. Sanahuja, T. Capell, C. Zhu, and P. Christou. 2010. When more is better: Multigene engineering in plants. *Trends Plant Sci* 15:48–56.

Naqvi, S., C. Zhu, G. Farre et al. 2009. Transgenic multivitamin corn through biofortification of endosperm with three vitamins representing three distinct metabolic pathways. *Proc Natl Acad Sci USA* 106:7762–7767.

Ohyanagi, H., T. Tanaka, H. Sakai et al. 2006. The Rice Annotation Project Database (RAP-DB): Hub for *Oryza sativa* spp. *japonica* genome information. *Nucleic Acids Res* 34:D741–D744.

Okazaki, K., K. Sakamoto, R. Kikuchi et al. 2007. Mapping and characterization of FLC homologs and QTL analysis of flowering time in *Brassica oleracea*. *Theor Appl Genet* 114:595–608.

Oliphant, A., D. L. Barker, J. R. Stuelpnagel, and M. S. Chee. 2002. BeadArray technology: Enabling an accurate, cost-effective approach to high-throughput genotyping. *Biotechniques* 32:S56.

Osborn, T. C., C. Kole, I. A. Parkin et al. 1997. Comparison of flowering time genes in *Brassica rapa*, *B. napus* and *Arabidopsis thaliana*. *Genetics* 146:1123–1129.

Ossowski, S., K. Schneeberger, R. M. Clark, C. Lanz, N. Warthmann, and D. Weigel. 2008. Sequencing of natural strains of *Arabidopsis thaliana* with short reads. *Genome Res* 18:2024–2033.

Ow, D. W. 2007. GM maize from site-specific recombination technology, what next? *Curr Opin Biotechnol* 18:115–120.

Paine, J. A., C. A. Shipton, C. S. Chaggar et al. 2005. Improving the nutritional value of Golden Rice through increased pro-vitamin A content. *Nat Biotechnol* 23:482–487.

Paterson, A. H. 2006. Leafing through the genomes of our major crop plants: Strategies for capturing unique information. *Nat Rev Genet* 7:174–184.

Paterson, A. H., J. E. Bowers, R. Bruggmann et al. 2009. The *Sorghum bicolor* genome and the diversification of grasses. *Nature* 457:551–556.

Paterson, A. H., J. E. Bowers, and B. A. Chapman. 2004. Ancient polyploidization predating divergence of the cereals, and its consequences for comparative genomics. *Proc Natl Acad Sci USA* 101:9903–9908.

Paterson, A. H., B. A. Chapman, J. C. Kissinger, J. E. Bowers, F. A. Feltus, and J. C. Estill. 2006. Many gene and domain families have convergent fates following independent whole-genome duplication events in *Arabidopsis*, *Oryza*, *Saccharomyces* and *Tetraodon*. *Trends Genet* 22:597–602.

Pertea, M. and S. L. Salzberg. 2002. Using GlimmerM to find genes in eukaryotic genomes. *Curr Protoc Bioinform* 11:44.

Pflieger, S., V. Lefebvre, and M. Causse. 2001. The candidate gene approach in plant genetics: A review. *Mol Breed* 7:275–291.

Podicheti, R., R. Gollapudi, and Q. Dong. 2009. WebGBrowse—A web server for GBrowse. *Bioinformatics* 25:1550–1551.

Rao, A. Q., A. Bakhsh, S. Kiani et al. 2009. The myth of plant transformation. *Biotech Adv* 27:753–763.

Remig, V., B. Franklin, S. Margolis, G. Kostas, T. Nece, and J. C. Street. 2010. Trans fats in America: A review of their use, consumption, health implications, and regulation. *J Am Diet Assoc* 110:585–592.

Rozen, S. and H. Skaletsky. 2000. Primer3 on the WWW for general users and for biologist programmers. *Methods Mol Cell Biol* 132:365–386.

Rutherford, K., J. Parkhill, J. T. Crook-Horsnell, P. Rice, M.-A. Rajandream, and B. Barrell. 2000. Artemis: Sequence visualisation and annotation. *Bioinformatics* 16:944–945.

Sanford, J. 2000. The development of the biolistic process. *In Vitro Cell Dev Biol-Plant* 36:303–308.

Sax, K. 1923. The association of sizes differences with seed coat pattern and pigmentation in *Phaseolus vulgaris*. *Genetics* 8:552–560.

Sayers, E. W., T. Tanya Barrett, D. A. Benson et al. 2009. Database resources of the National Center for Biotechnology Information. *Nucleic Acids Res* 37:5–15.

Schmutz, J., S. B. Cannon, J. Schlueter et al. 2010. Genome sequence of the palaeopolyploid soybean. *Nature* 463:178–183.

Schnable, P. S., D. Ware, R. S. Fulton et al. 2009. The B73 maize genome: Complexity, diversity, and dynamics. *Science* 326:1112–1115.

Schranz, M. E., P. Quijada, S. B. Sung, L. Lukens, R. Amasino, and T. C. Osborn. 2002. Characterization and effects of the replicated flowering time gene FLC in *Brassica rapa*. *Genetics* 162:1457–1468.

Schwab, R., S. Ossowski, M. Riester, N. Warthmann, and D. Weigel. 2006. Highly specific gene silencing by artificial microRNAs in *Arabidopsis*. *Plant Cell* 18:1121–1133.

Seoighe, C. and C. Gehring. 2004. Genome duplication led to highly selective expansion of the *Arabidopsis thaliana* proteome. *Trends Genet* 20:461–464.

Shewry, P. R., H. D. Jones, and N. G. Halford. 2008. Plant biotechnology: Transgenic crops. *Adv Bio Eng/Biotech* 111:149–186.

Srivastava, V. and D. Gidoni. 2010. Site-specific gene integration technologies for crop improvement. *In Vitro Cell Dev Biol-Plant* 46:219–232.

Stack, S. M., C. R. Clarke, W. E. Cary, and J. T. Muffly. 1974. Different kinds of heterochromatin in higher plant chromosomes. *J Cell Sci* 14:499–504.

Sternberg, N. and D. Hamilton. 1981. Bacteriophage P1 site-specific recombination. I. Recombination between loxP sites. *J Mol Biol* 150:467–486.

Stoesser, G., P. Sterk, M. A. Tuli, P. J. Stoehr, and G. N. Cameron. 1997. The EMBL nucleotide sequence database. *Nucleic Acids Res* 25:7–14.

Storozhenko, S., B. V. De, M. Volckaert et al. 2007. Folate fortification of rice by metabolic engineering. *Nat Biotechnol* 25:1277–1279.

Swarbreck, D., C. Wilks, P. Lamesch et al. 2008. The Arabidopsis Information Resource (TAIR): Gene structure and function annotation. *Nucleic Acids Res* 36:D1009–D1014.

Tabor, H. K., N. J. Risch, and R. M. Myers. 2002. Candidate-gene approaches for studying complex genetic traits: Practical considerations. *Nat Rev Genet* 3:391–397.

Tadege, M., C. C. Sheldon, C. A. Helliwell, P. Stoutjesdijk, E. S. Dennis, and W. J. Peacock. 2001. Control of flowering time by FLC orthologues in *Brassica napus*. *Plant J* 28:545–553.

Tang, H., J. E. Bowers, X. Wang, R. Ming, M. Alam, and A. H. Paterson. 2008a. Synteny and colinearity in plant genomes. *Science* 320:486–488.

Tang, H., J. E. Bowers, X. Wang, and A. H. Paterson. 2010. Angiosperm genome comparisons reveal early polyploidy in the monocot lineage. *Proc Natl Acad Sci USA* 107:472–477.

Tang, H., X. Wang, J. E. Bowers, R. Ming, M. Alam, and A. H. Paterson. 2008b. Unraveling ancient hexaploidy through multiply-aligned angiosperm gene maps. *Genome Res* 18:1944–1954.

Temnykh, S., G. DeClerck, A. Lukashova, L. Lippovich, S. Cartinhour, and S. McCouch. 2001. Computational and experimental analysis of microsatellites in rice (*Oryza sativa*); frequency, length variation, transposon associations, and genetic marker potential. *Genome Res* 11:1441–1452.

Teutonico, R. A. and T. C. Osborn. 1995. Mapping loci controlling vernalization requirement in *Brassica rapa*. *Theor Appl Genet* 91:1279–1283.

Thomas, B. C., B. Pedersen, and M. Freeling. 2006. Following tetraploidy in an *Arabidopsis ancestor*, genes were removed preferentially from one homolog leaving clusters enriched in dose-sensitive genes. *Genome Res* 16:934–946.

Thornsberry, J. M., M. M. Goodman, J. Doebley, S. Kresovich, D. Nielsen, and E. S. Buckler. 2001. Dwarf8 polymorphisms associate with variation in flowering time. *Nat Genet* 28:286–289.

Tung, C.-W., K. Zhao, M. Wright et al. 2010. Development of a research platform for dissecting phenotye-genotype associations in rice (*Oryza* spp.). *Rice* 3:205–217.

Tuskan, G. A., S. DiFazio, S. Jansson et al. 2006. The genome of black cottonwood, *Populus trichocarpa* (Torr. & Gray). *Science* 313:1596–1604.

UniProt Consortium. 2010. The Universal Protein Resource (UniProt) in 2010. *Nucleic Acids Res* 38:142–148.

Volfovsky, N., B. J. Haas, and S. L. Salzberg. 2001. A clustering method for repeat analysis in DNA sequences. *Genome Biol* 2:0027.

Waterhouse, P. M., M. W. Graham, and M. B. Wang. 1998. Virus resistance and gene silencing in plants can be induced by simultaneous expression of sense and antisense RNA. *Proc Natl Acad Sci USA* 95:13959–13964.

Weber, A. L., W. H. Briggs, J. Rucker et al. 2008. The genetic architecture of complex traits in teosinte (*Zea mays* ssp parviglumis): New evidence from association mapping. *Genetics* 180:1221–1232.

Wheeler, D. L., T. Barrett, D. A. Benson et al. 2009. Database resources of the National Center for Biotechnology Information. *Nucleic Acids Res* 37:D5–D15.

Winzeler, E. A., D. R. Richards, A. R. Conway et al. 1998. Direct allelic variation scanning of the yeast genome. *Science* 281:1194–1197.

Ye, X., S. Al-Babili, A. Kloti et al. 2000. Engineering the provitamin A (beta-carotene) biosynthetic pathway into (carotenoid-free) rice endosperm. *Science* 287:303–305.

Youens-Clark, K., B. Faga, and I. V. Yap. 2009. CMap 1.01: A comparative mapping application for the Internet. *Bioinformatics* 25:3040–3042.

Yu, J. M., J. B. Holland, M. D. McMullen, and E. S. Buckler. 2008. Genetic design and statistical power of nested association mapping in maize. *Genetics* 178:539–551.

Yu, J., S. N. Hu, J. Wang et al. 2002. A draft sequence of the rice genome (*Oryza sativa* L. spp indica). *Science* 296:79–92.

Yu, J., G. Pressoir, W. Briggs et al. 2005a. A unified mixed-model method for association mapping that accounts for multiple levels of relatedness. *Nat Genet* 38:203–208.

Yu, J., J. Wang, W. Lin et al. 2005b. The genomes of *Oryza sativa*: A history of duplications. *PLos Biol* 3:266–281.

Zhang, J. H., D. A. Wheeler, I. Yakub, S. Wei, R. Sood, and W. Rowe. 2005. SNP detector: A software tool for sensitive accurate SNP detection. *PLoS Comput Biol* 1:395–404.

Zhu, M. and S. Zhao. 2007. Candidate gene identification approach: Progress and challenges. *Int J Biol Sci* 3:420–427.

# 8 Genomics of Fruit Quality and Disorders

*Federico Martinelli, Carlos H. Crisosto,*
*and Abhaya Dandekar*

## CONTENTS

## 8.1 INTRODUCTION

Postharvest losses of fruits can be 5%–25% in developed countries and 20%–50% in developing countries, depending on the commodity. A recent survey carried out in the United Kingdom claims that an estimated 4.4 million apples, 5.5 million potatoes, 2.8 million tomatoes, 1.6 million bananas, and 1.2 million oranges are thrown in the trash every day due to deterioration problems. Based on those estimates, these five items alone add up to 525,000 t of food waste each year (www.lovefoodhatewaste.com). The U.S. Department of Agriculture's Economic Research Service estimates that 57% of fresh fruits by weight and 51% of fresh vegetables by weight were not consumed in 2005. Fresh and processed products derived from the *Rosaceae* plant family (almonds, apples, apricots, blackberries, peaches, pears, plums, sweet cherries, tart cherries, strawberries, raspberries, roses, and other ornamentals) provide vital contributions to human nutrition, health, and well-being and collectively constitute the economic backbone of many rural economies in the United States. Although current domestic production of these crops is valued above $7 billion and global per-capita production and consumption is expanding in both domestic and export markets, the U.S. rosaceous crop industries face many limitations to profitability and sustainability. Overcoming these barriers requires rapid development and deployment of new cultivars with improved characteristics to meet dynamic industry, market, and consumer preferences. The diversity of *Rosaceae* species provides extraordinary opportunities for using fundamental genomics research to improve crops through targeted breeding programs (www.bioinfo.wsu.edu/gdr/), (www.anla.org/research/floriculture.htm), and (www.nationalberrycrops.org/).

*Rosaceae* genetics and genomics information, and associated enabling technologies, are developing rapidly, leading to many discoveries with potential application. In 2010, genetic linkage maps were available for all major crop species; the apple, peach, and strawberry genomes were being sequenced; and more than 250 major genes and quantitative trait loci (QTLs) were identified (www.hrt.msu.edu/faculty/Iezzoni /RosBREED_Consortium.html).

Fruit quality traits (texture, flavor, color, and nutrition) are extremely important to the modern *Rosaceae* industry because they define consumer preference, which drives the market. These "consumer traits" are central to breeding programs. Important QTLs and major gene loci for fruit quality are known from genetic studies, but their utility for specific breeding programs is not yet established. QTLs identified within other members of the Maloideae subfamily such as wild *Malus* species or pear may also be useful for apple. Furthermore, QTLs in the extensively studied stone fruit crops (*Prunus* species, of the Amygdaloideae subfamily) may be transferable to apple. Breeders interested in improving the efficiency of cultivar development with modern genomics technologies would benefit from a simple protocol for assessing reported QTLs, including those identified in related crops, for validity and utility.

## 8.2 FRUIT: BOTANICAL DEFINITION AND COMPOSITION

The genus *Prunus* includes about 430 species of deciduous or evergreen trees and shrubs and is widespread throughout temperate regions. It belongs to subfamily Prunoideae of the *Rosaceae* family. While some ornamental species do not yield edible fruits, others are grown for commercial fruit and nut production, such as peach (*Prunus persica*), nectarine (*P. persica* var. nectarina), European plum (*Prunus domestica*), Japanese plum (*Prunus salicina*), apricot (*Prunus armeniaca*), mume or Japanese apricot (*Prunus mume*), sweet cherry (*Prunus avium*), sour cherry (*Prunus cerasus*), and almond (*Prunus amygdalus*). Most of these species originated in Asia or Southern Europe, and their fruits are botanically defined as drupes, from the Latin word *drupa* (Brady 1993). Drupes develop mostly from flowers with superior ovaries having a single carpel. The fruits usually have a clear ventral suture, do not retain floral residues next to the pedicel, and are characterized by a membranous exocarp with an outer fleshy mesocarp consisting mainly of parenchyma cells (Romani and Jennings 1971). The mesocarp surrounds a shell (the pit or stone) of hardened endocarp with a seed inside; thus, *Prunus* species bear "stone fruit." Unlike almonds, in which the seed within the pit is consumed, the edible part in most stone fruits is the mesocarp, and eventually the exocarp. Growth of stone fruits usually shows a double sigmoid pattern after fertilization, with an initial stage characterized by active cell division, followed by a phase in which all the parts of the ovary besides the embryo and endosperm grow. Later, whole fruit growth decelerates while seed development and endocarp lignification occur and finally, mesocarp expansion resumes (Romani and Jennings 1971).

Peach fruits are characteristically soft fleshed and highly perishable, with a limited potential market life. A peach fruit is ~87% water, with only 43 cal from carbohydrates, organic acids, pigments, phenolics, vitamins, volatiles, antioxidants, and trace amounts of proteins and lipids: a very attractive balance for consumers (Kader and Mitchell 1989b, USDA 2003). Immature peach fruit contains few or no starch grains that are rapidly converted into soluble sugars as the fruit matures and ripens. Consequently, there is no significant increase in soluble sugars during storage and ripening (Romani and Jennings 1971). In mature peach fruits, soluble sugars comprise ~7%–18% fresh weight (FW) and fiber, 0.3%. Sucrose, glucose, and fructose represent about 75% of soluble sugars, and malic acid is the predominant organic acid, followed by citric acid. These organic acids (0.4%–1.2% FW) are important because the ratio of soluble solids to titratable acidity, or soluble solids concentration (SSC):TA, determines consumer perception of most ripe peach cultivars. In most peach cultivars, acidity decreases about 30% during ripening. Peach fruit has little protein (0.5%–0.8% FW), but small proteins have an important function as enzymes catalyzing various chemical reactions responsible for compositional changes. Although lipids constitute only 0.1%–0.2% FW, they are critical components of surface wax, which contributes to fruit cosmetic appearance, and of cuticle, which protects fruit against water loss and pathogens. Lipids are also important constituents of cell membranes, which influence fruit physiology. Minerals in fruits include base-forming elements (calcium, magnesium, potassium, sodium) and acid-forming elements (phosphorus, chloride, sulfur). Calcium, associated with cell wall structure, is important in fruit softening, and calcium in the apoplast has been related to senescence. Postharvest changes in fruit mineral concentrations are small. Volatile compounds in very low concentrations include esters, alcohols, aldehydes, ketones, and acids and that provide the characteristic fruit aroma. Lactones may be important in peach flavor, but more detailed studies are needed on this topic.

## 8.3 ANTIOXIDANTS IN *ROSACEAE* SPECIES

The ORAC assay has been routinely applied to determine antioxidant capacity and currently there are databases available for different foods (USDA 2007a, Wu et al. 2004). Black currants and cranberries rate highest, with ORAC $\sim$ 10,000 mol TE/100 g. Blueberries, long recognized for their high antioxidant concentration, have ORAC comparable to plums. Almonds and cherries also have high ORAC (3361 and 4454 mol TE/100 g, respectively), similar to that found in strawberries. The ORAC reported for peach, nectarine, and apricot are usually lower than in other *Prunus* species (Wu et al. 2004). The distribution of antioxidants also varies within the fruit. In plum and cherry, TAC was always higher in the skin than in the flesh (Díaz Mula et al. 2008). In peach, removal of peel also results in a significant loss of total antioxidant capacity (Remorini et al. 2008).

## 8.4 PHYTONUTRIENTS (NUTRACEUTICALS)

Several groups of health-promoting, bioactive phytochemicals are present in peach and almonds. Stone fruits contain carotenoids, anthocyanins, and other phenolic compounds including hydroxycinnamates, flavan 3-ols, and flavonols. Chlorogenic acids, neochlorogenic acids, and anthocyanin and quercetin derivatives predominate (Kim et al. 2003, Tomas-Barberan et al. 2001). Similarly, almonds are rich in phytochemicals including phytoesterols, tannins, and flavonoids and the phenolic acids isohamnetin, catechin, epicatechin, and kaempferol and quercetin derivatives (Chen and Blumberg 2008, Garrido et al. 2008). Many of these compounds may help prevent chronic diseases such as cancer, cardiovascular disease, Alzheimer's, and metabolic syndrome (Chen and Blumberg 2008, Chen et al. 2007). For example, whole almonds and almond fractions reduced aberrant crypt foci in a rat model of colon carcinogenesis (Davis and Iwahashi 2001), while peach and plum phenolic compounds inhibit growth and induction of differentiation of colon cancer cells (Lea et al. 2008). Many of these diseases may originate in the presence of chronic inflammation (Middleton et al. 2000); thus, it is important to consider it as a tool for initial screening. Drs. Cisneros-Zevallos and Seeram have investigated the health-promoting properties of many crops using several approaches based on *in vitro* and *in vivo* bioassays, focusing on cancer and cardiovascular disease (Lea et al. 2008, Seeram et al. 2007). Bioassay-directed fractionation allows the discovery and chemical identification of bioactive compounds in a crop extract using HPLC-MS and NMR. Understanding the underlying mechanism by which the compound exerts its effect on the disease can increase the crop value, especially in alternative markets. It is important to initiate studies by screening varieties that express the appropriate bioactive compounds (Cevallos-Casals et al. 2006) and the genes associated with them. Such studies are the basis for selection of enhanced bioactive-enriched genotypes, for developing appropriate strategies for cultivation practices and postharvest handling procedures, and for selecting the proper alternative markets.

## 8.5 GENETIC FACTORS

There are large differences in total antioxidants, phenolics, and carotenoids among *Prunus* species and among varieties within any given species. Analysis of 37 apricot varieties showed a 10-fold difference in carotenoid accumulation (Ruiz et al. 2005). In another apricot study, total phenolics varied from 30.3 to 742 mg gallic acid equivalents per 100 g (Drogoudi et al. 2008). In plum, varieties with dark purple skins contained 200% more total phenolics than others. The plum cultivars Black Beauty and Angeleno are especially rich in phenolics (Tomás Barberán et al. 2001). In peach, fruit showing higher endocarp staining presented higher antioxidant capacity.

## 8.6 FRUIT QUALITY ATTRIBUTES AND FLAVOR

Quality is a group of attributes that give the peach its economic value at the sale and/ or consumption point. These attributes include production quality, flavor quality, postharvest quality (storage and shelf life), nutritional quality, and internal/external appearance. The fruit production and marketing industry seeks a fruit with no or few defects. Quality can be measured using fruit yield, fruit size distribution, background and red fruit color, internal breakdown (IB) incidence, sensory characteristics, consumer acceptance/preferences, storage/shipping potential, and shelf-life potential. The economic relevance of these components varies depending on which step of the fruit production and marketing process is assessed. A grower will be interested in harvest date, yield, red color, size distribution, disease resistance, ability to harvest, and number of defects. Fruit shippers, handlers, and receivers define quality primarily as fruit firmness, used to predict potential storage and quality. This is an erroneous and incomplete way to predict fruit postharvest potential market life for domestic distribution. In peaches, the main determinant for tasty cultivars is the lack of development of IB symptoms such as lack of flavor, off flavor, flesh mealiness, and flesh browning, although in some cultivars and/or long distance market situations, firmness also affects postharvest quality. Some California or Italian white-fleshed peach cultivars not susceptible to IB have a high rate of softening that limits distribution in Asian markets, which often lack facilities with good temperature control within their distribution systems. Retail store handlers historically have used fruit red color and size as a main component of their quality definition. There are some indications that flavor and ripeness stage ("ready to buy") are being included in a new quality definition (consumer quality). Fruit safety and antioxidant concentration are also expected by fruit consumers. These changes in definitions are being driven by retailer evaluations of consumer consumption trends. These changes in quality definition that focus on consumer demand for flavor and "ready to eat" stage fruit can increase peach consumption with proper marketing promotion and education programs.

Because consumer quality cannot be improved after harvest in fruits such as peach, it is important to understand how preharvest factors affect consumer acceptance and market life (Crisosto et al. 1997, Kader and Zagory 1988). Unfortunately, little research has been conducted on this topic. The effects of rootstocks on controlling plant development and production are well known (Caruso et al. 1996, 1997). In contrast, their influence on fruit bioactive compounds is quite variable, ranging from no pronounced differences (Drogoudi et al. 2007) to significant differences in the concentrations of phytochemicals (Giorgi et al. 2005, Remorini et al. 2008). Preharvest factors often interact in complex ways depending on cultivar, stage of development, and season. The orchard quality potential of a cultivar can be achieved only by understanding the role of preharvest factors in consumer acceptance and postharvest life potential.

## 8.7   MATURITY AND QUALITY

Harvest maturity controls the fruit's final flavor components, deterioration problems, market life, and ability to ripen. Delayed harvest can greatly improve fruit size and SSC, but its impact on fruit quality is restricted to cultivars that are adapted to this delay. Controlled delayed harvest, canopy manipulations for better light interception, and canopy growth competition control can maximize orchard flavor quality potential when correctly applied. In peaches, early studies associated consumer acceptance of fruit with high SSC (INFOS-CTIFL 1999). Based on these studies, a minimum quality index of 10% SSC was proposed for yellow-fleshed peaches and nectarines in California (Kader 1995). In France, where popular peach cultivars are more varied in color and acidity, a minimum of 10% SSC for peaches with low titratable acidity (<0.9% TA at maturity) and 11% SSC those with high acidity (TA > 0.9%) has been proposed as a quality standard (Hilaire 2003). In Californian and Chilean yellow-fleshed peaches, approximately 30% of the TA in a mature fruit at harvest will be lost during ripening. For white-fleshed peaches, this value varied (C.H. Crisosto, unpublished). In Italy, which grows a high proportion of yellow-fleshed cultivars, a minimum of 10% SSC for early season, 11% for mid season, and 12% for late season cultivars was proposed (Giovannini et al. 2000, Neri et al. 1996). As plantings of new peach cultivars with different sensory characteristics (low acid, high acid, high SSC, highly aromatic, nonmelting, etc.) expand and as new markets with consumers of different ethnic backgrounds expand (Crisosto et al. 2003, Liverani et al. 2002), it becomes more critical to understand the role of SSC, TA, and other flavor components in consumer acceptance and to segregate cultivars into different sensory categories prior to proposing any quality index (Crisosto 2002, Crisosto et al. 2003, Neri et al. 2003). Developing orchard techniques that increase the number of fruit that exceed the proposed quality index within each category is also necessary.

The potential role in consumer acceptance of flavor components such as TA, SSC:TA, volatiles, and texture to test cultivars representative of these different sensory groups using a trained panel and "in-store" consumer acceptance tests is being studied. For "Ivory Princess" (white-fleshed/low TA), "Elegant Lady," and "O'Henry" peaches (yellow-fleshed/high TA) and for "Spring Bright" (yellow-fleshed/high TA) and "Honey Kist" (yellow-fleshed/low TA) nectarines, consumer acceptance correlated with ripe soluble solids concentration (RSSC) or RSSC:RTA. However, this relationship was cultivar dependant and/or maturity dependent. A low RTA could compensate for a low RSSC within a given RSSC and RTA range; however, very low acidity reduced consumer acceptance. Thus, the relationship between RSSC:RTA and consumer acceptance is not linear. More reliable information on the relationship between sensory characteristics, consumer acceptance, and orchard factors from different cultivars is necessary to justify using RSSC by itself as a quality index within each flavor category. As a long-term solution, breeding programs should include these quality characteristics in their screening process. The creation of peach categories with their own quality indexes and sensory description may help marketing and promotion.

## 8.8  GENOTYPE

Genotype has an important role in flavor quality, nutrient composition, and postharvest life potential. SSC and acidity are determined by several factors such as cultivar (Byrne 2002, Crisosto et al. 1995, 1997, Liverani et al. 2002) and rootstock (Giovannini et al. 2003, Reighard 2002). Reduction of physiological disorders, decay, and insect losses can be achieved by choosing the correct genotype for the environmental conditions. Extensive harvest quality and postharvest storage potential evaluations have been carried out since 1970 in California (Tonini et al. 2000), Chile, South Africa, Italy, Spain, and France. Brown rot and gray mold resistance have not been successfully introduced into recently released cultivars. These are the main peach diseases, but other diseases have been investigated (Frecon et al. 2002, Reighard 2002). Current breeding programs are creating new cultivars with improved production and visual appearance attributes, but the ideal cultivar(s) that combine consumer quality attributes and domestic and long-distance shipping remain elusive.

## 8.9  FRUIT MATURATION AND RIPENING

Fruits are harvested mature or ripe, while vegetables and ornamentals are harvested over a wide range of physiological ages: Zucchini and cucumber are harvested before maturation has commenced. Postharvest fruit ripening is a dramatic transformation of a physiologically mature but inedible plant organ into a visually attractive fruit with high consumer acceptance. This is the result of a complex of biochemical and anatomical changes, many occurring independently of one another, that begin during the latter stages of growth and development and continue through the early stages of senescence, resulting in characteristic aesthetic and/or food quality changes in composition, color, texture, or other sensory attributes. During ripening, fruit undergoes many physiochemical changes that determine the quality of the fruit eventually purchased by the consumer. Ripening marks the completion of fruit development and the beginning of senescence and is normally irreversible. Fruits can be classified according to their ripening abilities. Some fruits do not continue ripening once removed from the plant: berries (blackberry, raspberry, and strawberry), cherry, citrus (grapefruit, lemon, lime, orange, mandarin, and tangerine), grape, lychee, pineapple, pomegranate, and tamarillo. Other fruits can be harvested mature and ripened "off" the plant, such as apple, pear, quince, persimmon, apricot, nectarine, peach, plum, kiwifruit, avocado, banana, mango, papaya, cherimoya, sapodilla, sapote, guava, and passion fruit. Fruits in the first group produce very small quantities of ethylene and do not respond to ethylene treatment except by degreening (removal of chlorophyll); these are picked when fully ripe to ensure good flavor quality. Fruits in the second group produce much larger quantities of ethylene during ripening, and, in some cases, exposure to ethylene will result in faster and more uniform ripening. Controlled ripening of peach, nectarine, plum, avocado, kiwifruit, mango, and pear fruits before marketing is increasingly used to provide consumers with the choice of purchasing "ready-to-eat" ripe fruits or mature fruits that can be ripened at home.

## 8.10 CHILLING INJURY SYMPTOMS

Temperature management during postharvest handling of fruits and vegetables is critical to maintain quality and reduce losses. Temperature management before, during, and after fruit ripening determines the final quality of the product. Initial produce quality is a critical part of establishing a reliable and successful fruit delivery program. Many tropical or subtropical commodities are sensitive to chilling injury (CI), which occurs when commodities such as poinsettia, bananas, and tomatoes are held at temperatures above their freezing points. Some important temperate-zone crops or cultivars are also susceptible to CI. For example, CI or IB of some peach, plum, and nectarine cultivars occurs below 50°F and is greatest at about 41°F. Unfortunately, the effect of chilling is cumulative in some commodities. Low temperatures in transit or in the field shortly before harvest add to the total chilling that occurs in cold storage. Some chilled fruits will appear sound while stored at low temperatures but CI symptoms develop upon transfer to warmer temperatures or during/after ripening. Thus, failure of mature fruits to ripen properly, lack of uniform ripening, and/or visual problems can be related to CI during postharvest handling prior to ripening at the production or distribution points.

No ice forms in the cells during CI development, but changes in the tissue's chemical composition, especially in the membrane phospholipids, lead to chilling damage. Many physiological and biochemical changes occur before CI symptoms are apparent such as cessation of cytoplasmic streaming, changes in membrane permeability, disorganization of cytoplasm, loss of mitochondrial activity, and alteration of respiratory metabolism ending in cellular dysfunction. At chilling temperatures, tissues are weakened by the inability to maintain normal metabolism. When chilling stress is prolonged, these cell alterations lead to development of CI symptoms. Failure of mature fruits to ripen, surface pitting, surface lesions, external and/or internal discoloration, appearance of water-soaked areas, development of necrotic areas, increased susceptibility to decay, shorter storage life, cessation of growth, loss of sprouting ability in propagules, and loss of characteristic flavor and aroma are associated with CI. Maturity at harvest and degree of ripeness can affect chilling sensitivity in some fruits like avocados, honeydew melons, and tomatoes. Riper fruit are less susceptible to CI. Injury will develop in these commodities after a period of exposure to chilling temperatures below 50°F–59°F, but well above freezing.

Expression of CI symptoms such as failure to ripen properly is a function of temperature and time. A fruit may be able to withstand temperatures just below the chilling threshold temperature. However, if produce is exposed to temperatures even further below its chilling threshold, the development of CI will be more severe and can affect ripening. A longer exposure results in irreversible damage that affects the ripening and final consumer quality. Thus, it is critical to store fruit at its optimum storage temperature and with proper handling practices throughout postharvest life. The time of exposure at a given temperature that triggers particular CI symptoms is specific to cultivar, maturity, production area, and other conditions. For example, skin pitting, scalding, and blackening are the main symptoms on mature-green avocados kept at 32°F–35°F for more than 7 days before transfer to warm temperatures. Avocados exposed to 37°F–41°F for more than 2 weeks may exhibit internal flesh browning, failure to ripen, and increased susceptibility to pathogen attack. Failure to ripen, surface discoloration, and dark brown sub-epidermal streaks result from exposing mature-green bananas for 1 h to 50°F, 5 h to 53°F, 24 h to 54°F, or 72 h to 55°F. Exposure of mature-green mangos to temperatures below 55°F and exposure of ripe mangos to temperatures below 50°F causes uneven ripening. In peach cultivars highly susceptible to IB, a 3-day exposure to the "killing" temperature range (36°F–46°F) can induce failure to ripen, off flavors, flesh browning, and mealiness. Failure to ripen, sunken surface areas, and pitting develop several days after storage at 35.5°F in cantaloupe and after storage at 45°F for honeydew melon and watermelons. Failure to ripen, lack of flavor, premature softening, and increased decay occur when tomatoes have been stored below 50°F for longer than 2 weeks or at 41°F for longer than 6–8 days.

Several treatments, including partial ripening (sometimes with ethylene) after harvest but before cold storage, exposure to high or low but nonchilling temperatures prior to cold storage, cold storage under controlled or modified atmospheres, or treatments with abscisic acid, methyl jasmonate, or other natural compounds, can reduce CI.

## 8.11   PEACH INTERNAL BREAKDOWN OR CHILLING INJURY, THE EXAMPLE

IB and CI in peach are genetically controlled and triggered by storage temperature. Symptoms include dry, mealy, woolly, or hard-textured fruit (not juicy), flesh or pit cavity browning, and flesh translucency usually radiating through the flesh from the pit. Development of an intense red color in the flesh ("bleeding"), usually radiating from the pit, may be associated with this problem in some peach cultivars. Recently released cultivars rich in skin red pigment showed flesh bleeding that does not affect fruit taste. The development of this symptom is associated with fruit maturity rather than storage temperature. In susceptible cultivars, flavor is lost before visual CI symptoms are evident (Crisosto and Labavitch 2002). There is large variability in IB susceptibility among peach cultivars (Crisosto et al. 1999c, Mitchell and Kader 1989). In general, mid-season and late-season peach cultivars are more susceptible to CI than early-season cultivars (Mitchell and Kader 1989), although as new cultivars are released from a new genetic pool, susceptibility to CI is becoming more random among new cultivars (Crisosto 2002, Crisosto et al. 1999c). Expression of CI symptoms develops faster and more intensely when susceptible fruit are stored at temperatures between 2.2°C and 7.6°C (killing temperature zone) than when stored at 0°C or below but above their freezing point (Harding and Haller 1934, Mitchell and Kader 1989). Therefore, market life is dramatically reduced when fruit are exposed to the killing temperature zone (Crisosto et al. 1999c). In addition, the severity of CI depends on the ripening stage at harvest: Higher incidence was reported for "Maycrest" peaches picked at more advanced ripening stages (Valero et al. 1997), although the opposite was found in other cultivars (Von Mollendorff et al. 1992).

Several treatments to delay and limit development of this disorder have been tested: controlled atmosphere (CA) environment, calcium applications, warming cold storage interruptions (Anderson 1979, Garner et al. 2001, Nanos and Mitchell 1991), plant growth regulators, and controlled delayed cooling. The major benefits of CA during storage/shipment are retention of fruit firmness and ground color. Conditions of 6% $O_2$ + 17% $CO_2$ at 0°C promote a modest reduction of IB during shipment of yellow-fleshed (Crisosto et al. 1999a) and white-fleshed cultivars (Garner et al. 2001). The CA efficacy depends on cultivar (Mitchell and Kader 1989), preharvest factors (Crisosto et al. 1997), temperature, fruit size (Crisosto et al. 1999a), marketing period, and shipping time (Crisosto et al. 1999c). Another tool that reduced CI in peach is modified atmosphere packaging (MAP). Thus, "Paraguayo," a flat type cultivar, had reduced CI severity when packed in polypropylene standard film with steady-state atmosphere of 12% $CO_2$ and 4% $O_2$, or in oriented polypropylene with 23% $CO_2$ and 2% $O_2$ (Fernández-Trujillo et al. 1998). A preconditioning treatment (Crisosto et al. 2004) prior to storage/shipment delayed IB symptoms and is successfully being used commercially on Californian and Chilean fruit shipped to U.S. and English markets (Crisosto et al. 2004). The "Paraguayo" cultivar subjected to intermittent warming cycles of 1 day at 20°C for every 6 days of storage at 2°C also showed fewer CI symptoms, although scald and translucency occurred (Fernández-Trujillo and Artés 1998).

## 8.12  BIOLOGICAL BASIS OF CHILLING INJURY

Numerous studies on the biochemical basis for mealiness have identified factors that may be important in the development of the symptoms, although considerable discrepancy exists among studies. Mealiness has been associated with pectin methylesterase (PME) activity that was reduced (Buescher and Furmanski 1978), increased (Ben-Arie and Sonego 1980), or unchanged (Obenland and Carroll 2000, Zhou et al. 2000c). Similarly, mealy fruit had reduced exo-polygalacturonase (exo-PG) activity in some studies (Zhou et al. 2000c), but not in others (Artes et al. 1996).

Reduced endo-PG activity during cold storage is commonly observed (Artes et al. 1996), although mealiness develops not in cold storage but during subsequent ripening at warm temperatures (Buescher and Furmanski 1978). If, on the other hand, the cold period exceeds a certain critical length, or the ripening period is short, no increase in endo-PG activity occurs during ripening and mealiness results (Ben-Arie and Sonego 1980). During ripening, fruit may develop mealiness with low extractable juice, but upon extended ripening become juicy (Von Mollendorff and de Villiers 1988, Von Mollendorff et al. 1989, 1993). However, this apparent restoration of free juice may be due to tissue breakdown and senescence. In mealy fruit, the most easily extractable cell wall pectins (those soluble in water or chelator) are less abundant and are of higher molecular weight and viscosity than in ripened, juicy fruit (Dawson et al. 1992, Lurie et al. 1994, Von Mollendorff and de Villiers 1988). The degree of methylesterification of pectin may also be altered (Ben-Arie and Lavee 1971, Lurie et al. 2003). Cell wall pectin participates in cell-to-cell adhesion through calcium cross-linking between partially de-methylesterified homogalacturonan in the middle lamella (Jarvis et al. 2003). Changes to pectin metabolism could cause mealiness either by cell fluids forming calcium-pectate gel complexes with high molecular weight pectin in the middle lamella (Ben-Arie and Lavee 1971, Zhou et al. 2000a) or through decreased intercellular adhesion in mealy fruit that reduces cell rupture during biting and chewing, preventing release of cellular contents (Brummell et al. 2004).

Other enzymes and cell wall proteins are being examined for links to the development of mealiness in peaches. Endo-1,4-glucanse activity and mRNA increases after chilling storage, unlike fruit from treatments that delayed the appearance of mealiness (Zhou et al. 2000b). Expansin protein and mRNA decreased as peaches became mealy (Obenland et al. 2003). Other enzymes, including endo-1,4-$\beta$-mannase, $\beta$-galactosidase, and $\alpha$-arabinosidase, were less active in mealy fruit than in ripe, juicy fruit (Brummell et al. 2004).

The other CI symptom that gives fruit a dry texture and uneven ripening is leatheriness. Some fruits remain firm and others become soft after a few days at 20°C following cold storage. In general, soft fruit with dry texture are mealy (woolly), while firm fruit with dry texture are leathery (Luza et al. 1992). Under the electron microscope, leathery fruit had consistently thicker cell walls than mealy or juicy fruit (Luza et al. 1992). A study of three "Huangjin" peach harvests, early, commercial, and late, found that early harvested fruit were most prone to leatheriness (Ju et al. 2000). These peaches did not soften as much as juicy or mealy fruit. The activities of ethylene synthesis pathway enzymes (ACC synthase and ACC oxidase) were lower in these fruit, as were the cell wall modifying enzymes PG and $\beta$-galactosidase, while insoluble pectin concentrations were higher than in juicy or mealy fruit. A more recent study examined cell wall polymer depolymerization, cell wall polysaccharide sugar composition, enzyme activity, and tissue physical characteristics during the development of leatheriness (Brummell et al. 2004). Increasing time of cold storage was used to induce increasingly severe CI symptoms and examine which changes in cell wall polymers or enzyme activities precede or accompany symptom developments. After 3 or 4 weeks in cold storage, some fruit developed a leathery texture. This was similar to mealiness, but with less free juice and more flesh browning, and the texture of the flesh was firm rather than grainy (Brummell et al. 2004). Fruit developing leatheriness had reduced chelator-soluble pectin concentrations and more tightly bound matrix PG, similar to mealy fruit. Leathery fruit showed a greater arrest of depolymerization than in mealy fruit, as indicated by the molecular weight distribution of chelator-soluble pectin. Leathery fruit possessed lower activities of exo-PG, endo-PG, endo-1,4-β-mannase, β-galactosidase, and α-arabinosidase than similar stored mealy fruit. The activities of PME and endo-1,4-β-glucanase were similar in fruits with both disorders (Brummell et al. 2004).

The appearance of brown discoloration in the fruit flesh, or flesh browning, occurs sooner at temperatures of 2°C–5°C than at the optimal storage temperature of 0°C. In fact, less flesh browning developed at −0.5°C than at +0.5°C (Ceretta et al. 2000). The disorder may be related to tissue deterioration or senescence, which alter membrane permeability, and to the interaction between phenols and polyphenol oxidase, which are generally found in separate compartments in the cell. The browning potential of peaches depended on the total concentration of phenolic compounds and on the polyphenol oxidase activity (Kader and Chordas 1984). The concentration of polyphenols differed among white-fleshed peach cultivars (Manabe et al. 1979). CA storage alleviated or prevented the development of this disorder in some cultivars (Ceretta et al. 2000, Crisosto et al. 1995). During normal air storage, a lack of juiciness indicative of either mealiness or leatheriness is observed before flesh browning develops to any degree (Crisosto et al. 1999b).

Many peach and nectarine cultivars have cells near the stone that contain anthocyanin. When fruit is halved, these appear as red rays extending out from the center that contains the pit (flesh bleeding). Following extended storage, these sharply delineated rays disappear and the whole area around the pit has a reddish appearance. This red color can extend throughout the flesh when the disorder is severe. There has been almost no research conducted on the causes of this disorder. It may be a consequence of tissue senescence, since it is inversely correlated with decreased organic acids in the tissue (S. Lurie, unpublished) and CA storage prevented its development (Lurie et al. 1992). Alternatively, it may be a consequence of the arrest of normal ripening, since the ethylene action inhibitor, 1-methylcyclopropene (1-MCP), greatly enhanced the development of this disorder (Dong et al. 2001). However, application of exogenous ethylene during 0°C storage for 30 days did not affect the development of internal reddening or flesh bleeding (Crisosto et al. 2001a).

## 8.13   GENOTYPE INFLUENCE ON CHILLING INJURY

There is a large variation among peach and nectarine selections and/or cultivars in susceptibility to CI when stored at either 0°C or 5°C (Mitchell and Kader 1989). This variation may allow geneticists and breeders to understand the genetic inheritance of CI, isolate the genes responsible, and develop stone fruit cultivars free of CI. In a large-scale study in California, 25 nectarine and 32 peach cultivars were evaluated for storage potential. Early season yellow-fleshed cultivars were less susceptible to CI than later-season cultivars (Crisosto et al. 1999a, S. Lurie, unpublished), but white-fleshed cultivars were not. Among newly released cultivars developed from a new genetic pool, susceptibility to CI is random (Crisosto et al. 1999a, Crisosto

2002,2003). In general, nectarine cultivars were less susceptible to CI than peach cultivars. Also, melting flesh peach cultivars were more susceptible than those with firmer, nonmelting flesh (Brovelli et al. 1998, Crisosto et al. 1999a). Nonmelting flesh cultivars have reduced endo-PG activity (Lester et al. 1996). The genetic locus for freestone appears to contain a cluster of endo-PG genes (Callahan et al. 2004).

## 8.14  FRUIT POSTHARVEST DISEASES

Worldwide, the most important pathogen of tree fruits is Botrytis rot, caused by the fungus *Botrytis cinerea*. It is a serious problem during wet spring weather and can occur during storage if fruits are contaminated through harvest and handling wounds. Avoiding mechanical injuries and good postharvest temperature management are effective controls. Brown Rot is caused by *Monilinia fructicola*, with infections beginning during flowering. It is the most important postharvest disease of peaches in California. Rhizopus Rot is caused by *Rhizopus stolonifer* and can occur in ripe or near-ripe peaches kept at 20°C–25°C. Keeping fruit below 5°C is an effective control. Good orchard sanitation practices and proper fungicide applications are essential to reduce these problems.

Postharvest fungicides are commonly applied to control these diseases. A Food and Drug Administration (FDA)-approved fungicide(s) is often incorporated into a fruit coating/wax for uniformity of application. Regulations regarding fruit coatings vary by country (CODEX). Careful handling to minimize fruit injury, sanitation of packing house equipment, and rapid, thorough cooling to 0°C as soon after harvest as possible are also important for effective disease suppression. Multidisciplinary programs to understand fruit disease resistance, identify genes responsible, and use marker-assisted selection for breeding program are ongoing in different countries.

## 8.15  TREE GENOMICS

Peach is a self-pollinated diploid species ($2n = 16$) with a small genome of approximately $5.9 \times 10^8$ base pairs/diploid nucleus, about twice the size of *Arabidopsis* (Arumuganathan et al. 1991). In spite of the small genome, progress in developing molecular markers has been very modest. The linkage maps in the diploid species peach and nectarine (*P. persica*, $2n = 2x = 16$), almond (*Prunus dulcis*, $2n = 2x = 16$), and sweet cherry (*P. avium*, $2n = 2x = 16$) are the most extensive (Arus et al. 1994, Chaparro et al. 1994, Dirlewanger and Bodo 1994, Foolad et al. 1995, Rajapakse et al. 1995, Stockinger et al. 1996, Viruel et al. 1995).

One linkage group postulated in *Prunus* is that of the *F* (freestone), *M* (melting), and *St* (soft) loci (Bailey and French 1949). *F* and *M* are an estimated 15 co units apart, *M* and *St* are about 30 co units apart). However, assignment of phenotypic classes based on subjective differences in fruit firmness has caused difficulties in assigning genotypes. Some have postulated that only one locus (*M*) with multiple alleles, rather than two loci, can account for the differences in fruit firmness and texture. These alternative hypotheses can be addressed using objective measures for fruit firmness like polygalacturonase (PG) activity, multiple sampling during fruit maturation, and examination of seedling genotypes on their own roots and on a standard rootstock. Recently, the *G* and *Cat-1* loci were located on linkage group 1 (F.A. Bliss et al., unpublished data). The *Y* locus controlling fruit flesh color was placed in linkage group 3 based on segregation of RAPDs and RFLP anchor loci (Warburton and Bliss 1996). Although a RAPD marker was linked to the *F* (free-stone) locus, it is not yet assigned to a linkage group (Warburton and Bliss 1996).

The phenotypic classes defined by the *M* (melting) and *St* (soft) loci were based originally on subjective observations or measurements of pressure resistance. A recent finding that an RFLP in a ripening-related PG peach gene cosegregated with the *M* locus provides evidence for the basis of melting flesh (Lester et al. 1996). Lesions in the *M* locus range from different restriction patterns to one cultivar that lacks the corresponding fragment, suggesting a deletion. The extent to which these differences affect the melting flesh phenotype deserves attention. In addition to endo-PG, two forms of exo-PG increase differentially between peach varieties during ripening (Downs and Brady 1990). While no strong relationships were found between the exo-PGs and free- or clingstone traits, the fruit softening effects controlled by the *M* and *St* loci have not been investigated fully. The *G* locus, which distinguishes peaches from nectarines by suppressing trichome development, is an example of the complex nature of some fruit organoleptic traits (FOTs) (Scorza and Sherman 1996). The mode of action of this gene (or possibly genes) is unclear and other phenotypic effects are associated with this locus.

Apart from the effects of major genes, there is considerable genetic variability among peach cultivars for different organic acids. The extent to which each of these is controlled by the *D* locus that distinguishes acidic (pH < 4.0) from nonacidic fruit (pH > 4.0) (Monet 1989) is not known. Although fruit concentrations of glucose, sucrose, fructose, and sorbitol vary, little is known about the genetic variation responsible. While understanding patterns of inheritance that control variation in each separate component is important to breeders, it is the SSC/acidity ratio that determines consumer acceptance. Quality, utility, and consumer acceptance depend on the expression of FOTs related to mealiness, flavor, aroma, texture, and appearance. To meet consumer demands, breeders of new peach cultivars must combine desirable traits by identifying, characterizing, and manipulating the genes that control the traits. Understanding the genetic control of FOT component traits allows critical genes to be identified, located in the genome, allelic differences characterized, important genetic interactions quantified, and linked markers (marker tags) developed for use in marker-aided selection to improve breeding efficiency. As a long-term solution, research on the genetic and biochemical basis of flavor, antioxidant pathways, and CI using available molecular genetics technologies is necessary. New information and techniques for breeding programs will lead to new peach cultivars with improved flavor, antioxidant attributes, and freedom from CI susceptibility.

A quantitative molecular genetic approach (Prioul et al. 1997) facilitates our ability to identify specific genes, gain knowledge of gene location, and develop molecular markers for marker-aided selection. The complex phenotypes characteristic of these FOTs are due to interactions among controlling genes, environmental factors, and physiological differences among fruits at different development stages. For genetic analyses to be meaningful, fruit from each tree in segregating progenies must be sampled several times during the development/ripening, trees must be evaluated growing on their own roots and on a standard commercial, and fruit measurements must be taken over several years. The resulting information, combining rigorous molecular genetic analysis with physiologically valid phenotypic measurements, will provide a solid basis for gene detection and development of marker tags to investigate gene action and improve breeding efficiency.

Peach fruit firmness and texture, related to the rate and degree of softening, and shelf life are key contributors to consumer satisfaction. They influence harvest and postharvest practices such as packing, transportation, storage, and processing. Peach fruits are generally classified into fresh market and canning based on firmness. Fresh market peaches are characterized by soft and juicy flesh that softens rapidly (melting) at the later stages of ripening. This melting phase coincides with the climacteric peak (Lester et al. 1996). Canning or processing peaches have nonmelting flesh. The fruit do not soften rapidly during ripening and remain firmer than the fresh market types throughout the ripening process.

Another trait associated with firmness is the adhesion of mesocarp (flesh) to the endocarp (stone). Fresh market fruit can be either freestone (FMF—freestone melting flesh) or clingstone (CMF—clingstone melting flesh), but all canning peach cultivars are clingstone (CNMF—clingstone nonmelting flesh). The canning industry will benefit from cultivars with a freestone nonmelting flesh (FNMF) fruit, a phenotype that has rarely, if ever, been found in breeding populations. Such FNMF cultivars would not require mechanical pitters for stone removal but would still maintain good texture, shape, and appearance after being canned. The ease of endocarp removal would also reduce the incidence of pit pieces in canned fruits, a safety issue for children. The fresh market industry can also benefit from FNMF fruit with improved firmness. When conventional fresh market fruit are left to ripen on the tree to achieve maximum fruit quality, they become susceptible to mechanical damage and decay during shipping and handling, and reduced postharvest life (Karakurt et al. 2000). A firmer fresh market fruit can be kept longer on the tree for better quality and taste without the traditional packing problems.

These two related traits (melting vs. nonmelting and freestone vs. clingstone) have been treated as monogenic, with melting and freestone being completely dominant. However, considerable variation exists within each of these phenotypes (Calahan et al. 2004, Karakurt et al. 2000, Peace et al. 2005, T. M. Gradziel, personal observation). Recent detailed genetic, biochemical, and physiological studies suggest involvement of other genes (unpublished observations). Some cultivars are classified as "semifreestone" or "semiclingstone," and the character can also vary according to seasonal conditions (Bailey and French 1949). Melting flesh and freestone are controlled by two linked loci, $M$ and $F$, respectively (Bailey and French 1949). Recent evidence suggests that $M$ and $F$ are the same locus with three major alleles: F, f, and f1 (Monet 1989, Peace et al. 2005). A gene encoding the cell wall–degrading enzyme endopolygalacturonase (endoPG) is encoded by the $F–M$ locus (Peace et al. 2005). A PCR test has been developed for endoPG to unambiguously distinguish FMF, CMF, and CNMF phenotypes (Morgutti et al. 2006, Peace et al. 2005). A simple sequence repeat (SSR) polymorphism was detected within the noncoding sequence of endoPG and used as a PCR-based marker for endoPG allelic diversity in *Prunus*. The SSR marker revealed that endoPG is a hyper-variable locus (Peace et al. 2007).

An SSR variant of the endoPG f1 allele is associated with subtle freestone/clingstone and melting/nonmelting variations among cling peach (CNFM) genotypes. There is need to convert the endoPG SSR marker to forms readily available for MAB of FNMF processing peach. A quantitative genetics approach to flesh texture and stone adhesion in diverse genetic backgrounds is required to unravel other genes influencing these important traits.

Fruit color is important for both nutrition and appearance. Peach and nectarine fruit flesh may be white, yellow, or (rarely) red; in canning peaches, intense yellow ("golden orange") is most desirable (Bellini et al. 1996a, b). Yellow/orange color is due to the presence of beta-carotene, a vitamin A precursor. Red color may be derived from anthocyanin-based compounds (Byrne et al. 2004). Brown color results from the oxidation of phenolic compounds, which, like anthocyanins, are known to have healthful antioxidant properties (Mathew and Parpia 1971, Mayer and Harel 1979). Selection for nonoxidizing phenolics could be a beneficial compromise between appearance and nutrition.

Pit bleeding (redness around the stone) is a genetic trait present in many fresh market peach and nectarine cultivars. It gives an attractive appearance to fresh fruit, but is detrimental for canning, as the redness becomes brown and unsightly, and can leak into canning syrup (Lurie and Crisosto 2005). This trait was mapped as single locus (*Cs*) to G3 of peach (Yamamoto et al. 2001). Redness may also spread through the flesh during normal ripening in susceptible varieties and confer an unexpected and unwanted appearance (Lurie and Crisosto 2005). In susceptible varieties, browning and bruising can occur after rough handling of less firm fruit (riper fruit of firm varieties, or fruit of softer varieties), or simply during normal ripening (Crisosto et al. 2001b). This is especially detrimental for fruit used as fresh-cut products, a rapidly growing segment of the industry. Fresh-cut products are a critical competitive strategy for retailers, and year-round availability is seen as a necessity by food service and retail buyers (Cook 2003).

Cold storage is a postharvest practice that is necessary to extend fruit shelf life but can damage fruit firmness, texture, and color (Crisosto et al. 1999a,b, 2006). Mealiness, browning, and bleeding are major symptoms of CI, a physiological disorder occurring during cold storage or after subsequent ripening. Genetic inheritance of these three symptoms is quantitative and several related QTLs have been localized (Ogundiwin et al. 2007, Peace et al. 2006). A major QTL controlling both mealiness and bleeding colocated with the endoPG gene (Ogundiwin et al. 2007, Peace et al. 2005, 2006). The progeny population (Pop-DG) used to localize this QTL had only FMF and CNMF individuals. EndoPG cosegregated with FMF/CNMF in this population. Mealiness was observed exclusively in FMF progeny, while cold-induced bleeding was observed almost exclusively in CNMF progeny. This segregation pattern showed colocalization of both the mealiness and bleeding major QTL with endoPG. A major QTL controlling cold-induced browning colocated with a gene encoding leucoanthocyanidin dioxygenase (PpLDOX), and enzyme in the anthocyanin biosynthesis pathway (Ogundiwin et al. 2008a).

Cold-induced browning originates from pit bleeding (Lurie and Crisosto 2005). Pit bleeding at maturity (without cold storage) will be measured as a quantitative trait in Pop-DG and two additional progeny populations to localize controlling QTLs.

The positions of the QTLs will indicate the location of other genes controlling pit bleeding. Cold-induced browning after storage at 5°C for 2 weeks will also be measured in the two new progeny populations as was done for Pop-DG. Pit bleeding QTL positions will be compared to the cold-induced browning QTLs. The PpLDOX marker and any other markers closely linked to pit bleeding will be converted to forms that are useful for MAB of browning- and pit bleeding–free peach cultivars.

A new peach genetic linkage map (Pop-DG) that is colineal with the *Prunus* reference "Texas" × "Earlygold" (T × E) map (Ogundiwin et al. 2007, Peace et al. 2005) has been developed. The genomic locations of over 50 fruit softening candidate genes have been determined either by fine mapping onto Pop-DG or by bin mapping onto the T × E reference map (Peace et al. 2006). Several QTLs controlling mealiness, flesh browning, flesh bleeding, flowering date, harvest date, fruit weight, skin blush, flesh total sugar content, acidity, bruising characteristics, browning potential, polyphenol oxidase activity, antioxidant capacity, and the *freestone, melting flesh,* and *flesh color* loci have been localized on Pop-DG linkage map (Ogundiwin et al. 2007). A molecular marker (endoPG) test that unambiguously distinguishes between FMF, CMF, and CNMF peach genotypes was developed for the UC Davis peach breeding program (Peace et al. 2005). PpLDOX has been identified as a candidate gene for cold storage browning in peach (Ogundiwin et al. 2008a).

An extensive database of expressed genes during mealiness development known as "ChillPeach" has been developed (Ogundiwin et al. 2008b). This database contains 8144 enriched, full-length expressed sequence tags (ESTs), out of which ~2000 are new to *Prunus*. All sequences have been deposited to GenBank and GDR. Seventy ChillPeach SSRs novel to *Prunus* were mapped directly to the expanded Pop-DG map or bin-mapped to the T × E reference map. A ChillPeach microarray containing around 4200 unigenes has been printed. This microarray has been used to identify genes differentially expressed between cold treated and normal peach mesocarp tissues (Ogundiwin et al. 2008b). Over 80 similarly differentially regulated ChillPeach unigenes were similarly mapped to the *Prunus* genome using Pop-DG and T × E maps (unpublished data). The positions of these mapped genes may coincide with known QTLs. A community-wide NimbleGen oligoarray platform is currently under construction by GDR for *Prunus* (Dorrie Main, personal communication). This will contain all available *Prunus* ESTs and the ChillPeach unigenes are an important component of this platform. The microarray platform will be useful to identify changes at the transcript level associated with important traits in peach.

## 8.16  MOLECULAR GENETIC MAPPING

At the beginning of the twentieth century, scientists discovered that the genes, the Mendelian factors controlling inheritance, were organized in linear order on structures called chromosomes. "Markers" are characters whose pattern of inheritance can be followed at the morphological, biochemical, or molecular level, and which can elicit information concerning the inheritance of less easily measured, but more critical, traits. Coinheritance of a gene of interest and a marker suggests that they are physically close together on the chromosome, or linked. Markers must be polymorphic, meaning that the two parents must carry different forms, so that chromosome inherited from one parent can be distinguished from that provided by the other. This polymorphism can be detected at three levels: differences in phenotype (morphological), in protein profile (biochemical), or in DNA nucleotide sequences (molecular). Markers can be associated with a physical place on the chromosome to construct a linkage map, a prerequisite for most genome sequencing projects. These maps are based on recombination frequencies between DNA sequences. Distance is measured in centimorgans (cM). The first molecular marker map developed mapped restriction length fragment polymorphisms (RFLP). Later, other molecular markers such as random amplified polymorphism DNA (RAPD) and amplified fragment length polymorphism (AFLP) were included. Briefly, the construction of RFLP genetic maps is based on the following steps: (1) Selection of parent plants that are genetically divergent enough to exhibit sufficient RFLP polymorphism but not so far distant that they lead to sterile progeny. (2) Production of a mapping population through crossing to produce a $F_1$ or $F_2$ generation, or by backcrossing the $F_1$ to one of the parents. (3) Scoring the RFLP in the mapping population by performing a linkage analysis, scoring the mapping population sequentially with probes from the library to construct a linkage map.

## 8.17   COMPARATIVE MAPPING

Comparative mapping is defined as the alignment of chromosomes of related species based on genetic mapping of common DNA markers. Comparative genetic mapping studies reveal similarities and differences in genes and gene order between genera or species belonging to different taxa. Maps constructed in one species can be compared with closely related species using common markers or single gene traits. These comparative maps show how the genome has rearranged through time and allow inferences about gene organization and repeated sequences in related species. Map-based cloning may be easier in species with a small genome like rice than in those with a massive genome, like wheat.

The first comparing mapping in fruit crops was performed between tomatoes and other species in the Solanaceae family such as tomato and potato (Tanksley et al. 1992) and tomato and eggplant (Doganlar et al. 2002). Apple (*Malus* × *domestica*), peach (*P. persica*), cherry (*P. avium* and *P. cerasus*), plum (*P. domestica* and *P. salicina*), apricot (*P. armeniaca*), almond (*P. dulcis*), pear (*Pyrus communis*), quince (*Cydonia oblonga*), and loquat (*Eriobotrya japonica*) belong to the *Rosaceae* family. Most of these species are large, woody perennial plants with a long juvenile phase that makes them poorly suited for traditional breeding. However, fruit trees have some advantageous features such as efficient methods of vegetative reproduction, a long life, the possibility of making interspecific crosses, and a small basic genome. In *Rosaceae*, comparative mapping was successfully used to construct a *Prunus* reference map with 562 molecular markers, allowing genome comparisons among 7 *Prunus* diploid (*x* = 8) species (almond, peach, apricot, cherry, *Prunus ferganensis*, *Prunus davidiana*, and *Prunus cerasifera*) (Dirlewanger et al. 2003). The *Rosaceae* also include other crops such as strawberry (*Fragaria* × *ananassa*) and rose (*Rosa* spp.). A high degree of synteny has been observed among rosaceous species, seen by comparing the apple and *Prunus* maps. Conserved genomic regions were detected between *Prunus* and *Arabidopsis*. Using data from different linkage maps anchored with the reference *Prunus* map, a general map with the position of 28 major genes controlling agronomic characters found in different species was made. Markers tightly linked to major genes expressing important traits (disease and pest resistances, fruit or nut quality, self-incompatibility, etc.) have been identified in apple and *Prunus* and are currently used for marker-assisted selection in breeding programs. Quantitative character dissection using linkage maps and candidate gene approaches has already started. Genomic tools such as the *Prunus* physical map, an increase in EST collections in both *Prunus* and *Malus*, and map positioning of many ESTs are required to better understand the *Rosaceae* genome and to foster additional research on fruit tree genetics.

A European project allowed the construction of a saturated linkage map of 246 markers (235 RFLPs and 11 isozymes) in an almond (cv. Texas) × peach (cv. Earlygold) $F_2$ progeny. This "T × E" map detected the expected eight linkage groups (G1–G8), with a total distance of 491 cM. A European consortium first constructed a detailed apple map using $F_1$ progeny of the cross cv. Prima × cv. Fiesta (the P × F map). Its 290 markers include 124 RFLPs, 10 SSRs, 17 isozymes, 133 RAPD, and 6 other markers distributed among 17 linkage groups. The high number of SSRs on this map will rapidly transfer this information to other apple-segregating populations, allowing its widespread use by *Malus* geneticists and breeders.

In *Prunus*, comparing the positions of anchor markers (RFLPs, SSRs, and isozymes) of the T × E map with those of 13 maps constructed with other *Prunus* populations showed that the genomes of the diploid ($2n = 16$) species peach, almond, apricot, cherry, *P. davidiana*, *P. cerasifera*, and *P. ferganensis*, are essentially colinear. Using 177 DNA probes to compare the *Prunus* map with the *Arabidopsis* genome, the 227 *Prunus* loci detected 703 loci in the *Arabidopsis* genome (Aranzana et al. 2003). In other plant families, genome evolution within a family consists of limited chromosome restructuring due to inversion and translocation events that lead to the conservation of large chromosomal fragments in the genomes of its constituent species. Results available so far in the *Rosaceae* indicate the same trend. The six members of the *Prunus* genus studied have a genome without any major chromosomal rearrangements, indicating their close relationship.

## 8.18   MARKER-ASSISTED SELECTION

Some important agronomic characters in fruit trees behave as major genes, including disease resistances and flower, vegetative, and fruit or nut quality traits. Their simple inheritance makes them obvious targets in the search for tightly linked markers for early selection, particularly for characters that require complex analysis, such as some pest or disease inoculation, or that cannot be evaluated until the plant matures, such as the self-incompatibility genotype. In almond and apricot, self-incompatibility is currently assessed using marker-assisted selection. Several species-specific or even allele-specific DNA markers were developed, allowing earlier and more accurate selection of the common self-incompatibility or self-compatibility alleles. Markers have been used to select genotypes resistant to important diseases in *Prunus* (Lecouls et al. 1999). Possible additional targets include a major gene involved in Sharka (plum pox virus) resistance and a major gene for shell hardness in almond (Arus et al. 1998).

## 8.19   MAPPING QTLs

Quantitatively inherited characters constitute most of the variability selected during the breeding process in fruit trees, as in most cultivated species. Characters related to plant growth and architecture, yield, blooming and harvesting times, and fruit quality are usually quantitative traits, and they have been analyzed with the help of molecular markers in several fruit species. Several major genes obtained from Asian *Malus* species confer race-specific resistance of apple to scab. QTLs for blooming, ripening, and fruit quality characters have been identified in both peach (Dirlewanger et al. 1999) and apple (King et al. 2001). An international consortium led by the Clemson University (Clemson, SC) has developed tools to characterize the *Prunus* genome. Using RFLPs on the T × E map and a BAC library of peach cv. Nemared, a physical map has been partially assembled. A *Rosaceae* database (www.genome.clemson.edu/gdr) has recently been created with the objective of assembling this information and making it available worldwide to researchers.

The progress made during the last decade on the genetics of cultivated *Rosaceae* species, particularly peach, is enormous. However, to use this new information to breed improved cultivars, some important topics need to be addressed in the near future. Detailed comparative mapping among the most important genera of this family like *Prunus*, *Malus*, *Pyrus*, *Fragaria*, and *Rosa*, should be undertaken. Some of these genera, like *Prunus* or *Malus*, include a large number of intercompatible species; this exotic germplasm represents an enormous gene pool available for fruit breeding. Little use has been made of this variability because of the slowness of the classical breeding methods. Genomic methods may make it possible to discover genes of interest from exotic materials in well characterized existing germplasm collections (www.ecpgr.cgiar.org/workgroups/prunus/prunus.htm) and to introgress them into cultivated species with methods already proposed and in use in annual species, but adapted to the characteristics of woody perennials.

## 8.20   GENOMIC DATABASES

Genomic databases are a collection of data arranged in a systematic way to be publicly searchable. Biological database design, development, and long-term management are core areas of the discipline of bioinformatics. Genomic data include nucleic acid and protein sequence variants (including neutral polymorphisms, susceptibility alleles to various phenotypes, and pathogenic mutations) and polymorphic haplotypes. The information comes from genomics, proteomics, metabolomics, microarray gene expression, and phylogenetics. It includes gene function, structure, localization (both cellular and chromosomal), clinical effects of mutations, similarities of biological sequences and structures, gene sequences, textual descriptions, attributes and ontology classifications, citations, and tabular data. These are often described as semi-structured data, and can be represented as tables, key delimited records, and XML structures. Cross-references among databases using accession numbers are common.

The Genome Database for *Rosaceae* (GDR) is a curated and integrated web-based relational database supported by the NSF Plant Genome Program and by the USDA Specialty Crop Research Initiative. It contains comprehensive data on the genetically anchored peach physical map, an annotated peach EST database, *Rosaceae* maps and markers, and all publicly available *Rosaceae* sequences. It contains annotations of ESTs include contig assembly, putative function, SSRs, and anchored position to the peach physical map where applicable. An integrated map viewer allows graphical interface to the genetic, transcriptome, and physical mapping information. ESTs, BACs, and markers can be queried by category and the search result sites are linked to the integrated map viewer. Users can browse and query the database, then compare their sequences with annotated GDR sequences via a dedicated sequence similarity server running either the BLAST or FASTA algorithm. The goals of establishing the GDR were (1) to develop an organized and integrated web resource for peach genomics data to facilitate gene discovery in other *Prunus* species through comparative mapping, (2) to collect and integrate all *Rosaceae* genomics data, and (3) to develop online tools and resources for the *Rosaceae* community. GDR will be expanded to include whole genome sequences and annotations for apple, peach, and strawberry, transcript data, metacyc pathways, large scale phenotype and genotype data, breeding data, controlled vocabularies, and new analysis tools, all implemented within the open source infrastructure. Data to be added in the near future include apple ESTs, strawberry ESTs, rose ESTs, and apricot map/marker data. Future efforts will focus on improving the tools and functionality of the web interface such as an advanced search site with options for search/display categories, full sequence processing facilities for *Rosaceae* researchers, a newsgroup for the *Rosaceae* community, a site for *Rosaceae* literature, and more analysis tools such as an interactive contig viewer and a comparative map viewer.

## 8.21    GENOMIC AND GENE DISCOVERY

Genomics can identify all genes in a plant, and transcriptomic and proteomic techniques can determine which genes are on or off in a particular plant cell or organ experiencing a particular growth stage or stress condition. Connecting genomics, transcriptomics, or proteomics with metabolomics using a systems biology approach allows the biochemical machinery of plants to be explored, highlighting new pathways for predictive metabolic engineering. A crucial prerequisite is the availability of gene sequences, or a complete genome. Two fundamentally different approaches are currently being used to examine gene function. A forward genetics approach begins with observing a unique phenotype and seeks to identify the gene(s) responsible. In contrast, reverse genetics begins with a candidate gene and examines the mutant phenotypes that result upon its disruption. Despite the fact that small genomes render forward genetics a potentially useful strategy for gene discovery, currently there are few forward-genetic populations available for rosaceous crops.

One approach to generating mutant plant phenotypes for both forward and reverse genetics is to inactivate a gene by inserting foreign DNA via *Agrobacterium*-mediated transformation (Krysan et al. 1999). An advantage of using this technique is that all mutations are tagged by a T-DNA sequence, enabling rapid direct identification of the gene related to the observed phenotype. In plants with completely sequenced genomes, identification of a short sequence of genomic DNA flanking the T-DNA insertion allows unambiguous identification of the mutated gene and its location on the chromosome. For plants that have not been completely sequenced, molecular tools such as EST collections and BAC libraries may allow successful cloning and characterizing of a gene of interest.

The apple genome, 750 Mb, is approximately the same size as that of tomato (*Solanum lycopersicum*) (Tatum et al. 2005). Over 300,000 apple ESTs have been generated from different tissues, conditions, and genotypes (Newcomb et al. 2006). Over 22,600 EST clones from nine cDNA libraries made from apples subjected to temperature or drought stress were clustered, annotated, and used to study gene expression in response to abiotic stress (Wisniewski et al. 2008). Apple EST sequences available in public databases were analyzed using statistical algorithms to identify genes associated with flavor and aroma components in mature fruit (Park et al. 2006). ESTs generated from young Fuji apples, peels of mature fruit, and carpels showed that most ESTs isolated from young fruit were preferentially expressed in reproductive organs, suggesting their importance during reproductive organ development (Sung et al. 1998).

Two bacterial artificial chromosome (BAC) libraries were constructed (Xu et al. 2001) and used for map-based positional cloning of a cluster of receptor-like genes within the scab resistance *Vf* locus in apple. Molecular studies have clarified ethylene perception and signal transduction pathways in rose by taking advantage of knowledge in *Arabidopsis* (Lavid et al. 2002). cDNA libraries from petals of the tetraploid *Rosa hybrida* cultivars "Fragrant Cloud" and "Golden Gate" have been constructed and over 3000 cDNA clones sequenced from these libraries. An annotated petal EST database of approximately 2100 unique genes has been generated and used to create a microarray. As genomic resources continue to develop for strawberry and rose, their applicability to each other and other *Rosaceae* crops will be more clearly defined.

## 8.22 FROM ESTs TO GENES CONTROLLING KEY QUALITY ATTRIBUTES

ESTs are used extensively and effectively in many fruit species as a tool for rapid gene discovery and for global gene expression pattern analysis of highly expressed genes. Novel cDNAs encoding enzymes involved in secondary metabolic pathways, such as essential oil and carotenoid biosynthesis, have been identified in EST libraries of various plant species. ESTs enable gene and marker discovery, aid genome annotation and gene structure identification, guide single nucleotide polymorphism characterization, and aid proteome analysis (Nagaraj et al. 2007). Over 400,000 ESTs are currently available for *Rosaceae* species via the National Center for Biotechnology Information (NCBI) dbEST and the GDR (www.rosaceae.org). Over 104,000 apple EST sequences have been produced, and a 40,000 unigene set has been identified. Another ~150,000 apple ESTs have been deposited in the NCBI by HortResearch in New Zealand (Newcomb et al. 2006). In apple, over 260,000 EST sequences are publicly available, resulting in a 17,000 unigene set.

EST sequencing projects in peach are being conducted in several laboratories worldwide, many focused on fruit development. All publicly available peach ESTs have been downloaded from NCBI and housed in GDR. There are currently ~87,751 ESTs with a unigene set comprised of 23,721 different sequences. These ESTs have come predominantly from laboratories of the *Prunus* Genome Mapping consortium, supported by the USDA Initiative for Future Agricultural and Food Systems program, ESTree (Parco Tecnologico Padano, Italy), and the Chile Consortium.

Some 50,000 EST sequences from *Fragaria vesca* and several thousand from *Fragaria ananassa* have been deposited in GenBank by several contributing laboratories. *F. vesca* cDNA libraries have been constructed from cold-, heat-, and salt-stressed seedlings and flower buds. These sequences are invaluable for annotation of *Fragaria* genomic sequences and as a source of candidate genes and random clones for reverse genetics. Nevertheless, given the EST sequence resources, development of libraries and sequencing in strawberry has lagged behind other major fruit crops and warrants further investment in genomic resource development. Cultivated strawberry represents a potential diverse source of alleles with relevance to selected traits of interest. Furthermore, examining alleles may further illuminate the ancient diploid contributors to the octoploid strawberry genome.

Papaya (*Carica papaya* L.) is the only species within the genus *Carica* and the most economically important within the family Caricaceae. *C. papaya* is a climacteric fruit crop that bears continuously throughout its 5–10 year life cycle. Fruit are ready to harvest 5–6 months after flowering, which can occur within 8 months of seed germination. The distribution of genes in two papaya fruit cDNA libraries using EST sequencing focused on putative genes involved in fruit ripening: softening, aroma production, and color development (Devitt et al. 2007). Identification, characterization, and expression analysis of newly identified genes will contribute to the understanding of fruit ripening and help identify candidate genes for future genetic improvements through marker-assisted breeding or genetic engineering. To identify genes involved in papaya fruit ripening, 1171 ESTs were generated from randomly selected clones of two independent fruit cDNA libraries derived from yellow and red-fleshed fruit varieties. The most abundant sequences encoded were chitinase, 1-aminocyclopropane-1-carboxylic acid (ACC) oxidase, catalase, and methionine synthase. DNA sequence comparisons identified ESTs with significant similarity to genes for cell wall hydrolases, cell membrane hydrolases, and ethylene synthesis and regulation that were associated with fruit softening, aroma, and color biosynthesis. Expressed papaya genes identified and associated with fruit aroma included isoprenoid biosynthesis and shikimic acid pathway genes and proteins associated with acyl lipid catabolism. Putative fruit color genes were identified from similarity to carotenoid and chlorophyll biosynthesis genes from other plant species.

In olive (*Olea europaea* L.), a species in which molecular biology studies are rare, several projects have allowed the isolation of EST involved in fruit development and response to biotic stress using cDNA subtractive libraries and next-generation sequencing technologies (Galla et al. 2009).

## 8.23 TRANSCRIPTOME

Genomics and the development of high throughput technologies for large-scale analyses of transcriptomes represent powerful tools for unraveling the molecular mechanisms of complex processes such as fruit ripening and for clarifying, on a large-scale basis, the role and effects of endogenous and/or exogenous factors.

Microarray analyses has been used for transcriptome profiling of the transition between pre-climacteric and climacteric stages and the role of ethylene in ripening in tomato (Alba et al. 2005) and peach (Trainotti et al. 2006) fruit. Apple has the largest collection of ESTs and microarrays and will provide the foundation for rosaceous microarray and gene expression analyses. Several apple microarrays are currently available or under construction for different platforms, including Nimblegen, Invitrogen, and Affymetrix. Field microarray experiments have successfully measured seasonal changes in gene expression during apple bud development. Some early plant microarray experiments were performed in strawberry. Using custom arrays, transcripts associated with ripening (Schwab et al. 2001), stress- and auxin-induced gene expression, volatile production, fruit development, and flavor were identified (Aharoni et al. 2002). These seminal studies represent well-designed and highly productive approaches that answered fundamental questions in plant biology. More importantly, research suggests that contemporary studies with larger probe sets may lead to important discoveries regarding a multitude of plant responses.

Limitations to the microarray technique include the inability to analyze genes not represented on the array. A complete disease response to any specific pathogen or pest is represented in the complexity of the RNA population, including both coding (mRNA) and noncoding (small RNA) sequences. This can now be analyzed to an unprecedented depth using new DNA sequencing methods such as next-generation sequencing technology that reveal very rare mRNA, splice variants, allelic variants, and SNPs. This technology, already applied in plants (Donaire et al. 2009), relies on the presence of extensive bioinformatics knowledge in the organism investigated. For plant species that lack whole genome sequence information, an extensive EST database can be used. These novel transcriptome tools have been used to capture and quantify almost all transcripts at a specific stage in grape berry development (Iandolino et al. 2008). In citrus, next-generation sequencing identified early differentially regulated genes in fruits and leaves at different stage of *Candidatus liberibacter* infection (F. Martinelli et al., unpublished data).

Sequence-based approaches to the study of gene expression have the advantage of querying both known and unknown RNAs in a sample. The only requirement is the ability to make cDNA copies of all RNA present in the sample, sequence them, map the sequences back to a reference genome, and deduce the structure using bioinformatic tools. This is in contrast to microarrays, which require prior knowledge that an RNA is present to design an oligonucleotide to detect its presence. If an RNA has not been annotated, it cannot be studied using expression microarrays.

## 8.24   METABOLOMICS

At least 270,000 and possibly more than 400,000 plant species exist worldwide, with an estimated 200,000–1,000,000 metabolites (Dixon and Strack 2003). Metabolomics is a rapidly emerging field of postgenome research. A metabolome (the complete set of small molecules in an organism) represents the ultimate phenotype of cells, deduced by perturbations in gene expression and modulations in protein function, caused by the environment or mutations. The metabolome can also influence gene expression and protein function. Therefore, metabolomics is used to understand cellular systems and decode gene functions. The procedure consists of chemical analysis of a plant sample using chromatography–mass spectrometry (MS), nuclear magnetic resonance (NMR), or Fourier transform infrared spectrometry (FTIR) to produce metabolite profile subsets covering a range of the metabolome. These multiple datasets from different analytical pipelines are integrated either before or after chemometric analysis. The combined data are investigated by multivariate and correlation analyses for functional genomics to study the systems biology of plant metabolism.

Rich research resources for *Arabidopsis*, such as an array of insertion mutants for reverse genetics, full-length cDNA collections for reverse biochemistry, and analytical informatics tools, makes the systematic investigation of *Arabidopsis* more feasible than that of other model plants. Systematic analyses of the transcriptome and metabolome and correlation of gene expression patterns with accumulation patterns of metabolites are possible ways to deduce gene functions. Software that enables projection of both transcriptome and metabolome data onto maps supports these systematic analyses. A set of genes (or proteins and metabolites) involved in a certain biological process is generally coregulated and thus coexpressed under the control of a shared regulatory system (Schauer and Fernie 2006). Therefore, if an unknown gene is coexpressed with known genes of a particular biological process, researchers assume that this unknown gene may be involved in this process. This co-occurrence principle can be extended to link metabolite accumulation with the expression of genes in the particular pathway in which the metabolite is involved.

With the exception of *Arabidopsis*, publicly available research resources and tools for nonmodel plants, crops, and medicinal plants are still under development. Thus, transcriptome and metabolome platforms for such plants must be established independently. Research in Solanaceous plants is relatively advanced because several major crops belong to this family, making the application of these data a reasonable possibility. Pioneering efforts have been made in tomato plants during their development and diurnal cycles (Carrari et al. 2006). These studies focus on central primary metabolism to clarify metabolite-to-metabolite and gene-to-metabolite networks. Metabolomic analysis of tomatoes has identified changes in fruit metabolism induced by parthenocarpy (Martinelli et al. 2009). To identify genes involved in production of volatiles, comprehensive gene expression analysis was combined with GC-MS-based metabolome analysis to annotate genes of different accessions and introgression lines of wild tomato (Tieman et al. 2006). Similarly, genes for synthesis of volatile compounds during developmental changes were isolated in strawberry (Aharoni et al. 2000). Most agriculturally important traits are under the control of QTL. Recent technical progress has made it possible to map putative genome regions of QTLs by determining trait values in a set of experimental lines generated by crossing two parents with distinctive natural variations. Genes related to traits such as yield and flowering time were identified by QTL analyses (Nonoue et al. 2008). Metabolite concentrations in plant tissues (m-trait) are also a quantitative trait and QTL analysis of m-traits such as seed vitamin E revealed the QTLs responsible for the control of its concentration and its genetic principles (Gilliland et al. 2006). Recently, metabolome QTL (mQTL) analyses of m-traits have been conducted to clarify their genetic background (Wentzell et al. 2007).

Regression analysis of metabolome data for *Arabidopsis* biomass traits demonstrated that seedling growth rate is to some extent predictable from the metabolome signature. These pioneering studies suggest that the interactions between metabolite composition and other traits may be predictable through advanced metabolome analysis in the future, although simple correlation and regression models cannot easily deal with this problem.

Rosaceous plants are extremely rich in specialized metabolites, many of which have documented utility in human health and nutrition. The chemistry and metabolism of flavonoids, anthocyanins, and phenolics have been studied extensively in rosaceous fruits with targeted analytical assays. Recent developments in metabolomics allow global analysis and interrogation of metabolic networks. An untargeted metabolomics approach based on Fourier transform ion cyclotron MS was used to study four consecutive stages of strawberry fruit development and identified novel information on the metabolic transition from immature to ripe fruit. Metabolomic profiles of apple fruit revealed changes provoked by UV–white light irradiation and cold storage in primary and secondary pathways associated with ethylene synthesis, acid metabolism, flavonoid pigment synthesis, and fruit texture (Rudell et al. 2008). Broader use of metabolomics in *Rosaceae* will speed the discovery of novel gene functions in primary and secondary metabolism and will provide comprehensive data sets necessary to model metabolic networks related to human health-promoting metabolites.

Metabolomics, combined with allergenicity and toxicity tests, can aid public acceptance of GM crops by providing data necessary for risk management. Following the acquisition of metabolome data from the tissues of GM plants, untransformants, and other cultivars, similarities in metabolic profiles were evaluated using multivariate analyses such as principal component analysis (PCA) and hierarchical clustering analysis.

## 8.25  TRANSFORMATION AND REGENERATION

Conventional breeding of temperate fruit trees is constrained by long reproductive cycles, extended juvenile periods, complex reproductive biology, and high heterozygosity. While commercial production of transgenic annual crops is a reality in many parts of the world, it is unclear whether genetic engineering of fruit trees will find commercial applications because of market resistance. There are several inherent advantages to using gene transfer for fruit tree improvement. Once a useful transformant is isolated (assuming stable transgene expression), normal vegetative propagation techniques provide unlimited production of the desired transgenic line. Fixation through the sexual cycle is unnecessary and inconvenient if commercially accepted cultivars are transformed. Since production is based on only a few cultivars in most fruit tree species, the impact of transforming one could be substantial.

The technique used for transformation must also be evaluated. For instance, before using *Agrobacterium*-mediated transformation, the virulence of various *Agrobacterium* strains in the target fruit species must be determined. Different environmental factors like pH, temperature, and osmotic conditions stimulate expression of vir genes. Adding phenolic compounds like acetosyringone to the culture medium stimulates transcription of virulence genes (Cervera et al. 1998). In nature, *Agrobacterium* infects host plants where there is liberation of phenolic compounds due to injury. Together with the gene of interest, other genes required for transformation are transferred, including marker genes that allow selection of transformed cells. Among the most commonly used selection genes are those for neomycin phosphotransferase (nptII), which confers resistance to aminoglycoside antibiotics, and phosphinothricin acetyl transferase, which confers resistance to the herbicide phosphinothricin (Miki and McHugh 2004). Public concern about introducing antibiotic resistance genes into food has led to methods to eliminate them from transformed plants and strategies that avoid selection of transformed cells with antibiotics (Zuo et al. 2002). However, these new methodologies have yet to be applied to transformed fruit trees.

Important advances have been produced with juvenile *Citrus* material, usually germinated apomictic seeds of a given cultivar, allowing the effect of different transgenes on transformed elite cultivars identical to the mother plant to be studied. However, *Citrus* cultivars have very long juvenile periods and transformation of adult material would be advisable. Genotype is a major determinant for transformation and procedures developed for one cultivar are often not suitable for others. This is the most serious hindrance to the application of gene transfer technologies to fruit crops. For species with cultivars that can be reliably transformed, usually only a few genotypes of a particular species are being transformed, which may not be commercially important. Development of genotype-independent transformation procedures will be very difficult to achieve with current technology. Meristem transformation may eliminate the need for regeneration in production of transgenic plants, allowing genetic manipulation of established cultivars. However, high explant mortality and difficulties controlling *Agrobacterium* growth have limited the development of this methodology (Scorza et al. 1995a,b).

## 8.26   TRANSGENIC PLANTS

The total area dedicated to GM plants increased 40-fold from 1996 to 2003, from 1.7 to 67.7 million ha. This represents an estimated market value of $4500 million, or 15% of total production (James 2003). Currently, the only transgenic tree fruit being commercially produced is papaya (*C. papaya* L.) resistant to PRSV (Papaya ringspot virus). Microprojectile bombardment has been used to transform papaya, but disarmed and genetically engineered *Agrobacterium* strains are more commonly used to transfer foreign DNA into the plant cells.

### 8.26.1   *APPLES*

Transgenic apples expressing the lytic peptide attacin E have been produced, and tests indicate that some transformants are more resistant to fire blight (*Erwinia amylovora*) (Ko et al. 2000). Scab (*Venturia inaequalis*) resistance has been incorporated into apple by introducing chitinase genes (Bolar et al. 2000), a wheat puroindoline B (pin B) gene coding a protein with antifungal activity (Faize et al. 2004). Delayed ripening in apple was obtained by suppressing the expression of ACC synthase

(ACS) or ACC oxidase (ACO) with the suppressed plants maintaining firmness for longer period of time with no effect on sugar-acid balance (Dandekar et al. 2004). Transgenic apple plants with alterations in their ability to synthesize sorbitol showed significant changes in sugar-acid balance in their fruit (Teo et al. 2006). Fruit aroma in apples was shown to be highly regulated in transgenic apple plants suppressed for the synthesis of ethylene especially the synthesis of fruity esters (Defilippi et al. 2004, 2005a, b). Plant growth has been modified by introducing the rol B gene from *Agrobacterium rhizogenes* into apple rootstocks, producing shorter internodes and better rooting (Welander et al. 1998).

### 8.26.2 *Apricots*

Little is known about transformation of *P. armeniaca*, but Sharka (plum pox virus) resistance is a crucial transformation objective. Sharka affects plums, peaches, and apricots, producing losses in fruit quality and quantity and weakening infected trees. It is probably the most important disease in *Prunus*. Expression of viral proteins in transgenic plants may confer immunity against the virus and much work has been done to produce this acquired resistance. Procedures for regeneration and transformation of commercial apricot cultivars have been published (Petri et al. 2004), but regeneration of transformed plants has not been reported yet.

### 8.26.3 *Almonds*

Efficient procedures transforming almond seedling tissues have been developed. The first almond plant expressing marker genes was obtained by transforming leaves from micropropagated almond seedlings (Miguel and Oliveira 1999). One major goal is eliminating self-incompatibility in important cultivars through antisense technology.

### 8.26.4 *Cherries*

*Agrobacterium rhizogenes* has been used to transform various species, including the cherry rootstock "Colt" (*P. avium* x *P. pseudocerasus*) (Gutierrez-Pesce et al. 1998). Adventitious roots were produced from transformed shoots. Transformation with an afp gene (antifreeze protein) cloned from an arctic fish (*Pseudopleuronectes americanus*) reduced the freezing temperature if transformed tobacco plants by 3°C–5°C. Cold resistance is difficult to obtain and identifying resistant individuals is very costly due to the time necessary for field evaluations.

### 8.26.5 *Citrus*

Major objectives of *Citrus* transformation have been resistance to *Citrus tristeza* virus (CTV) mediated by pathogen-derived genes (Domınguez et al. 2002), resistance to *Phytophthora citrophthora* using antifungal proteins (Fagoaga et al. 2001), and tolerance to salinity from the HAL2 yeast-derived genes (Cervera et al. 2000). Parthenocarpic citrus Carrizo plants have been obtained (A.M. Dandekar et al., unpublished data). *Arabidopsis* floral genes such as LEAFY (LFY) or APETALA1 (AP1), constitutively expressed in citrus seedlings from apomictic seeds, shortened the juvenile phase and promoted precocious flowering. Transgenic plants produced normal, fertile flowers that set fruits with seeds. Citrus plants expressing bovine lysozyme and snowdrop lectin are being evaluated in the greenhouse and in the field for resistance to citrus canker (*Xanthomonas axonopodis* pv. *citri*) and insects, respectively (Mirkov et al., unpublished data).

Mexican lime plants transformed with the sequences of the *Citrus tristeza* virus (CTV) genome in sense, antisense, and intron-hairpin formats were obtained and analyzed for transgene-derived transcript and short interfering RNA (siRNA) accumulation and for CTV resistance (Lopez et al. 2010). Transgenic grapefruit (*Citrus paradisi*) plants transformed with several constructs derived from the *Citrus tristeza* virus (CTV) genome were tested for resistance to CTV disease.

### 8.26.6 *GRAPES*

Various table and wine grape cultivars have been transformed with different objectives. Embryogenic callus of "Neo Muscat" was transformed with the RCC2 gene coding for chitinases that confer resistance to pathogenic fungi, and somatic embryos obtained from "Thomson Seedless" leaves were transformed with a lytic peptide coding gene and tomato ringspot virus coat protein gene (Scorza et al. 1996). Other *Vitis vinifera* cultivars have been transformed with cpGFLV (grape fanleaf virus) and antifreezing proteins, genes coding for antimicrobial peptides (Vidal et al. 2003), or the gene DefH9-iaaM, which induces parthenocarpy in flowers of several species (Mezzetti et al. 2002). Somatic embryos of *Vitis rupestris* have been transformed with the GVA (grapevine virus A) gene coding for the virus movement protein (Martinelli et al. 2002). Transgenic grape plants expressing polygalacturonase inhibiting protein gene (PGIP) were resistant to *Xylella fastidiosa* (Aguero et al. 2005, 2006).

### 8.26.7 *JAPANESE PERSIMMONS*

Leaves from the Japanese persimmon cultivar "Jiro" have been transformed with a synthetic cryIA(c) construct encoding the insecticidal crystal protein of *Bacillus thuringiensis* (Tao et al. 1997). Commercial kiwifruit cultivars have been transformed with the genes rol A, B, and C from *A. rhizogenes* to obtain plants with better rooting ability. Kiwifruit has been transformed with a soybean b-1,3-endoglucanase cDNA for increased resistance to gray mould disease (*Botrytis cinerea*) and with a stilbene synthase gene from *Vitis* to produce piceid (resveratrol-glucoside), which may confer beneficial effects on human health to the transformed kiwifruits.

## 8.26.8 OLIVES

Although there are no published reports of olive transformation in the literature, under the entries B/IT/98/30 and 31 (http://gmoinfo.jrc.it/) are recorded two deliberate releases of GM olives transformed with genes coding for rol product(s) and pathogenesis-related proteins, respectively.

## 8.26.9 PAPAYAS

Somatic embryos from seeds of the papaya cultivar "Sunset" were transformed by particle bombardment (Fitch et al. 1992). Transgenic papaya carrying the coat protein gene of PRSV was resistant to virus infection, remaining symptom free and ELISA-negative for 24 months after inoculation with virus strains under field conditions.

## 8.26.10 PEARS

Like apples, pears are affected by fire blight (*E. amylovora*) and several breeding programs are trying to obtain resistant cultivars. Transgenic pears expressing the gene attacin E from *Hyalophora cecropia* have higher resistance to the disease than nontransformed controls. Recently, it has been demonstrated that integration of D5C1, an artificial gene with similar activity to attacin E, also affects *Psylla pyri*, a pear insect pest (Puterka et al. 2002).

## 8.26.11 PEACHES

"Shooty mutants" strains of *Agrobacterium tumefaciens* have been used to make transformed peach trees with a high production of endogenous cytokinin, greater branching, and shorter internodes (Smigocki and Hammerschlag 1991). Transformation of peach tissues with the ipt gene allowed selection of transformed shoots on a medium with low concentrations of growth regulators; these were the first transformed peaches reported.

## 8.26.12 PLUMS

Transforming plum hypocotyls produced transformed plants containing the gene coding for cpPPV. The same group also produced transformed seedlings expressing the coat protein of PRSV and challenged them with the Sharka virus (Scorza et al. 1995a, b). Adult plum tissue has also been transformed with marker genes, but a dramatic reduction in the regeneration rates was observed after culturing leaves in a selective medium with kanamycin. A progressive increase in the selection pressure allowed regeneration of transformed plants for two genotypes tested (Yancheva et al. 2002).

## 8.26.13 WALNUTS

The apple worm (*Cydia pomonella*) is a pest of this species and completely resistant transgenic plants have been obtained from somatic embryos by expression of the gene cryIAc (Dandekar et al. 1998).

## REFERENCES

Aguero, C. B., C. P. Meredith, A. M. Dandekar et al. 2006. Genetic transformation of *Vitis vinifera* L. cvs Thompson Seedless and Chardonnay with the pear PGIP and GFP encoding genes. *Vitis* 45:1–8.

Aguero, C. B., S. L. Uratsu, L. C. Greve et al. 2005. Evaluation of tolerance to Pierce's disease and Botrytis in transgenic plants of *Vitis vinifera* L. Expressing the pear PGIP gene. *Mol Plant Pathol* 6:43–51.

Aharoni, A., L. C. P. Keizer, H. C. Van den Broeck et al. 2002. Novel insight into vascular, stress, and auxin-dependent and -independent gene expression programs in strawberry, a non-climacteric fruit. *Plant Physiol* 129:1019–1031.

Aharoni, A. and A. Oconnell. 2000. Strawberry on chips: From gene expression to metabolic pathways. *Abstr Pap Am Chem Soc Natl Meet* 219:267.

Alba, R., P. Payton, Z. J. Fei et al. 2005. Transcriptome and selected metabolite analyses reveal multiple points of ethylene control during tomato fruit development. *Plant Cell* 17:2954–2965.

Anderson, R. E. 1979. Influence of storage-temperature and warming during storage on peach and nectarine fruit-quality. *J Am Soc Hortic Sci* 104:459–461.

Artes, F., A. Cano, and J. P. Fernandez-Trujillo. 1996. Pectolytic enzyme activity during intermittent warming storage of peaches. *J Food Sci* 61:311–312.

Arumuganathan, K. and E. D. Earle. 1991. Nuclear DNA content of some important plant species. *Plant Mol Biol Rep ISPMB* 9:208–218.

Arus, P., J. Ballester, B. Jauregui et al. 1998. The European *Prunus* mapping project: Update on marker development in almond. *Acta Hortic* 484:331–336.

Bailey, J. S. and A. P. French. 1949. The inheritance of certain fruit and foliage characteristics in the peach. *Mass Agric Exp Sta Bull* 452.

Bellini, E., E. Giordani, I. Sabbatini et al. 1996a. Peach genetic improvement: Breeding program carried on at Florence to obtain white flesh nectarines. *Acta Hortic* 374:9–20.

Bellini, E., E. Giordani, I. Sabbatini et al. 1996b. Peach genetic improvement: Breeding program carried on at Florence University to obtain canning nectarines. *Acta Hortic* 374:21–32.

Ben-Arie, R. and S. Lavee. 1971. Pectic changes occurring in Elberta peaches suffering from woolly breakdown. *Phytochemistry* 10:531–538.

Ben-Arie, R. and L. Sonego. 1980. Pectolytic enzyme activity involved in woolly breakdown of stored peaches. *Phytochemistry* 19:2553–2555.

Bolar, J. P., J. L. Norelli, K. W. Wong et al. 2000. Expression of endochitinase from *Trichoderma harzianum* in transgenic apple increases resistance to apple scab and reduces vigor. *Phytopathology* 90:72–77.

Brady, P. L. 1993. Canning fruit pie fillings. *FSHED* 89:89–91.

Brovelli, E. A., J. K. Brecht, W. B. Sherman et al. 1998. Anatomical and physiological responses of melting- and nonmelting-flesh peaches to postharvest chilling. *J Am Soc Hortic Sci* 123:668–674.

Brummell, D. A., V. Dal Cin, S. Lurie et al. 2004. Cell wall metabolism during the development of chilling injury in cold-stored peach fruit: Association of mealiness with arrested disassembly of cell wall pectins. *J Exp Bot* 55:2041–2052.

Buescher, R. W. and R. J. Furmanski. 1978. Role of pectinesterase and polygalacturonase in the formation of woolliness in peaches. *J Food Sci* 43:264–266.

Byrne, D., M. Vizzotto, L. Cisneros-Zevallos et al. 2004. Antioxidant content of peach and plum genotypes. *HortScience* 39:798.

Callahan, A. M., R. Scorza, C. Bassett et al. 2004. Deletions in an endopolygalacturonase gene cluster correlate with non-melting flesh texture in peach. *Funct Plant Biol* 31:159–168.

Carrari, F., C. Baxter, B. Usadel et al. 2006. Integrated analysis of metabolite and transcript levels reveals the metabolic shifts that underlie tomato fruit development and highlight regulatory aspects of metabolic network behavior. *Plant Physiol* 142:1380–1396.

Caruso, T., D. Giovannini, and A. Liverani. 1996. Rootstock influences the fruit mineral, sugar and organic acid content of a very early ripening peach cultivar. *J Hortic Sci* 71:931–937.

Caruso, T., P. Inglese, M. Sidari et al. 1997. Rootstock influences seasonal dry matter and carbohydrate content and partitioning in above-ground components of 'Flordaprince' peach trees. *J Am Soc Hortic Sci* 122:673–679.

Ceretta, M., P. L. Antunes, A. Brackmann et al. 2000. Controlled atmosphere storage of the peach cultivar Eldorado. *Cienc Rural* 30:73–79.

Cervera, M., J. A. Pina, J. Juarez et al. 1998. Agrobacterium-mediated transformation of citrange: Factors affecting transformation and regeneration. *Plant Cell Rep* 18:271–278.

Cervera, M., J. A. Pina, J. Juarez et al. 2000. A broad exploration of a transgenic population of citrus: Stability of gene expression and phenotype. *Theor Appl Genet* 100:670–677.

Cevallos-Casals, B. A., D. Byrne, W. R. Okie et al. 2006. Selecting new peach and plum genotypes rich in phenolic compounds and enhanced functional properties. *Food Chem* 96:273–280.

Chaparro, J. X., D. J. Werner, D. Omalley et al. 1994. Targeted mapping and linkage analysis of morphological isozyme, and RAPD markers in peach. *Theor Appl Genet* 87:805–815.

Chen, C. Y. O. and J. B. Blumberg. 2008. In vitro activity of almond skin polyphenols for scavenging free radicals and inducing quinone reductase. *J Agric Food Chem* 56:4427–4434.

Chen, C. Y., P. E. Milbury, S. K. Chung et al. 2007. Effect of almond skin polyphenolics and quercetin on human LDL and apolipoprotein B-100 oxidation and conformation. *J Nutr Biochem* 18:785–794.

Cook, W. E. 2003. *Foodwise: Understanding What We Eat and How It Affects Us. The Story of Human Nutrition*. Herndon, VA: SteinerBooks, Anthroposophic Press.

Crisosto, C. H. 2002. How do we increase peach consumption? *Acta Hortic* 592:601–605.

Crisosto, C. H. 2003. Searching for consumer satisfaction: New trend in the California peach industry. In *Proceedings of the First Mediterranean Peach Symposium*, Agrigento, Italy, F. Marra and F. Sottile (eds.), pp. 113–118.

Crisosto, C. H., G. M. Crisosto, and K. R. Day. 2008. Market life update for peach, nectarine, and plum cultivars grown in California. *Adv Host Sci* 22(3):201–204.

Crisosto, C. H., G. M. Crisosto, G. Echeverria et al. 2006. Segregation of peach and nectarine (*Prunus persica* (L.) Batsch) cultivars according to their organoleptic characteristics. *Postharvest Biol Technol* 39:10–18.

Crisosto, C. H., D. Garner, H. L. Andris et al. 2004. Controlled delayed cooling extends peach market life. *HortTechnology* 14:99–104.

Crisosto, C. H., D. Garner, L. Cid et al. 1999a. Peach size affects storage, market life. *Calif Agric* 53:33–36.

Crisosto, C. H., G. Gugliuzza, D. Garner et al. 2001a. Understanding the role of ethylene in peach cold storage life. *Acta Hortic* 553:287–288.

Crisosto, C. H., R. S. Johnson, T. Dejong et al. 1997. Orchard factors affecting postharvest stone fruit quality. *HortScience* 32:820–823.

Crisosto, C. H. and J. M. Labavitch. 2002. Developing a quantitative method to evaluate peach (*Prunus persica*) flesh mealiness. *Postharvest Biol Technol* 25:151–158.

Crisosto, C. H., F. G. Mitchell, and S. Johnson. 1995. Factors in fresh market stone fruit quality. *Postharvest News Inform* 6:17–21.

Crisosto, C. H., F. G. Mitchell, and Z. Ju. 1999b. Susceptibility to chilling injury of peach, nectarine, and plum cultivars grown in California. *HortScience* 34:1116–1118.

Crisosto, C. H., D. Slaughter, D. Garner et al. 2001b. Stone fruit critical bruising thresholds. *J Am Pomol Soc* 55:76–81.

Dandekar, A. M., G. H. McGranahan, P. V. Vail et al. 1998. High levels of expression of full-length cryIA(c) gene from *Bacillus thuringiensis* in transgenic somatic walnut embryos. *Plant Sci* 131:181–193.

Dandekar, A. M., G. Teo, B. G. Defilippi et al. 2004. Effect of down-regulation of ethylene biosynthesis on fruit flavor complex in apple fruit. *Transgenic Res* 13:373–384.

Davis, P. A. and C. K. Iwahashi. 2001. Whole almonds and almond fractions reduce aberrant crypt foci in a rat model of colon carcinogenesis. *Cancer Lett* 165:27–33.

Dawson, D. M., L. D. Melton, and C. B. Watkins. 1992. Cell wall changes in nectarines (*Prunus persica*). Solubilization and depolymerization of pectic and neutral polymers during ripening and in mealy fruit. *Plant Physiol* 100:1203–1210.

Defilippi, B. G., A. M. Dandekar, and A. A. Kader. 2004. Regulation of fruit flavor metabolites in ethylene suppressed apple fruit. *J Agric Food Chem* 52:5694–5701.

Defilippi, B. G., A. M. Dandekar, and A. A. Kader. 2005a. Relationship of ethylene biosynthesis to aroma production, aroma-related enzymes and precursor availability in apple peel and flesh tissues. *J Agric Food Chem* 53:3133–3141.

Defilippi, B. G., A. A. Kader, and A. M. Dandekar. 2005b. Apple aroma: Alcohol acyltransferase, a rate limiting step for ester biosynthesis, is regulated by ethylene. *Plant Sci* 68:1199–1210.

Devitt, L. C., R. G. Dietzgen, and T. A. Holton. 2007. Genes associated with fruit colour in *Carica papaya*: Identification through expressed sequence tags and colour complementation. *Acta Hortic* 740:133–140.

Diaz-Mula, H. M., P. J. Zapata, F. Guillen et al. 2008. Changes in physicochemical and nutritive parameters and bioactive compounds during development and on-tree ripening of eight plum cultivars: A comparative study. *J Sci Food Agric* 88:2499–2507.

Dirlewanger, E. and C. Bodo. 1994. Molecular-genetic mapping of peach. *Euphytica* 77:101–103.

Dirlewanger, E., P. Cosson, C. Poizat et al. 2003. Synteny within the *Prunus* genomes detected by molecular markers. *Acta Hortic* 622:177–187.

Dirlewanger, E., A. Moing, C. Rothan et al. 1999. Mapping QTLs controlling fruit quality in peach (*Prunus persica* (L.) Batsch). *Theor Appl Genet* 98:18–31.

Dixon, R. A. and D. Strack. 2003. "Phytochemistry meets genome analysis, and beyond. *Phytochemistry* 62:815–816.

Doganlar, S., A. Frary, M. C. Daunay et al. 2002. A comparative genetic linkage map of eggplant (*Solanum melongena*) and its implications for genome evolution in the Solanaceae. *Genetics* 161:1697–1711.

Dominguez, A., A. H. de Mendoza, J. Guerri et al. 2002. Pathogen-derived resistance to *Citrus tristeza* virus (CTV) in transgenic Mexican lime (*Citrus aurantifolia* (Christ.) Swing.) plants expressing its p25 coat protein gene. *Mol Breed* 10:1–10.

Donaire, L., Y. Wang, D. Gonzalez-Ibeas et al. 2009. Deep-sequencing of plant viral small RNAs reveals effective and widespread targeting of viral genomes. *Virology* 392:203–214.

Dong, L., H. W. Zhou, L. Sonego et al. 2001. Ethylene involvement in the cold storage disorder of 'Flavortop' nectarine. *Postharvest Biol Technol* 23:105–115.

Downs, C. G. and C. J. Brady. 1990. Two forms of exopolygalacturonase increase as peach fruits ripen. *Plant Cell Environ* 13:523–530.

Drogoudi, P. D. and C. G. Tsipouridis. 2007. Effects of cultivar and rootstock on the antioxidant content and physical characters of clingstone peaches. *Sci Hortic* 115:34–39.

Drogoudi, P. D., S. Vemmos, G. Pantelidis et al. 2008. Physical characters and antioxidant, sugar, and mineral nutrient contents in fruit from 29 apricot (*Prunus armeniaca* L.) cultivars and hybrids. *J Agric Food Chem* 56:10754–10760.

Fagoaga, C., I. Rodrigo, V. Conejero et al. 2001. Increased tolerance to *Phytophthora citrophthora* in transgenic orange plants constitutively expressing a tomato pathogenesis related protein PR-5. *Mol Breed* 7:175–185.

Faize, M., S. Sourice, F. Dupuis et al. 2004. Expression of wheat puroindoline-b reduces scab susceptibility in transgenic apple (*Malus* × *domestica* Borkh.). *Plant Sci* 167:347–354.

Febres, V. J., R. F. Lee, G. A. Moore et al. 2008. Transgenic resistance to *Citrus tristeza* virus in grapefruit. *Plant Cell Rep* 27:93–104.

Fernandez-Trujillo, J. P. and F. Artes. 1998. Effect of intermittent warming and modified atmosphere packaging on color development of peaches. *J Food Qual* 21:53–69.

Fernandez-Trujillo, J. P., A. Cano, and F. Artes. 1998. Physiological changes in peaches related to chilling injury and ripening. *Postharvest Biol Technol* 13:109–119.

Foolad, M. R., S. Arulsekar, V. Becerra et al. 1995. A genetic-map of *Prunus* based on an interspecific cross between peach and almond. *Theor Appl Genet* 91:262–269.

Frecon, J. L., R. Belding, and G. Lokaj. 2002. Evaluation of white-fleshed peach and nectarine varieties in New Jersey. *Acta Hortic* 592:467–477.

Galla, G., G. Barcaccia, A. Ramina et al. 2009. Computational annotation of genes differentially expressed along olive fruit development. *BMC Plant Biol* 9:128.

Garner, D., C. H. Crisoto, and E. Otieza. 2001. Controlled atmosphere storage and aminoethoxyvinyl-glycine postharvest dip delay post cold storage softening of 'Snow King' peach. *HortTechnology* 11:598–602.

Garrido, I., M. Monagas, C. Gomez-Cordoves et al. 2008. Polyphenols and antioxidant properties of almond skins: Influence of industrial processing. *J Food Sci* 73:C106–C115.

Gilliland, L. U., M. Magallanes-Lundback, M. Hemming et al. 2006. Genetic basis for natural variation in seed vitamin E levels in *Arabidopsis thaliana. Proc Natl Acad Sci USA* 103:18834–18841.

Giorgi, M., F. Capocasa, J. Scalzo et al. 2005. The rootstock effects on plant adaptability, production, fruit quality, and nutrition in the peach (cv. 'Suncrest'). *Sci Hortic* 107:36–42.

Giovannini, D., A. Liverani, and F. Brandi. 2000. Indagine sulla qualità commerciale delle pesche prodotte in Romagna: Metodi di valutazione e possibilità di miglioramento. In *Proceedings of the XXIV Convegno Peschicolo*, Cesena, Italy, pp. 145–151.

Giovannini, D., M. Merli, and B. Marangoni. 2003. Integrated and conventional peach orchard management: Influence on tree productivity and soil fertility (Speciale: pesco). *Riv Fruttic Ortofloric* 65:39–48.

Gutierrez-Pesce, P., K. Taylor, R. Muleo, and E. Rugini. 1998. Somatic embryogenesis and shoot regeneration from transgenic roots of the cherry rootstock Colt (*Prunus avium* × *P.-pseudocerasus*) mediated by pRi 1855 T-DNA of agrobacterium rhizogenes. *Plant Cell Rep* 17:574–580.

Harding, P. L. and M. H. Haller. 1934. Peach storage with special reference to breakdown. *Proc Am Soc Hortic Sci* 32:160–163.

Iandolino, A., K. Nobuta, F. G. da Silva et al. 2008. Comparative expression profiling in grape (*Vitis vinifera*) berries derived from frequency analysis of ESTs and MPSS signatures. *BMC Plant Biol* 8:53.

Jarvis, M. C., S. P. H. Briggs, and J. P. Knox. 2003. Intercellular adhesion and cell separation in plants. *Plant Cell Environ* 26:977–989.

Ju, Z., Y. Duan, and Z. Ju. 2000. Leatheriness and mealiness of peaches in relation to fruit maturity and storage temperature. *J Hortic Sci Biotechnol* 75:86–91.

Kader, A. A. and A. Chordas. 1984. Evaluating the browning potential of peaches. *Calif Agric* 38:14–15.

Kader, A. A. and D. Zagory. 1988. Quality maintenance in fresh fruits and vegetables by controlled atmospheres. *Abstr Pap Am Chem Soc* 196:101–103.

Karakurt, Y., D. J. Huber, and W. B. Sherman. 2000. Quality characteristics of melting and non-melting flesh peach genotypes. *J Sci Food Agric* 13:1848–1853.

Kim, D. O., O. K. Chun, Y. J. Kim et al. 2003. Quantification of polyphenolics and their antioxidant capacity in fresh plums. *J Agric Food Chem* 51:6509–6515.

King, G. J., J. R. Lynn, C. J. Dover et al. 2001. Resolution of quantitative trait loci for mechanical measures accounting for genetic variation in fruit texture of apple (*Malus pumila* Mill.). *Theor Appl Genet* 102:1227–1235.

Ko, K. S., J. L. Norelli, J. P. Reynoird et al. 2000. Effect of untranslated leader sequence of AMV RNA 4 and signal peptide of pathogenesis-related protein 1b on attacin gene expression, and resistance to fire blight in transgenic apple. *Biotechnol Lett* 22:373–381.

Krysan, P. J., J. C. Young, M. R. Sussman et al. 1999. T-DNA as an insertional mutagen in *Arabidopsis*. *Plant Cell* 11:2283–2290.

Lavid, N., J. H. Wang, M. Shalit et al. 2002. O-methyltransferases involved in the biosynthesis of volatile phenolic derivatives in rose petals. *Plant Physiol* 129:1899–1907.

Lea, M. A., C. Ibeh, C. Desbordes et al. 2008. Inhibition of growth and induction of differentiation of colon cancer cells by peach and plum phenolic compounds. *Anticancer Res* 28:2067–2076.

Lecouls, A. C., M. J. Rubio-Cabetas, J. C. Minot et al. 1999. RAPD and SCAR markers linked to the Ma1 root-knot nematode resistance gene in Myrobalan plum (*Prunus cerasifera* Ehr.). *Theor Appl Genet* 99:328–335.

Lee, K. Y., P. Lund, K. Lowe et al. 1990. Homologous recombination in plant cells after Agrobacterium-mediated transformation. *Plant Cell* 2:415–425.

Lester, D. R., W. B. Sherman, and B. J. Atwell. 1996. Endopolygalacturonase and the melting flesh (M) locus in peach. *J Am Soc Hortic Sci* 121:231–235.

Liverani, A., D. Gionvannini, and F. Brandi. 2002. Increasing fruit quality of peaches and nectarines: The main goals of ISF-FO. *Acta Hortic* 592:507–514.

Lurie, S. and C. H. Crisosto. 2005. Chilling injury in peach and nectarine. *Postharvest Biol Technol* 37:195–208.

Lurie, S., A. Levin, L. C. Greve et al. 1994. Pectic polymer changes in nectarines during normal and abnormal ripening. *Phytochemistry* 36:11–17.

Lurie, S., H. W. Zhou, A. Lers et al. 2003. Study of pectin esterase and changes in pectin methylation during normal and abnormal peach ripening. *Physiol Plant* 119:287–294.

Luza, J. G., R. Vangorsel, V. S. Polito et al. 1992. Chilling injury in peaches—A cytochemical and ultrastructural cell-wall study. *J Am Soc Hortic Sci* 117:114–118.

Manabe, M., K. Nakamichi, R. Shingai et al. 1979. Effects of the temperature in post-harvest ripening and storage on quantitative changes of anthocyanin and polyphenol in white peaches. *J Jpn Soc Food Sci Technol* 26:175–179.

Martinelli, L., E. Candioli, D. Costa et al. 2002. Stable insertion and expression of the movement protein gene of grapevine virus A (GVA) in grape (*Vitis rupestris* S.). *Vitis* 41:189–193.

Martinelli, F., S. L. Uratsu, R. L. Reagan et al. 2009. Gene regulation in parthenocarpic tomato fruit. *J Exp Bot* 60:3873–3890.

Mathew, A. G. and H. A. B. Parpia. 1971. Food browning as a polyphenol reaction. *Adv Food Res* 19:175–201.

Mayer, A. M. and E. Harel. 1979. Polyphenol oxidases in plants. *Phytochemistry* 18:193–215.

Mezzetti, B., T. Pandolfini, O. Navacchi et al. 2002. Genetic transformation of *Vitis vinifera* via organogenesis. *BMC Biotechnol* 2:18.

Middleton, E., C. Kandaswami, and T. C. Theoharides. 2000. The effects of plant flavonoids on mammalian cells: Implications for inflammation, heart disease, and cancer. *Pharmacol Rev* 52:673–751.

Miguel, C. M. and M. M. Oliveira. 1999. Transgenic almond (*Prunus dulcis* Mill.) plants obtained by Agrobacterium-mediated transformation of leaf explants. *Plant Cell Rep* 18:387–393.

Miki, B. and S. McHugh. 2004. Selectable marker genes in transgenic plants: Applications, alternatives and biosafety. *J Biotechnol* 107:193–232.

Mitchell, F. G. and A. A. Kader. 1989. Factors affecting deterioration rate. In *Peaches, Plums and Nectarines—Growing and Handling for Fresh Market*, J. H. Larue and R. S. Johnson (eds.), pp. 165–178. Publication 3331. UCDavis Davis, CA: University of California Division of Agriculture and Natural Resources.

Monet, R. 1989. Peach genetics: Past present and future. *Acta Hortic* 254:49–57.

Morgutti, S., N. Negrini, F. F. Nocito et al. 2006. Changes in endopolygalacturonase levels and characterization of a putative endo-PG gene during fruit softening in peach genotypes with nonmelting and melting flesh fruit phenotypes. *New Phytol* 171:315–328.

Nagaraj, S. H., N. Deshpande, R. B. Gasser et al. 2007. ESTExplorer: An expressed sequence tag (EST) assembly and annotation platform. *Nucleic Acids Res* 35:W143–W147.

Nanos, G. D. and F. G. Mitchell. 1991. High-temperature conditioning to delay internal breakdown development in peaches and nectarines. *HortScience* 26:882–885.

Neri, F., G. C. Pratella, and S. Brigati. 2003. Definition of quality standards: Maturation indicators for optimizing the organoleptic quality of fruit. *Riv Fruttic Ortofloric* 65:20–24.

Newcomb, R. D., R. N. Crowhurst, A. P. Gleave et al. 2006. Analyses of expressed sequence tags from apple. *Plant Physiol* 141:147–166.

Nonoue, Y., K. Fujino, Y. Hirayama et al. 2008. Detection of quantitative trait loci controlling extremely early heading in rice. *Theor Appl Genet* 116:715–722.

Obenland, D. M. and T. R. Carroll. 2000. Mealiness and pectolytic activity in peaches and nectarines in response to heat treatment and cold storage. *J Am Soc Hortic Sci* 125:723–728.

Obenland, D. M., C. H. Crisosto, and J. K. C. Rose. 2003. Expansin protein levels decline with the development of mealiness in peaches. *Postharvest Biol Technol* 29:11–18.

Ogundiwin, E. A., C. Martc, J. Forment et al. 2008a. Development of ChillPeach genomic tools and identification of cold-responsive genes in peach fruit. *Plant Mol Biol* 68:379–397.

Ogundiwin, E. A., C. P. Peace, T. M. Gradziel et al. 2007. Molecular genetic dissection of chilling injury in peach fruit. *Acta Hortic* 738:633–638.

Ogundiwin, E. A., C. P. Peace, C. M. Nicolet et al. 2008b. Leucoanthocyanidin dioxygenase gene (PpLDOX): A potential functional marker for cold storage browning in peach. *Tree Genet Genomes* 4:543–554.

Palou, L. and C. H. Crisosto. 2003. The influence of exogenous ethylene application during cold storage on stone fruit quality and brown rot development. *Acta Hortic* 628:269–276.

Park, S., N. Sugimoto, M. D. Larson et al. 2006. Identification of genes with potential roles in apple fruit development and biochemistry through large-scale statistical analysis of expressed sequence tags. *Plant Physiol* 141:811–824.

Peace, C. P., A. Callahan, E. A. Ogundiwin et al. 2007. Endopolygalacturonase genotypic variation in *Prunus*. *Acta Hortic* 738:639–646.

Peace, C. P., C. H. Crisosto, D. T. Garner et al. 2006. Genetic control of internal breakdown in peach. *Acta Hortic* 713:489–496.

Peace, C. P., C. H. Crisosto, and T. M. Gradziel. 2005. Endopolygalacturonase: A candidate gene for Freestone and Melting flesh in peach. *Mol Breed* 16:21–31.

Petri, C., N. Alburquerque, S. Garcia-Castillo et al. 2004. Factors affecting gene transfer efficiency to apricot leaves during early Agrobacterium-mediated transformation steps. *J Hortic Sci Biotechnol* 79:704–712.

Prioul, J. L., S. Quarrie, M. Causse et al. 1997. Dissecting complex physiological functions through the use of molecular quantitative genetics. *J Exp Bot* 48:1151–1163.

Puterka, G. J., C. Bocchetti, P. Dang et al. 2002. Pear transformed with a lytic peptide gene for disease control affects nontarget organism, pear psylla (Homoptera: Psyllidae). *J Econ Entomol* 95:797–802.

Rajapakse, S., L. E. Belthoff, G. He et al. 1995. Genetic-linkage mapping in peach using morphological, Rflp and Rapd markers. *Theor Appl Genet* 90:503–510.

Reighard, G. L. 2002. Current directions of peach rootstock programs worldwide. *Acta Hortic* 592:421–427.

Remorini, D., S. Tavarini, E. Degl'innocenti et al. 2008. Effect of rootstocks and harvesting time on the nutritional quality of peel and flesh of peach fruits. *Food Chem* 110:361–367.

Reynoird, J. P., F. Mourgues, J. Norelli et al. 1999. First evidence for improved resistance to fire blight in transgenic pear expressing the attacin E gene from *Hyalophora cecropia*. *Plant Sci* 149:23–31.

Romani, R. J. and W. G. Jennings. 1971. Stone fruits. In *The Biochemistry of Fruits and Their Products*, Vol. 2, A. C. Hulme (ed.), pp. 411–436. New York: Academic Press.

Rudell, D. R., J. P. Mattheis, F.A. Curry et al. 2008. Prestorage ultraviolet-white light irradiation alters apple peel metabolome. *J Agric Food Chem* 56:1138–1147.

Ruiz, D., J. Egea, F. A. Tomas-Barberan et al. 2005. Carotenoids from new apricot (*Prunus armeniaca* L.) varieties and their relationship with flesh and skin color. *J Agric Food Chem* 53:6368–6374.

Schauer, N. and A. R. Fernie. 2006. Plant metabolomics: Towards biological function and mechanism. *Trends Plant Sci* 11:508–516.

Schwab, W., A. Aharoni, T. Raab et al. 2001. Cytosolic aldolase is a ripening related enzyme in strawberry fruits (*Fragaria × ananassa*). *Phytochemistry* 56:407–415.

Scorza, R., J. M. Cordts, D. J. Gray et al. 1996. Producing transgenic 'Thompson Seedless' grape (*Vitis vinifera* L) plants. *J Am Soc Hortic Sci* 121:616–619.

Scorza, R., J. M. Cordts, D. W. Ramming et al. 1995a. Transformation of grape (*Vitis inifera* L.) zygotic-derived embryos and regeneration of transgenic plants. *Plant Cell Rep* 14:589–592.

Scorza, R., L. Levy, V. Damsteegt et al. 1995b. Transformation of plum with the papaya ringspot virus coat protein gene and reaction of transgenic plants to plum pox virus. *J Am Soc Hortic Sci* 120:943–952.

Scorza, R. and W. B. Sherman. 1996. Peaches. In *Fruit Breeding*. Volume I: *Tree and Tropical Fruits*, J. Janick and J. N. Moore (eds.), pp. 352–440. London, U.K.: John Wiley & Sons.

Seeram, N. P., W. J. Aronson, Y. Zhang et al. 2007. Pomegranate ellagitannin-derived metabolites inhibit prostate cancer growth and localize to the mouse prostate gland. *J Agric Food Chem* 55:7732–7737.

Smigocki, A. C. and F. A. Hammerschlag. 1991. Regeneration of plants from peach embrio cells infected with a shooty mutant strain of agrobacterium. *J Am Soc Hortic Sci* 116:1092–1097.

Stockinger, E. J., C. A. Mulinix, C. M. Long et al. 1996. A linkage map of sweet cherry based on RAPD analysis of a microspore-derived callus culture population. *J Hered* 87:214–218.

Sung, S. K., D. H. Jeong, J. M. Nam et al. 1998. Expressed sequence tags of fruits, peels, and carpels and analysis of mRNA expression levels of the tagged cDNAs of fruits from the fuji apple. *Mol Cells* 8:565–577.

Tanksley, S. D., M. W. Ganal, J. P. Prince et al. 1992. High-density molecular linkage maps of the tomato and potato genomes. *Genetics* 132:1141–1160.

Tao, R., A. M. Dandekar, S. L. Uratsu et al. 1997. Engineering genetic resistance against insects in Japanese persimmon using the cryIA(c) gene of *Bacillus thuringiensis*. *J Am Soc Hortic Sci* 122:764–771.

Tatum, T. C., S. Stepanovic, D. P. Biradar et al. 2005. Variation in nuclear DNA content in *Malus* species and cultivated apples. *Genome* 48:924–930.

Tieman, D. M., M. Zeigler, E. A. Schmelz et al. 2006. Identification of loci affecting flavour volatile emissions in tomato fruits. *J Exp Bot* 57:887–896.

Tomas-Barberan, F. A., M. I. Gil, P. Cremin et al. 2001. HPLC-DAD-ESIMS analysis of phenolic compounds in nectarines, peaches, and plums. *J Agric Food Chem* 49:4748–4760.

Tonini, G., A. M. Menniti, R. Zanoli et al. 2000. *Monilinia laxa* postharvest rot control on peach and nectarine. *Att, Giorn Fitopatol Perugia* 2:63–68.

Trainotti, L., C. Bonghi, F. Ziliotto et al. 2006. The use of microarray mu PEACH1.0 to investigate transcriptome changes during transition from pre-climacteric to climacteric phase in peach fruit. *Plant Sci* 170:606–613.

Valero, D., M. Serrano, M. C. Martinezmadrid et al. 1997. Polyamines, ethylene, and physicochemical changes in low-temperature-stored peach (*Prunus persica* L. cv. Maycrest). *J Agric Food Chem* 45:3406–3410.

Vidal, J. R., J. R. Kikkert, P. G. Wallace et al. 2003. High-efficiency biolistic co-transformation and regeneration of 'Chardonnay' (*Vitis vinifera* L.) containing npt-II and antimicrobial peptide genes. *Plant Cell Rep* 22:252–260.

Viruel, M. A., R. Messeguer, M. C. Vicente et al. 1995. A linkage map with RFLP and isozyme markers for almond. *Theor Appl Genet* 91:964–971.

Von Mollendorff, L. J. and O. T. de Villiers. 1988. Role of pectolytic enzymes in the development of wooliness in peaches. *J Hortic Sci* 63:53–58.

Von Mollendorff, L. J., O. T. de Villiers, and G. Jacobs. 1989. Effect of time of examination and ripening temperature on the degree of woolliness in nectarines. *J Hortic Sci* 64:443–447.

Von Mollendorff, L. J., O. T. de Villiers, G. Jacobs et al. 1993. Molecular characteristics of pectic constituents in relation to firmness, extractable juice and woolliness in nectarines. *J Am Soc Hortic Sci* 118:77–80.

Von Mollendorff, L. J., G. Jacobs, and O. T. de Villiers. 1992. The effects of storage temperature and fruit size on firmness, extractable juice, woolliness and browning in two nectarine cultivars. *J Hortic Sci* 67:647–654.

Warburton, M. L. and F. A. Bliss. 1996. Genetic diversity in peach (*Prunus persica* L. Batch) revealed by randomly amplified polymorphic DNA (RAPD) markers and compared to inbreeding coefficients. *J Am Soc Hortic Sci* 121:1012–1019.

Welander, M., N. Pawlicki, P. G. Wallace et al. 1998. Genetic transformation of the apple rootstock M26 with the RolB gene and its influence on rooting. *J Plant Physiol* 153:371–380.

Wisniewski, M., C. Bassett, J. Norelli et al. 2008. Expressed sequence tag analysis of the response of apple (*Malus* × *domestica* 'Royal Gala') to low temperature and water deficit. *Physiol Plant* 133:298–317.

Wu, X. L., L. W. Gu, J. Holden et al. 2004. Development of a database for total antioxidant capacity in foods: A preliminary study. *J Food Compos Anal* 17:407–422.

Xu, M. L. and S. S. Korban. 2002. A cluster of four receptor-like genes resides in the Vf locus that confers resistance to apple scab disease. *Genetics* 162:1995–2006.

Xu, M. L., J. Q. Song, Z. K. Cheng et al. 2001. A bacterial artificial chromosome (BAC) library of Malus floribunda 821 and contig construction for positional cloning of the apple scab resistance gene Vf. *Genome* 44:1104–1113.

Yamamoto, T., T. Shimada, T. Imai et al. 2001. Characterization of morphological traits based on a genetic linkage map in peach. *Breed Sci* 51:271–278.

Yancheva, S. D., P. Druart, B. Watillon et al. 2002. Agrobacterium—Mediated transformation of plum (*Prunus domestica* L.). *Acta Hortic* 517:215–217.

Zhou, H. W., R. Ben-Arie, and S. Lurie. 2000a. Pectin esterase, polygalacturonase and gel formation in peach pectin fractions. *Phytochemistry* 55:191–195.

Zhou, H. W., S. Lurie, A. Lers et al. 2000b. Delayed storage and controlled atmosphere storage of nectarines: Two strategies to prevent woolliness. *Postharvest Biol Technol* 18:133–141.

Zhou, H., L. Sonego, A. Khalchitski et al. 2000c. Cell wall enzymes and cell wall changes in 'Flavortop' Nectarines: mRNA abundance, enzyme activity, and changes in pectic and neutral polymers during ripening and in woolly fruit. *J Am Soc Hortic Sci* 125:630–637.

Zuo, K.-J., X.-L. Zhang, Y. C. Nie et al. 2002. Sequence analysis of Bt insertion flanking fragments in transgenic Bt cotton. *Yi Chuan Xue Bao* 29:735–740.

# 9 Systems Biology Approaches Reveal New Insights into Mechanisms Regulating Fresh Fruit Quality

*Claudio Bonghi and George A. Manganaris*

## CONTENTS

## 9.1 FRUIT RIPENING AND QUALITY

Fruit quality is defined by traits such as fruit size and composition and is the result of a complex network of biological processes, involving exchanges (transpiration, respiration, photosynthesis, phloem and xylem fluxes, and ethylene emission) between the fruit and its environment, tissue differentiation, and cell functioning (Genard et al. 2007). The quality of horticultural products can be defined using a number of descriptors and is measured by several physicochemical parameters; a further quality evaluation occurs during or following consumption, when properties such as flavor and texture are considered (Struik et al. 2005). Although the genetic regulation of fruit development and ripening is well documented in some cases (Giovannoni 2004), fruit should also be examined through a system and a process-based modeling approach (Genard et al. 2007).

Fruit ripening is a peculiar phase of development with direct implications for a large component of the food supply and related areas of human health and nutrition, in which a coordinated series (or syndrome) of developmental and biochemical events lead to changes in color, texture, aroma, and nutritional quality (reviewed in Alexander and Grierson 2002, Barry and Giovannoni 2007) (Figure 9.1). The color change during fruit ripening is mainly due to the degradation of chlorophyll and dismantling of the photosynthetic apparatus that allows the unmasking of pigments, and the neosynthesis of different types of anthocyanins as well as of carotenoids such as β-carotene, xanthophyll esters, xanthophylls, and lycopene. The increase in flavor and aroma during fruit ripening is attributed to the production of a complex mixture of volatile compounds and degradation of bitter principles, flavanoids, tannins, and related compounds (reviewed in Defilippi et al. 2009, Prasanna et al. 2007). The taste development is due to a general increase in sweetness, which is the result of increased gluconeogenesis, hydrolysis of polysaccharides, especially starch, decreased acidity, and accumulation of sugars and organic acids, resulting in

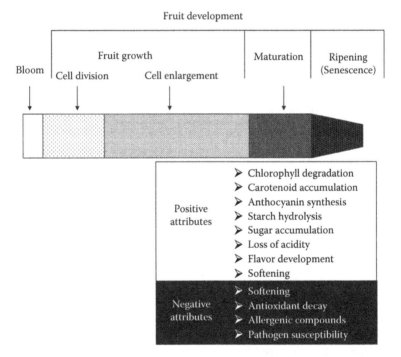

**FIGURE 9.1** Main stages of fleshy fruit development. Maturity is a state achieved by the fruit at the end of maturation. Only mature fruits, when detached from the tree, can complete the ripening phase. The latter involves changes that transform the mature fruit into one that is ready to eat (positive attributes). However, these changes can also negatively affect some quality traits (negative attributes).

an excellent sugar/acid blend. The major textural change is the softening of fruit that implies an increase of susceptibility to pathogens and a lower tolerance to mechanical damage that may quickly render the fruit unmarketable.

Tissue softening of fleshy fruits is a developmentally programed process that involves cell wall disassembly and the coordinated and interdependent action of an array of hydrolytic enzymes (Brummell et al. 2004b). The role of individual cell wall–modifying enzymes in fruit softening and the composition of polymers in the fruit cell wall may differ between fruit species, leading to many different textures associated with ripe fruit even within cultivars of the same species (e.g., melting, nonmelting, and stony hard peaches). Modifications of the cell wall are believed to underlie changes in firmness and texture, but the type and magnitude of the alterations carried out during ripening may vary considerably. Pectin solubilization, depolymerization and demethylesterification, hemicellulose depolymerization, and neutral sugar loss are some common ripening-related cell wall modifications; however, other cell wall processes occur to very different extents or are absent in certain species (Vicente et al. 2007). Indicatively, the depolymerization of ionically bound pectin during ripening is almost undetectable in strawberry, banana, and apple; relatively slight in melon; moderate in tomato; and dramatic in avocado and watermelon, while the extent of pectin solubilization is high in kiwifruit, tomato, and plum and almost absent in apple and watermelon (reviewed in Brummell et al. 2004a).

Based on ripening mechanisms, fruits are characterized as climacteric and nonclimacteric. In the former, ripening is accompanied by a peak in respiration rate and a concomitant burst of ethylene, while in the latter, respiration shows no dramatic change and ethylene production remains at a very low level. As confirmed by biotechnology approaches, such as antisense (reverse genetics) technology, specific isoforms of 1-aminocyclopropane-1-carboxylic acid (ACC) synthase and ACC oxidase, the key enzymes of ethylene biosynthesis, control ethylene production during the initiation and subsequent autocatalytic phase of ethylene production at fruit ripening (Lin et al. 2009). The complexity of ethylene action during ripening is confirmed by the activation of multiple receptors and signal transduction components. At the present time, the block of receptors, obtained by using substances such as 1 methylcyclopropene (1-MCP), proved to be a powerful tool in both basic (elucidation of fruit ripening syndrome) and applied aspects (extension of postharvest life) of fresh produce quality (reviewed in Huber 2008). However, although ethylene is the dominant trigger for ripening in climacteric fruit, both ethylene-dependent and ethylene-independent gene regulation pathways coexist to coordinate the process. For example, the suppression of ethylene production by antisense ACC oxidase RNA in "Charentais" melon has shown that, while many ripening pathways were ethylene regulated (e.g., aroma synthesis, climacteric rise of respiration rate and degreening of the rind), some were ethylene-independent (e.g., initiation of climacteric, sugar accumulation, loss of acidity, and pulp coloration) (Pech et al. 2008). These facts stimulated a reevaluation of the role of other hormones, besides ethylene, or their interactions in the ripening of climacteric fruit. Within this context, the ethylene/auxin cross-talk is becoming a critical point in the ripening regulatory network (Trainotti et al. 2007). Similarly, for nonclimacteric fruit, ethylene action has been deeply revised (Chervin et al. 2008, Maihlac and Chervin 2006), and its regulatory function is dependent on

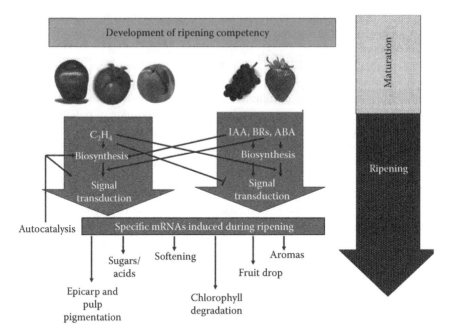

**FIGURE 9.2** Model of interaction between factors involved in the ripening regulation of climacteric (apple, tomato, and peach) and nonclimacteric (grape and strawberry) fruits. Ripening competency is gained during the first phase of syndrome (maturation) that must be completed on the plant. Action of each hormone (ethylene, $C_2H_4$; auxin, IAA; brassinolides, BR; and ABA) and their interactions occur during the second phase (ripening) that can regularly proceed, also in the postharvest phase, as long as the fruit possesses the ripening competency.

the interaction with abscissic acid (ABA). In addition to ethylene, auxin, and ABA, significant involvement has also been proposed for jasmonates and brassinosteroids in climacteric (Ziosi et al. 2008) and nonclimacteric fruits (Symons et al. 2006), respectively. These results pointed out that all the hormone categories are directly or indirectly involved in the ripening of climacteric and nonclimacteric fruits, thus supporting the hypothesis of a model common for both fruit categories (Giovannoni 2001) (Figure 9.2). Furthermore, recent advances in ripening research have given insights regarding developmental signals responsible for the acquisition of the ripening competence (i.e., the state at which a mature fruit is capable of ripening in response to endogenous or exogenous hormones) mediated by transcription factors common to a number of fruit species (Martel and Giovannoni 2007).

In fruits, the transition from the immature to the mature stage is a crucial step involving the acquisition of edible traits and organoleptic quality. Due to the economic importance of fruit crop species, fruit ripening has received a substantial amount of attention from horticulturists, plant physiologists, biochemists, and molecularly oriented developmental biologists, having important practical and economical implications. Many fruits are harvested in the unripe (but about ready to ripe) state in order to assure good survival of storage and shipping conditions.

## 9.2 "OMICS" TECHNOLOGIES TO INVESTIGATE THE MOLECULAR AND ANALYTICAL BASIS OF FRESH FRUIT QUALITY

Quality traits are seldom subjected to modeling, since they are usually a result of poorly understood chain of processes, with only partly known, complex underlying mechanisms (Struik et al. 2005). The study of complex biological processes, such as fruit ripening, through comparative genomic studies is rapidly expanding, offering improved opportunities for gene identification and characterization (reviewed in Rose and Saladie 2005). The employment of state-of-the art techniques is particularly useful in defining processes that affect fruit quality.

Genomic technologies are currently being used in a range of crops coupled with other technologies such as genetic marker development and breeding lines in order to improve the quality of fruits and vegetables (Granell et al. 2007). Emerging genomic tools and approaches are rapidly providing new clues and candidate genes that are expanding the known regulatory circuitry of ripening (Adams-Phillips et al. 2004). Genomics are classically divided into two basic areas: (1) the characterization of the physical nature of whole genomes (structural genomics) and (2) the characterization of overall patterns of gene expression, usually indicated as transcriptomics. Besides RNA, targets of functional genomic studies are also proteins (proteomics) and metabolites (metabolomics). A multidisciplinary (systems biology) approach, including the coordinated approaches of transcriptomics, proteomics, and metabolomics, is instrumental for elucidating complex interplaying mechanisms that affect postharvest performance, taste, and flavor life of the horticultural commodities (Figure 9.3).

Transcriptome analysis represents an important approach that, in combination with other techniques, allows the elucidation and better understanding of complex physiological processes, as well as their genetic regulation (Blencowe et al. 2009, Forrest and Carninci 2009). The first works on transcriptome analysis were oriented to the alignments of expressed sequence tags (ESTs). *In silico* EST analyses have extensively been used to study fruit development and ripening and, to a less extent, the postharvest behavior and responses to different storage conditions. The *in silico* expression analysis is based on comparisons of tag frequencies in different libraries corresponding to an exact digital representation of the copy number of a transcript into the examined tissue. Large EST collections have been produced from many cDNA libraries of different tissues of several fruit species including apple, grape, melon, and tomato, where specific analyses of the sequence pool have been performed in relation to fruit development and, more specifically, to the ripening process. These analyses provide the primary tool for gene discovery especially for rapid screening of candidate genes related to interested quality traits. Usually candidate genes are isolated by studying associations between genes involved in relevant metabolic pathways and major genes or quantitative trait loci (QTLs) (Salvi and Tuberosa 2005). This strategy can be very time consuming and has been successful only infrequently. The comparison between ESTs obtained from mutant and wild individual with similar genetic background can make the identification of candidate genes easier (Eveland et al. 2008, Shi and Wang 2008).

Systems of high-throughput analysis of the transcriptome have appeared, thus providing more rapid and reproducible information on a large number of RNA sequences.

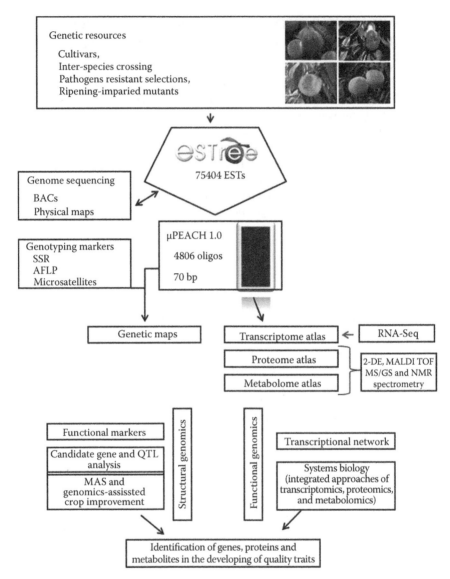

**FIGURE 9.3** Diagram of genomic project for studying fruit development and ripening in fleshy fruits. The illustrated diagram refers to peach. In this species, genetics and genomic resources as well as tools, such as platform for transcriptome analysis, have been developed. These platforms can be employed to profile the transcriptome of other *Prunus* species taking into account the high levels of synteny present in this genus.

These studies can produce larger amounts of data in terms of gene expression and provide a good alternative for new transcriptomic studies in relation to candidate gene analysis and EST development. This is a crucial point for studying fruit physiology considering that most postharvest phenotypes are genetic traits associated with one or more genes. Therefore, the unraveling of the genetic determinants that confer quality traits in fruits and other commodities is of prime importance for the development of new postharvest technologies. Among the tools developed for large-scale gene expression analysis, cDNA biochips (microarrays) are rapidly and successfully spreading because of their features and advantages mainly represented by the possibility of carrying out a massive gene analysis with a single experiment, thus avoiding the limits of the traditional single-gene approaches (Schena et al. 1995). Currently, most microarray profiling systems employ glass slides containing thousands of anchored sequences of interest (Bonghi and Trainotti 2006). The development of custom microarrays with probe sets designed to detect individual exons or using combinations of probes specific to exon and splice junction sequences was the strategy used by many groups whose research goal was the study of fruit ripening process (Bonghi and Trainotti 2006). Two different microarray hybridization strategies have been developed. The first, named two-channel microarrays (e.g., cDNA array), is performed by using a mixture of cDNAs prepared from two samples to be compared (e.g., treated tissue versus control tissue) and that are labeled with two different fluorophores. The second, named single-channel microarray (e.g., Affymetrix), provides intensity data for each probe or probe set indicating a relative level of hybridization with the labeled target. The comparison of two conditions for the same gene requires two separate single-dye hybridizations. Independently from the hybridization strategy adopted, the major drawback of microarray approach is that profiling coverage is strictly limited by the probe sets available for specific hybridization in each species. In some species, this limitation has been overcome thanks to the availability of the full genome sequence that allowed the development of new microarray platforms such as genomic tilling arrays based on a set of overlapping oligonucleotide probes representing the whole genome at very high resolution (Bertone et al. 2004). This approach could be very useful to investigate less known species at a molecular level belonging to a genus for which a full genome sequence is available and which is suitable as a reference. In addition, the sensitivity and specificity of this technology are limited by the fact that detection is indirect, generally measured by using a fluorescent signal, and is thus subject to a variety of confounding noise variables (Wechter et al. 2007). An alternative to microarrays approach is the massive (high-throughput) sequencing of transcriptome (RNA-Seq), allowed by a lowering of the costs thanks to the next-generation DNA sequencing platforms (Morozova and Marra 2008). Moreover, Wang et al. (2009) indicated that RNA-Seq, in contrast to tiling microarrays, has very low, if any, background signal because DNA sequences can be unambiguously mapped to unique regions of the genome.

The RNA-Seq approach yields a comprehensive view of both the transcriptional structure (e.g., identification of exons and introns and transcription start sites) and the expression levels of all the genes quantifying the number and density of reads corresponding to RNA from each exon (Nagalakshmi et al. 2008, Wang et al. 2009). With enough sequenced and mapped reads, it can detect and measure rare, yet physiologically relevant, species of transcripts (Mortazavi et al. 2008). In addition, RNA-Seq can be combined with other genomic and proteomic investigations to provide an integrated view of gene regulation (Fu et al. 2009, Hawkins et al. 2010). Furthermore, Werner (2010) indicated the great potential contribution of this technology to functional genomics with a special focus on gene regulation by transcription factor–binding rates as well as other regulatory molecules such as small RNAs (sRNAs). The latter are small (19–24 nt) noncoding RNAs, organized into two classes named microRNAs (miRNAs) and short interfering RNAs (siRNAs), that play important roles in the regulation of various cellular processes by inhibiting gene expression at the posttranscriptional level (Jones-Rhoades et al. 2006). To date, large-scale analysis of expression of plant sRNAs and associated prediction of precursor sequences has been restricted to a small number of fruit species taking into account that extensive genomic information is required.

The study of complex biological processes, such as fruit ripening, through comparative proteomics is becoming increasingly attractive as the rapidly expanding plant genomic and EST sequence databases provide improved opportunities for protein identification (Rose and Saladié 2005). Numerous proteins involved in various metabolic pathways have already been reported for tomato, pepper, strawberry, grape, banana, apple, and pear. Better quantitative analyses and higher throughput proteomic technologies will further improve proteomic research in horticultural products, thus having significant impact on future breeding programs coupled with novel postharvest technologies in order to improve nutritional and eating quality (Song and Braun 2008).

As transcriptomics and proteomics aim to study the products of gene transcription and translation, metabolomic approaches aim at the quantification and the identification of all metabolites present within the cell under a given set of conditions; such approaches have emerged as a methodology that makes an important contribution to the understanding of complex molecular interaction in biological systems. Metabolites in plants function in many resistance and stress responses and contribute to color, taste, and aroma development. The employment of high-throughput techniques (gas [GC] or liquid [LC] chromatography coupled with mass spectrometry [MS] methods, nuclear magnetic resonance [NMR] spectroscopy, etc.) equipped with computer hardware and software that allow the interpretation of large datasets lead to the quantification molecules that govern quality attributes of horticultural products. Although only recently such high-throughput methods have been developed, metabolomic applications in plant biology and horticultural produce are rapidly increasing (Saito and Matsuda 2010).

Overall, genomic tools are commonly used in plant science to increasingly understand the biological basis of fruit ripening, both on- and off-tree. This chapter focuses on the molecular and analytical aspects of the main climacteric and nonclimacteric fruits in which systems biology approaches have been applied in the recent past.

## 9.3 MOLECULAR AND ANALYTICAL ASPECTS OF CLIMACTERIC FRUIT RIPENING

### 9.3.1 TOMATO (*SOLANUM LYCOPERSICUM*)

Tomato is characterized as a model fruit for the ripening of climacteric fruits, where the most advanced functional genomic and proteomic tools for studying fruit ripening and quality traits have been applied. Currently, a combination of transcriptomic, proteomic, and metabolomic approaches has been applied in order to identify gene regions/QTLs relevant to tomato fruit quality (reviewed in Granell et al. 2007).

Positional cloning of genes defined by ripening defect mutations in tomato fruit system have led to the identification of novel ethylene signal transduction components, as well as to the elucidation of the function of unique transcription factors, affecting ripening-related ethylene production (reviewed in Barry and Giovannoni 2007). Tomato ripening mutations include (a) never ripe (*Nr*), (b) ripening inhibitor (*rin*), (c) colorless nonripening (*Cnr*), and (d) no ripening (*nor*). *Nr* phenotype, characterized by an ethylene insensitivity, is due to a dominant mutation in a member of the ethylene receptor gene family. The *rin* and *Cnr* mutations are recessive and dominant mutations, respectively, that effectively block the ripening process: *rin* encodes a partially deleted MADS-box protein of the SEPALLATA clade, whereas *Cnr* is an epigenetic change that alters the promoter methylation of a SQAMOSA promoter binding (SPB) protein. The *nor* locus harbors a gene with structural features suggestive of a transcription factor, although not a member of the MADS-box family. Fruit homozygous for either *rin* or *nor* or carrying a dominant *Cnr* allele undergoes complete fruit expansion and yields mature seed, yet fails to proceed in any significant way to ripening. However, both *rin* and *nor* are capable of ethylene synthesis in response to wounding, suggesting that the lack of ethylene-mediated ripening is attributed to the deficiency of appropriate developmental signals. These results, besides the fact that application of endogenous ethylene does not restore ripening to *rin*, *Nr*, or *Cnr* fruit but does result in the induction of ethylene-regulated genes, suggest that these mutants have a broader influence on aspects of climacteric ripening than those aspects controlled solely by ethylene (Giovannoni 2007).

Toward a better understanding of tomato gene expression in a plant system, a tomato functional genomics database (TFGD) has been recently generated (Fei et al. 2011). The TFGD includes all the tomato functional genomics resources organized in three major data components: gene expression, metabolite profiles, and sRNAs. Gene expression repertoire contains data obtained by using three microarray platforms (TOM1 cDNA array, TOM2 oligonucleotide array, and Affymetrix genome array) for a total of 1,308 hybridizations from 43 experiments. The employment of the TOM1 cDNA array platform showed that the *Nr*, which reduces ethylene sensitivity and inhibits ripening, altered the expression of 37% out of a total of 869 genes (Alba et al. 2005). The same research group also showed that the *Nr* affected fruit morphology, seed number, ascorbate accumulation, carotenoid biosynthesis, and ethylene evolution. Such data indicated the central role of ethylene on multiple aspects of development both prior to and during tomato fruit ripening, thus providing new insights into the molecular basis of ethylene-mediated ripening. The TOM1 cDNA array has also been employed for comparative transcriptomic studies with related Solanaceae species (pepper and eggplant fruit), and genes with central role in fruit ripening and development were identified (Moore et al. 2005).

A screening for genes, whose expression varied between lines genetically close but differing in fruit quality, showed that 39% of the unigenes corresponded to proteins that had never been isolated in fruit or with functions in fruit that were not clear or unknown. Since the BLAST comparison revealed that 41% of the unigenes were not included in this set, results revealed that some genes would not have been identified with commercially available microarrays and constitute new targets for fruit quality control (Page et al. 2008).

For metabolites, in addition to TFGD database (in which a total of more than 60 flavor and nutrition-related metabolites are collected), another database (MoToDB) was already available containing compounds that were detected in ripe tomato fruits of 96 cultivars using LC-MS (Grennan 2009, Moco et al. 2006). These databases appear to be of great help in studying the dynamics of metabolome to elucidate mutants and gene function based on differential metabolic profiles and to decipher the biological relevance of each metabolite. From this point of view, correlation analysis carried out between either the primary metabolites or the volatile organic compounds and organoleptic properties revealed a number of interesting associations such as aroma–guaiacol and sourness–alanine (Zanor et al. 2009). Furthermore, TFGD provides a central repository with tools for several large-scale tomato sRNA data sets (Fei et al. 2011, Itaya et al. 2008, Moxon et al. 2008, Pilcher et al. 2007). Among these, several conserved miRNAs showed fruit-specific expression, which, combined with target gene validation results, suggests that miRNAs may play a role in fleshy fruit development (Moxon et al. 2008).

The first characterization of the tomato fruit proteome and description of its variation during maturation included a comparative proteomic investigation on tomato fruits from a regional and commercial elite ecotype and specific proteins were recognized in each ecotype as differentially expressed during ripening (Rocco et al. 2006). A comparative analysis of the fruit pericarp proteome allowed 1,791 well-resolved spots to be selected, showing differential accumulation during cell division, cell expansion, and fruit-ripening stages (Faurobert et al. 2007). Ninety spots have been identified and most of these, showing an increasing accumulation at ripening, are related to carbohydrate metabolism or oxidative processes. A comparison between protein accumulation and expression profile of corresponding mRNA carried out on ripe tomatoes, using cDNA TOM1 microarray, indicated the presence of discrepancies between transcriptomic and proteomic data (Alba et al. 2005). Indicatively, 40% of the 90 identified varying spots corresponded to sequences present on TOM1 that had been classified as unchanged. These differences should be attributed to posttranscriptional and translational processes that modulate the quantity, temporal expression, and localization of proteins. As support to this fact, some results have shown that, even though a strong relationship between ripening-associated transcripts and specific metabolite groups (organic acids and sugar phosphates) was observed, posttranslational mechanisms dominate metabolic regulation during tomato fruit development (Carrari and Fernie 2006).

### 9.3.2 APPLE (*MALUS × DOMESTICA* BORKH.) AND RELATED SPECIES

Apple and pear fruit ripening involves complex biochemical and physiological changes and production of human health–promoting metabolites for which many molecular and genetic approaches have been undertaken to understand the associated cellular mechanisms.

The release of the apple ESTs into a public database has made possible large-scale expression studies, allowing the identification and characterization of genes with potential roles in fruit development, particularly those related to aroma production and protein degradation during ripening. Apple cDNA and oligonucleotide microarrays have been generated for more comprehensive examinations. Such tools are powerful means for elucidating the molecular events involved in metabolite bio-synthesis and physiological changes and may also enable researchers to understand how to control the ripening process (Seo and Kim 2009). For example, a gene expression analysis, using a microarray spotted with 6,253 cDNAs, showed that apple fruit development depends on the tight regulation of the expression of a number of genes, which are also expressed in other organs (Lee et al. 2007). Furthermore, an array designed from apple ESTs, representing approximately 13,000 genes, has been used to study gene expression during fruit development, and 1,955 genes showed significant changes in expression over this time course (Janssen et al. 2008). Intriguingly, the employment for comparative purposes of tomato microarrays during fruit development indicated that 16 genes showed similar pattern in apple and tomato; these genes may play fundamental roles in fruit development (Janssen et al. 2008). In addition, accumulating information about the involvement of some sRNAs in the apple fruit ripening process provides a better definition of the regulatory mechanism of expression operating in this process. In particular, sRNAs having target transcription factors such as AP2, TIR, SBP, and the ARF family, which are actively involved in the control of ripening, have been identified (Yu et al. 2011).

Taking into account that aroma governs apple fruit quality, the transcriptome approach has been used to analyze the expression of gene involved in (or related to) the aroma evolution. For this purpose, a transgenic line of "Royal Gala" apple was generated using an antisense ACC oxidase, harboring apples with no ethylene-induced ripening attributes including typical apple aroma volatile compounds such as terpenes. The comparison via microarray of untransformed and antisense ACC oxidase plants allowed the description of the expression profile of a repertoire of 179 candidate genes that might be involved in the production of aroma compounds. Among these, only 17 were typically affected by ethylene and most of them control the aroma biosynthesis, suggesting that only certain points (often the first and in all pathways the last steps) of this pathway are regulated by the hormone (Schaffer et al. 2007). The relation between ethylene and aroma was further investigated by Zhu et al. (2008). This research group examined the expression patterns of alcohol acyltransferase ($AAT$) and ACC synthase gene family members in two apple cultivars characterized by different levels of volatile ester production. The results pointed out that the climacteric expression of $ACS1$ greatly enhanced the expression levels of two alcohol acyltransferase ($AAT1$ and $AAT2$) genes that could be responsible for the emission of aromatic volatile esters. It was also suggested that the expression of $ACS3$ might play a role on induction of $AAT$ gene expression during early fruit development as it is expressed prior to $ACS1$.

The complexity of the genetic control of important fruit quality traits has been confirmed by the analysis of apple genome (Velasco et al. 2010). In apple, as observed in other genomes, numerous events of duplication regarding genes involved in metabolism of anthocyanins and flavonoids, isoflavones and isoflavonones, terpenes, and carbohydrates occurred. For the latter, compared with other plant genomes, apple has considerably more copies of key genes related to sorbitol metabolism (71 in apple; while in other species, the number ranges between 9 and 43).

The availability of the full apple genome sequence with its synteny to the pear genome (Celton et al. 2009) has opened the way to efficient localization of a number of genes involved in pear ripening. This aspect is of paramount importance in pear industry considering that fruits ripened on-tree generally do not develop the characteristic buttery and juicy texture required for marketing and consumption. Most European pears, unlike other climacteric fruits, possess varying degrees of resistance to ripening at harvest even when harvested at the appropriate maturity and require a period of chilling and/or ethylene exposure to ripen properly. This resistance to ripening poses a number of practical challenges for the pear industry in preparing the fruit for the market (Villalobos and Mitcham 2008).

The length of cold storage after harvest has a significant relationship with ethylene biosynthesis and the minimum chilling period required for normal ripening varies among pear cultivars. Pear ripening is associated with a burst of autocatalytic ethylene production. Some late pear cultivars such as Passe Crassane require a long (80 days) chilling treatment before the fruit will produce autocatalytic ethylene and ripen; therefore, cold requirement is linked to the capacity to respond to ethylene. Late ripening pears require several weeks at low temperatures and will then ripen rapidly at higher temperatures. In a few genotypes such as Passe Crassane, unchilled fruit will generally not ripen normally. In all cases, cold treatment stimulates ethylene biosynthesis that leads to ripening (Villalobos and Mitcham 2008).

Preclimacteric "Rocha" pears, stored under chilling conditions, had a larger increase of ACO activity and softened faster than those treated with ethylene. Nontreated fruit did not ripen or soften, acquired a rubbery texture, and showed barely detectable levels of ACO activity (Fonseca et al. 2005).

A collection of more than 25,000 ESTs from various tissues of the Japanese pear (*Pyrus pyrifolia* Nakai) cultivar "Housui," focusing on fruit tissues at several developmental stages have been put together from 11 different cDNA libraries. Several ESTs showing homology to genes involved in cell wall formation, phytohormone response and metabolism, transcriptional regulation, and other functions were also obtained (Nishitani et al. 2009).

Other "omics" approaches have been carried out in cultivars characterized by excellent organoleptic features in order to thoroughly investigate their genetic potential. An apple cultivar (cv Annurca), characterized by crispness, excellent taste, and long shelf life, was analyzed at the proteomic level. The results indicated 44 spots that were identified and associated to 28 different species. They were related to important physiological processes such as energy production, ripening, and stress response (Guarino et al. 2007). A metabolomic approach to characterize changes occur in an apple cultivar susceptible to superficial scald (cv. "Granny Smith") after 1-MCP or DPA treatment showed differentiation between treated and nontreated fruits within 1 week following storage initiation. α-farnese oxidation products with known associations to scald were associated with presymptomatic as well as scalded control fruit. The results demonstrate that extensive metabolomic changes associated with scald precede actual symptom development (Rudell et al. 2009).

### 9.3.3 Peach (*Prunus persica*) and Related Species

Among *Prunus* species, peach is becoming the model for molecular studies considering the huge amount of information regarding the ripening processes and especially the availability of molecular tools (microarray platforms) and, recently, the release of genome sequence (IPGI consortium; see at http://services.appliedgenomics.org/projects/drupomics/).

To date, the largest collection of ESTs (79,580 out of 107,973 *Prunus* EST) has been generated in peach mainly starting from mesocarp at different development stages, and more than 28,000 putative unigenes (20,682 contigs and 7,709 singlets) have been detected. This information is compiled in the ESTree database (http://www.itb.cnr.it/estree), where ~200 ESTs have been selected for mapping on a physical framework map. A total of 33,189 single nucleotide polymorphisms (SNPs) have also been identified, and further analysis concentrated on a subset of different SNPs representing genes putatively involved in important aspects of secondary metabolism (Lazzari et al. 2008). Additional genes associated with other quality traits were identified with a candidate gene approach (Etienne et al. 2002, Ogundiwin et al. 2009) and comparative EST approaches (Trainotti et al. 2003, Vizoso et al. 2009). The EST repertoire was used for developing the first peach microarray (μPEACH1.0) and was initially used to identify genes differentially transcribed during the transition of nectarine fruit from preclimacteric to climacteric phase (Trainotti et al. 2006). A significant number (~30%) of these genes were not ethylene regulated (Trainotti et al. 2007) (Figure 9.4). The results indicated a dramatic upregulation of genes encoding transcription factors, belonging to several families including MADS-box, Aux/IAA, bZIP, bHLH, HD, and Myb, and enzymes involved in ethylene biosynthesis and action.

In climacteric peach and tomato fruits, it has been shown that, concomitant with ethylene production, increases in the amount of auxin can also be measured. A genomic approach has been used in order to understand if auxin affects peach climacteric ripening. The results showed that auxin plays a role of its own during peach ripening, having the ability to regulate the expression of a number of different genes, and the hypothesis that a cross talk between auxin and ethylene exist has been supported (Trainotti et al. 2007). A large-scale transcriptome analysis has been also conducted using μPEACH1.0 microarray on nectarine fruit treated with 1-MCP. This compound maintains flesh firmness but did not block ethylene biosynthesis. Microarray comparison of this sample with untreated fruit 24 h after harvest revealed that about 45% of the genes affected by 1-MCP at the end of the incubation period changed their expression during the following 48 h in air. Among these genes, an ethylene receptor (*ETR2*) and three ethylene-responsive factors (*ERFs*) were present, together with other transcription factors and ethylene-dependent genes involved in quality parameter changes (Ziliotto et al. 2008).

Peach has been also chosen as a model fruit to shed light on the physiological role of Jasmonates (JAs) during ripening. Results showed that exogenous JAs led to a ripening delay due to an interference with ripening- and stress/defense-related genes, as reflected in the transcriptome of treated fruit at harvest (Ziosi et al. 2008).

Peach fruit undergoes a rapid softening process that involves a number of metabolic changes. Storing fruits at low temperatures has been widely used to extend their postharvest life. However, this leads to undesired changes, such as mealiness (woolliness) and flesh browning, thus affecting the quality of the fruit (Manganaris et al. 2006). Transcriptomic studies have been extensively employed over the recent past in order to elucidate the molecular basis of the incidence of chilling injury (CI)

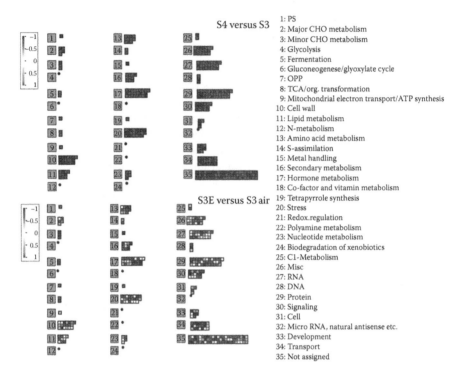

**FIGURE 9.4** Among genes differentially expressed during the transition between preclimacteric (S3 stage) and climacteric stage (S4 stage) only a subset is controlled by ethylene. Data from Trainotti et al. (2007) were recomputed and visualized by using the Mapman platform. The overview pathway shows each category (listed on the right) of genes up- and downregulated during S4/S3 transition (above) and the effect of ethylene treatment, performed at S3 stage, on their transcription (below). The grayscale heat map shows changes in gene expression, calculated as $\log_2$ ratio in the S4/S3 and S3E (ethylene)/S3 air comparisons. Up- ($\log_2$ ratio $>1$) and downregulated ($\log_2$ ratio $<-1$) genes are displayed in light gray and dark gray, respectively, while those unchanged ($\log_2$ ratio between $-1$ and $1$) in white. Only 50% of genes differentially expressed at S4/S3 transition are controlled by ethylene.

symptoms in peach fruit. The ChillPeach database was developed to facilitate the identification of genes controlling CI, a global-scale postharvest physiological disorder in peach. Microarray slides containing 4,261 ChillPeach unigenes were printed and used in a pilot experiment to identify differentially expressed genes in cold-treated compared to control mesocarp tissues, and in vegetative compared to mesocarp tissues. The microarray and qRT-PCR analyses indicated that ChillPeach is rich in putative fruit-specific and novel cold-induced genes and a web site (http://bioinfo.ibmcp.upv.es/genomics/ChillPeachDB) was created that has detailed information on the ChillPeach database (Ogundiwin et al. 2008). Other candidate genes for CI tolerance have been identified by using the µPEACH 1.0 platform. Falara et al. (2011) by comparing the transcriptome of peach fruit from "Morettini N°2" and "Royal Glory," two cultivars showing sensitivity and tolerance to CI, respectively, found that a β-D-xylosidase and PR-4B precursor could be related to the difference in tolerance to CI.

In addition, a comparative proteomic approach with 2-D DIGE allowed to point out differentially accumulated proteins in peach fruit during normal softening as well as under conditions that led to fruit CI proteins such as endopolygalacturonase, catalase, NADP-dependent isocitrate dehydrogenase, pectin methylesterase, and dehydrins, which were found to be very important for distinguishing between healthy and chilling-injured fruits (Nilo et al. 2009). A significant proportion of the proteins identified had not been associated with softening, cold storage, or CI–altered fruits before; thus, comparative proteomics has proven to be a valuable tool for understanding fruit softening and postharvest behavior.

The μPEACH1.0 was also used in comparative studies of fruit development of apricot and peach (Manganaris et al. 2011). When applied to μPEACH1.0, apricot target cDNAs showed significant hybridization with an average of 43% of spotted probes validating the use of μPEACH1.0 to profile the transcriptome of apricot fruit. Microarray analyses, carried out separately on peach and apricot fruits to profile transcriptome changes during fruit development, showed that 71% of genes had the same expression pattern in both species. Such data indicate that the transcriptome is quite similar in apricot and peach fruit, but also highlighted the presence of species-specific transcript changes. A similar comparative approach was used to dissect common and/or diverse mechanisms regulating plum (*Prunus salicina*) fruit ripening in genotypes characterized by different patterns of ethylene production (Manganaris et al. 2010).

## 9.4 MOLECULAR AND ANALYTICAL ASPECTS OF NONCLIMACTERIC FRUIT RIPENING

Notwithstanding the economic importance of nonclimacteric fruits like grape, citrus fruit, and strawberry, little is known about the mechanisms that regulate their ripening. Up to date, no growth regulator has emerged with a primary role similar to that played by ethylene in the ripening of the climacteric fruits. Strawberries can produce ethylene, although in limited amounts. Overall, similarities between nonclimacteric and climacteric fruit ripening exist and certain ethylene-dependent events in climacteric fruits are observed, apparently in the absence of or with extremely low levels of ethylene, in nonclimacteric fruits. Identification of additional components involved in ethylene signal transduction, the further characterization of ripening mutants, and additional studies on the biochemistry of ripening are essential for complete understanding of the ripening process. Therefore, understanding what controls these processes in nonclimacteric ripening may prove pertinent in gaining a full understanding of climacteric fruit ripening and vice versa (Alexander and Grierson 2002).

### 9.4.1 CITRUS FRUIT (*CITRUS* SPP.)

Citrus includes orange (*Citrus sinensis*), mandarin (*Citrus nobilis*), *Citrus aurantiumm*, *Citrus bergamina*, *Citrus grandis*, lemon (*Citrus limon*), *Citrus medica*, grapefruit (*Citrus paradisii*), as well as many interspecific hybrids. The major commercial traits in citrus include improved fruit quality, higher yield, and tolerance to environmental stresses (Terol et al. 2007). In terms of postharvest citrus fruit performance, the existence of differential preformed mechanisms as well as inducible responses to cold temperature storage has been revealed with the employment of microarray analysis. These tools and analysis provide valuable information to design postharvest protocols and to introduce those candidate genes in the plant breeding programs (Granell et al. 2007).

The first functional genomic projects, initiated to approach the molecular characterization of the main biological and agronomical traits of citrus fruits, consisted in the generation of ESTs from different fruit tissues (Forment et al. 2005) or from cultivars with different ripening properties (Terol et al. 2007). The main positive effect of these projects was the development of cDNA platforms to profile changes in the transcriptome of fruit (whole or its tissues separately) during development and ripening or postharvest phase. A custom microarray platform, based on 366 genes of interest in peel pericarp and endocarp during three developmental stages of "Washington Navel" orange fruit, was used to profile peel-specific genes. Most highly differentially expressed genes were those involved in the modification of the cell wall architecture during growth and in the development of color and aroma (Goudeau et al. 2008).

In-house citrus microarrays have been developed to identify candidate for fruit quality genes and to study the impact of genetic background and environment on gene expression (reviewed in Granell et al. 2007). A Citrus GeneChip microarray, developed by using the Affymetrix technology, was employed to gain insight into the molecular mechanisms involved in the responses of citrus fruit to low-temperature storage (Maul et al. 2008). Exposure to chilling, besides the well-known gene dataset including those associated with cell wall turnover; pathogen defense; photosynthesis; respiration; and protein, nucleic acid, and secondary metabolism, enhanced the transcript levels of genes related to membranes; lipid, sterol, and carbohydrate metabolism; stress stimuli; hormone biosynthesis; and modifications in DNA binding and transcription factors as adaptive mechanism (Maul et al. 2008).

A RNA-Seq approach was used to identify and quantitatively profile small RNAs involved in the posttranscriptional mechanism responsible for the higher lycopene accumulation in the red-flesh sweet orange mutant (MT) in comparison to its wild type (WT). Comparative profiling revealed that 60 miRNAs exhibited significant expression differences between MT and WT. Among their target predictions, those implicated in carotenogenesis were present suggesting that this pathway is deeply altered in the red-flesh sweet orange mutant (Xu et al. 2010).

Proteomics can be used to study processes strictly related to fruit quality. Within this context, Katz et al. (2007) showed that in mature juice-sac cells, the decline in acidity is a consequence of the use of citric acid for the synthesis of amino acid and sugar. This process, together with the increase in invertase activity and sugar transporters, is part of a mechanism that maintains juice-sac cell sugar homeostasis. A combination of 2-DE and LC-MS/MS approaches was used to identify the differentially expressed proteome of a pigmented sweet orange (cv Moro) compared to a common cultivar (cv Cadenera) at the ripening stage. The comparison of the protein patterns of the 2 cultivars showed 64 differentially expressed protein spots. Most of the proteins related to sugar metabolism were overexpressed in "Moro" fruit, while those related to stress responses were overexpressed in "Cadenera" fruit. Proteomic results were compared with the known variations of the same fruits at transcript level, outlining the existence of many discrepancies. Therefore, the necessity to associate both proteomic and transcriptomic approaches in order to achieve a more complete characterization of the biological system is essential (Muccilli et al. 2009).

## 9.4.2 GRAPE (*VITIS* SPP.)

In the recent past, grape ripening was studied with holistic approaches based mainly on microarray chips obtained selecting suitable probes from the large EST collection present in the public databases (Deluc et al. 2007, Grimplet et al. 2007, Pilati et al. 2007). However, the availability of extended genome sequence (Jaillon et al. 2007) facilitated the analysis of transcriptomic data, rendering grape as a model fruit for studying the nonclimacteric ripening. Recently, the massively parallel sequencing technologies have been applied to dissect the wide range of transcriptional responses that are associated with berry development in *Vitis vinifera* cv "Corvina" (Zenoni et al. 2010). Through this approach, 17,324 genes (out of 30,434 protein-coding genes predicted in the genome) were expressed during berry development, and about 30% of these showed a stage-specific expression, suggesting a significant complexity in terms of transcriptional regulatory mechanisms. Among these mechanisms an important role is played by sRNA, thus an RNA-Seq approach, via 454 technology, was performed to identify sRNA actively transcribed during berry development (Carra et al. 2009). Stage-specific expression was observed for sRNA, 53 at green phase, 42 at veraison (the point where growth ends and ripening begins), and 40 at fully-ripe stage. Among miRNAs upregulated at the fully-ripe stage, an abundance of miR169 family members was observed. Li et al. (2008) showed that the transcription factor NFYA5 is targeted by miR169 and that overexpression of miR169 leads to excessive water loss through leaves and hypersensitivity to drought stress in *Arabidopsis thaliana*. In this light, the upregulation of miR169 family members might represent a system leading to a reduction in cell turgor, an event positively associated to the initiation of softening (Saladiè et al. 2007). In grape, the kinetic of water losses is also important in the postharvest phase when grape berries are subjected to withering, a technique used for the production of dessert and fortified wines. The molecular processes that occur during withering are poorly understood, so a detailed postharvest transcriptomic analysis of grape berries was carried out by AFLP-transcriptional profiling (AFLP-TP) analysis (Zamboni et al. 2008) as well as a microarray approach (Rizzini et al. 2009). These two approaches pointed out that genes involved in transcriptional regulation; hormone, carbohydrate, and secondary metabolism; transport; and stress responses are particularly affected by dehydration, demonstrating that grape berries are metabolically reactive to water stress even after harvest. Among the different secondary metabolic processes, those concerning the phenylpropanoid pathway are of paramount relevance in terms of quality properties in particular for red wines (Figure 9.5). Associated to withering, other postharvest treatments can be performed for modulating the metabolism of important molecules associated with grape berry quality traits. Among these, particular attention was paid to transcriptome changes induced by $CO_2$ (Becatti et al. 2010) or ethylene (Rizzini et al. 2010) application. In $CO_2$-treated berries, functional categorization and gene

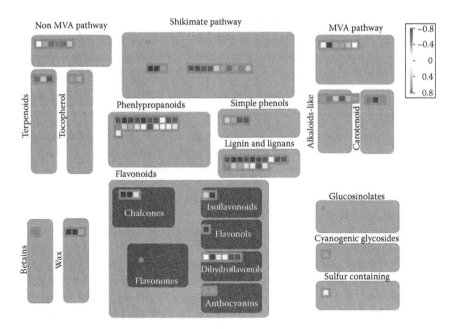

**FIGURE 9.5** Expression of genes involved in secondary metabolism in the skin of dehy-drated grape berries. Data adapted from Rizzini et al. (2009) were recomputed and visualized by using the Mapman platform. In the secondary metabolism pathway, genes involved in phenylpropanoids are significantly affected by dehydration (30% of water loss). The grayscale heat map shows changes in gene expression, calculated as $\log_2$ ratio in the dehydrated versus control berry skin comparison. Up-($\log_2$ ratio >0.8) and downregulated ($\log_2$ ratio <−0.8) genes are displayed in light gray and dark gray, respectively, while those unchanged ($\log_2$ ratio between −0.8 and 0.8) in white.

enrichment analyses pointed out that epicarp cells, in comparison to mesocarp ones, undergo more pronounced changes in transcript profiling at the end of the incubation period. In the skin, highly represented categories were fermentation, CHO metabo-lism, and redox regulation, while in both tissues the categories were those related to protein, stress, transcript, RNA, and hormone (ethylene, ABA) metabolism. Ethylene application affected the transcription of the majority of genes involved in phenyl-propanoid biosynthetic pathway with the exception of the UDP-glucose:flavonoid 3-$O$-glucosyltransferase (*UFGT*) gene. This result is in contrast with the observa-tion of El-Kereamy et al. (2003) who reported an upregulation induced at veraison by ethylene, suggesting that UFGT is differentially regulated during fruit develop-ment and ripening. Among upregulated targets by ethylene treatment, there are also some present that correspond to cell wall hydrolases. Considering their role in cell wall structure and architecture, the upregulation could be related to the increased extractability of polyphenols induced by ethylene and, consequently, to the different characteristics observed in the resulting wines.

Recently, grape berries have been studied throughout the integration of transcrip-tomic, proteomic, and metabolomic data achieved using a hierarchical clustering strategy based on the multivariate bidirectional orthogonal projections to latent structures technique (Zamboni et al. 2010). This technique identified stage-specific functional networks of linked transcripts, proteins, and metabolites. In the case of ripening and withering, the characteristic accumulation of secondary metabolites such as acylated anthocyanins was confirmed. The accumulation pattern of this compound is strictly related to that of a BEACH transcript that encodes a protein that could facilitate the compartmentalization of anthocyanins through membrane trafficking. It was also pointed out that withering involves the activation of specific osmotic and oxidative stress response genes and the specific production of stilbenes and taxifolin.

To date, grape is probably the species in which "omics" technologies have been fully integrated in the dissection of genomic basis of fruit quality, thus providing a compendium of strategies for other species.

### 9.4.3 STRAWBERRY (*FRAGARIA* × *ANANASSA*)

Following the pioneering work of Aharoni et al. (2000) who identified a novel alcohol acyltransferase (SAAT) gene responsible for flavor biogenesis in ripening strawberry using a cDNA microarray, some other cDNA-based arrays have been produced and used for transcript profiling during strawberry ripening. Using cDNA microarrays, containing 1,701 probes obtained mainly from red fruit, a comprehensive investigation of gene expression was carried out in strawberry fruit in order to understand the flow of events associated with its maturation (Aharoni et al. 2002, Aharoni and O'Connell 2002). In particular, the hormonal control of nonclimacteric fruit ripening and the differences in terms of transcripts between receptacle and achene tissues was dissected. The results emphasized the role of auxin and oxidative stress condition as regulatory elements of the ripening process. Gene sets specific for achene and the receptacle were different, for an enrichment of genes involved in the desiccation tolerance in the achene, while in receptacle tissue genes associated with the metabolism of ripening related compounds (pigments, cell wall components, fatty acids, volatile flavor, etc.) were largely represented. No further efforts have been reported for the improvement of microarray platform in strawberry. This could be important for further elucidation of the ripening biology of this nonclimacteric fruit since, as previously mentioned, the original 1,700 probes were all coming from ripe fruit. Furthermore, the microarray developed by Carbone et al. (2005) has the same bias toward ripening associated mRNAs, since it contains about 1,800 probes all derived from red fruit. New insights concerning valuable horticultural traits have been obtained after the completion of *Fragaria vesca* genome sequence (Shulaev et al. 2010). In particular, many structural genes responsible for the flavor production (acyltransferases, the terpene synthases, and small molecule *O*-methyltransferases) as well as transcription factors involved in their transcriptional regulatory mechanism have been identified.

## 9.5 FUTURE PERSPECTIVES

Taking into account the great variability that occurs within cultivars of the same species, the integration of genomic, metabolomic, and proteomic data will be indispensable for future molecular and analytical characterization and hence full exploitation of the peculiar organoleptic, nutritional, and agronomic traits of produce from cultivars with diverse properties. Moreover, genomic approaches are expanding the gene pools available for crop improvement and increasing the precision and efficiency with which superior individuals can be identified and selected. Nevertheless, efforts are still required for full exploitation of existing bioinformatics platforms and for developing new ones that enable large-scale data sets to be meaningfully managed. In particular, methods for integrating large datasets from different biological systems or provided through different "omics" approaches need to be developed.

## REFERENCES

Adams-Phillips, L., C. Barry, and J. Giovannoni. 2004. Signal transduction systems regulating fruit ripening. *Trends Plant Sci* 9:331–338.

Aharoni, A., L. C. Keizer, H. J. Bouwmeester et al. 2000. Identification of the SAAT gene involved in strawberry flavor biogenesis by use of DNA microarrays. *Plant Cell* 5:647–662.

Aharoni, A. and A. P. O'Connell. 2002. Gene expression analysis of strawberry achene and receptacle maturation using DNA microarrays. *J Exp Bot* 53:2073–2087.

Aharoni, A. and O. Vorst. 2001. DNA microarray for functional plant genomics. *Plant Mol Biol* 48:99–118.

Alba, R., P. Payton, Z. J. Fei et al. 2005. Transcriptome and selected metabolite analyses reveal multiple points of ethylene control during tomato fruit development. *Plant Cell* 17:2954–2965.

Alexander, L. and D. Grierson. 2002. Ethylene biosynthesis and action in tomato: A model for climacteric fruit ripening. *J Exp Bot* 53:2039–2055.

Barry, C. S. and J. J. Giovannoni. 2007. Ethylene and fruit ripening. *J Plant Growth Regul* 26:143–159.

Becatti, E., L. Chkaiban, P. Tonutti et al. 2010. Short-term postharvest carbon dioxide treatments induce selective molecular and metabolic changes in grape berries. *J Agric Food Chem* 58:8012–8020.

Bertone, P., V. Stolc, T. E. Royce et al. 2004. Global identification of human transcribed sequences with genome tiling arrays. *Science* 306:2242–2246.

Blencowe, B. J., S. Ahmad, and L. J. Lee. 2009. Current-generation high-throughput sequencing: Deepening insights into mammalian transcriptomes. *Gene Dev* 23:1379–1386.

Bonghi, C. and L. Trainotti. 2006. Genomic tools for a better understanding of the fruit ripening process. *Stewart Postharvest Rev* 2:1–10.

Brummell, D. A., V. Dal Cin, C. H. Crisosto, and J. M. Labavitch. 2004a. Cell wall metabolism during maturation, ripening and senescence of peach fruit. *J Exp Bot* 55:2029–2039.

Brummell, D. A., V. Dal Cin, S. Lurie, C. H. Crisosto, and J. M. Labavitch. 2004b. Cell wall metabolism during the development of chilling injury in cold-stored peach fruit: Association of mealiness with arrested disassembly of cell wall pectins. *J Exp Bot* 55:2041–2052.

Carbone, F., F. Mourgues, C. Rosati et al. 2005. Microarray and real time-PCR analysis of fruit transcriptome in strawberry elite genotypes and correlation with PTR-MS spectra of volatile compounds. *Acta Hortic* 682:269–275.

Carra, A., E. Mica, G. Gambino et al. 2009. Cloning and characterization of small non-coding RNAs from grape. *Plant J* 59:750–776.

Carrari, F. and A. R. Fernie. 2006. Metabolic regulation underlying tomato fruit development. *J Exp Bot* 57:1883–1897.

Celton, J.-M., D. Chagné, S. D. Tustin et al. 2009. Update on comparative genome mapping between *Malus* and *Pyrus. BMC Res Notes* 2:182.

Chervin, C., A. Tira-umphona, N. Terrier, M. Zouine, D. Severacc, and J. P. Roustan. 2008. Stimulation of the grape berry expansion by ethylene and effects on related gene transcripts, over the ripening phase. *Physiol Plant* 134:534–546.

Defilippi, B. G., D. Manríquez, K. Luengwilai, and M. González-Agüero. 2009. Aroma volatiles: Biosynthesis and mechanisms of modulation during fruit ripening. *Adv Bot Res* 50:1–37.

Deluc, L. G., J. Grinplet, M. D. Wheatley et al. 2007. Transcriptomic and metabolite analyses of Cabernet Sauvignon grape berry development. *BMC Genomics* 8:429.

El-Kereamy, A., C. Chervin, J. P. Roustan et al. 2003. Exogenous ethylene stimulates the long-term expression of genes related to anthocyanin biosynthesis in grapeberries. *Physiol Plant* 119:175–182.

Etienne, C., C. Rothan, A. Moing et al. 2002. Candidate genes and QTLs for sugar and organic content in peach [*Prunus persica* (L.) Batsch]. *Theor Appl Genet* 105:145–159.

Eveland, A. L., D. R. McCarty, and K. E. Koch. 2008. Transcript profiling by 3′-untranslated region sequencing resolves expression of gene families. *Plant Physiol* 146:32–44.

Falara, V., G. A. Manganaris, F. Ziliotto et al. 2011. A β-D-xylosidase and a PR-4B precursor identified as genes in accounting for differences in peach cold storage tolerance. *Funct Integr Genomics* 11, 357–368.

Faurobert, M., C. Mihr, N. Bertin et al. 2007. Major proteome variations associated with cherry tomato pericarp development and ripening. *Plant Physiol* 143:1327–1346.

Fei, Z., J.-G. Joung, X. Tang et al. 2011. Tomato functional genomics database: A comprehensive resource and analysis package for tomato functional genomics. *Nucleic Acids Res* 39:1156–1163.

Fonseca, S., L. Monteiro, M. G. Barreiro, and M. S. Pais. 2005. Expression of genes encoding cell wall modifying enzymes is induced by cold storage and reflects changes in pear fruit texture. *J Exp Bot* 56:2029–2036.

Forment, J., J. Gadea, L. Huerta et al. 2005. Development of a citrus genome-wide EST collection and cDNA microarray as resources for genomic studies. *Plant Mol Biol* 57:375–391.

Forrest, A. R. R. and P. Carninci. 2009. Whole genome transcriptome analysis. *RNA Biol* 6:107–112.

Fu, X., N. Fu, S. Guo et al. 2009. Estimating accuracy of RNA-Seq and microarrays with proteomics. *BMC Genomics* 10:161.

Genard, M., N. Bertin, C. Borel et al. 2007. Towards a virtual fruit focusing on quality: Modelling features and potential uses. *J Exp Bot* 58:917–928.

Giovannoni, J. J. 2001. Molecular regulation of fruit ripening. *Annu Rev Plant Physiol Plant Mol Biol* 52:725–749.

Giovannoni, J. J. 2004. Genetic regulation of fruit development and ripening. *Plant Cell* 16:170–180.

Giovannoni, J. J. 2007. Fruit ripening mutants yield insights into ripening control. *Curr Opin Plant Biol* 10:283–289.

Goudeau, D., S. L. Uratsu, K. Inoue et al. 2008. Tuning the orchestra: Selective gene regulation and orange fruit quality. *Plant Sci* 174:310–320.

Granell, A., C. Pons, C. Marti et al. 2007. Genomic approaches-innovative tools to improve quality of fresh cut produce. *Acta Hortic* 746:203–211.

Grennan A. K. 2009. MoToZanoe DB: A metabolic database for tomato. *Plant Physiol* 151:1701–1702.

Grimplet, J., L. G. Deluc, R. L. Tillett et al. 2007. Tissue-specific mRNA expression profiling in grape berry tissues. *BMC Genomics* 8:187.

Guarino, C., S. Arena, L. De Simone et al. 2007. Proteomic analysis of the major soluble components in Annurca apple flesh. *Mol Nutr Food Res* 51:255–262.

Hawkins, R. D., G. C. Hon, and B. Ren. 2010. Next-generation genomics: An integrative approach. *Nat Rev Genet* 11:476–486.

Huber, D. J. 2008. Suppression of ethylene responses through application of 1-methylcyclopropene: A powerful tool for elucidating ripening and senescence mechanisms in climacteric and nonclimacteric fruits and vegetables. *HortScience* 43:106–111.

Itaya, A., R. Bundschuh, A. J. Archual et al. 2008. Small RNAs in tomato fruit and leaf development. *Biochim Biophys Acta* 1779:99–107.

Jaillon, O., J.-M. Aury, B. Noel et al. 2007. The grapevine genome sequence suggests ancestral hexaploidization in major angiosperm phyla. *Nature* 449:463–467.

Janssen, B. J., K. Thodey, R. J. Schaffer et al. 2008. Global gene expression analysis of apple fruit development from the floral bud to ripe fruit. *BMC Plant Biol* 8:16.

Jones-Rhoades, M. W., D. P. Bartel, and B. Bartel. 2006. MicroRNAs and their regulatory roles in plants. *Annu Rev Plant Biol* 57:19–53.

Katz, E., M. Fon, Y. J. Lee, B. S. Phinney, A. Sadka, and E. Blumwald. 2007. The citrus fruit proteome: Insights into citrus fruit metabolism. *Planta* 226:989–1005.

Lazzari, B., A. Caprera, A. Vecchietti et al. 2008. Version VI of the ESTree db: An improved tool for peach transcriptome analysis. *BMC Bioinform* 9:S9.

Lee, Y. P., G. H. Yu, Y. S. Seo et al. 2007. Microarray analysis of apple gene expression engaged in early fruit development. *Plant Cell Rep* 26:917–926.

Li, W. X., Y. Oono, J. Zhu et al. 2008. The Arabidopsis NFYA5transcription factor is regulated transcriptionally and posttranscriptionally to promote drought resistance. *Plant Cell* 20:2238–2251.

Lin, Z., S. Zhong, and S. D. Grierson. 2009. Recent advances in ethylene research. *J Exp Bot* 60:3311–3336.

Maihlac, N. and C. Chervin. 2006. Ethylene and grape berry ripening. *Stewart Postharvest Rev* 2:7–10.

Manganaris, G. A., A. Jajo, V. Ziosi et al. 2010. Comparative transcriptomic analysis of plum fruit treated with 1-MCP. *Acta Hortic* 887:1105–1110.

Manganaris, G. A., A. Rasori, D. Bassi, A. Ramina, P. Tonutti, and C. Bonghi. 2011. Comparative transcript profiling of apricot (*Prunus armeniaca* L.) fruit development and on-tree ripening. *Tree Genet Genomes* 7, 609–616.

Manganaris, G. A., M. Vasilakakis, G. Diamantidis, and I. Mignani. 2006. Cell wall physicochemical aspects of peach fruit related to internal breakdown symptoms. *Postharvest Biol Technol* 39:69–74.

Martel, C. and J. J. Giovannoni. 2007. Fruit ripening. In *Plant Cell Separation and Adhesion*, J. Roberts and Z. Gonzalez-Carranzas (eds.), pp. 164–176, Oxford, U.K.: Blackwell Publishing Ltd.

Maul, P., G. T. McCollum, M. Popp, C. L. Guy, and R. Porat. 2008. Transcriptome profiling of grapefruit flavedo following exposure to low temperature and conditioning treatments uncovers principal molecular components involved in chilling tolerance and susceptibility. *Plant Cell Environ* 31:752–768.

Moco, S., R. J. Bino, O. Vorst et al. 2006. A liquid chromatography–mass spectrometry-based metabolome database for tomato. *Plant Physiol* 141:1205–1218.

Moore, S., P. Payton, M. Wright, S. Tanksley, and J. Giovannoni. 2005. Utilization of tomato microarrays for comparative gene expression analysis in the Solanaceae. *J Exp Bot* 56:2885–2895.

Morozova, O. and M. A. Marra. 2008. Applications of next-generation sequencing technologies in functional genomics. *Genomics* 92:255–264.

Mortazavi, A., B. A. Williams, K. McCue, L. Schaeffer, and B. Wold. 2008. Mapping and quantifying mammalian transcriptomes by RNA-Seq. *Nat Methods* 5:621–628.

Moxon, S., R. Jing, G. Szittya et al. 2008. Deep sequencing of tomato short RNAs identifies microRNAs targeting genes involved in fruit ripening. *Genome Res* 18:1602–1609.

Muccilli, V., C. Licciardello, D. Fontanini, D. M. P. M. P. Russo, V. Cunsolo, R. Saletti, G. R. Recupero, and S. Foti. 2009. Proteome analysis of *Citrus sinensis* L. (Osbeck) flesh at ripening time. *Proteomics* 73:134–152.

Nagalakshmi, U., Z. Wang, K. Waern et al. 2008. The transcriptional landscape of the yeast whole genome defined by RNA sequencing. *Science* 320:1344–1349.

Nilo, R., C. Saffie, K. Lilley et al. 2009. Proteomic analysis of peach fruit mesocarp softening and chilling injury using difference gel electrophoresis (DIGE). *BMC Genomics* 11:43.

Nishitani, C., T. Shimizu, H. Fujii, S. Terakami, and T. Yamamoto. 2009. Analysis of expressed sequence tags from Japanese pear 'Housui'. *Acta Hortic* 814:645–650.

Ogundiwin, E. A., C. Marti, and J. Forment. 2008. Development of ChillPeach genomic tools and identification of cold-responsive genes in peach fruit. *Plant Mol Biol* 68:379–397.

Ogundiwin, E. A., C. P. Peace, T. M. Gradziel, F. A. Bliss, D. E. Parfitt, and C. H. Crisosto. 2009. A fruit quality gene map of *Prunus*. *BMC Genomics* 10:587.

Page, D., I. Marty, J. P. Bouchet, B. Gouble, and M. Causse. 2008. Isolation of genes potentially related to fruit quality by subtractive selective hybridization in tomato. *Postharvest Biol Technol* 50:117–124.

Pech, J. C., M. Bouzayen, and A. Latche. 2008. Climacteric fruit ripening: Ethylene-dependent and independent regulation of ripening pathways in melon fruit. *Plant Sci* 175:114–120.

Pilati, S., M. Perazzolli, A. Malossini et al. 2007. Genome-wide transcriptional analysis of grapevine berry ripening reveals a set of genes similarly modulated during three seasons and the occurrence of an oxidative burst at veraison. *BMC Genomics* 8:428.

Pilcher, R. L., S. Moxon, N. Pakseresht et al. 2007. Identification of novel small RNAs in tomato (*Solanum lycopersicum*). *Planta* 226:709–717.

Prasanna, V., T. N. Prabha, and R. N. Tharanathan. 2007. Fruit ripening phenomena—An overview. *Crit Rev Food Sci Nutr* 47:1–19.

Rizzini, F. M., C. Bonghi, L. Chkaiban, F. Martinelli, and P. Tonutti. 2010. Effects of postharvest partial dehydration and prolonged treatments with ethylene on transcript profiling in skins of wine grape berries. *Acta Hortic* 877:1099–2004.

Rizzini, F. M., C. Bonghi, and P. Tonutti. 2009. Postharvest water loss induces marked changes in transcript profiling in skins of wine grape berries. *Postharvest Biol Technol* 52:247–253.

Rocco, M., C. D' Ambrosio, S. Arena, M. Faurobert, A. Scaloni, and M. Marra. 2006. Proteomic analysis of tomato fruits from two ecotypes during ripening. *Proteomics* 6:3781–3791.

Rose, J. K. C. and M. Saladié. 2005. Proteomic analysis and fruit ripening. *Acta Hortic* 682:211–224.

Rudell, D. R., J. P. Mattheis, and M. L. A. T. M. Hertog. 2009. Metabolomic change precedes apple superficial scald symptoms. *J Agric Food Chem* 57:8459–8466.

Saito, K. and F. Matsuda. 2010. Metabolomics for functional genomics, systems biology, and biotechnology. *Annu Rev Plant Biol* 61:463–489.

Saladié, M., A. J. Matas, T. Isaacson et al. 2007. A reevaluation of the key factors that influence tomato fruit softening and integrity. *Plant Physiol* 144:1012–1028.

Salvi, S. and R. Tuberosa. 2005. To clone or not to clone plant QTLs: Present and future challenges. *Trends Plant Sci* 10:297–304.

Schaffer, R. J., E. N. Friel, E. J. F. Souleyre et al. 2007. A genomics approach reveals that aroma production in apple is controlled by ethylene predominantly at the final step in each biosynthetic pathway. *Plant Physiol* 144:1899–1912.

Schena, M., D. Shalon, R. W. Davis, and P. O. Brown. 1995. Quantitative monitoring of gene-expression patterns with a complementary-DNA microarray. *Science* 270:467–470.

Seo, Y. S. and W. T. Kim. 2009. A genomics approach using expressed sequence tags and microarrays in ripening apple fruit (*Malus domestica* Borkh.). *J Plant Biol* 52:35–40.

Shi, B. J. and G. L. Wang. 2008. Comparative study of genes expressed from rice fungus-resistant and susceptible lines during interactions with *Magnaporthe oryzae*. *Gene* 427:80–85.

Shulaev, V., D. J. Sargent, R. N. Crowhurst et al. 2010. The genome of woodland strawberry (*Fragaria vesca*). *Nat Genet* 43:109–116.

Song, J. and G. Braun. 2008. Application of proteomic techniques to fruits and vegetables. *Curr Proteomics* 5:191–201.

Struik, P. C., X. Y. Yin, and P. de Visser. 2005. Complex quality traits: Now time to model. *Trends Plant Sci* 10:513–516.

Symons, G. M., C. Davies, Y. Shavrukov, I. B. Dry, J. B. Reid, and M. R. Thomas. 2006. Grapes on steroids. Brassinosteroids are involved in grape berry ripening. *Plant Physiol* 140:150–158.

Terol, J., A. Conesa, J. M. Colmenero et al. 2007. Analysis of 13000 unique Citrus clusters associated with fruit quality, production and salinity tolerance. *BMC Genomics* 8:31.

Trainotti, L., C. Bonghi, F. Ziliotto et al. 2006. The use of microarray μPEACH1.0 to investigate transcriptome changes during transition from pre-climacteric to climacteric phase in peach fruit. *Plant Sci* 170:606–613.

Trainotti, L., A. Tadiello, and G. Casadoro. 2007. The involvement of auxin in the ripening of climacteric fruits comes of age: The hormone plays a role of its own and has an intense interplay with ethylene in ripening peaches. *J Exp Bot* 58:3299–3308.

Trainotti, L., D. Zanin, and G. Casadoro. 2003. A cell wall-oriented genomic approach reveals a new and unexpected complexity of the softening in peaches. *J Exp Bot* 54:1821–1832.

Velasco, R., A. Zharkikh, J. Affourtit et al. 2010. The genome of the domesticated apple (*Malus × domestica* Borkh.). *Nat Genet* 42:833–841.

Vicente, A. R., M. Saladie, J. K. C. Rose, and J. M. Labavitch. 2007. The linkage between cell wall metabolism and fruit softening: Looking to the future. *J Sci Food Agric* 87:1435–1448.

Villalobos, M. and E. J. Mitcham. 2008. Ripening of European pears: The chilling dilemma. *Postharvest Biol Technol* 49:187–200.

Vizoso, P., L. A. Meisel, A. Tittarelli et al. 2009. Comparative EST transcript profiling of peach fruits under different post-harvest conditions reveals candidate genes associated with peach fruit quality. *BMC Genomics* 10:423.

Wang, Z., M. Gerstein, and M. Snyder. 2009. RNA-Seq: A revolutionary tool for transcriptomics. *Nat Rev Gen* 10:57–63.

Wechter, W. P., A. Levi, D. A. Kluepfel, E. T. Gonzalez, and G. Presting. 2007. Microarray analysis: Uses and limitations. *HortScience* 42:477.

Werner, T. 2010. Next generation sequencing in functional genomics. *Brief Bioinformatics* 11:499–511.

Xu, Q., Y. Liu, A. Zhu, X. Wu, J. Ye, K. Yu, W. Guo, and X. Deng. 2010. Discovery and comparative profiling of microRNAs in a sweet orange red-flesh mutant and its wild type. *BMC Genomics* 17:246.

Yu, H., C. Song, Q. Jia et al. 2011. Computational identification of microRNAs in apple expressed sequence tags and validation of their precise sequences by miR-RACE. *Physiol Plant* 141:56–70.

Zamboni, A., M. Di Carli, F. Guzzo et al. 2010. Identification of putative stage-specific grapevine berry biomarkers and omics data integration into networks. *Plant Physiol* 154:1439–1459.

Zamboni, A., L. Minoia, A. Ferrarini et al. 2008. Molecular analysis of post-harvest withering in grape by AFLP transcriptional profiling. *J Exp Bot* 59:4145–4159.

Zanor, M. I., J.-L. Rambla, J. Chaïb et al. 2009. Metabolic characterization of loci affecting sensory attributes in tomato allows an assessment of the influence of the levels of primary metabolites and volatile organic contents. *J Exp Bot* 60:2139–2154.

Zenoni, S., A. Ferrarini, E. Giacomelli et al. 2010. Characterization of transcriptional complexity during berry development in *Vitis vinifera* using RNA-Seq. *Plant Physiol* 152:1787–1795.

Zhu, Y., D. R. Rudell, and J. Mattheis. 2008. Characterization of cultivar differences in alcohol acyltransferase and 1-aminocyclopropane-1-carboxylate synthase gene expression and volatile ester emission during apple fruit maturation and ripening. *Postharvest Biol Technol* 49:330–339.

Ziliotto, F., M. Begheldo, A. Rasori, C. Bonghi, and P. Tonutti. 2008. Transcriptome profiling of ripening nectarine (*Prunus persica* L. Batsch) fruit treated with 1-MCP. *J Exp Bot* 59:2781–2791.

Ziosi, V., C. Bonghi, A. M. Bregoli et al. 2008. Jasmonate-induced transcriptional changes suggest a negative interference with the ripening syndrome in peach fruit. *J Exp Bot* 59:563–573.

# 10 Coffee Genomics

*Sarada Krishnan and Tom A. Ranker*

## CONTENTS

## 10.1 INTRODUCTION

Coffee is one of the most economically important crops produced in about 80 tropical countries with an annual production of nearly 7 million tons of green beans (Musoli et al. 2009). It is the second most valuable commodity exported by developing countries with over 75 million people depending on it for their livelihood (Pendergrast 2009). *Coffea* (family Rubiaceae, subfamily Ixoroideae, and tribe Coffeeae) consists of 103 species distributed in Africa, Madagascar, the Comoros, and the Mascarene Islands (La Réunion and Mauritius) (Davis and Rakotonasolo 2008). Of these, three species are economically important for the production of the beverage coffee: *Coffea arabica* (Arabica coffee), *C. canephora* (Robusta coffee), and, to a lesser extent, *C. liberica* (Liberian or Liberica coffee, or Excelsa coffee) (Davis et al. 2006). Higher beverage quality is associated with *C. arabica*, which accounts for about 70% of the world's coffee production (Lashermes et al. 1999). *C. arabica* is a tetraploid ($2n = 4x = 44$ chromosomes) and is self-fertile, whereas all other *Coffea* species are diploid ($2n = 2x = 22$ chromosomes) and mostly self-sterile (Pearl et al. 2004).

It is thought that people took coffee to Yemen from its origins in Ethiopia around the sixth century (Pendergrast 1999). From Yemen, two genetic bases spread giving rise to most of the present commercial cultivars of Arabica coffee grown world-wide (Anthony et al. 2002). The two subpopulations of wild coffee introduced from Ethiopia to Yemen underwent successive reductions in genetic diversity (Figure 10.1) with the first reduction occurring with the introduction of coffee to Yemen 1500 to 300 years ago (Anthony et al. 2002). Introduction of coffee to Java, Amsterdam, and La Réunion at the beginning of the eighteenth century led to further reductions in genetic diversity (Anthony et al. 2002). Several authors indicate that the Typica

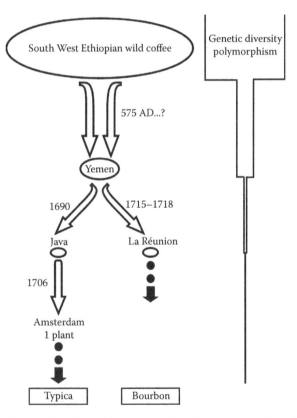

**FIGURE 10.1**  History of coffee cultivation revealing loss of genetic diversity. (Reprinted with kind permission from Springer Science+Business Media: *Theor. Appl. Genet.*, The origin of cultivated *Coffea arabica* L. varieties revealed by AFLP and SSR markers, 104, 2002, 894, Anthony, F., Combes, M. C., Astorga, C., Bertrand, B., Graziosi, G., and Lashermes, P.)

genetic base originated from a single plant cultivated in Amsterdam in the early eigh-teenth century, introduced from Java, whereas the Bourbon genetic base originated from coffee trees introduced to La Réunion (then Bourbon Island) from Mocha, Yemen, in 1715 and 1718 (Anthony et al. 2002). Coffee then spread rapidly to the Americas and Indonesia from self-fertilized seeds with intense reduction in genetic diversity (Anthony et al. 2002). Anthony et al. (2002) detected few polymorphisms within Typica and Bourbon genetic bases using AFLP markers and none using SSR markers, with higher polymorphisms in the Bourbon genetic base indicating that the descendents of this genetic base may have been derived from several individuals compared to the derivation of the Typica genetic base from just a single individual.

## 10.2   DIVERSITY AND PHYLOGENY

*Coffea* comprises 103 species with 41 endemic to Africa, 59 endemic to Madagascar, and 3 endemic to the Mascarenes (Davis et al. 2006). The genus is classified into two subgenera: subgenus *Coffea* (95 species) and subgenus *Baracoffea* (8 species) (Davis et al. 2006). *Coffea* subgenus *Coffea* occurs throughout the natural range of the genus in Africa, Madagascar, and the Mascarenes, whereas *Coffea* subgenus *Baracoffea* is restricted to the dry forests of Western Madagascar (Davis et al. 2006). Differing greatly in morphology, size, and ecological adaptation, all species are perennial woody shrubs or trees (Anthony et al. 2010). Generally occurring in humid, ever-green forests, *Coffea* species in Africa and Madagascar inhabit diverse forest types, which may correlate with the high species diversity of this genus (Davis et al. 2006).

Phylogenetic analysis of plastid DNA sequences (*trnL–trnF* intergenic spacer) revealed strong geographical distinction distributed in five clades (Cros et al. 1998). More recent phylogenetic analysis of *Coffea* subgenus *Coffea* using the same and different plastid DNA sequences (*trnL-F, trnT-L*, and *atpB–rbcL* intergenic spacers) revealed two lineages: clade A-IO (Africa-Indian Ocean) spanning the entire geograph-ical range and clade G-C restricted to the Guineo-Congolian region (Anthony et al. 2010). Species within these clades were further resolved into geographically defined subclades (Figure 10.2) as EA (East Africa), E-CA (East-Central Africa), C (Congolia), LG (Lower Guinea), and UG (Upper Guinea) (Anthony et al. 2010). Nucleotide sequence diversity was highest in west equatorial Africa, suggesting that Lower Guinea could be the center of origin and initial radiation of *Coffea* subgenus *Coffea* (Anthony et al. 2010). The creation of a savannah barrier between Upper Guinea and Lower Guinea by the Dahomey Gap and fragmentation of the rain forest in the Guineo-Congolian region have played significant roles in the evolution of species in this region (Anthony et al. 2010, Maurin et al. 2007). The presence of distinct genetic groups of *C. canephora* in Upper Guinea and Central Africa suggests the colonization of coffee in Upper Guinea before the formation of the Dahomey Gap (Anthony et al. 2010).

Anthony et al. (2010) suggested a recent origin of *Coffea* subgenus *Coffea* due to the low number of insertions and deletions required for plastid sequence align-ment and due to low sequence divergence within *Coffea* species compared to diver-gence between *Coffea, Rubia,* and other Rubiaceae species. The sequences from the Madagascan species when compared to species from surrounding islands and from East Africa showed high similarities, suggesting a common origin (Anthony et al. 2010).

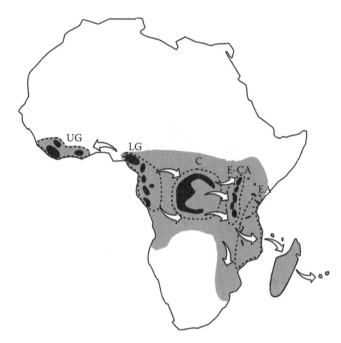

**FIGURE 10.2** Reconstruction of dispersal of *Coffea* subgenus *Coffea* from its center of origin in Lower Guinea to other identified biogeographic regions: *UG*, Upper Guinea; *LG*, Lower Guinea; *C*, Congolia; *E-CA*, East-Central Africa; and *EA*, East Africa. Gray areas represent actual distribution and black areas represent putative forest refuges during the last major arid phase. (Reprinted with kind permission from Springer Science+Business Media: *Plant Syst. Evol.*, Adaptive radiation on *Coffea* subgenus *Coffea* L. (Rubiaceae) in Africa and Madagascar, 285, 2010, 51, Anthony F., Diniz, L. E. C., Combes, M.-C., and Lashermes, P.)

Due to limited ranges of Madagascan species, Davis et al. (2006) suggested radial and rapid speciation of these species as well as recent origins (Cros et al. 1998). Colonization of volcanic islands of the Indian Ocean such as the Comoros Islands, La Réunion, and Mauritius most likely occurred through long-distance dispersals (Cros et al. 1998).

From its center of origin in Lower Guinea, coffee is likely to have spread radially to Upper Guinea and eastward toward Central Africa (Figure 10.2), with a single dispersal event from the African mainland leading to colonization of Madagascar followed by insular speciation (Anthony et al. 2010, Maurin et al. 2007). High similarity between species from Grand Comore and North Madagascar indicate colonization of Grand Comore from North Madagascar (Maurin et al. 2007) in one step after crossing the Mozambique channel (Anthony et al. 2010). Detection of a common origin between species from the Mascarenes with East African and Madagascan species indicate rapid colonization of Mauritius and La Réunion from Madagascar (Anthony et al. 2010). Variations in gene-expression mechanisms rather than the nucleotide composition of the genes themselves have been suggested as the origin of the high adaptive capacity of *Coffea* subgenus *Coffea* species (Anthony et al. 2010).

## 10.3   GENOME ANALYSIS

The core aims of genome science are as follows: (1) to establish an integrated web-based database and research interface; (2) to assemble physical and genetic maps of the genome; (3) to generate and categorize genomic and expressed gene sequences; (4) to identify and annotate the complete set of genes encoded within a genome; (5) to characterize DNA sequence diversity; (6) to compile atlases of gene expression; (7) to accumulate functional data, including phenotypic and biochemical properties of genes; and (8) to provide resources for comparison with other genomes (Gibson and Muse 2009).

Development of cytogenetic research in the genus *Coffea* has been complicated due to the small size of the chromosomes and the uniform karyotypes of the species (Pinto-Maglio 2006). In recent years, there has been a dramatic increase in tools available for molecular and genomic research of cultivated *Coffea* species (De Kochko et al. 2010). Techniques such as fluorescent *in situ* hybridization (FISH) and genomic *in situ* hybridization (GISH) have been used for identification of small and morphologically similar chromosomes (Pinto-Maglio 2006). These techniques are based on the presence or absence of specific DNA sequences and their number and location in the compliment rather than the size and shape of the chromosome (Pinto-Maglio 2006). The GISH technique has been used to elucidate the genomic organization of interspecific hybrids (De Kochko et al. 2010). Techniques such as fluorescent banding with DAPI (4'-6-diamidino-2-phenyllindole), CMA (chromomycin A), and FISH were used to characterize 14 *Coffea* species and 3 species of the closely related *Psilanthus* (Pinto-Maglio 2006). The FISH technique offers an important alternative for cytogenetic characterization of *Coffea* and for future DNA-specific sequence mapping (Pinto-Maglio 2006).

Genetic marker and cytogenetic techniques have been used in understanding the organization and evolution of the *Coffea* genome (Lashermes et al. 1999). The main focus of cytological research in coffee has been the origin of the species *C. arabica*, the only polyploid species in the genus (Pinto-Maglio 2006). *C. arabica* was identified as an amphidiploid formed by hybridization between *C. eugenioides* as the female parent and *C. canephora*, or related ecotypes, as the other parent (Lashermes et al. 1999). By employing GISH, Lashermes et al. (1999) demonstrated that the *C. arabica* genome arose from association of chromosomes belonging to two distinct ancestral genomes, namely, the canephoroid and eugenioides groups with *C. canephora* and *C. eugenioides* as being the two extant species most similar to these genomic groups, respectively. Chloroplast DNA from *C. arabica* appeared similar to chloroplast DNA from *C. eugenioides* and *Coffea* sp. Moloundou, providing strong support for the hypothesis that species related to *C. eugenioides* and *Coffea* sp. Moloundou as maternal progenitors (Cros et al. 1998). Other researchers have reported a segmental allopolyploid nature of *C. arabica*, where a segmental allopolyploid is defined as a type of intermediate between allopolyploids and autopolyploids with differentiation of the progenitor genome insufficient for effective allopolyploidy (Clarindo and Carvalho 2008). Using improved cytogenetic protocols, Clarindo and Carvalho (2008) identified distinct chromosomes that suggest that *C. arabica* is not a segmental allopolyploid, but a true amphidiploid originating from different species exhibiting similar and distinct chromosomes.

## 10.3.1   GENOME SIZE

The first genome size evaluation of 12 diploid species of *Coffea* by Cros et al. (1995) (as cited in Noirot et al. 2003) revealed a broad size range, from 2C = 0.95 pg in *C. racemosa* to 2C = 1.78 pg in *C. humilis*. This study conducted genome size evaluation using flow cytometry with propidium iodide (PI) as dye and *Oryza sativa* ssp. *japonica* as the external standard. Since then, a more reliable and accurate flow cytometry method was developed using *Petunia hybrida* (2.85 pg) as an internal standard and better statistical control of stoichiometric error (Barre et al. 1996). Using flow cytometry, Clarindo and Carvalho (2009) measured the mean genome size of *C. canephora* and *C. arabica* to be 2C = 1.41 pg and 2C = 2.62 pg, respectively.

Environmental variation is one of the main consequences of stoichiometric error leading to within-species genome size variations (Noirot et al. 2005). Intraspecific and interspecific genome size variations in coffee could be explained by the presence of phenolic compounds such as caffeine and chlorogenic acids (CGAs) with caffeine increasing dye accessibility and CGA decreasing it (Noirot et al. 2003). This leads to pseudo-genome size variations within and between species, and hence all genome size variations should be carefully interpreted in phenol-rich species (Noirot et al. 2005). Correlations between genome size and abiotic factors such as geographic gradient and soil water deficit have also been reported (Noirot et al. 2003).

## 10.3.2   EXPRESSED SEQUENCE TAGS

The term expressed sequence tag (EST) describes a single sequence representing a partial sequence of a complementary DNA (cDNA) (Gibson and Muse 2009). Instead of sequencing a whole genome, by extracting mRNA and reverse transcribing it into cDNA, many of the expressed genes can be sequenced (Barker and Wolf 2010). By clustering EST sequences into a condensed set of contiguous sequences (contigs), bioinformatic tools can be used to identify unique, nonoverlapping sequences (singletons). These, when pooled together, form a collection of unique genes or unigenes (Barker and Wolf 2010). This method provides a broad sampling of an organism's transcriptome regardless of its genome complexity (Barker and Wolf 2010). Large-scale ESTs are used to provide gene repertoires of a given species; to identify composition of genes; to study gene expression under specific conditions or in particular tissues; and in comparative genetics such as phylogenetic studies, genetic mapping, and investigation of gene and genome duplications (De Kochko et al. 2010).

GenBank (http://www.ncbi.nlm.nih.gov/genbank/) has a listing of 100,191 *Coffea* ESTs with the following breakdown: 56,231 *C. canephora*, 43,619 *C. arabica*, 145 *C. canephora* × *C. congensis*, 108 *C. arabica* × *C. canephora*, 24 *Coffea* hybrid cultivars, and 64 other taxa (National Center for Biotechnology Information GenBank). Sequences are available for 13,686 ESTs at the CoffeeDNA database (http://www.coffeedna.net/). The Brazilian Coffee Genome Project has sequenced 130,792, 12,381, and 10,566 EST sequences for *C. arabica*, *C. canephora*, and *C. racemosa*, respectively (Vieira et al. 2006). These resources combined with many other nonpublic ESTs developed by private organizations represent a valuable resource for analysis of the *Coffea* genome.

### 10.3.3 Bacterial Artificial Chromosome Libraries

Bacterial artificial chromosome (BAC) libraries have become an important tool in the development of diverse genomic applications in plants such as comparative genomics, construction of physical maps, map-based gene cloning, identification of quantitative trait loci (QTLs) genes, integration of cytogenetic and physical maps, and facilitation of chromosome and whole genome-sequencing projects (De Kochko et al. 2010, Leroy et al. 2005, Noir et al. 2004). The first reported construction and characterization of BAC genomic library in *Coffea* species was by Noir et al. (2004) for the *C. arabica* cultivar IAPAR 59. This BAC library, combining the two subgenomes of *C. canephora* and *C. eugenioides*, offers the opportunity to better investigate the speciation mechanism in *C. arabica* by reconstructing the phylogeny of homoeologous loci in this allotetraploid genome (Noir et al. 2004). The first BAC library for Robusta coffee (*C. canephora*) was constructed by Leroy et al. (2005) with the aim of developing molecular resources to study the genome structure and evolution of this species. The specific aim of this study was to gain insights into the structure and evolution of genes coding for enzymes involved in sucrose metabolism and demonstrates the use of BAC libraries as powerful tools for further genomic studies in coffee. In addition, BAC libraries will be valuable in coffee for improvement through cloning of genes for important agronomic traits such as resistance to diseases and nematodes, fructification time, and other important economic traits (De Kochko et al. 2010, Leroy et al. 2005).

### 10.3.4 Conserved Ortholog Set

Conserved ortholog set (COS) markers, single-copy orthologous genes among plant genomes, have become a promising new source of markers for comparative plant genomics (Fulton et al. 2002). Though studies on species within families linked by a common set of orthologous genes have progressed well, little has been done to study comparative genomics among divergent species belonging to different plant families until recently (Fulton et al. 2002). These markers will be valuable in the identification of a subset of genes that have remained stable in sequence and copy numbers since radiation of flowering plants from their last common ancestor, which would facilitate taxonomic and phylogenetic studies (Fulton et al. 2002).

Wu et al. (2006) used COSII markers for comparative mapping across the plant families Solanaceae (tomato) and Rubiaceae (coffee). This study identified 2869 COS markers (COSII) common to most euasterid plant families, which includes one-quarter of all flowering plants and *Arabidopsis* and provided evidence that ancestral species that gave rise to Solanaceae and Rubiaceae had a basic chromosome number of $x = 11$ or 12 and that a whole genome duplication event (polyploidization) did not occur immediately prior to or after the radiation of either Solanaceae or Rubiaceae.

### 10.3.5 Whole Genome Sequencing

The development of molecular markers in coffee, the first step in genomics, has led to the assessment of genetic diversity within the two main cultivated species, *C. arabica* and *C. canephora*; analysis of diversity of wild *Coffea* species and their phylogenetic relationships within the genus; identification of quantitative trait loci (QTLs); characterization of major genes of interest; and detection of introgressions (De Kochko et al. 2010). Being a perennial plant, genetic mapping of *Coffea* species is time consuming and costly, taking 5–7 years, which in association with low genetic diversity of *C. arabica* has delayed the construction of a genetic map for this important crop species (Pearl et al. 2004). Using AFLP markers, Pearl et al. (2004) constructed a preliminary genetic linkage map of *C. arabica*. Construction of a draft sequence of the *C. canephora* genome is currently in the developmental stage, which once developed will be used to map the Arabica genome (De Kochko et al. 2010). In addition, to assemble the Arabica genome, a high-density map of *C. eugenioides* will also be needed (De Kochko et al. 2010). Sequencing the *C. canephora* and *C. eugenioides* genomes will provide a better understanding of the evolutionary dynamics of the *C. arabica* genome after the hybridization event between the two progenitor species (De Kochko et al. 2010).

## 10.4  MOLECULAR MARKERS AND GENETIC DIVERSITY

During the last three decades, molecular techniques based on polymorphisms in proteins or DNA have played a key role in the evaluation of genetic variability, catalyzing research in a variety of disciplines such as phylogenetics, taxonomy, ecology, genetics, and breeding (Weising et al. 2005). Properties making a specific molecular marker desirable include the following: (1) moderately to highly polymorphic, (2) codominant inheritance, (3) unambiguous assignment of alleles, (4) frequent occurrence in the genome, (5) even distribution throughout the genome, (6) selectively neutral, (7) easy access, (8) easy and fast assay, (9) high reproducibility, (10) easy exchange of data between laboratories, and (11) low cost for both marker development and assay (Weising et al. 2005). Though no single marker will fulfill all of these criteria, based on the particular application, there are many marker systems to choose from combining many of the desirable characteristics.

Molecular marker techniques have been used in coffee to assess genetic diversity of the species, construct genetic maps, and identify QTLs (De Kochko et al. 2010). The development and use of molecular methods has expanded the possibilities and tools available for genetic analysis for efficient conservation and use of coffee genetic resources (Philippe et al. 2009). The following sections give an overview of the different molecular marker systems that have been used in coffee molecular studies.

### 10.4.1  Isozymes and Allozymes

Isozymes are enzymes that convert the same substrate, though they are not necessarily products of the same gene (Weising et al. 2005). Allozymes are isozymes that convert the same substrate that are encoded by orthologous genes, differing by one or more amino acids due to allelic differences (Weising et al. 2005). Though allozymes have been used extensively in the past for discriminating genotypes, DNA markers have replaced their use due to the higher level of polymorphism detection by DNA markers (Weising et al. 2005).

The earliest molecular genetic data reported for coffee was by Berthou et al. (1980) (as cited in De Kochko et al. 2010) using isozymes from 18 populations of wild coffee. Another study by Berthaud in 1986 (as cited in Ky et al. 2001) using nine isozyme loci in *C. canephora* showed high polymorphism with an average of 3.5 alleles per locus.

## 10.4.2 Restriction Fragment Length Polymorphism

Restriction fragment length polymorphism (RFLP) analysis involves cutting (restricting) DNA with one or more restriction enzymes (endonucleases), resulting in fragments that separate according to molecular weight during gel electrophoresis (Avise 2004). Reproducible fragments of defined lengths are produced by digestion of a particular DNA molecule with a particular restriction enzyme (Weising et al. 2005). Polymorphism between different genotypes is detected through altered patterns of restricted fragments, which results from point mutations within the recognition sequence as well as insertions or deletions between two recognition sites (Weising et al. 2005).

Using RFLP analysis of the chloroplast genome and sequence analysis of the *atpB–rbcL* intergenic region of 52 samples belonging to 25 different *Coffea* taxa and 2 species of *Psilanthus*, Lashermes et al. (1996a) observed low-sequence divergence suggesting that *Coffea* is a young genus. They also found exclusive maternal inheritance of cpDNA in interspecific hybrids between *C. arabica* and *C. canephora*, and in intraspecific progeny of *C. canephora* (Lashermes et al. 1996a). RFLP markers in combination with GISH were used to investigate the origin of *C. arabica*, and the results supported the hypothesis that *C. arabica* is an amphidiploid formed through hybridization between the two diploid species, *C. eugenioides* and *C. canephora* or ecotypes related to these two species (Lashermes et al. 1999). This study also confirmed the relatively recent speciation of *C. arabica*.

## 10.4.3 Random Amplified Polymorphic DNA

The random amplified polymorphic DNA (RAPD) technique involves the use of short single primers with about 10 nucleotides of arbitrary sequence to amplify anonymous genomic sequences to uncover DNA-level polymorphisms (Avise 2004). RAPDs are mainly used in the identification of cultivars and clones, genetic mapping, marker-assisted selection (MAS), population genetics, and molecular systematics at the species level (Weising et al. 2005). In recent years, the RAPD technique has been replaced by other more informative codominant markers such as microsatellites (Avise 2004).

Using 19 coffee samples representing 8 species (*C. arabica*, *C. canephora*, *C. congensis*, *C. eugenioides*, *C. liberica*, *C. resinosa*, *C. stenophylla*, and *C. pseudozanguebariae*), RAPDs were used to estimate inter- and intraspecific variation and genetic relationships between accessions (Cros et al. 1993). Extensive interspecific variation and intraspecific variation in *C. canephora* and *C. liberica* were observed (Cros et al. 1993). Interspecific relationships inferred from hierarchical clustering analysis of RAPD marker variation were consistent with previous studies based on morphological and cytological studies (Cros et al. 1993). RAPD markers were used to analyze the genetic diversity among cultivated and subspontaneous accessions of *C. arabica*, and the results confirmed the narrow genetic base of commercial cultivars (Lashermes et al. 1996b). Results from this study also indicated an east–west differentiation in Ethiopia, the primary center of diversification of *C. arabica* and a relatively large genetic diversity within the germplasm collection, emphasizing the importance of germplasm collecting missions (Lashermes et al. 1996b). Another study using RAPD markers compared genetic diversity among 119 *C. arabica* individuals representing 88 accessions derived from spontaneous and subspontaneous trees in Ethiopia, 6 cultivars grown locally in Ethiopia, and 2 accessions derived from genetic populations of Typica and Bourbon, which concluded the relevant use of RAPD markers in fingerprinting coffee accessions (Anthony et al. 2001).

### 10.4.4 Amplified Fragment Length Polymorphism

Amplified fragment length polymorphism (AFLP) analysis uses a combination of both RFLP-based and polymerase chain reaction (PCR)-based methods (Weising et al. 2005). In this method, restriction fragments are produced by digestion of genomic DNA by two restriction endonucleases, one with a 4 bp and the other with a 6 bp recognition site. A subset of restriction fragments from this complex mixture of fragments is linked to adapter sequences and biotinylated and following PCR, polymorphisms are scored as differences in lengths of amplified fragments (Avise 2004).

The AFLP technique has been used successfully in coffee genetic studies with excellent repeatability (Steiger et al. 2002). Genetic diversity of 61 *C. arabica* accessions belonging to 6 cultivars, Typica, Bourbon, Catimor, Catuai, Caturra, and Mokka Hybrid, was assessed using AFLP markers with 6 *Eco*RI-*Mse*I primer combinations (Steiger et al. 2002). Of these six cultivars, Catimor had the highest level of genetic diversity and Caturra showed the lowest (Steiger et al. 2002). In addition, diversity of *C. arabica* was compared with that of the two diploid species, *C. canephora* and *C. liberica*, with results suggesting that *C. arabica* is more closely related to *C. canephora* than to *C. liberica* (Steiger et al. 2002). Using AFLPs, a genetic linkage map was constructed for *C. arabica* on a pseudo-F$_2$ population (Pearl et al. 2004). Molecular marker linkage maps in many crop species, including coffee, are being used successfully for directed germplasm improvement (Pearl et al. 2004).

### 10.4.5 Simple Sequence Repeats

Simple sequence repeats (SSRs), also known as microsatellites or short tandem repeats (STRs), are tandemly reiterated short sequences (usually di-, tri-, or tetra-nucleotide motifs) at a particular locus, with variation in repeat copy number leading to allelic polymorphism (Avise 2004, Weising et al. 2005). SSRs have become the most popular and powerful of current molecular methods for identifying polymorphic Mendelian markers due to their codominant inheritance, high abundance, high allelic diversity, and ease of accessing size variation by PCR with pairs of flanking primers (Weising et al. 2005).

Numerous microsatellite markers have been developed for coffee and their cross-compatibility across various *Coffea* species have been tested with great success. Combes et al. (2000) describe 11 microsatellite primer pairs that were used to PCR amplify microsatellite fragments across 11 *Coffea* species and 2 *Psilanthus* species. Of the 11 microsatellite loci, only 5 appeared to be polymorphic in *C. arabica*, illustrating the low genetic diversity of this species. The transferability of SSRs across different *Coffea* species and their high levels of polymorphisms have been demonstrated by many authors (Baruah et al. 2003, Coulibaly et al. 2003, Hendre et al. 2008, Poncet et al. 2004, 2007). Microsatellites have also become valuable in analysis of genetic diversity and structure in various coffee species and identification of cultivars (Cubry et al. 2008, Maluf et al. 2005, Moncada and McCouch 2004, Prakash et al. 2005, Silvestrini et al. 2007). SSRs derived from ESTs also have potential for use as markers in coffee for genome analysis (Aggarwal et al. 2007, Poncet et al. 2006).

### 10.4.6 INTER-SIMPLE SEQUENCE REPEAT

Developed from common SSR motifs, inter-simple sequence repeats (ISSRs) are amplification products of the interrepeat region, within amplifiable distance of one another (Wolfe and Liston 1998). The design of the oligonucleotide primers does not require sequencing (Zietkiewicz et al. 1994), but rather primers developed for SSRs themselves can be used with or without a 5′- or 3′-anchor sequence (Wolfe and Liston 1998). Use of ISSRs has applications in taxonomic and phylogenetic comparisons and as a mapping tool in a wide variety of organisms (Zietkiewicz et al. 1994).

Though not widely used as markers in coffee (De Kochko et al. 2010), ISSRs have been used to analyze genetic variation in populations of *C. arabica* and *C. canephora*. Using 11 ISSR primers, Aga et al. (2005) analyzed genetic variation of *C. arabica* from four regions of Ethiopia. The results showed low genetic diversity and based on partitioning of populations, strategies for *in situ* conservation were made (Aga et al. 2005). Genetic variation study in a *C. robusta* founder gene pool from the Democratic Republic of Congo using ISSRs revealed high variability (Tshilengr et al. 2009). Compared to RAPDs, the ISSRs detected fewer polymorphic loci (95% vs. 52%), but when used conjointly, these two markers can target a larger portion of the genome (Tshilengr et al. 2009).

Molecular markers are powerful tools in various biological applications and their uses have been widespread in coffee genomic studies. In phylogenetic studies, markers such as RFLPs, RAPDs, AFLPs, and SSRs have been valuable in determining the relationships between various coffee species and cultivars and in interpreting historical biogeographical events. The different marker technologies have confirmed the recent origin of the genus *Coffea* and the amphidiploid nature of *C. arabica*. In addition, parentage assignment and confirmation of the low genetic diversity of *C. arabica* have been consistent regardless of the marker system used. All the different marker systems have also been used in determining genetic diversity and structure within and among various coffee species and cultivars with great implications for developing germplasm conservation strategies and germplasm improvement through breeding.

## 10.5   MOLECULAR BREEDING

Conventional breeding of coffee offers limitations due to the long regeneration time of the coffee tree (i.e., approximately 5 years), the high cost of field trials (Lashermes et al. 2000b), and dependence on environmental conditions. In cases where back-crossing is done over 5 generations, a minimum of 25 years after initial hybridization will be required to ensure that the desirable trait for improved quality or disease or pest resistance has been assimilated in the progeny (Lashermes et al. 2000b). The development of MAS provides an alternative to overcome the limitations of conventional coffee breeding (Lashermes et al. 2000b). The general principle of MAS is the use and selection of an identified molecular marker linked to a gene for a specific trait rather than selection for the trait itself and reduces the number of backcrosses required (Lashermes et al. 2000b).

The low genetic diversity of *C. arabica* is attributed to its origin, reproductive biology, and evolution (Lashermes et al. 1999), which limit the potential for germ-plasm improvement (Pearl et al. 2004). Enlarging the genetic base and improvement of Arabica cultivars, characterized by homogeneous agronomic behavior with high susceptibility to pests and diseases, have become high priorities for research-ers (Lashermes et al. 2000b). Though *C. canephora* has been utilized in breeding programs, utilization of other taxa such as *C. eugenioides*, *C. congensis*, or *Coffea* sp. Moloundou has been neglected as desirable gene sources (Lashermes et al. 1999). Many of the resistance traits to diseases and pests such as coffee leaf rust (*Hemileia vastatrix*), coffee berry disease caused by *Colletotrichum kahawae*, and root-knot nematode (*Meloidogyne* sp.) not found in *C. arabica* have been found in *C. canephora* (Lashermes et al. 2000b). *Coffea racemosa* also constitutes a promis-ing source of coffee leaf miner (*Perileucoptera coffeella*) resistance (Guerreiro Filho et al. 1999).

Intensive breeding research programs gained importance in the early 1950s with increased commercial importance of coffee (Pinto-Maglio 2006). Most breeding programs between 1950 and 1978 involved intraspecific and interspecific hybrid-ization between the two cultivated species, *C. arabica* and *C. canephora*, with the use of some wild species of coffee (Pinto-Maglio 2006). Spontaneous inter-specific hybrids that occur occasionally have also been widely used for improv-ing disease and pest resistance in Arabica coffee (Pearl et al. 2004). An example is the Timor Hybrid, a spontaneous interspecific cross between *C. arabica* and *C. canephora*, discovered in the Island of Timor, which has been used inten-sively in coffee breeding programs for disease resistance such as coffee leaf rust (Lashermes et al. 2000b, Pearl et al. 2004). Introgressed lines of *C. liberica* from a spontaneous interspecific hybrid between *C. arabica* and *C. liberica* has been used as a main source of rust resistance in breeding programs in India (Prakash et al. 2002).

Molecular markers have been used in coffee for introgression assessment, deter-mination of mode of inheritance of disease and pest resistance, assessment of bever-age quality, and analysis of QTLs, all of which have great implications for future breeding. Using AFLP markers, introgressed genotypes derived from the Timor

Hybrid were evaluated and compared to parental genotypes of *C. arabica* and *C. canephora* to estimate the amount of introgression present to gain insights into the mechanism of introgression in *C. arabica* (Lashermes et al. 2000a). These researchers concluded that AFLP is an extremely efficient technique for DNA marker generation in coffee and offers an efficient way of distinguishing and finger-printing coffee germplasm collections. In early breeding programs in India, S.26, a putative natural hybrid between *C. arabica* and a diploid species has been used as a main source of rust resistance (Prakash et al. 2002). Using AFLP markers, Prakash et al. (2002) deduced that the polymorphism identified in this natural hybrid and its derivatives was a consequence of introgressive hybridizations involving *C. liberica*. De Brito et al. (2010) amplified 176 AFLP primer combinations using bulked segre-gant analysis (BSA) in the Timor Hybrid and its derivatives and identified 3 markers linked to a coffee leaf rust resistance gene, of which 2 were distributed on either side flanking the resistant gene, with great implications for future MAS in coffee breeding programs.

In a study examining the phenotypic and genetic differentiation between *C. liberica* and *C. canephora* using AFLP, ISSR, and SSR markers relative to 16 quantitative traits, 15 of them were found to be significantly different with 8 QTLs associated with variation in petiole length, leaf area, number of flowers per inflorescence, fruit shape, fruit disk diameter, seed shape, and seed length detected (N'Diaye et al. 2007). Using $F_2$ progeny derived from a cross between a root-knot nematode (*Meloidogyne exigua*)-resistant introgression line T2296 and a susceptible accession Et6, segregation data analysis was performed showing that resistance to *M. exigua* is controlled by a simply inherited major gene designated as the *Mex*-1 locus with 14 AFLP markers associated with the resistance (Noir et al. 2003). In another study to identify the genetic basis and host resistance and identification of molecular markers associated with coffee berry disease caused by *C. kahawae*, eight AFLP and two microsatellite markers were identified to be tightly linked to the resistant phenotypes, which were mapped to one unique chromosomal fragment introgressed from *C. canephora* (Gichuru et al. 2008). Three RAPD markers were also found to be closely associated with resistance to coffee berry disease in Arabica coffee controlled by the *T* gene found in the varieties Hibrido de Timor and Catimor (Agwanda et al. 1997). In one of the first attempts to develop PCR-based sequence specific markers linked to partial resis-tance to coffee leaf rust (*Hemileia vastatrix*), five AFLP and two SSR markers exhibiting significant association with partial resistance were identified (Herrera et al. 2009).

Efficient use of the genetic variation in wild species involves the genetic deter-mination of the desirable trait and the ability to introgress the desirable DNA seg-ments from wild species to the genome of the cultivated species (Prakash et al. 2004) without affecting quality traits (Herrera et al. 2002). The identification of markers linked to specific traits represents an important starting point for early selection of seedlings with these specific traits through enhanced backcross breeding programs and will allow conversion of these to PCR-specific markers, making them suitable for MAS (Noir et al. 2003).

## 10.6  GENOMICS AND QUALITY OF COFFEE

Of the two main cultivated coffees, Robusta coffee (*C. canephora*) is characterized as a weak-flavored, neutral coffee with occasional strong and pronounced bitterness and the Arabica coffee (*C. arabica*) is a milder and fruit-flavored acidulous beverage (Bertrand et al. 2003). AFLP analysis of the amount of *C. canephora* genetic material accumulated in *C. arabica* through introgressive breeding gave estimates of approximately 8%–27% of the *C. canephora* genome present (Lashermes et al. 2000a). This could involve, in addition to transfer of desirable traits such as disease resistance, also the incorporation of undesirable traits such as lower beverage quality (Bertrand et al. 2003). Some of the factors affecting the beverage quality of coffee are biochemical contents such as CGAs, caffeine, sucrose, and trigonelline.

### 10.6.1  CHLOROGENIC ACIDS

CGAs are phenolic compounds found in green coffee beans and their presence modifies cup taste with the quality of the beverage increasing when CGA content decreases (Ky et al. 1999). A major phenolic secondary metabolite found in the plant kingdom, CGA control germination and cell growth, provide defense mechanisms against phytopathogens, or act as lignin precursors (Ky et al. 1999). As a complex trait involved in attributes such as aroma, physiology, and genetics, CGA should be studied in relation to other traits such as morphology, phenology, and biochemistry for better breeding program planning (Ky et al. 1999). Utilization of molecular tools in identifying markers near QTLs will be helpful in developing MAS (Ky et al. 1999).

### 10.6.2  CAFFEINE

Caffeine, an alkaloid, is a secondary metabolite of great interest in coffee because of its impact on beverage quality, with higher caffeine content increasing the bitterness of the drink (Campa et al. 2005). The caffeine content in green coffee beans varies between species and within species with 0% dry matter basis (dmb) in *C. pseudozanguebariae* to 3.3% dmb in *C. canephora* (Campa et al. 2005). One of the main aims of breeding *C. canephora* has been for a lower caffeine content to improve cup quality (Campa et al. 2005). Akaffou et al. (2003) studied the impact of fructification time (the period from flowering to fruit ripening) on caffeine content in the interspecific hybrid between *C. pseudozanguebariae* and *C. liberica* var. Dewevrei. The major gene *Ft1* was identified to be involved in fructification time, which had an indirect effect on caffeine content implying the importance in breeding programs through MAS (Akaffou et al. 2003).

### 10.6.3  SUCROSE

Sucrose is one of the compounds in raw coffee bean responsible for coffee cup quality and is an important precursor of flavor and aroma (Geromel et al. 2006). Of the free sugars, although glucose, fructose, and sucrose are present in young coffee beans, only sucrose is present in mature beans with higher sucrose levels in mature

Arabica than in Robusta endosperm (Rogers et al. 1999), giving the Arabica coffee a better cup quality (Geromel et al. 2006). Sucrose content in *C. arabica* varies from 7% to 11% dmb compared to lower values in *C. robusta* ranging from 4% to 7% dmb (Ky et al. 2001). The enzyme sucrose synthase plays a significant role in sucrose metabolism during sucrose accumulation in the coffee fruit, and two full-length cDNAs (*CaSUS1* and *CaSUS2*) have been identified. The complete gene sequence of *CaSUS2* has been isolated (Geromel et al. 2006), which has great implications in the development of MAS breeding programs.

### 10.6.4 TRIGONELLINE

Trigonelline is an alkaloid and an aroma precursor in coffee with higher levels in *C. arabica* ranging from 0.88% to 1.77% dmb and 0.75% to 1.24% dmb in *C. canephora* (Ky et al. 2001). Trigonelline and other biochemical compounds are quantitatively inherited in coffee trees, and hence there is considerable potential for biochemical improvement in *C. arabica* (Ky et al. 2001).

Increasing Robusta cup quality has been one of the targets of several breeding programs. Achieving this would involve increasing sucrose and trigonelline contents while decreasing CGA and caffeine contents (Ky et al. 2001). Evaluation of biochemical polymorphism and inheritance indicate that plants can be bred to decrease CGA and caffeine contents and increase sucrose contents (Ky et al. 2001). Future breeding programs based on introgression at the diploid level should include a biochemical evaluation of all *Coffea* genetic resources to identify suitable parental species (Ky et al. 2001) to improve beverage quality of coffee.

## 10.7   CONSERVATION GENETICS

Due to the narrow genetic base of cultivated coffee (*C. arabica*), utilization of wild species of coffee in future breeding programs for crop improvement is imperative. With many wild species being lost due to habitat destruction, there is an urgent need for the conservation of these valuable genetic resources. Coffee seeds are recalcitrant or exhibit intermediate storage behavior, making preservation of germplasm through seed banking problematic. With forests being lost at a fast pace, conserving these species in ex situ germplasm becomes vital. To meaningfully conserve the genetic diversity of a taxon, knowing the genetic structure of the population is essential and hence this should become one of the principal strategies in the conservation efforts of species to ensure success (Gole et al. 2002, Shapcott et al. 2007). To make progress in coffee improvement, detecting and quantifying genetic diversity becomes key for effective conservation of coffee genetic resources (Moncada and McCouch 2004).

Using microsatellite markers, Moncada and McCouch (2004) analyzed allelic diversity of 5 diploid species and 23 wild and cultivated accessions of *C. arabica* from Africa, Indonesia, and South America, with the 5 diploid species exhibiting more allelic diversity than the 23 tetraploid genotypes. The wild tetraploids on average exhibited 55% of the alleles not shared with cultivated genotypes, supporting the importance of utilizing wild tetraploid ancestors from Ethiopia as a source of novel genetic variation for crop improvement and expansion of the gene pool of *C. arabica* germplasm. Utilization of wild coffee species with significantly lower natural levels of caffeine than *C. arabica* and *C. canephora* in breeding programs will be critical in meeting the increasing demand for decaffeinated coffee (Mazzafera et al. 1991). Genetic diversity studies of *C. canephora* from Uganda showed significant population structure, with this population being genetically distinct from other diversity groups such as Guinean and Congolese groups (Musoli et al. 2009). The identification of this distinct genetic group from Uganda leads to a new conservation strategy definition for *C. canephora* (Musoli et al. 2009).

Ex situ field genebanks offer an alternative to conserve genetic resources of crop plants for preserving germplasm of taxa that are difficult to conserve as seed (Duloo et al. 1998). One of the big drawbacks of plants held in ex situ collections is that they are grown in monoculture leading to susceptibility to pests and diseases and the growing of plants in ecological conditions not suitable for their growth, leading to strong selection pressure and genetic erosion (Duloo et al. 1998). One way to combat that is by setting up a core collection with accessions chosen to represent diverse genetic variability and duplicating the collection in diverse ecogeographic sites (Duloo et al. 1998). To achieve this, there is an urgent need to assess the extent of genetic variability of plants held in existing ex situ collections and initiating new collecting programs to fill gaps in these field collections (Duloo et al. 1998). In addition, *in situ* conservation of wild species and landraces should also be emphasized. Molecular tools utilizing DNA markers should be utilized to increase our understanding of coffee genetic diversity and to develop strategies for conservation of coffee genetic resources with wide genetic representation.

## 10.8 CONCLUSION

In an attempt to quantify the economic value of *C. arabica* genetic resources in Ethiopian highland forests, Hein and Gatzweiler (2006) conducted a valuation based on an assessment of the potential benefits and costs of the use of *C. arabica* genetic information in breeding programs for developing enhanced coffee cultivars with increased pest and disease resistance, low caffeine contents, and increased yields. The resulting valuation of coffee genetic resources based on comparing costs and benefits for a 30-year discounting period was U.S.$1458 million and $420 million at discount rates of 5% and 10%, respectively, demonstrating the potential economic importance of Ethiopian coffee genetic resources.

The development of genomic technologies has broadened our scope of understanding of how organisms function at the genome level, which has improved our knowledge of vast disciplines such as phylogenetics, taxonomy, evolutionary biology, ecology, genetics, and breeding. The development of molecular marker technologies in coffee has paved the way for a better understanding of the origin and phylogeny of cultivated coffee and wild species; for genetic diversity of cultivated and wild coffee; for the identification of QTLs and their utilization in MAS in breeding programs to improve quality, yield, and pest and disease resistance; and for prioritizing conservation of valuable genetic resources. With many livelihoods in developing countries dependent on coffee cultivation, advances in coffee genomics will lead to sustainable coffee production with great economic and ecological implications.

# REFERENCES

Aga, E., E. Bekele, and T. Bryngelsson. 2005. Inter-simple sequence repeat (ISSR) variation in forest coffee trees (*Coffea arabica* L.) populations from Ethiopia. *Genetica* 124:213–221.

Aggarwal, R. K., P. S. Hendre, R. K. Varshney, P. R. Bhat, V. Krishnakumar, and L. Singh. 2007. Identification, characterization and utilization of EST-derived genic microsatellite markers for genome analyses of coffee and related species. *Theor Appl Genet* 114:359–372.

Agwanda, C. O., P. Lashermes, P. Trouslot, M. C. Combes, and A. Charrier. 1997. Identification of RAPD markers for resistance to coffee berry disease, *Colletotrichum kahawae*, in arabica coffee. *Euphytica* 97:241–248.

Akaffou, D. S., C. L. Ky, P. Barre, S. Hamon, J. Louarn, and M. Noirot. 2003. Identification and mapping of a major gene (*Ft1*) involved in fructification time in the interspecific cross *Coffea pseudozanguebariae* × *C. liberica* var. Dewevrei: Impact on caffeine content and seed weight. *Theor Appl Genet* 106:1486–1490.

Anthony, F., B. Bertrand, O. Quiros et al. 2001. Genetic diversity of wild coffee (*Coffea arabica* L.) using molecular markers. *Euphytica* 118:53–65.

Anthony, F., M. C. Combes, C. Astorga, B. Bertrand, G. Graziosi, and P. Lashermes. 2002. The origin of cultivated *Coffea arabica* L. varieties revealed by AFLP and SSR markers. *Theor Appl Genet* 104:894–900.

Anthony F., L. E. C. Diniz, M.-C. Combes, and P. Lashermes. 2010. Adaptive radiation on *Coffea* subgenus *Coffea* L. (Rubiaceae) in Africa and Madagascar. *Plant Syst Evol* 285:51–64.

Avise, J. C. 2004. *Molecular Markers, Natural History, and Evolution*. Second Edition. Sunderland, MA: Sinauer Associates, Inc.

Barker, M. S. and P. G. Wolf. 2010. Unfurling fern biology in the genomics age. *BioScience* 60:177–185.

Barre, P., M. Noirot, J. Louarn, C. Duperray, and S. Hamon. 1996. Reliable flow cytometric estimation of nuclear DNA content in coffee trees. *Cytometry* 24:32–38.

Baruah, A., V. Naik, P. S. Hendre, R. Rajkumar, P. Rajendrakumar, and R. K. Aggarwal. 2003. Isolation and characterization of nine microsatellite markers from *Coffea arabica* L., showing wide cross-species amplifications. *Mol Ecol Notes* 3:647–650.

Berthaud, J. 1986. *Les resources génétiques pour l'amélioration des caféiers africains diploïdes*. Paris, France: Coll. Trav. & Doc. ORSTOM.

Berthou, F., P. Trouslot, S. Hamon, F. Vedel, and F. Quetier. 1980. Analyse en électrophorèse du polymorphisme biochimique des caféiers: Variation enzymatique dans dix-huit populations sauvages. *Café Cacao Thé* 24:313–326.

Bertrand, B., B. Guyot, F. Anthony, and P. Lashermes. 2003. Impact of the *Coffea canephora* gene introgression on beverage quality of *C. arabica*. *Theor Appl Genet* 107:387–394.

Campa, C., S. Doulbeau, S. Dussert, S. Hamon, and M. Noirot. 2005. Diversity in bean Caffeine content among wild *Coffea* species: Evidence of a discontinuous distribution. *Food Chem* 91:633–637.

Clarindo, W. R. and C. R. Carvalho. 2008. First *Coffea arabica* karyogram showing that this species is a true allotetraploid. *Plant Syst Evol* 274:237–241.

Clarindo, W. R. and C. R. Carvalho. 2009. Comparison of the *Coffea canephora* and *C. arabica* karyotype based on chromosomal DNA content. *Plant Cell Rep* 28:73–81.

Combes, M. C., S. Andrzejewski, F. Anthony et al. 2000. Characterization of microsatellite loci in *Coffea arabica* and related coffee species. *Mol Ecol* 9:1178–1180.

Coulibaly, I., B. Revol, M. Noirot et al. 2003. AFLP and SSR polymorphism in a *Coffea* interspecific backcross progeny [(*C. heterocalyx* × *C. canephora*) × *C. canephora*]. *Theor Appl Genet* 107:1148–1155.

Cros, J., M. C. Combes, N. Chabrillange, C. Duperray, A. Monnot des Angles, and S. Hamon. 1995. Nuclear DNA content in the subgenus *Coffea* (Rubiaceae): Inter- and intra-specific variation in African species. *Can J Bot* 73:14–20.

Cros, J., M. C. Combes, P. Trouslot et al. 1998. Phylogenetic analysis of chloroplast DNA variation in *Coffea* L. *Mol Phylogenet Evol* 9(1):109–117.

Cros, J., P. Lashermes, P. Marmey, F. Anthony, S. Hamon, and A. Charrier. 1993. Molecular analysis of genetic diversity and phylogenetic relationships in *Coffea*. In *15th Conference of ASIC*. Montpellier, France.

Cubry, P., P. Musoli, H. Legnate et al. 2008. Diversity in coffee assessed with SSR markers: Structure of the genus *Coffea* and perspectives for breeding. *Genome* 51:50–63.

Davis, A. P., R. Govaerts, D. M. Bridson, and P. Stoffelen. 2006. An annotated taxonomic conspectus of the genus *Coffea* (Rubiaceae). *Bot J Linn Soc* 152:465–512.

Davis, A. P. and F. Rakotonasolo. 2008. A taxonomic revision of the *Baracoffea* alliance: Nine remarkable *Coffea* species from western Madagascar. *Bot J Linn Soc* 158:355–390.

De Brito, G. G., E. T. Caixeta, A. P. Gallina et al. 2010. Inheritance of coffee leaf rust resistance and identification of AFLP markers linked to the resistance gene. *Euphytica* 173:255–264.

De Kochko, A., S. Akaffou, A. C. Andrade et al. 2010. Advances in coffee genomics. In *Advances in Botanical Research* (Volume 53), Kader, J.-C. and M. Delseny (eds.), pp. 23–63. London, U.K.: Academic Press.

Dulloo, M. E., L. Guarino, F. Engelmann et al. 1998. Complementary conservation strategies for the genus *Coffea*: A case study of Mascarene *Coffea* species. *Genet Resour Crop Evol* 45:565–579.

Fulton, T. M., R. Van der Hoeven, N. T. Eannetta, and S. D. Tanksley. 2002. Identification, analysis, and utilization of conserved ortholog set markers for comparative genomics in higher plants. *Plant Cell* 14:1457–1467.

Geromel, C., L. P. Ferreira, S. M. C. Guerreiro et al. 2006. Biochemical and genomic analysis of sucrose metabolism during coffee (*Coffea arabica*) fruit development. *J Exp Bot* 57:3243–3258.

Gibson, G. and S. V. Muse. 2009. *A Primer of Genome Science*. Third Edition. Sunderland, MA: Sinauer Associates, Inc. Publishers.

Gichuru, E. K., C. O. Agwanda, M. C. Combes et al. 2008. Identification of molecular markers linked to a gene conferring resistance to coffee berry disease (*Colletotrichum kahawae*) in *Coffea* arabica. *Plant Pathol* 57:1117–1124.

Gole, T. W., M. Denich, D. Teketay, and P. L. G. Vlek. 2002. Human impacts on *Coffea arabica* genepool in Ethiopia and the need for its in situ conservation. In *Managing Plant Genetic Diversity*, Engels, J. M. M., Rao, V. R., Brown, A. H. D. and Jackson, M. T. (eds.), pp. 237–247. New York: CABI Publishing.

Guerreiro Filho, O., M. B. Silvarolla, and A. B. Eskes. 1999. Expressions and mode of inheritance of resistance in coffee to leaf miner *Perileucoptera coffeella*. *Euphytica* 105:7–15.

Hein, L. and F. Gatzweiler. 2006. The economic value of coffee (*Coffea arabica*) genetic resources. *Ecol Econ* 60:176–185.

Hendre, P. S., R. Phanindranath, V. Annapurna, A. Lalremruata, and R. K. Aggarwal. 2008. Development of new genomic microsatellite markers from robusta coffee (*Coffea canephora* Pierre ex A. Froehner) showing broad cross-species transferability and utility in genetic studies. *BMC Plant Biol* 8:51–69.

Herrera, P. J. C., A. G. Alvarado, G. H. A. Cortina, M. C. Combes, G. G. Romero, and P. Lashermes. 2009. Genetic analysis of partial resistance to coffee leaf rust (*Hemileia vastatrix* Berk & Br.) introgressed into the cultivated *Coffea arabica* L. from the diploid *C. canephora* species. *Euphytica* 167:57–67.

Herrera, J. C., M. C. Combes, F. Anthony, A. Charrier, and P. Lashermes. 2002. Introgression into the allotetraploid coffee (*Coffea arabica* L.): Segregation and recombination of the *C. canephora* genome in the tetraploid interspecific hybrid (*C. arabica* × *C. canephora*). *Theor Appl Genet* 104:661–668.

Ky, C. L., J. Louarn, S. Dussert, B. Guyot, S. Hamon, and M. Noirot. 2001. Caffeine, triogonelline, chlorogenic acids and sucrose diversity in wild *Coffea arabica* L. and *C. canephora* P. accessions. *Food Chem* 75:223–230.

Ky, C. L., J. Louarn, B. Guyot, A. Charrier, S. Hamon, and M. Noirot. 1999. Relations between and inheritance of chlorogenic acid contents in an interspecific cross between *Coffea pseudozanguebariae* and *Coffea liberica* var 'dewevrei'. *Theor Appl Genet* 98:628–637.

Lashermes, P., S. Andrzejewski, B. Bertrand et al. 2000a. Molecular analysis of introgressive breeding in coffee (*Coffea arabica* L.). *Theor Appl Genet* 100:139–146.

Lashermes, P., M.-C. Combes, J. Robert et al. 1999. Molecular characterization and origin of the *Coffea Arabica* L. genome. *Mol Gen Genet* 261:259–266.

Lashermes, P., M. C. Combes, P. Topart, G. Graziosi, B. Bertrand, and F. Anthony. 2000b. Molecular breeding in coffee (*Coffea arabica* L.). In *Coffee Biotechnology and Quality*, Sera, T., Soccol, C. R., Pandey, A. and Roussos, S. (eds.), pp. 101–112. Amsterdam, the Netherlands: Kluwer Academic Publishers.

Lashermes, P., J. Cros, M. C. Combes et al. 1996a. Inheritance and restriction fragment length polymorphism of chloroplast DNA in the genus *Coffea* L. *Theor Appl Genet* 93:626–632.

Lashermes, P., P. Trouslot, F. Anthony, M. C. Combes, and A. Charrier. 1996b. Genetic diversity for RAPD markers between cultivated and wild accessions of *Coffea arabica*. *Euphytica* 87:59–64.

Leroy, T., P. Marraccini, M. Dufour et al. 2005. Construction and characterization of a *Coffea canephora* BAC library to study the organization of sucrose biosynthesis genes. *Theor Appl Genet* 111:1032–1041.

Maluf, M. P., M. Silvestrini, L. M. C. Ruggiero, O. G. Filho, and C. A. Colombo. 2005. Genetic diversity of cultivated *Coffea arabica* inbred lines assessed by RAPD, AFLP, and SSR marker systems. *Sci Agric* 62:366–373.

Maurin, O., A. P. Davis, M. Chester, E. F. Mvungi, Y. Jaufeerally-Fakim, and M. F. Fay. 2007. Towards a phylogeny for *Coffea* (Rubiaceae): Identifying well-supported lineages based on nuclear and plastid DNA sequences. *Ann Bot* 100:1565–1583.

Mazzafera, P., A. Crozier, and A. C. Magalhaes. 1991. Caffeine metabolism in *Coffea arabica* and other species of coffee. *Phytochemistry* 30:3913–3916.

Moncada, P. and S. McCouch. 2004. Simple sequence repeat diversity in diploid and tetraploid *Coffea* species. *Genome* 47:501–509.

Musoli, P., P. Cubry, P. Aluka et al. 2009. Genetic differentiation of wild and cultivated populations: Diversity of *Coffea canephora* Pierre in Uganda. *Genome* 52:634–646.

N'Diaye, A., M. Noirot, S. Hamon, and V. Poncet. 2007. Genetic basis of species differentiation between *Coffea liberica* Hiern and *C. canephora* Pierre: Analysis of an interspecific cross. *Genet Resour Crop Evol* 54:1011–1021.

Noir, S., F. Anthony, B. Bertrand, M. C. Combes, and P. Lashermes. 2003. Identification of a major gene (*Mex*-1) from *Coffea canephora* conferring resistance to *Meloidogyne exigua* in *Coffea arabica*. *Plant Pathol* 52:97–103.

Noir, S., S. Patheyron, M. C. Combes, P. Lashermes, and B. Chalhoub. 2004. Construction and characterization of a BAC library for genome analysis of the allotetraploid coffee species (*Coffea arabica* L.). *Theor Appl Genet* 109:225–230.

Noirot, M., P. Barre, C. Duperray, S. Hamon, and A. De Kochko. 2005. Investigation on the causes of stoichiometric error in genome size estimation using heat experiments: Consequences on data interpretation. *Ann Bot* 95:111–118.

Noirot, M., V. Poncet, P. Barre, P. Hamon, S. Hamon, and A. De Kochko. 2003. Genome size variations in diploid African *Coffea* species. *Ann Bot* 92:709–714.

Pearl, H. M., C. Nagai, P. H. Moore, D. L. Steiger, R. V. Osgood, and R. Ming. 2004. Construction of a genetic map for arabica coffee. *Theor Appl Genet* 108:829–835.

Pendergrast, M. 1999. *Uncommon Grounds: The History of Coffee and How It Transformed Our World*. New York: Basic Books.

Pendergrast, M. 2009. Coffee second only to oil? *Tea Coffee Trade J* April:38–41.

Philippe, L., B. Benoît, and E. Harvé. 2009. Breeding coffee (*Coffea arabica*) for sustainable production. In *Breeding Plantation Tree Crops: Tropical Species*, Jain, S. M. and Priyadarshan, P. M. (eds.), pp. 525–543. New York: Springer Science+Business Media. LLC.

Pinto-Maglio, C. A. F. 2006. Cytogenetics of coffee. *Braz J Plant Physiol* 18(1):37–44.

Poncet, V., M. Dufor, P. Hamon, S. Hamon, A. De Kochko, and T. Leroy. 2007. Development of genomic microsatellite markers in *Coffea canephora* and their transferability to other coffee species. *Genome* 50:1156–1161.

Poncet, V., P. Hamon, J. Minier, C. Carasco, S. Hamon, and M. Noirot. 2004. SSR cross-amplification and variation within coffee trees (*Coffea* spp.). *Genome* 47:1071–1081.

Poncet, V., M. Rondeau, C. Tranchant et al. 2006. SSR mining in coffee tree EST databases: Potential use of EST-SSRs as markers for the *Coffea* genus. *Mol Genet Genomics* 276:436–449.

Prakash, N. S., M. C. Combes, S. Dussert, S. Naveen, and P. Lashermes. 2005. Analysis of genetic diversity in Indian robusta coffee genepool (*Coffea canephora*) in comparison with a representative core collection using SSRs and AFLPs. *Genet Resour Crop Evol* 52:333–343.

Prakash, N. S., M. C. Combes, N. Somanna, and P. Lashermes. 2002. AFLP analysis of introgression in coffee cultivars (*Coffea arabica* L.) derived from a natural interspecific hybrid. *Euphytica* 124:265–271.

Prakash, N. S., D. V. Marques, V. M. P. Varzea, M. C. Silva, M. C. Combes, and P. Lashermes. 2004. Introgression molecular analysis of a leaf rust resistance gene from *Coffea liberica* into *C. arabica* L. *Theor Appl Genet* 109:1311–1317.

Rogers, W. J., S. Michaux, M. Bastin, and P. Bucheli. 1999. Changes to the content of sugars, sugar alcohols, myo-inositol, carboxylic acids and inorganic anions in developing grains from different varieties of Robusta (*Coffea canephora*) and Arabica (*C. arabica*) coffees. *Plant Sci* 149:115–123.

Shapcott, A., M. Rakotoarinivo, R. J. Smith, G. Lysakova, M. F. Fay, and J. Dransfield. 2007. Can we bring Madagascar's critically endangered palms back from the brink? Genetics, ecology and conservation of the critically endangered palm *Beccariophoenix madagascariensis*. *Bot J Linn Soc* 154:589–608.

Silvestrini, M., M. G. Junqueira, A. C. Favarin et al. 2007. Genetic diversity and structure of Ethiopian, Yemen and Brazilian *Coffea arabica* L. accessions using microsatellite markers. *Genet Resour Crop Evol* 54:1367–1379.

Steiger, D. L., C. Nagai, P. H. Moore, C. W. Morden, R. V. Osgood, and R. Ming. 2002. AFLP analysis of genetic diversity within and among *Coffea arabica* cultivars. *Theor Appl Genet* 105:209–215.

Tshilengr, P., K. K. Nkongolo, M. Mehes, and A. Kalonji. 2009. Genetic variation in *Coffea canephora* L. (Var. Robusta) accessions from the founder gene pool evaluated with ISSR and RAPD. *Afr J Biotechnol* 8(3):380–390.

Vieira, L. G. E., A. C. Andrade, C. A. Colombo et al. 2006. Brazilian coffee genome project: An EST-based genomic resource. *Braz J Plant Physiol* 18:95–108.

Weising, K., H. Nybom, K. Wolff, and G. Kahl. 2005. *DNA Fingerprinting in Plants: Principles, Methods, and Applications*. Second Edition. Boca Raton, FL: CRC Press.

Wolfe, A. D. and A. Liston. 1998. Contributions of PCR-based methods to plant systematic and evolutionary biology. In *Plant Molecular Systematic II*, Soltis, D. E., Soltis, P. S. and Doyle, J. J. (eds.), pp. 43–86. Boston, MA: Kluwer Academic Publishers.

Wu, F., L. A. Mueller, D. Crouzillat, V. Petiard, and S. D. Tanksley. 2006. Combining bioinformatics and phylogenetics to identify large sets of single-copy orthologous genes (COSII) for comparative, evolutionary and systematic studies: A test case in the euasterid plant clade. *Genetics* 174:1407–1420.

Zietkiewicz, E., A. Rafalski, and D. Labuda. 1994. Genome fingerprinting by simple sequence repeat (SSR)-anchored polymerase chain reaction amplification. *Genomics* 20:176–183.

## INTERNET RESOURCES

A listing of some of the coffee resources available on the Internet:

The Brazilian Coffee Genome Project: http://www.lge.ibi.unicamp.br/cafe/

The Coffee Science Information Center: http://www.cosic.org/

International Coffee Organization: http://www.ico.org/

TropGene Database: http://tropgenedb.cirad.fr/en/coffee.html

CCMB Coffee Database: http://www.ccmb.res.in/coffeegermplasm/index.htm

Cenicafe Database: http://bioinformatics.cenicafe.org/

MoccaDB: http://moccadb.mpl.ird.fr/

CoffeeDNA: http://www.coffeedna.net/

Association for Science and Information on Coffee (ASIC): http://www.asic-cafe.org/htm/eng/about_history.php

# 11 Omics Approaches to Meat Quality Management

*Ruth M. Hamill, Begonya Marcos,*
*Dilip K. Rai, and Anne Maria Mullen*

## CONTENTS

## 11.1 INTRODUCTION

Meat quality is not one single value, but encompasses a diverse array of characteristics relating to eating quality, nutritional level, and technological performance; broader definitions can also include safety aspects. For the consumer, sensory characteristics including appearance, color, and palatability (tenderness, texture, juiciness, and flavor) are key (McIlveen and Buchanan 2001, Verbeke et al. 2009), while nutritive aspects include composition, protein content, fatty acid profile, and mineral level (Leheska et al. 2008, Scollan et al. 2005). In terms of sensory acceptability, which attribute is most important depends on geographic location (Aaslyng et al. 2007), but tenderness is usually considered the biggest driver (Aaslyng 2009). When most products are tender, juiciness and flavor play bigger roles in liking (Miller et al. 2001). The technological aspects of quality center round the ability of muscle to interact with processing conditions to produce optimal fresh and processed products. The ability of the muscle to bind water, the pH in the early postmortem period, and the ultimate post-rigor pH are valuable indicators of technological performance (Poso and Puolanne 2005).

The biological processes and pathways important for meat quality development are still not fully understood. This is exemplified by the fact that selection for production gains such as rapid lean growth and increased muscle mass has, in many cases, had antagonistic effects on product quality. Enabling the meat industry to deliver uniform high-quality meat and meat products to consumers on a consistent basis, without compromising production gains, is therefore a persistent challenge. One of the main reasons for this is that because routine assessment of meat quality outside a research setting is rarely carried out, it has not been possible to develop selection programs for quality traits. This is compounded by a lack of financial incentives to stakeholders at all stages of the chain toward improvements in quality (Simm et al. 2009). While grading based on consumer assessment of quality has recently begun to be implemented in some markets, it requires a whole chain approach such as the Meat Standards Australia model (Polkinghorne et al. 2008, Watson et al. 2008). Indirect methods to predict meat quality are therefore desirable.

It is known that many aspects of meat quality are heritable, quantitative traits. These reflect underlying muscle biology, for example, fiber characteristics (Choi and Kim 2009, Hambrecht et al. 2005) and the metabolic pathways, in particular energy metabolism, active in life and in postmortem muscle (Poso and Puolanne 2005), modulated by environmental factors (Hocquette et al. 2007b, Pethick et al. 2007). Genomic, proteomic, and metabolomic approaches are therefore highly relevant to determine the influence of the animal genetic makeup, physiology in life and *postmortem* muscle metabolism on ultimate functionality and quality of meat produced (Elsik et al. 2009, Hocquette et al. 2007b, Hollung et al. 2007). Emanating from this research is a small but growing number of biological markers of meat quality, including DNA polymorphisms, transcript signatures, and protein markers. It is clear that the further development of such marker systems would be hugely advantageous for the industry with a wide range of potential applications spanning animal production via genome-assisted selection programs and grading and meat management systems for processors. In this chapter, we outline the most important quality traits for which markers are being sought and describe some of the recent progresses in -omics fields toward increasing our understanding of palatability and technological quality keeping in focus the potential for application in the industrial setting.

## 11.2  KEY MEAT QUALITY TRAITS FOR BEEF AND PORK

### 11.2.1  Tenderness

Of the three most important palatability attributes, that is, flavor, juiciness, and tenderness, many authors including Ouali (1990), Warkup et al. (1995), and Szczesniak (1998) determined that beef tenderness was the primary driver of sensory satisfaction among beef consumers. The value of this trait is recognized by consumers, for example, Norwegian beef consumers stated they were prepared to pay 50% more for very tender beef and 25% more for tender beef compared with less tender beef (Alfnes et al. 2005). Therefore, providing consistently tender beef should be a key priority for the beef industry. Numerous sources contribute to the variation in tenderness of meat: differences in muscle fiber characteristics (size and type and oxidative and glycolytic capacities); glycogen content; collagen (content and solubility); protease activities; heat shock proteins; and postmortem processes, including proteolysis and interactions of soluble muscle proteins, intracellular pH, and ion transport during the early postmortem phase (Bendixen 2005, Bouley et al. 2004, Zapata et al. 2009). Connective tissue amount and quality, sarcomere length, and the rate and extent of postmortem proteolysis of key structural proteins are considered to be primary components contributing to explainable tenderness variation (King et al. 2009). The heritability of tenderness is known to be lower than that for other traits such as intramuscular fat (IMF). However, determining the genetic and genomic signatures associated with tenderness has been a goal of the meat genomics research community in recent years (Hocquette et al. 2007a).

### 11.2.2  Intramuscular Fat Content

Important quality traits such as flavor and juiciness are closely linked to the proportion of fat in the meat, and IMF has been shown to contribute 10%–15% of the variance in palatability of beef (Dikeman 1987). IMF is an important determinant of carcass value in the Japanese market (Oka et al. 2002). For pork, consumer perception of texture and taste as well as juiciness is enhanced with increased IMF levels (Fernandez et al. 1999). However, in recent years, intensive genetic selection for increased lean growth has resulted in a dramatic reduction in the proportion of fat throughout the carcass, including a reduction in IMF in commercially important cuts. Because a certain minimum amount of fat is desirable within the muscle for flavor, very low IMF levels in both lean beef and pork are having adverse effects on palatability. Because IMF and overall fat content are only partially correlated (Suzuki et al. 2009), in theory, selection for higher IMF without leading to waste in fatter carcasses should be possible and is the focus of research at present.

The nutritional quality as well as the quantity of IMF in muscle has high relevance for human coronary health. The total monounsaturated and long-chain unsaturated fat content and particularly the ratio of saturated versus unsaturated FA and $n - 6/n - 3$ FA influence the nutritive and health value. Fatty acid profile varies from species to species and is generally more favorable in pork, compared with beef (Wood et al. 2008). While the overall fat content in beef muscle is quite low (less than 5%), the saturated content and $n - 6/n - 3$ FA ratio are dependent on the diet of the animals and therefore can be modulated (Scollan et al. 2005). More favorable fatty acid ratios are observed in the muscle of grass-fed than that of concentrate-fed cattle (Scollan et al. 2005). It has also been shown that cattle fed modified diets produce beef enriched with even higher levels of polyunsaturated fatty acids and conjugated linoleic acid (Noci et al. 2007).

### 11.2.3 WATER-HOLDING CAPACITY AND COLOR

A key attribute of fresh beef and in particular pork for both processors and consumers is the ability of meat to retain water (known as water-holding capacity [WHC] or drip loss) (Huff-Lonergan and Lonergan 2005). Pork with low WHC is unappealing to consumers, often less tender, flavorsome, and juicy and results in unsatisfactory cooking losses (Mullen and Troy 2005). For processors, pork with low WHC has poor color and consistency and is not amenable to processing, and drip loss results in a loss of between 1% and 10% of fresh pork weight annually (Offer and Knight 1988). In processed meat, variation in WHC leads to variation in product quality, for example, color, binding ability in comminuted products, and sliceability in hams. The biochemical, physiological, and postmortem structural changes that modulate the amount and distribution of water within muscle/meat are complex and not fully understood (Schellander 2007).

While palatability is key in consumer acceptability of beef and pork, the appearance and color of the product remains the most important aspect regarding decision to purchase (Aaslyng 2009). However, consumer preference for color is highly variable among consumer markets. For pork, the consumer preference for meat color (e.g., dark- versus light-colored pork) varies from country to country (Ngapo et al. 2007). In beef, most consumers prefer to visually select lean beef with low marbling and bright cherry-red color, though some prefer well-marbled and dark beef (Killinger et al. 2004). In the same study, consumers who preferred high marbling seemed to desire products with high eating quality, whereas consumers with a preference for low marbling seemed to desire lean products. The lean cover is also visually important, and for pork, most consumers will select a lean-looking piece of meat with low fat cover, although consumers in some regions prefer well-marbled pork (Ngapo et al. 2007). Various metabolic pathways are known to influence product color. In beef, lipid and protein oxidation negatively influence color, metmyoglobin-reducing activity affects myoglobin status, and natural antioxidants such as dietary vitamin E can be beneficial in maintaining a desirable color (Mohamed et al. 2008).

Metabolic factors affecting color in beef include glycogen depletion in the peri-mortem period, which can cause dark, firm, and dry (DFD) meat (Hambrecht et al. 2005), and in pork, the appearance of pale, soft, and exudative (PSE) meat is scored poorly by consumers (Nam et al. 2009).

## 11.3  GENETIC VARIATION AND MEAT QUALITY

The search for genetic variation relevant to meat quality has proceeded via quantitative trait loci (QTL) mapping, candidate gene analysis, and in the genomics arena by genome-wide association study (GWAS) approaches. A large database of meat quality QTL for farm animal species is located at http://www.genome.iastate.edu/cgi-bin/QTLdb/index. The application of GWAS is a relatively new -omics approach and is facilitated by massively parallel SNP arrays (Pant et al. 2010, Snelling et al. 2010). Once QTL regions have been identified, candidate genes in the interval can be examined by sequencing phenotypically divergent individuals at candidate loci. This may lead to the identification of individual single-nucleotide polymorphisms (SNPs) or haplotypes that are causative for traits of interest. Haplotypes may also be used in genome-assisted selection (Hayes et al. 2009).

### 11.3.1  DNA MARKERS FOR TENDERNESS

Heritability of tenderness in beef and pork is relatively low, for example, $h^2$ of Warner–Bratzler shear force was $0.14 \pm 0.15$ (Wheeler et al. 2004) and despite extensive studies, there are few genetic markers that have thus far been definitively associated with genetic variation in tenderness. The polymorphisms that have been linked to tenderness mainly lie in genes relevant to postmortem proteolysis. The calpain enzyme family of calcium-dependent cysteine proteases, members of which are responsible for muscle turnover in life and postmortem proteolysis, has been shown to be a source of important genetic variation influential on beef tenderness. These enzymes break down the fibers of meat, increasing tenderness in particular mu- and m-calpain. Significant associations with shear force (an objective measure of tenderness) were identified for three SNPs at the mu-calpain locus (Page et al. 2002, 2004, White et al. 2005). The 316 and 4751 polymorphisms in particular have been validated in a number of independent populations (Corva et al. 2007, Costello et al. 2007, Curi et al. 2009, Franke et al. 2007, Gill et al. 2009, Morris et al. 2006). An SNP in the calpain 3 gene has also been patented for association with tenderness (Barendse 2007). It is known that calpastatin activity in the postmortem muscle is highly related to meat tenderness via the inhibition of the endogenous cysteine peptidases, the calpains (Koohmaraie et al. 1991, Sentendreu et al. 2002). Four polymorphisms in the CAST gene region have been found to be associated with shear force in *longissimus* muscle (Barendse 2002, Casas et al. 2006a,b, Schenkel et al. 2006). Three of these have been validated in multiple independent populations (e.g., Curi et al. 2009, Van Eenennaam et al. 2007). The calpain and calpastatin polymorphisms have been shown to have largely independent effects on toughness (Casas et al. 2006a). Several companies are currently marketing commercial tests for beef tenderness in beef production based on these SNPs including Igenity® Merial and Pfizer.

Two non-synonymous SNPs in the calpastatin gene have also been associated with texture traits in pork, including sensory tenderness, chewiness, and firmness as well as shear force (Ciobanu et al. 2004), and commercial genotyping of these SNPs is offered by Geneseek and Landmark Genetics. Recently, associations have been identified between individual SNPs and haplotypes in the bovine ankyrin 1 gene promoter region and instrumental and sensory tenderness of beef (Aslan et al. 2010).

### 11.3.2 DNA MARKERS OF INTRAMUSCULAR FAT CONTENT AND NUTRITIVE VALUE

In contrast to tenderness, heritability of IMF is moderate (Wheeler et al. 2004), and according to a recent review of the genetic and genomic influences on IMF in beef (Pannier et al. 2010a), there are QTL for IMF on 20 of the 29 bovine somatic chromosomes including a large number of QTL for marbling and other important traits (e.g., milk quality) on chromosome 14 (Wibowo et al. 2008). Polymorphisms in a number of candidate genes underlying bovine QTL have been investigated for associations with IMF or marbling content in resource populations, and in some studies significant associations have been identified, for example, thyroglobulin (Barendse et al. 2004), diacylglycerol-O-acyltransferase (DGAT1) (Thaller et al. 2003), corticotrophin-releasing hormone (Buchanan et al. 2005), and adipocyte fatty acid–binding protein (FABP4) (Michal et al. 2006), though these associations could not all be confirmed in independent populations (e.g., Casas et al. 2005, Pannier et al. 2010b). The somatotropic axis consists of growth hormones, insulin-like growth factors I and II, and interacting hormones such as leptin and their receptors and ligands, for example, ghrelin (Renaville et al. 2002). Key genes in this pathway have been found to harbor genetic variation influential on IMF in beef. For example, SNPs in the growth hormone gene have been shown to be associated with carcass fat (Tatsuda et al. 2008) and marbling (Barendse et al. 2006) in *Bos taurus* populations. Additionally, several recent studies report a correlation between a polymorphism in the growth hormone receptor gene and marbling score (Han et al. 2009) and IMF (Reardon et al. 2010) in beef. Two polymorphisms have been identified on the bovine leptin gene with associations identified with carcass fatness (Buchanan et al. 2002, Schenkel et al. 2005) though it seems likely that there is among-population variability in the relationship of these SNPs with IMF (Barendse et al. 2005, Pannier et al. 2009).

An important functional candidate gene for fatty acid profile and, in particular, unsaturated fatty acid content is the stearoyl CoA desaturase (SCD) gene, which is a protein complex involved in monounsaturated fatty acid (MUFA) synthesis. The A allele at an SNP at position 702 in the open reading frame of the cDNA was found to contribute to higher MUFA percentage and lower melting point in IMF in muscle from Japanese Black cattle (Taniguchi et al. 2004). The association with IMF was found to extend to European *Bos taurus* cattle (Reardon et al. 2010). DNA polymorphisms in the thioesterase (TE) domain of bovine fatty acid synthase gene have been found to be associated with beef fatty acid composition (Zhang et al. 2008). Cattle with the g.17924GG genotype had fatty acids more favorable to human health than other genotypes, with lower total saturated fatty acid and greater MUFA ($P < 0.01$) compared to those with the g.17924AA genotype

(Zhang et al. 2008). The urotensin gene is a novel candidate gene for beef marbling and monounsaturated fat content (Jiang and Michal 2009).

For pork, 57 QTL are currently presented in QTLdb (Hu et al. 2007). For example, a recent study in pork has identified two significant QTL on SSC5 and X chromosome for both IMF and marbling score in the *longissimus* muscle and three QTL on SSC1 and SSC9 for IMF (Ma et al. 2009). Genes in the fatty acid synthesis pathway have also been investigated, for example, polymorphisms in the pig acetyl CoA carboxylase alpha gene is associated with fatty acid composition in a Duroc commercial line (Gallardo et al. 2009).

### 11.3.3  POLYMORPHISMS ASSOCIATED WITH WATER-HOLDING CAPACITY AND COLOR

While, in beef, dark-cutting meat can present problems, in general WHC is a more serious issue in pork. Much research has focused on the search for genetic variation underpinning drip loss, pale color, and poor texture related to poor WHC. In pork, 936 QTL for drip loss have been reported according to AnimalQTLdb. Two SNPs have been identified that have major effects on WHC, and the effects on the muscle proteome of these two key mutations are reviewed in Section 11.5.4. The recessive mutation at the ryanodine receptor (HAL gene) that governs $Ca^{++}$ transport across muscle cell membranes results in susceptibility to stress-induced death in pigs or porcine stress syndrome (Fujii et al. 1991). A dominant mutation in the AMP-activated protein kinase, γ-3 subunit, PRKAG3 gene, also known as the rendement napole (RN) gene, results in poor meat quality that has a low pH, poor color and taste, as well as high drip and cooking losses (Milan et al. 2000, Skrlep et al. 2010, van der Steen et al. 2005). Several SNP alleles in the PRKAG3 gene have, however, been shown to have positive effects on pork quality traits including ultimate pH, meat color, WHC, drip loss, tenderness, and cooking loss (Ciobanu et al. 2001). PRKAG3 is also expressed in bovine skeletal muscle, and its expression levels have been shown to correlate significantly with sensory flavor and juiciness (Bernard et al. 2007). Recent studies in beef indicate that a mutation in bovine PRKAG3 is also associated with WHC and pH-related traits (Reardon et al. 2010).

While coding mutations in these key signaling genes negatively impact WHC, significant variability remains when these are controlled for (Borchers et al. 2007). It is likely that a number of other genes contribute to quantitative variation in this trait. In pork, calpastatin haplotypes have been found to be positively correlated with several WHC traits, including cooking loss, juiciness, and cured ham moisture content (Ciobanu et al. 2004, Skrlep et al. 2010), and these associations have been patented (Rothschild and Ciobanu 2003) and commercialized. In beef, the calpastatin–calpain axis is also important. Casas et al. (2006b) identified an association between an SNP in the 3′ untranslated region of CAST and juiciness in a U.S. *Bos taurus* population, whereas an SNP in the CAST gene (Schenkel et al. 2006) was found to be significantly associated with ultimate pH color in loin and ham muscles (Reardon et al. 2010). In the latter study, although the ultimate pH values were within the acceptable range, GG genotype animals may be more likely to produce dark-cutting beef, compared with other genotypes. Other genes for which associations with pH have been reported include myogenin (Kim et al. 2009), PKM2 (Sieczkowska et al. 2010), and troponin I (Yang et al. 2010). PKM2 and CYP21 are associated with drip loss and DECR1 has been associated with glycolytic potential (Kaminski et al. 2010, Sieczkowska et al. 2010).

### 11.3.4 GENOME-WIDE ASSOCIATION STUDIES AND GENOMIC SELECTION

Through the bovine genome sequencing project, millions of SNP in all major breeds of cattle have been identified (Van Tassell et al. 2008). A number of high-throughput SNP genotyping platforms have been subsequently developed including the Affymetrix GeneChip® Bovine 25 K chip and the Illumina Infinium® Bovine SNP50 BeadChip™ genotyping system, which permit interrogation of 25,000 and 54,000 SNP, respectively. The Illumina Infinium® BovineHD BeadChip™ features more than 777,000 SNPs that uniformly span the entire bovine genome (www.illumina.com). One of the major applications of these arrays is in GWASs. Several economically important traits in livestock have been studied using this approach including growth, milk production, reproduction, and disease susceptibility (Settles et al. 2009, Snelling et al. 2010, Stoop et al. 2009, Wang et al. 2009c), and some studies focused on meat quality, for example, IMF (Barendse et al. 2009).

For the industry, the significance of these markers lies in the enhancement of breeding programs via genomic selection (Goddard and Hayes 2007, Hayes et al. 2009). Genomic selection refers to the making of selection decisions based on genomic estimated breeding values (gEBVs) calculated as the sum of the effects of marker haplotypes across the entire genome, which can potentially capture the effects of all QTL that contribute to trait variation (Hayes et al. 2009, Meuwissen et al. 2001). Challenges include achieving sufficient numbers of genotyped and phenotyped individuals, accounting for breed and family structure, the potential for loss of linkage disequilibrium between marker and trait over time, and the development of appropriate statistical methods (Hayes et al. 2009). Genome-wide selection requires a large set of DNA markers, hence is becoming feasible with larger SNP chips (Wiggans et al. 2009). While the approach needs to be robustly tested and validated in multiple populations, it is expected to increase the rate of genetic improvement twofold per year in many livestock systems (Goddard and Hayes 2009) and is currently being applied in a dairy context in several countries (Berry et al. 2009, Luan et al. 2009, Pryce et al. 2010, VanRaden et al. 2009). Substantial genetic progress for important meat quality traits via whole genome association and genomic selection approaches is likely to be viable as long as appropriate methodologies are applied (Allan and Smith 2008).

## 11.4 TRANSCRIPTOMIC ANALYSIS OF MEAT QUALITY

Progress in both bovine and porcine genomics has accelerated the ability of researchers to investigate the functional regulation of meat quality, and many recent studies have been directed at uncovering the genes regulating the key attributes of beef eating quality: tenderness, flavor, and juiciness, and technological traits such as WHC. Knowledge of the transcripts expressed in bovine/porcine skeletal muscle is expanding (e.g., Band et al. 2002, Bai et al. 2003, Couture et al. 2009, Fahrenkrug et al. 2002, Sudre et al. 2005, Tuggle et al. 2003) and it is becoming possible to identify those genes differentially regulated as a consequence of nutritional status, breed, age, animal handling, and carcass management, which may in turn affect the overall eating quality of the meat (Hocquette et al. 2009). The ultimate quality of fresh meat is dictated by the biological characteristics of the muscle, reflecting the function in the living animal and defined by developmental patterns and associated characteristic of gene expression profiles. Resources that have been explored in meat quality transcriptomics include muscle of divergent breeds, for example, Piedmontese-cross versus Wagyu-cross cattle and embryos (Lehnert et al. 2007, Wang et al. 2005); natural extremes of quality within breeds (Bernard et al. 2007, Canovas et al. 2010); developmental stage (Wimmers et al. 2007); and manipulation of production regimes, such as dietary restriction of protein (Hamill et al. 2009). These have been investigated by application of several platforms, including commercial oligonucleotide arrays and muscle- and developmental stage–specific cDNA microarrays for both pork and beef muscles (e.g., Bai et al. 2003, Lehnert et al. 2004). Most of the expression changes that underpin divergence in meat quality traits are relatively small, typically less than twofold (Liu et al. 2009, McBryan et al. 2010), yet these small changes cumulatively act to have a powerful influence on phenotype. It is therefore important that appropriate normalization factors and the most stable housekeeping genes are selected for validation of microarray studies (McBryan et al. 2010).

Recent research has indicated the important role played by microRNAs in regulating muscle biology, and consequently meat quality as reviewed by McDaneld (2009). miRNA plays critical roles in modulation of gene expression during skeletal muscle development and adipogenesis (McDaneld et al. 2009). Recent studies indicate that miR-1 and miR-133 contribute to hypertrophy in mice (McCarthy and Esser 2007) and miR-206 to hypertrophy in Texel sheep (Clop et al. 2006). Several miRNAs have been associated with major muscle-wasting diseases (Eisenberg et al. 2007). MiR-1 is associated with calcium signaling in heart muscle and in relation to regulation of a major gene for meat quality, the ryanodine receptor (Terentyev et al. 2009). Exploration of the role of these important regulatory mechanisms in the development of meat quality is likely to be a fruitful area of enquiry.

### 11.4.1 GENOMIC REGULATION OF TENDERNESS

Of the sensory traits, tenderness is the one thought to be least influenced by premortem factors and most by the postmortem environment (Sinclair et al. 2001, Sorheim et al. 2001, Thompson et al. 2006). However, there are several biological mechanisms that are postulated to have an influence on tenderness, in particular, postmortem proteolysis during meat aging (Koohmaraie and Geesink 2006). With a view of understanding the molecular mechanisms controlling tenderness, several studies have been carried out, in which a group of animals divergent for quality were profiled using microarrays. Bernard et al. (2007) examined 14 Charolais bull calves that were divergent for sensory quality and identified 146 genes greater than 1.4-fold differentially expressed in relation to beef sensory tenderness. One gene in particular, DNAJA1, which was downregulated in the most tender compared with the most tough beef samples, was found to explain 63% of the observed variability in tenderness. This gene, DNAJA1, encodes a member of the 40 kDa heat shock protein family, which plays a role in protein folding and mitochondrial protein import. The protein is a co-chaperone of the 70 kDa heat shock protein (HSP70), which has been highlighted by several studies to be relevant to muscle biology and meat quality (Bai et al. 2003). Bernard et al. (2007) cite the hypothesis of Ouali et al. (2006), which proposes that apoptosis plays an important role in the early postmortem aging of beef. This protein family is known to have an anti-apoptotic role, hence may be protective of the muscle cell against aging *postmortem*. Lobjois et al. (2008) also examined the gene expression pathways associated with tenderness in pork. Gene expression levels were measured using microarrays for *longissimus* muscle samples selected to represent a range of values for Warner–Bratzler shear force, an objective measure of tenderness. After excluding the very tender samples, linear regression modeling revealed gene expression was correlated with shear force for a number of genes. Many of the genes mapped to three key functional networks, that is, cell cycle, energy metabolism, and muscle development, are thus relevant to variability in toughness. Interestingly, 12 out of the 22 genes that could be mapped to the pig genome were located in chromosomal regions known to harbor QTL affecting pig meat tenderness (chromosomes 2, 6, and 13).

## 11.4.2 GENOMIC REGULATION OF INTRAMUSCULAR FAT CONTENT AND NUTRITIVE VALUE

In order to improve IMF, it is first necessary to obtain a comprehensive understanding of the biological processes and pathways controlling IMF accumulation (Du et al. 2010). Interestingly, both muscle and adipocyte cells are derived from mesenchymal stem cells, which are present in high numbers in developing muscle but decrease with age. It is therefore important to consider both early and late developmental stages in order to gain a complete understanding of IMF deposition (Du et al. 2010, Hausman et al. 2009). With this in mind, several studies have focused on skeletal muscle differentiation in early development in cattle and pigs. Seven important stages of myogenesis (days 14, 21, 35, 49, 63, 77, and 91 postconception) were studied in two breeds, Pietrain and Duroc, which differ greatly in muscle structure and muscularity using differential display RT-PCR (Murani et al. 2007). Forty-three transcripts showed stage-associated and 37 showed breed-associated expression changes. The most frequent functional categories represented genes encoding myofibrillar proteins, genes involved in cell adhesion, cell–cell signaling and extracellular matrix synthesis/remodeling, regulation of gene expression, and metabolism. Prenatal muscle tissue expression profiles of Duroc and Pietrain have also been compared using microarrays (Cagnazzo et al. 2006).

A recent study investigated gene expression profiles of pigs with divergent phenotypes for a number of fatness-related traits using the Affymetrix porcine array (Canovas et al. 2010). It was found that both lipogenic and lipolytic genes were upregulated in higher fat content muscle, suggesting that a cycle of triacylglycerol synthesis and degradation may be upregulated in high fat content muscle and the phenotypic consequences may arise due to a tip in the balance between synthesis and degradation. Real-time PCR studies of these animals for several candidate genes in a group of pigs that have been selected for decreased backfat thickness at constant IMF revealed that both SCD and acetyl CoA carboxylase were reduced in expression in reduced backfat animals (Canovas et al. 2009). The researchers found there was a positive relationship between muscle SCD protein expression and IMF ($r - 0.48$, $P < 0.05$). The involvement of SCD in the specific control of IMF is significant and suggests its potential as a biomarker of IMF.

Bovine resources that have been explored in meat quality transcriptomics include muscle of divergent breeds, for example, Piedmontese-cross versus Wagyu-cross cattle and embryos (Lehnert et al. 2007, Wang et al. 2005). The Japanese Black breed of cattle is known for high IMF, which appears to be mainly due to an increased number of adipocytes and a high monounsaturated fat content compared to Western breeds. Wang et al. (2005) investigated differential gene expression in the LD muscle of Japanese Black (JB) and Holstein (HOL) cattle at 11.5 months of age in order to provide insight into the genes regulating this characteristic. In a similar experiment, it was found that the muscle transcriptome of animals with high marbling potential (Wagyu × Hereford cross) could be reliably distinguished from less marbled animals (Piedmontese × Hereford cross) when the animals were as young as 7 months of age (Wang et al. 2009a). This is significant as at such an early stage, it is not possible to identify meaningful differences in IMF deposition. Real-time PCR studies have also provided insight into IMF metabolism in the bovine. SCD enzyme activity has been shown to correlate with fatty acid composition in a survey of bovine adipose tissue (Yang et al. 1999).

### 11.4.3 GENOMIC REGULATION OF WATER-HOLDING CAPACITY AND COLOR

WHC is a particularly important trait for pork, and the trait has been shown to be affected by differential expression of muscle genes and their protein products. It has been suggested by Hambrecht et al. (2005) that different muscle fiber types reacted differently to stress and after intense physical activity and/or high psychological stress levels preslaughter, and this has consequent effects on the incidence of poor-quality pork. For example, glycolytic muscle types may be more likely to promote PSE development, whereas oxidative muscle types tended to produce DFD pork. Gene expression studies also indicate that fiber type is very important in defining muscle characteristics. The relative expression of myosin heavy-chain type IIb was greater in pigs with large loin muscle areas and was associated with the difference between large and small muscle areas (Wimmers et al. 2008). Bai et al. (2003) developed a muscle-specific porcine cDNA array and applied it to identify differentially expressed genes between red and white muscles. As might be expected, genes in functional categories involved in anaerobic glycolysis and fast isoforms of fiber proteins were upregulated in white muscle, whereas mitochondrial genes with functions in oxidative phosphorylation were more expressed in red muscle. Novel pathways highlighted in this experiment include the casein kinase 2 signaling pathway that is involved in growth, and the role of heat shock proteins (in this case, HSP70) in characterizing divergent muscle characteristics was also found to be important.

Differences in transcript abundance have been described between porcine muscle samples in relation to divergence in WHC (Davoli et al. 2007, Ponsuksili et al. 2008).

Highlighted pathways relevant for WHC include glycolysis, calcium signaling, and myogenesis (e.g., Bernard et al. 2009, Davey et al. 2008). Ponsuksili et al. (2008) identified a significant overrepresentation of genes related to receptor and signal transducer activity, non-membrane-bound organelles, cytoskeleton, plasma membrane, and cell communication and signaling in genes whose expression was associated with poor WHC in pigs. The pathways "extracellular matrix receptor interaction" and "calcium signaling pathway" were also significantly overrepresented. Genes that were positively correlated with WHC included mitochondrial genes, protein metabolism, and electron and ion transporter activity. Notably, 20 genes in the KEGG pathway "oxidative phosphorylation" were significantly negatively correlated with drip loss, again emphasizing the fundamental role of aerobic versus anaerobic metabolic pathways in influencing meat quality. Several genes have been shown to be correlated with drip loss using real-time PCR studies. Expression of COL1A1 increased significantly with increasing drip loss, while expression of CAST decreased significantly with increasing drip loss (McBryan et al. 2010). This is consistent with previous research in which the expression of *COL1A1* was shown to correlate positively with drip loss in a population of 74 animals of Pietrain and Duroc background (Ponsuksili et al. 2008).

Through genetical genomics, researchers aim to identify genomic regions containing candidate genes for the regulation of expression of genes influencing phenotype (Wimmers and Ponsuksili 2010). These expressions or eQTL ultimately control complex traits. Mapping of eQTL to the region of the gene itself indicates that *cis* genetic variation is responsible for the changes in expression levels, whereas when an eQTL is found to map distantly from the position of its corresponding gene, this indicates that the gene is regulated in *trans*. In an experiment mapping eQTL for drip loss–related gene expression profiles of 1279 genes in pork, 897 eQTL were identified with 104 significant eQTL having been detected in previously identified QTL regions for drip loss on SSC 2–6, and 18 (Ponsulksili et al. 2009).

### 11.4.4 NEXT-GENERATION SEQUENCING AND MEAT QUALITY

While great insight into the pathways and processes regulating meat quality have been provided by methods such as microarrays, suppressive subtractive hybridization, and differential display analysis, even more depth of information is now possible with next-generation sequencing methods that can provide absolute, quantitative expression measurements through RNA-seq (Shendure 2008, Wang et al. 2009b, Wilhelm and Landry 2009). Advantages of these approaches include greatly increased transcriptome coverage; increased accuracy; the possibility to study weakly transcribing genes such as transcription factors that are expressed at low levels; and the ability to assess the contribution of novel transcripts, alternative transcripts, and small RNAs (Shendure 2008). Where a well-developed genome scaffold is in place, it is possible to detect and quantify RNAs from all biologically relevant abundance classes and to map RNA splice variants for transcripts of moderate and high abundance using a technology known as RNA-seq (Mortazavi et al. 2008, Wang et al. 2009b). This new technological advance has the potential to provide unprecedented levels of detail on the genomic control of meat quality, provided appropriate bioinformatic protocols are developed.

## 11.5 PROTEOMICS AND MEAT QUALITY

The genome only represents the first step in the complexity of understanding biological function. The shift in thinking from genomics to proteomics comes from the fact the proteome is dynamic and changes with the physiological state of the organism. Hence, it is necessary to determine the protein expression levels directly. The proteome of the cell will reflect the immediate environment of the protein (Dhingra et al. 2005). Proteomics can be defined as the systematic determination of protein sequence, quantity, modification state, interaction partners, activity, subcellular localization, and structure in a given cell type at a particular time (Campbell 2003). Proteome analysis is a direct measurement of proteins in terms of their presence and relative abundance (Wilkins et al. 1996). Neither genomic DNA code nor the amount of mRNA that is expressed for each protein yields an accurate picture of the state of a cell. This is because genes may be present but not transcribed, and the number of mRNA copies does not always reflect the number of functional proteins present (Celis et al. 2000). The aim of proteomics is to obtain information about cellular protein expression and hence to reveal the function of genes, with the ultimate goal of explaining how heredity and environment interact to control cellular functions (Bendixen 2005). When applied to meat science, even if the genetic background is determinant, a major contribution to meat quality development comes from environmental conditions and meat processing. Therefore, proteomics can provide more information than genomics alone. Moreover, the possibility to realize an integrated approach of genomics and proteomics is essential to obtain a complete picture of the molecular mechanisms behind meat quality. Proteomics offers a powerful tool to identify the specific gene products that may be involved in (and indicative of) meat quality alterations (Carbonaro 2004). Proteomic techniques can be used to identify molecular markers that can be used as an indirect measure of a quality attribute. With this purpose it becomes necessary to establish the relationships between changes at the proteome level and changes in meat quality. Identification of protein markers predictive of meat quality traits would offer a powerful tool to be transferred to the meat industry for improved assurance of meat quality.

A big challenge for the meat industry is to obtain reliable information on meat quality throughout the production process, which would provide a guaranteed quality of meat products for consumers (Damez and Clerjon 2008). Meat characteristics depend directly on the muscle biology of live animals, which is regulated by genetic, nutritional, and rearing factors. However, it is well known that quality attributes depend to a great extent on *postmortem* factors like temperature, pH, and proteolysis that degrades muscle proteins during the postmortem aging of meat (Maltin et al. 2003). A prerequisite for the improvement of meat quality is a sound knowledge of the mechanisms influencing meat quality development in the postmortem period. In the following sections, advances in proteomic research to understand the development of key meat quality traits and to address critical meat quality problems are presented. Moreover, a detailed description of the proteins involved in meat quality changes can be found in Table 11.1.

**TABLE 11.1**

**Proteins Involved in the Variability of Meat Quality Attributes**

| Quality Trait | Species/Muscle | Proteins Involved in Quality Changes | References |
|---|---|---|---|
| Texture (WBSF) | Pig *Longissimus dorsi* | Actin fragments, MHC fragment, MLC II, glycolytic enzyme triose phosphate isomerase I | Lametsch et al. (2003) |
| Texture (WBSF) | Bovine *Longissimus dorsi* | MHC, MLC, actin, troponin C, desmin, and tubulin or their fragments, HSPβ6, cysteine- and glycine-rich proteins, α- and β-hemoglobin | Zapata et al. (2009) |
| Tenderness (sensory analysis) | Bovine *Longissimus thoracis* | Succinate dehydrogenase, actin, MyBPH, HSP27, α-crystallin | Morzel et al. (2008) |
| Texture (WBSF) | Bovine *Longissimus thoracis* | Peroxiredoxin 6 | Jia et al. (2009) |
| Texture (WBSF) | Pig *Longissimus* | Adipocyte fatty acid–binding protein, acyl CoA–binding protein, enoyl CoA hydratase, aldose reductase, triosephosphate isomerase, initiation factor elf-3β, chaperonin subunit 2, profilin II | Laville et al. (2007) |
| Texture (WBSF) Color (L*) WHC (drip loss) | Pig *Longissimus dorsi* | MLC I, desmin, troponin T, cofilin 2, F-actin capping protein β subunit, ATP synthase, carbonate dehydratase, triosephosphate isomerase, actin and its relevant peptides, peroxiredoxin 2, α-β crystallin and HSP 27 kDa | Hwang et al. (2005) |
| Texture (WBSF) Color (L*) WHC (drip loss) | Pig *Semimembranosus* | Triosephosphate isomerase, phosphoglucomutase, pyruvate dehydrogenase, succinyl CoA ligase and dihydropilamide succinyltransferase, ubiquinol cytochrome c reductase, ubiquinone oxidoreductase, mitochondrial ATP synthase, HSP 27, Rβ-C, HSP 71, HSP70/HSP90 | Laville et al. (2009) |

**TABLE 11.1 (continued)**
**Proteins Involved in the Variability of Meat Quality Attributes**

| Quality Trait | Species/Muscle | Proteins Involved in Quality Changes | References |
|---|---|---|---|
| Color (L*) | Pig *Semimembranosus* | ATP synthase β subunit, NADH dehydrogenase, succinate dehydrogenase, enolase 1, enolase 3, glycerol-3-phosphate dehydrogenase, hemoglobin α- and β-chain, transferring, HSP27, RB-crystallin, glucose-regulated protein 58 kDa, low-molecular-weight protein tyrosine phosphatase, S-transferase ω, cyclophilin D | Sayd et al. (2006) |
| Color (L*) WHC (drip loss) | Pig *Longissimus dorsi* | Cofilin 2, troponin T, α-β crystallin, HSP27 kDa, group chain A aldehyde dehydrogenase, glycerol-3 phosphate dehydrogenase, hemoglobin α-chain, DJ-1 protein | Hwang (2004) |
| Color (L*, a*, b*) WHC (drip loss, EM) | Pig *Longissimus dorsi* | α-β crystallin, HSP 27, HSP 70, HSP 90 | Yu et al. (2009) |
| WHC (drip loss) | Pig *Longissimus dorsi* *Biceps femoris* | Creatine phosphokinase M-type, desmin, SWI/SNF-related matrix-associated actin-dependent regulator of chromatin a 1 isoform b | Van de Wiel and Zhang (2007) |
| Color (L*, a*, b) WHC (drip loss) | Pig *Longissimus lumborum* | Myoglobin isoform, HSP72, CKM, a calcium-binding protein, cytosolic glycerol-3-phosphate dehydrogenase, dimeric dihydrodiol dehydrogenase, isoform M1 of pyruvate kinase | Kwasiborski et al. (2008) |

WBSF, Warner–Bratzler shear force; EM, expressible moisture; MLC, myosin light chain; MHC, myosin heavy chain; HSP, heat shock protein; CKM, creatine kinase.
En blau els no comprobats.

## 11.5.1 PROTEOMICS AND TENDERNESS DEVELOPMENT

It is well established that meat tenderizes during *postmortem* aging due to degradation of structural proteins such as troponin T, nebulin, titin, vinculin, desmin, and dystrophin. However, the exact biochemical and physiochemical mechanisms underlying the tenderization processes are still a matter of dispute (Lametsch et al. 2003, van de Wiel and Zhang 2007). Over the last decade, proteomic studies relating changes in the proteome with changes in meat texture have contributed to gain understanding of the mechanisms controlling beef tenderness. Lametsch et al. (2003) investigated *postmortem* changes related to tenderness in pork *longissimus dorsi* (LD) muscle. Three actin fragments, a myosin heavy-chain fragment, myosin light chain II, and the glycolytic enzyme triose phosphate isomerase I, were correlated to texture values measured as shear force. They concluded that the results demonstrate that *postmortem* degradation of actin and myosin heavy chain is highly related to meat tenderness.

Early predictors for tenderness of bovine *m. longissimus thoracis* were investigated with two-dimensional electrophoresis (2-DE) and mass spectrometry (MS) (Morzel et al. 2008). The best common predictor of initial and overall tenderness was found to be succinate dehydrogenase. Structural (actin, MyBPH) and chaperone (HSP27, α-crystallin) proteins were identified as targets of *postmortem* proteolysis during aging. The existence of an underlying HSP27-related cellular mechanism, with consequences on tenderness development, was suggested. Another study described the association of texture measurements with structural proteins: myosin heavy and light chains, actin, desmin, and tubulin or their fragments (Zapata et al. 2009). Degradation of the thick filament components at 36h postmortem was found to be predictive of future tenderness in beef. Interesting association between metabolic, developmental, and chaperone function proteins and tenderization. The authors stressed the importance of further investigating the participation of proteins other than structural proteins in meat tenderization processes. In this sense, Laville et al. (2007) investigated the role of sarcoplasmic proteins in cooked pork texture variability. Protein expression between two meat groups (tough and tender) was compared in order to improve understanding of protein-related metabolic pathways underlying meat tenderness, other than proteolysis. Protein involved in lipid traffic and in the control of gene expression regulating cell proliferation and differentiation, and proteins indirectly related to lipid metabolism were overrepresented in the tender group. The tender group was further characterized by increased levels of proteins involved in protein folding and polymerization. The authors suggested that the lower post-cooking shear force could at least in part be related to muscle adipogenetic and/or myogenetic status.

## 11.5.2 Proteomics and Water-Holding Capacity

Loss of water and soluble constituents occurs during storage of meat at different levels. Formation of drip is generally considered as a result of denaturation of contractile proteins and shrinkage of myofibrils during rigor development (Bertram et al. 2004b, Offer et al. 1989). Proteome analysis of porcine muscle by 2-DE has identified candidate protein markers highly relevant to the process of drip loss (van de Wiel and Zhang 2007). The most clearly identified proteins were creatine phosphokinase M-type, desmin, and a transcription activator. In another study, Hwang et al. (2005) identified three proteins: adenylate kinase, substrate protein of mitochondrial ATP-dependent proteinase SP-22, and troponin T slow-type isoform, correlated with changes in meat drip loss. In a recent study, the correlation between meat quality and heat shock protein expression in *m.* LD of pigs was investigated with a proteomic approach (Yu et al. 2009). The four heat shock proteins tested (α-β crystallin,

HSP27, HSP70, and HSP90) by ELISA in the LD tissue of pigs tended to decrease after transportation. Yu et al. (2009) found a relationship between the decline in heat shock protein expression and increased drip loss in LD muscle, pointing at this mechanism as a possible cause resulting in poor meat quality in the LD.

Finally, the relationship between changes on the proteome with changes on WHC induced by meat-processing technologies can also be addressed with a proteomic approach. Marcos and Mullen (2009) have investigated the effects of high-pressure processing LD muscle. They confirmed a relationship between pressure-induced sarcoplasmic protein denaturation onto the myofibrils and WHC.

### 11.5.3 PROTEOMICS AND MEAT COLOR

The color of raw meat is a combination of the influence of myoglobin content and the changes in reflection due to protein denaturation (Aaslyng 2002, Miller 2002). Thus, proteomic approaches can help in understanding changes on meat color. Sayd et al. (2006) investigated the biochemical mechanisms responsible for variation in meat color. With this purpose, a differential proteome analysis was performed on the sarcoplasmic protein fraction of *semimembranosus* pig muscles, characterized by high or low L* (lightness) values. Twenty-two proteins or fragments were differentially expressed. Muscles leading to darker meat had a more oxidative metabolism, indicated by more abundant mitochondrial enzymes of the respiratory chain, hemoglobin, and chaperone or regulator proteins (HSP27, α-β crystallin, and glucose-regulated protein 58 kDa). Conversely, enzymes of glycolysis were overexpressed in the lighter group. Such samples were also characterized by higher levels of glutathione S-transferase ω, which can activate the RyR calcium channels, and higher levels of cyclophilin D. This protein pattern is likely to have severe implications on postmortem metabolism, namely, acceleration of ATP depletion and pH fall and subsequent enhanced protein denaturation, which are well known to induce discoloration. Their proteomic study successfully provided new insights into the development of regulator proteins in meat color development.

Kwasiborski et al. (2008) used a proteomic approach to assess the effects of premortem factors on the color coordinates of pig *longissimus* muscle. One myoglobin isoform and 72 kDa heat shock protein (HSP72), and a HSP70 isoform were found to explain an 84% variability in L*. Proteins retained in the model for redness involved proteins related to *postmortem* oxidative activity. The influence of heat shock proteins on pork color was further studied by Yu et al. (2009). A decrease in heat shock proteins in the LD muscle was suggested to be disadvantageous for maintaining muscle cell integrity and repairing denatured proteins, such as desmin, and sarcoplasmic and myofibrillar proteins, which could subsequently lead to reduced meat color.

### 11.5.4 PROTEOMIC APPROACHES TO ASSESS MEAT QUALITY DEFECTS

#### 11.5.4.1 Differences in Pig Muscle Proteome Related to HAL Gene

PSE pork is a cause of considerable economic losses. The development of PSE pork is related to an increased rate of early postmortem glycolysis and pH decline. A greater understanding of postmortem metabolism during the conversion of muscle to meat and the mechanisms of enhanced and extended glycolysis are critical to characterizing pork quality development (Scheffler and Gerrard 2007).

The production of PSE pork meat has been closely related with porcine stress syndrome, a condition synonymous with malignant hyperthermia. Malignant hyperthermia is a heritable trait resulting from a mutation on the ryanodine receptor (RYR1) gene known as the halothane gene present in some porcine populations (Fujii et al. 1991). This gene encodes a protein of the sarcoplasmic reticulum responsible for calcium release. It is responsible for sudden increases in calcium levels in the cytoplasm during challenges such as stress (Michelson et al. 1988). This mutation has important consequences for production and quality traits, as it may be a cause of mortality during transport or of reduced meat quality, as it becomes PSE when occurring before slaughter (Sybesma and Eikelenboom 1969).

Proteome research has provided advanced knowledge on the relationship between protein denaturation, aggregation, and precipitation and the development of the PSE meat quality defect. Laville et al. (2005) used a proteomic approach to characterize PSE zones in pig *semimembranosus* muscles. 2-DE showed that troponin T, myosin light chain I, and α-crystallin were less proteolysed in defective muscles, while fragments of creatine kinase were more represented. It was also noted that heat shock protein HSP27 was absent in the PSE meat. In another study, Laville et al. (2009) studied the sarcoplasmic protein fraction obtained from *semimembranosus* muscles from pigs of different HAL genotypes. The results indicated that the faster pH decline in nn pigs was not explained by higher abundance of glycolytic enzymes. They also observed that nn muscles contained fewer proteins of the oxidative metabolic pathway, fewer antioxidants, and more protein fragments. The authors concluded that compared to NN and/ or Nn muscles, nn are less oxidative and have less antioxidative and repair capabilities. Further research would be needed to confirm the proteins of the cellular protective system as markers for meat quality traits. Hwang (2004) described a model that successfully classified PSE meat from Korean native black pigs. Twelve proteins were related to hunter L* value, which included contractile apparatus and related proteins such as alpha actin, myosin light chain 1, cofilin 2, and troponin T, and chaperone proteins of α-β crystallin. Four proteins (troponin T, adenylate kinase, ATP-dependent proteinase SP-22, and DJ-1 protein) were related to drip loss.

### 11.5.4.2   Differences in Pig Muscle Proteome Related to RN⁻ Gene

A single-point mutation, rendement napole (RN⁻), is responsible for elevated muscle glycolytic potential in pork (Monin and Laborde 1985). Greater availability of glycogen contributes to an extended pH decline by providing additional substrate for glycolysis. Thus, the mutant RN⁻ genotype generates pork of inferior technological quality (PSE) by increasing the glycolytic potential and extending postmortem pH decline, resulting in pork with a low pHu (Scheffler and Gerrard 2007). Hedegaard et al. (2004) studied the effects of this mutation on protein expression patterns in skeletal muscle. The results revealed that the key enzyme in the synthesis of glycogen, UDP-glucose pyrophosphorylase, was significantly upregulated in RN⁻ carriers. They also reported differences in the expression patterns of enzymes related to glycolysis and the citric acid cycle, suggesting that hyperaccumulation of glycogen mediated by the RN⁻ mutation is due to an increased synthesis of glycogen.

### 11.5.4.3 Differences in Pig Muscle Proteome Related to Boar Taint

There are a number of chemical substances responsible for boar taint, of which skatole and androstenone are judged to be the primary compounds. Skatole and androstenone, when present in fatty tissues separately or together, give rise to off-odor from meat of pigs (Dijksterhuis et al. 2000). van de Wiel et al. (2006) pointed proteomics as a highly effective tool for the purpose of identifying candidate marker genes for boar taint. Proteomes from Duroc pigs presenting a range of androstenone levels in back fat were studied. The authors identified four candidate marker proteins for boar taint after MS/MS Maldi-TOF analysis; however, the specific proteins affected are not reported.

## 11.6 METABOLOMICS

The completion of genome sequencing of human, bovine, and other species has led to exponential growth of transcriptomics, proteomics, and metabolomics. These -omics technologies in conjunction with powerful bioinformatic and chemometric tools have enabled us to understand more about the roles of various genes and their interactions in a biological system. Metabolomics, which in essence was in practice since the mid-1960s, has now been widely applied to areas including disease biomarkers, drug intervention or environmental stress, nutrigenomics, personal health assessment, clinical diagnostics, mode of action studies, and metabolic engineering. However, metabolomics has been intermittently applied in meat science. The advent of metabol(n)omics in tandem with other "-omics" has great potential to lead to identification and establishment of new phenotypic markers that could be exploited genetically and/or external management of animals for better meat quality. This section reviews current and potential applications for metabolomics in predicting and monitoring meat quality.

### 11.6.1 METABOLOMICS VERSUS METABONOMICS

"Metabolomics" and "metabonomics" are loosely used in defining metabolite profiling and in recent times have been rechristened to a single term "metabol(n)omics" (Nicholson et al. 1999). Nevertheless, efforts have been made to define and distinguish metabonomics from metabolomics. Metabolomics covers the *comprehensive* analysis of all chemical compounds that participate as substrates, intermediates, or by-products in the cellular metabolic process within a defined physiological condition (Wind and Hu 2006). The chemical species in a biological living system range from low molecular weight polar volatiles such as ethanol to a relatively high-molecular-weight polar *sugars*, *amino acids*, nonpolar *amino acids*, *lipids*, and inorganic species with varying concentrations ($10^{-15}$–$10^{-6}$ M). Metabonomics, on the other hand, is the *quantitative* measurement of changes of metabolic profiles of a living system in response to pathophysiological stimuli or genetic modification (Nicholson et al. 1999).

Metabolomics can be performed in two different approaches, that is, holistic and/or targeted metobolomics. In the holistic approach, the metabolite profiles are processed with pattern recognition to determine *similarities or differences* which may indicate disease or mode of action. Targeted metabolomics focus on specific metabolites formed during the cellular anabolic or catabolic reactions. Currently, the most commonly used tools for metabolomic experiments are nuclear magnetic resonance (NMR) spectroscopy and MS techniques on which the subsequent sections will be based on. The former technology is generally associated with the holistic metabolomics approach, while the MS is almost always associated with the targeted metabolomics.

### 11.6.2 Metabolomics of Tenderness

Meat tenderness is an attribute of meat quality that has been comprehensively studied by NMR spectroscopy (Choi et al. 2007, Fontanesi et al. 2008, Kemp et al. 2010, Ryu and Kim 2005). In most of the earlier studies on meat tenderness, $^{31}$P-NMR spectroscopy was mostly employed to obtain the information on the levels of phosphorylated metabolites and their postmortem changes in meat muscles from beef, pork, and lamb (Lahucky et al. 1993, 2002, Lundberg et al. 1987, Miri et al. 1992, Moesgaard et al. 1995, Vogel et al. 1985). This is because of the fact that under the anaerobic condition following slaughter, replenishment of the cell energy (adenosine triphosphate [ATP] from adenosine diphosphate [ADP]) occurs primarily via degradation of glycogen (glycolysis), sugar phosphates such as glucose-6-phosphate (G-6-P), and from the use of creatine phosphate. The rate of postmortem degradation of phosphorus metabolites (ATP/ADP, phosphomonoesters that are mainly sugar phosphates, inorganic phosphates, and creatine phosphate) was higher in animals stunned by captive bolt pistol followed by electrical stunning and least with anesthesia (Bertram et al. 2002c). This correspondingly correlated to the muscle glycolysis rates in the same order, that is, captive bolt pistol > electrical > anesthesia, and thereby pointing the lowest meat quality in the captive bolt pistol stunned animals. In pork, the $^{31}$P-NMR spectroscopy revealed that the high phosphomonoesters and low phosphocreatinine concentrations associate with PSE-prone meat, while high inorganic phosphate and low phosphomonoesters indicate a DFD-prone meat (Miri et al. 1992). $^{31}$P-NMR was also extensively used to show that the pigs with malignant hyperthermia syndrome suffer from impaired muscle metabolism resulting in poor meat quality traits (Lahucky et al. 1993, 2002, Moesgaard et al. 1995). In the muscle-to-meat conversion process in carcasses, the rate of pH decline is reflected by the rate of glycolysis among other characteristics such as animal species, preslaughter handling, and postmortem temperature (Bertram et al. 2002c, 2006a, Jones et al. 1993, Josell et al. 2000). The rate of glycolysis and its stage in the LD muscle is determined by the content of muscle glycogen and G-6-P. For instance, rapid rate of postmortem glycolysis is associated with low level of glycogen and high level of G-6-P, suggesting an increased phosphorylase activity (Moesgaard et al. 1995).

### 11.6.3 Metabolomics of Water-Holding Capacity

WHC is by far the most widely studied aspect of meat quality using the metabol(n) omic platform since the mid-1980s (Bertram and Andersen 2007, Bertram et al. 2001a,b, 2002b, Hertzman et al. 1993, Renou et al. 1985). The mechanism of

WHC is based on the proteins (i.e., myofibrillar proteins) and muscle structures that bind and entrap water (Huff-Lonergan and Lonergan 2005). Bertram et al. (2002b) have shown that the WHC is depended on the structural features of meat affecting the sarcomere lengths from the low-field NMR analysis of porcine *longissmus* muscles. The drip loss from the meat was found to be lower for samples with longer sarcomere lengths than in the cold-induced contracted sarcomeres (Bertram et al. 2001a, 2002a,b, Honikel et al. 1986). This led them to conclude that the highly organized myofibrillar protein structures such as actins and myosins are involved in water mobility and distribution. Although chilling improved WHC, it could also induce shortening of muscle cells if the temperature drops sharply which would explain the higher toughness of meat with rapid chilling than the conventional chilled meat (Jones et al. 1993, van der Wal et al. 1995). Further NMR studies on the effect of heating porcine muscles on their WHC reconfirmed the association of myofibrillar proteins and water mobility (Bertram et al. 2006a,b, Straadt et al. 2007). The heat denaturing experiments revealed major changes in water mobility occurred within a narrow temperature window, that is, between 40°C and 50°C, possibly due to continual denaturation of myosin heads. At 53°C–58°C, myosin rod denaturation occurred and induced changes in myofibrillar water characteristics; at 70°C–74°C, collagen denaturation generally takes place and it has a lesser impact on myofibrillar water than the denaturation of myosin. Closer to the boiling point of water, at 80°C–82°C, denaturation of actin and expulsion of water from the meat occurred. In addition, the changes in pH and ionic strength in the meat–water milieu can also affect the WHC, which will be of importance to the meat-processing industries (Bertram et al. 2004a). This would mean that adding salt to meat causes more water to be tightly bound to the myofibrillar matrix, while the rest becomes less tightly bound (Bertram et al. 2001c).

As the studies on WHC gained momentum, research activities were also focused on the association of slaughter environment and the effects of dietary supplements to WHC (Andersen et al. 2005, Bertram et al. 2002c, Maurizio et al. 2004, Young et al. 2005). For example, Bertram et al. (2002c) found no drip loss difference between animals stunned by captive bolt pistol and electrocution, although the pH was lower in animals that were electrically stunned compared to $CO_2$ stunning (or anesthesia). In the study of influence of season by Bianchi et al. (2004), a significant deterioration of WHC was observed in turkey flocks slaughtered during summer compared to those samples collected in winter (Maurizio et al. 2004). The rapid loss of water in summer could possibly be due to accelerated postmortem muscle metabolism.

In a recent high-resolution NMR study of porcine plasma, lactate and acetate were the two important metabolites found to be related to preslaughter exercise-stressed pigs and meat quality (Bertram et al. 2010). Pigs slaughtered immediately after exercise-induced stress had a high level of lactate as a result of anaerobic metabolism of muscular glycogen breakdown. The combined effect of decreasing pH (lactate accumulation) and increasing temperature denatured myosins and ultimately reduced the WHC (Bertram et al. 2001b). Likewise acetate, an important cofactor in carbohydrate and fat metabolism, was elevated in the exercise-stressed pigs.

This study further substantiated that the resting period before slaughter can reverse the stress-induced changes of the metabolite profile, which could impart beneficial effects on meat quality.

### 11.6.4 METABOLOMICS IN RELATION TO TRACEABILITY

The geographical origin of beef was confirmed by characterizing the fatty acid contents of animal's diet using [1]H-MAS NMR (Brescia et al. 2002, Renou et al. 2004). A similar approach on 23 raw-dried beef of certified origin from 4 different continents also proved to be useful in tracing the origin and thereby determining the meat quality (Shintu et al. 2007). In a recent large-scale survey (533 samples) aiming to carry out an age-wise classification of Australian sheep meat collected over 4–6 months period, GC-MS was deployed to determine the branched-chain fatty acid contents in sheep fat (Watkins et al. 2010). The distinction of lamb from hogget or mutton was only possible with the background knowledge of animal nutrition that would be impractical as the preslaughter information dilutes along the meat supply chain.

MS, both GC-MS and LC-MS, have been applied to determine the gender of meat origin by analyzing the hormonal characteristics, in particular, assessing the ratio of progesterone to pregnenolone (Draisci et al. 2000). Male beef meat had a significantly higher level of progesterone:pregnenolone than the female beef. In this case, LC-MS has the advantage over GC-MS, as the male hormones and their metabolites can be better detected and quantified.

## 11.7  CONCLUSION

It is clear that our understanding of the biological pathways and processes underpinning meat quality are being greatly accelerated by the application of -omics approaches. Currently, just a small number of DNA markers are being marketed to improve quality in beef and pork. However, given the technological breakthroughs currently underway in the areas of next-generation sequencing and SNP chips, it is likely that progress in the identification of QTL and causative mutations for quality will accelerate in the next 2–3 years. In parallel, functional genomic and proteomic markers and metabolite profiles associated with quality also have potential to be incorporated into meat quality management programs. The application of the knowledge for industry is the critical next step and requires extensive consideration. Genome-assisted selection (Allan and Smith 2008) and palatability-assured critical control points (PACCPs) systems are potential mechanisms for application of genetic information for industry (Mullen et al. 2006). Potential models have also been proposed for genomic and proteomic markers (e.g., Goldberg and Goldberg 2010, Lewin et al. 2009), while there is great potential for the application of current metabolomics tools, such as MS and NMR spectroscopy to routine low-cost analysis of metabolomic markers of meat quality as well as marker discovery. Using the wealth of information being generated, it is feasible that meat quality can become an important part of future animal selection and meat quality management systems to ensure an increase in consumer satisfaction and industry profitability as long as appropriate models are applied.

# REFERENCES

Aaslyng, M. D. 2002. Quality indicators for raw meat. In: *Meat processing, Improving Meat Quality*, J. P. Kerry, J. Kerry, and D. A. Ledward (eds.), pp. 157–174. Cambridge, U.K.: Woodhead Publishing Ltd.

Aaslyng, M. D. 2009. Trends in meat consumption and the need for fresh meat and meat products of improved quality. In: *Improving the Sensory and Nutritional Quality of Fresh Meat*, J. Kerry, and D. A. Ledward (eds.), pp. 3–18. Cambridge, U.K.: Woodhead Publishing Ltd.

Aaslyng, M. D., M. Oksama, E. V. Olsen et al. 2007. The impact of sensory quality of pork on consumer preference. *Meat Sci* 76:61–73.

Allan, M. F. and T. P. L. Smith. 2008. Present and future applications of DNA technologies to improve beef production. *Meat Sci* 80:79–85.

Andersen, H. J., N. Oksbjerg, J. F. Young, and M. Therkildsen. 2005. Feeding and meat quality—A future approach. *Meat Sci* 70:543–554.

Aslan, O., T. Sweeney, A. M. Mullen, and R. M. Hamill. 2010. Regulatory polymorphisms in the bovine Ankyrin 1 gene promoter are associated with tenderness and intra-muscular fat content. *BMC Genet* 11:111.

Bai, Q., C. McGillivray, N. da Costa et al. 2003. Development of a porcine skeletal muscle cDNA microarray: Analysis of differential transcript expression in phenotypically distinct muscles. *BMC Genomics* 4:8.

Barendse, W. 2007. DNA marker for meat tenderness in cattle. United States Patent Application 20090148844. what document?

Barendse, W., R. J. Bunch, and B. E. Harrison. 2005. The leptin C73T missense mutation is not associated with marbling and fatness traits in a large gene mapping experiment in Australian cattle. *Anim Genet* 36:86.

Barendse, W., R. J. Bunch, B. E. Harrison, and M. B. Thomas. 2006. The growth hormone 1 GH1:c.457C > G mutation is associated with intramuscular and rump fat distribution in a large sample of Australian feedlot cattle. *Anim Genet* 37:211–214.

Barendse, W., R. Bunch, M. Thomas et al. 2004. The TG5 thyroglobulin gene test for a marbling quantitative trait loci evaluated in feedlot cattle. *Aust J Exp Agric* 44:669–674.

Barendse, W., B. E. Harrison, R. J. Bunch, M. B. Thomas, and L. B. Turner. 2009. Genome wide signatures of positive selection: The comparison of independent samples and the identification of regions associated to traits. *BMC Genomics* 10:178.

Bendixen, E. 2005. The use of proteomics in meat science. *Meat Sci* 71:138–149.

Bernard, C., I. Cassar-Malek, M. Le Cunff et al. 2007. New indicators of beef sensory quality revealed by expression of specific genes. *J Agric Food Chem* 55:5229–5237.

Bernard, C., I. Cassar-Malek, G. Renand, and J. F. Hocquette. 2009. Changes in muscle gene expression related to metabolism according to growth potential in young bulls. *Meat Sci* 82:205–212.

Berry, D. P., J. F. Kearney, and B. L. Harris. 2009. Genomic selection in Ireland. *Interbull Bull* 39:29–34.

Bertram, H. C. and H. J. Andersen. 2007. NMR and the water-holding issue of pork. *J Anim Breed Genet* 124 (Suppl. 1):35–42.

Bertram, H. C., H. J. Andersen, and A. H. Karlsson. 2001a. Comparative study of low-field NMR relaxation measurements and two traditional methods in the determination of water holding capacity of pork. *Meat Sci* 57:125–132.

Bertram, H. C., S. Donstrup, A. H. Karlsson, H. J. Andersen, and H. Stodkilde-Jorgensen. 2001b. Post mortem energy metabolism and pH development in porcine *M. longissimus dorsi* as affected by two different cooling regimes. A (31)P-NMR spectroscopic study. *Magn Reson Imaging* 19:993–1000.

Bertram, H. C., A. H. Karlsson, M. Rasmussen et al. 2001c. Origin of multiexponential T(2) relaxation in muscle myowater. *J Agric Food Chem* 49:3092–3100.

Bertram, H. C., A. Kohler, U. Bocker, R. Ofstad, and H. J. Andersen. 2006a. Heat-induced changes in myofibrillar protein structures and myowater of two pork qualities. A combined FT-IR spectroscopy and low-field NMR relaxometry study. *J Agric Food Chem* 54:1740–1746.

Bertram, H. C., M. Kristensen, and H. J. Andersen. 2004a. Functionality of myofibrillar proteins as affected by pH, ionic strength and heat treatment—A low-field NMR study. *Meat Sci* 68:249–256.

Bertram, H. C., N. Oksbjerg, and J. F. Young. 2010. NMR-based metabonomics reveals relationship between pre-slaughter exercise stress, the plasma metabolite profile at time of slaughter, and water-holding capacity in pigs. *Meat Sci* 84:108–113.

Bertram, H. C., P. P. Purslow, and H. J. Andersen. 2002a. Relationship between meat structure, water mobility, and distribution: A low-field nuclear magnetic resonance study. *J Agric Food Chem* 50:824–829.

Bertram, H. C., M. Rasmussen, H. Busk et al. 2002b. Changes in porcine muscle water characteristics during growth—An in vitro low-field NMR relaxation study. *J Magn Reson* 157:267–276.

Bertram, H. C., H. Størdkilde-Jørgensen, A. H. Karlsson, and H. J. Andersen. 2002c. Post mortem energy metabolism and meat quality of porcine *M. longissimus dorsi* as influenced by stunning method—A 31P NMR spectroscopic study. *Meat Sci* 62:113–119.

Bertram, H. C., A. K. Whittaker, W. R. Shorthose, H. J. Andersen, and A. H. Karlsson. 2004b. Water characteristics in cooked beef as influenced by ageing and high-pressure treatment—An NMR micro imaging study. *Meat Sci* 66:301–306.

Bertram, H. C., Z. Wu, F. van den Berg, and H. J. Andersen. 2006b. NMR relaxometry and differential scanning calorimetry during meat cooking. *Meat Sci* 74:684–689.

Bouley, J., C. Chambon, and B. Picard. 2004. Mapping of bovine skeletal muscle proteins using two-dimensional gel electrophoresis and mass spectrometry. *Proteomics* 4:1811–1824.

Brescia, M. A., A. C. Jambrenghi, V. di Martino et al. 2002. High resolution nuclear magnetic resonance spectroscopy (NMR) studies on meat components: Potentials and prospects. *Ital J Anim Sci* 1:151–158.

Buchanan, F. C., C. J. Fitzsimmons, A. G. Van Kessel et al. 2002. Association of a missense mutation in the bovine leptin gene with carcass fat content and leptin mRNA levels. *Genet Sel Evol* 34:105–116.

Buchanan, F. C., T. D. Thue, P. Yu, and D. C. Winkelman-Sim. 2005. Single nucleotide polymorphisms in the corticotrophin-releasing hormone and pro-opiomelancortin genes are associated with growth and carcass yield in beef cattle. *Anim Genet* 36:127–131.

Campbell, P. 2003. A cast of thousands. *Nat Biotechnol* 21:213 [Editorial].

Canovas, A., J. Estany, M. Tor, R. N. Pena, and O. Doran. 2009. Acetyl-CoA carboxylase and stearoyl-CoA desaturase protein expression in subcutaneous adipose tissue is reduced in pigs selected for decreased backfat thickness at constant intramuscular fat content. *J Anim Sci* 87:3905–3914.

Canovas, A., R. Quintanilla, M. Amills, and R. Pena. 2010. Muscle transcriptomic profiles in pigs with divergent phenotypes for fatness traits. *BMC Genomics* 11:372.

Carbonaro, M. 2004. Proteomics: Present and future in food quality evaluation. *Trends Food Sci Technol* 15:209–216.

Casas, E., S. N. White, D. G. Riley et al. 2005. Assessment of single nucleotide polymorphisms in genes residing on chromosomes 14 and 29 for association with carcass composition traits in Bos indicus cattle. *J Anim Sci* 83:13–19.

Casas, E., S. White, T. Wheeler et al. 2006a. Testing for interactions between Calpastatin and M-Calpain markers in beef cattle on tenderness traits. *J Anim Sci* 84:135–136.

Casas, E., S. White, T. L. Wheeler et al. 2006b. Effects of calpastatin and mu-calpain markers in beef cattle on tenderness traits. *J Anim Sci* 84:520–525.

Celis, J. E., M. Kruhoffer, I. Gromova et al. 2000. Gene expression profiling: Monitoring transcription and translation products using DNA microarrays and proteomics. *FEBS Lett* 480:2–16.

Choi, Y. M. and B. C. Kim. 2009. Muscle fiber characteristics, myofibrillar protein isoforms, and meat quality. *Livest Sci* 122:105–118.

Choi, Y. M., Y. C. Ryu, and B. C. Kim. 2007. Influence of myosin heavy- and light chain isoforms on early postmortem glycolytic rate and pork quality. *Meat Sci* 76:281–288.

Ciobanu, D. C., J. W. M. Bastiaansen, S. M. Lonergan et al. 2004. New alleles in calpastatin gene are associated with meat quality traits in pigs. *J Anim Sci* 82:2829–2839.

Ciobanu, D., J. Bastiaansen, M. Malek et al. 2001. Evidence for new alleles in the protein kinase monophospate-activated y3-subunit gene associated with low glycogen content in pig skeletal muscle and improved meat quality. *Genetics* 159:1151–1162.

Clop, A., F. Marcq, H. Takeda et al. 2006. A mutation creating a potential illegitimate microRNA target site in the myostatin gene affects muscularity in sheep. *Nat Genet* 38:813–818.

Corva, P., L. Soria, A. Schor et al. 2007. Association of CAPN1 and CAST gene polymorphisms with meat tenderness in *Bos taurus* beef cattle from Argentina. *Genet Mol Biol* 30:1064–1069.

Costello, S., E. O'Doherty, D. J. Troy et al. 2007. Association of polymorphisms in the *calpain I*, *calpain II* and growth hormone genes with tenderness in bovine *M. longissimus dorsi*. *Meat Sci* 75:551–557.

Curi, R. A., L. A. L. Chardulo, M. C. Mason et al. 2009. Effect of single nucleotide polymorphisms of CAPN1 and CAST genes on meat traits in Nellore beef cattle (*Bos indicus*) and in their crosses with *Bos taurus*. *Anim Genet* 40:456–462.

Damez, J.-L. and S. Clerjon. 2008. Meat quality assessment using biophysical methods related to meat structure. *Meat Sci* 80:132–149.

Davey, G., C. McGee, A. Di Luca et al. 2008. Gene expression profiling of animals from an Irish pig herd divergent in meat quality attributes. In: *Pig Genome II. Second European Conference on Pig Genomics*, Abstracts' book, p. 17.

Davoli, R., M. Colombo, S. Schiavina et al. 2007. Transcriptome analysis of porcine skeletal muscle: Differentially expressed genes in Italian Large White pigs with divergent values for glycolytic potential. *Ital J Anim Sci* 6:113–115.

Dhingra, V., M. Gupta, T. Andacht, and Z. F. Fu. 2005. New frontiers in proteomics research: A perspective. *Int J Pharm* 299:1–18.

Dijksterhuis, G. B., B. Engel, P. Walstra et al. 2000. An international study on the importance of androstenone and skatole for boar taint: II. Sensory evaluation by trained panels in seven European countries. *Meat Sci* 54:261–269.

Dikeman, M. 1987. Fat reduction in animals and the effect on palatability and consumer acceptance of meat products. In: *Proceedings of 40th Annual Reciprocal Meat Conference*, vol. 40. Chicago, IL, pp. 93–103.

Draisci, R., L. Palleschi, E. Ferretti, L. Lucentini, and P. Cammarata. 2000. Quantitation of anabolic hormones and their metabolites in bovine serum and urine by liquid chromatography-tandem mass spectrometry. *J Chromatogr A* 870:511–522.

Du, M., J. Yin, and M. J. Zhu. 2010. Cellular signaling pathways regulating the initial stage of adipogenesis and marbling of skeletal muscle. *Meat Sci* 86:103–109.

Eisenberg, I., A. Eran, I. Nishino et al. 2007. Distinctive patterns of microRNA expression in primary muscular disorders. *Proc Natl Acad Sci USA* 104:17016–17021.

Elsik, C. G., R. L. Tellam, K. C. Worley et al. 2009. The genome sequence of taurine cattle: A window to ruminant biology and evolution. *Science* 324:522–528.

Fernandez, X., G. Monin, A. Talmant, J. Mourot, and B. Lebret. 1999. Influence of intramuscular fat content on the quality of pig meat—2. Consumer acceptability of *M. longissimus lumborum. Meat Sci* 53:67–72.

Fontanesi, L., R. Davoli, L. Nanni Costa et al. 2008. Investigation of candidate genes for glycolytic potential of porcine skeletal muscle: Association with meat quality and production traits in Italian Large White pigs. *Meat Sci* 80:780–787.

Franke, D. E., D. H. Fischer, M. G. Thomas, and T. D. Bidner. 2007. Calpastatin and calpain genetic marker influences on shear force in Brahman steers. *J Anim Sci* 85:3.

Fujii, J., K. Otsu, F. Zorzato et al. 1991. Identification of a mutation in porcine ryanodine receptor associated with malignant hyperthermia. *Science* 253:448–451.

Gallardo, D., R. Quintanilla, L. Varona et al. 2009. Polymorphism of the pig acetyl-coenzyme A carboxylase alpha gene is associated with fatty acid composition in a Duroc commercial line. *Anim Genet* 40:410–417.

Gill, J. L., S. C. Bishop, C. McCorquodale, J. L. Williams, and P. Wiener. 2009. Association of selected SNP with carcass and taste panel assessed meat quality traits in a commercial population of Aberdeen Angus-sired beef cattle. *Genet Sel Evol* 41:36.

Goddard, M. E. and B. J. Hayes. 2007. Genomic selection. *J Anim Breed Genet* 124:323–330.

Goddard, M. E. and B. J. Hayes. 2009. Mapping genes for complex traits in domestic animals and their use in breeding programmes. *Nat Rev Genet* 10:381–391.

Goldberg, D. B. and M. Goldberg, (Boulder, CO, US). 2010. Measurement of protease activity in post-mortem meat samples. United States Patent Application 201002099.

Hambrecht, E., J. J. Eissen, D. J. Newman et al. 2005. Preslaughter handling effects on pork quality and glycolytic potential in two muscles differing in fiber type composition. *J Anim Sci* 83:900–907.

Hamill, R., A. Aslan, T. Sweeney et al. 2009. Gene expression analysis of porcine muscle divergent in intramuscular fat content. In: *Book of Abstracts, Pig Genome III*, p. 48.

Han, S. H., I. C. Cho, J. H. Kim et al. 2009. A GHR polymorphism and its associations with carcass traits in Hanwoo cattle. *Genes Genomics* 31:35–41.

Hausman, G. J., M. V. Dodson, K. Ajuwon et al. 2009. The biology and regulation of preadipocytes and adipocytes in meat animals. *J Anim Sci* 87:1218–1246.

Hayes, B. J., P. J. Bowman, A. J. Chamberlain, and M. E. Goddard. 2009. Invited review: Genomic selection in dairy cattle: Progress and challenges. *J Dairy Sci* 92:433–443.

Hedegaard, J., H. Per, R. Lametsch et al. 2004. UDP-glucose pyrophosphorylase is upregulated in carriers of the porcine RN-mutation in the AMP-activated protein kinase. *Proteomics* 4:2448–2454.

Hertzman, C., U. Olsson, and E. Tornberg. 1993. The influence of high temperature, type of muscle and electrical stimulation on the course of rigor, ageing and tenderness of beef muscles. *Meat Sci* 35:119–141.

Hocquette, J. F., S. Lehnert, W. Barendse, I. Cassar-Malek, and B. Picard. 2007a. Recent advances in cattle functional genomics and their application to beef quality. *Animal* 1:159–173.

Hocquette, J. F., H. Leveziel, G. Renand, and A. Malafosse. 2007b. The genomics revolution and its benefits to the beef industry. *Cah Agric* 16:457–463.

Hollung, K., E. Veiseth, X. H. Jia, E. M. Faergestad, and K. I. Hildrum. 2007. Application of proteomics to understand the molecular mechanisms behind meat quality. *Meat Sci* 77:97–104.

Honikel, K. O., C. J. Kim, R. Hamm, and P. Roncales. 1986. Sarcomere shortening of prerigor muscles and its influence on drip loss. *Meat Sci* 16:267–282.

Hu, Z. L., E. R. Fritz, and J. M. Reecy. 2007. AnimalQTLdb: A livestock QTL database tool set for positional QTL information mining and beyond. *Nucleic Acids Res* 35:D604–D609.

Huff-Lonergan, E. and S. M. Lonergan. 2005. Mechanisms of water-holding capacity of meat: The role of postmortem biochemical and structural changes. *Meat Sci* 71:194–204.

Hwang, I. 2004. Proteomics approach in meat science: A model study for Hunter L* value and drip loss. *Food Sci Biotechnol* 13:208–214.

Hwang, I. H., B. Y. Park, J. H. Kim, S. H. Cho, and J. M. Lee. 2005. Assessment of postmortem proteolysis by gel-based proteome analysis and its relationship to meat quality traits in pig longissimus. *Meat Sci* 69:79–91.

Jiang, Z. P. (WA, US) and J. J. Michal (Albion, WA, US). 2009. Urotensin 2 and its receptor as candidate genes for beef marbling score, ribeye area and fatty acid composition. USPTO Patent Application 20090254388.

Jones, S. D. M., L. E. Jeremiah, and W. M. Robertson. 1993. The effects of spray and blast-chilling on carcass shrinkage and pork muscle quality. *Meat Sci* 34:351–362.

Josell, Å., L. Martinsson, C. Borggaard, J. R. Andersen, and E. Tornberg. 2000. Determination of RN-phenotype in pigs at slaughter-line using visual and near-infrared spectroscopy. *Meat Sci* 55:273–278.

Kaminski, S., M. Kocwin-Podsiadla, H. Sieczkowska et al. 2010. Screening 52 single nucleotide polymorphisms for extreme value of glycolytic potential and drip loss in pigs. *J Anim Breed Genet* 127:125–132.

Kemp, C. M., P. L. Sensky, R. G. Bardsley, P. J. Buttery, and T. Parr. 2010. Tenderness—An enzymatic view. *Meat Sci* 84:248–256.

Killinger, K. M., C. R. Calkins, W. J. Umberger, D. M. Feuz, and K. M. Eskridge. 2004. Consumer visual preference and value for beef steaks differing in marbling level and color. *J Anim Sci* 82:3288–3293.

Kim, J. M., B. D. Choi, B. C. Kim, S. S. Park, and K. C. Hong. 2009. Associations of the variation in the porcine myogenin gene with muscle fibre characteristics, lean meat production and meat quality traits. *J Anim Breed Genet* 126:134–141.

King, D. A., T. L. Wheeler, S. D. Shackelford, and M. Koohmaraie. 2009. Fresh meat texture and tenderness. In: *Improving the Sensory and Nutritional Quality of Fresh Meat*, J. P. Kerry, and D. A. Ledward (eds.), pp. 61–83. Abington, Cambridge, U.K.: Woodhead Publishing.

Koohmaraie, M. and G. H. Geesink. 2006. Contribution of postmortem muscle biochemistry to the delivery of consistent meat quality with particular focus on the calpain system. *Meat Sci* 74:34–43.

Kwasiborski, A., T. Sayd, C. Chambon et al. 2008. Pig *Longissimus lumborum* proteome: Part II: Relationships between protein content and meat quality. *Meat Sci* 80:982–996.

Lahucky, R., U. Baulain, M. Henning et al. 2002. In vitro 31P NMR studies on biopsy skeletal muscle samples compared with meat quality of normal and heterozygous malignant hyperthermia pigs. *Meat Sci* 61:233–241.

Lahucky, R., J. Mojto, J. Poltarsky et al. 1993. Evaluation of halothane sensitivity and prediction of post-mortem muscle metabolism in pigs from a muscle biopsy using 31P NMR spectroscopy. *Meat Sci* 33:373–384.

Lametsch, R., A. Karlsson, K. Rosenvold et al. 2003. Postmortem proteome changes of porcine muscle related to tenderness. *J Agric Food Chem* 51:6992–6997.

Laville, E., T. Sayd, V. Santé-Lhoutellier et al. 2005. Characterisation of PSE zones in semimembranosus pig muscle. *Meat Sci* 70:167–172.

Laville, E., T. Sayd, C. Terlouw et al. 2007. Comparison of sarcoplasmic proteomes between two groups of pig muscles selected for shear force of cooked meat. *J Agric Food Chem* 55:5834–5841.

Laville, E., T. Sayd, C. Terlouw et al. 2009. Differences in pig muscle proteome according to HAL genotype: Implications for meat quality defects. *J Agric Food Chem* 57:4913–4923.

Leheska, J. M., L. D. Thompson, J. C. Howe et al. 2008. Effects of conventional and grass-feeding systems on the nutrient composition of beef. *J Anim Sci* 86:3575–3585.

Lehnert, S. A., Y. H. Wang, and K. A. Byrne. 2004. Development and application of a bovine cDNA microarray for expression profiling of muscle and adipose tissue. *Aust J Exp Agric* 44:1127–1133.

Lewin, H. A. (IL, US), Liu, Zonglin (Peoria, IL, US), Rodriguez-zas, Sandra (IL, US), Everts, Robin E. (IL, US). 2009. Gene expression profiles that identify genetically elite cattle. United States Patent No. 7638275.

Liu, J. S., M. Damon, N. Guitton et al. 2009. Differentially-expressed genes in pig *Longissimus* muscles with contrasting levels of fat, as identified by combined transcriptomic, reverse transcription PCR, and proteomic analyses. *J Agric Food Chem* 57:3808–3817.

Lobjois, V., L. Liaubet, M. SanCristobal et al. 2008. A muscle transcriptome analysis identifies positional candidate genes for a complex trait in pig. *Anim Genet* 39:147–162.

Luan, T., J. A. Woolliams, S. Lien et al. 2009. The accuracy of genomic selection in Norwegian red cattle assessed by cross-validation. *Genetics* 183:1119–1126.

Lundberg, P., H. J. Vogel, S. Fabiansson, and H. Ruderus. 1987. Post-mortem metabolism in fresh porcine, ovine and frozen bovine muscle. *Meat Sci* 19:1–14.

Ma, J., J. Ren, Y. Guo et al. 2009. Genome-wide identification of quantitative trait loci for carcass composition and meat quality in a large-scale White Duroc x Chinese Erhualian resource population. *Anim Genet* 40:637–647.

Maltin, C., D. Balcerzak, R. Tilley, and M. Delday. 2003. Determinants of meat quality: Tenderness. *Proc Nutr Soc* 62:337–347.

Marcos, B. and A. M. Mullen. 2009. High pressure processing of beef: Correlation between meat quality and proteomic profile. In: *55th International Congress of Meat Science and Technology* (ICoMST), Copenhagen, Denmark. August 16–21, 2009.

Maurizio, B., C. Francesco, A. C. Mauro et al. 2004. Influence of the season on the relationships between NMR transverse relaxation data and water-holding capacity of turkey breast meat. *J Sci Food Agric* 84:1535–1540.

McBryan, J., R. Hamill, G. Davey, P. Lawlor, and A. Mullen. 2010. Identification of suitable reference genes for gene expression analysis of pork meat. *Meat Sci* 86:436–439.

McCarthy, J. J. and K. A. Esser. 2007. MicroRNA-1 and microRNA-133a expression are decreased during skeletal muscle hypertrophy. *J Appl Physiol* 102:306–313.

McDaneld, T. G. 2009. MicroRNA: Mechanism of gene regulation and application to livestock. *J Anim Sci* 87:E21–E28.

McDaneld, T. G., T. P. L. Smith, M. E. Doumit et al. 2009. MicroRNA transcriptome profiles during swine skeletal muscle development. *BMC Genomics* 10:77.

McIlveen, H. and J. Buchanan. 2001. The impact of sensory factors on beef purchase and consumption. *Nutr Food Sci* 31:286–292.

Meuwissen, T. H. E., B. J. Hayes, and M. E. Goddard. 2001. Prediction of total genetic value using genome-wide dense marker maps. *Genetics* 157:1819–1829.

Michal, J. J., Z. W. Zhang, C. T. Gaskins, and Z. Jiang. 2006. The bovine fatty acid binding protein 4 gene is significantly associated with marbling and subcutaneous fat depth in Wagyu x Limousin F-2 crosses. *Anim Genet* 37:400–402.

Michelson, J., E. Gallant, L. Litterer et al. 1988. Abnormal sarcoplasmic reticulum ryanodine receptor in malignant hyperthermia. *J Biol Chem* 263:9310–9315.

Milan, D., J. T. Jeon, C. Looft et al. 2000. A mutation in PRKAG3 associated with excess glycogen content in pig skeletal muscle. *Science* 288:1248–1251.

Miller, R. K. 2002. Factors affecting the quality of raw meat. In: *Meat Processing, Improving Meat Quality*, J. P. Kerry, and D. A. Ledward (eds.), pp. 27–63. Cambridge, U.K.: Woodhead Publishing Ltd.

Miller, M. F., M. A. Carr, C. B. Ramsey, K. L. Crockett, and L. C. Hoover. 2001. Consumer thresholds for establishing the value of beef tenderness. *J Anim Sci* 79:3062–3068.

Miri, A., A. Talmant, J. P. Renou, and G. Monin. 1992. 31P NMR study of post mortem changes in pig muscle. *Meat Sci* 31:165–173.

Moesgaard, B., B. Quistorff, V. G. Christensen, I. Therkelsen, and P. F. Jørgensen. 1995. Differences of post-mortem ATP turnover in skeletal muscle of normal and heterozygote malignant-hyperthermia pigs: Comparison of 31P-NMR and analytical biochemical measurements. *Meat Sci* 39:43–57.

Mohamed, A., B. Jamilah, K. A. Abbas, and R. A. Rahman. 2008. A review on some factors affecting colour of fresh beef cuts. *J Food Agric Environ* 6:181–186.

Monin, G. and D. Laborde. 1985. Water holding capacity of pig muscle proteins: Interaction between the myofibrillar proteins and sarcoplasmic compounds. *Sci Aliment* 5:341–345.

Morris, C. A., N. G. Cullen, S. M. Hickey et al. 2006. Genotypic effects of calpain 1 and calpastatin on the tenderness of cooked *M. longissimus dorsi* steaks from Jersey x Limousin, Angus and Hereford-cross cattle. *Anim Genet* 37:411–414.

Mortazavi, A., B. A. Williams, K. McCue, L. Schaeffer, and B. Wold. 2008. Mapping and quantifying mammalian transcriptomes by RNA-Seq. *Nat Methods* 5:621–628.

Morzel, M., C. Terlouw, C. Chambon, D. Micol, and B. Picard. 2008. Muscle proteome and meat eating qualities of Longissimus thoracis of "Blonde d'Aquitaine" young bulls: A central role of HSP27 isoforms. *Meat Sci* 78:297–304.

Mullen, A. M., P. C. Stapleton, D. Corcoran, R. M. Hamill, and A. White. 2006. Understanding meat quality through the application of genomic and proteomic approaches. *Meat Sci* 74:3–16.

Mullen, A. M. and D. Troy. 2005. Current and emerging technologies for the prediction of meat quality. In: *Indicators of Milk and Beef Quality*, J. F. Hocquette and S. Gigli (eds.), pp. 179–190. Wageningen, the Netherlands: Academic Publishers.

Murani, E., M. Muraniova, S. Ponsuksili, K. Schellander, and K. Wimmers. 2007. Identification of genes differentially expressed during prenatal development of skeletal muscle in two pig breeds differing in muscularity. *BMC Dev Biol* 7:109.

Nam, Y. J., Y. M. Choi, D. W. Jeong, and B. C. Kim. 2009. Comparison of postmortem meat quality and consumer sensory characteristic evaluations, according to porcine quality classification. *Food Sci Biotechnol* 18:307–311.

Ngapo, T. M., J. F. Martin, and E. Dransfield. 2007. International preferences for pork appearance: I. Consumer choices. *Food Qual Prefer* 18:26–36.

Nicholson, J. K., J. C. Lindon, and E. Holmes. 1999. 'Metabonomics': Understanding the metabolic responses of living systems to pathophysiological stimuli via multivariate statistical analysis of biological NMR spectroscopic data. *Xenobiotica* 29:1181–1189.

Noci, F., P. French, F. J. Monahan, and A. P. Moloney. 2007. The fatty acid composition of muscle fat and subcutaneous adipose tissue of grazing heifers supplemented with plant oil-enriched concentrates. *J Anim Sci* 85:1062–1073.

Offer, G. and P. Knight. 1988. Drip losses. In: *Developments in Meat Science*, R. Lawrie (ed.), pp. 173–243. London, U.K.: Elsevier.

Offer, G., P. Knight, R. Jeacocke et al. 1989. The structural basis of the water-holding, appearance and toughness of meat and meat products. *Food Microstruct* 8:151–170.

Oka, A., F. Iwaki, T. Dohgo et al. 2002. Genetic effects on fatty acid composition of carcass fat of Japanese Black Wagyu steers. *J Anim Sci* 80:1005–1011.

Ouali, A., C. H. Herrera-Mendez, G. Coulis et al. 2006. Revisiting the conversion of muscle into meat and the underlying mechanisms. *Meat Sci* 74:44–58.

Page, B. T., E. Casas, M. P. Heaton et al. 2002. Evaluation of single-nucleotide polymorphisms in CAPN1 for association with meat tenderness in cattle. *J Anim Sci* 80:3077–3085.

Page, B. T., E. Casas, R. L. Quaas et al. 2004. Association of markers in the bovine CAPN1 gene with meat tenderness in large crossbred populations that sample influential industry sires. *J Anim Sci* 82:3474–3481.

Pannier, L., R. M. Hamill, A. M. Mullen, and T. Sweeney. 2010a. Functional genomic approaches to understand the biological pathways underpinning intramuscular fat in beef. *Perspect Agric Vet Sci Nutr Nat Resour* 5:1–11.

Pannier, L., A. M. Mullen, R. M. Hamill, P. C. Stapleton, and T. Sweeney. 2010b. Association analysis of single nucleotide polymorphisms in DGAT1, TG and FABP4 genes and intramuscular fat in crossbred *Bos taurus* cattle. *Meat Sci* 85:515–518.

Pannier, L., T. Sweeney, R. M. Hamill et al. 2009. Lack of an association between single nucleotide polymorphisms in the bovine leptin gene and intramuscular fat in *Bos taurus* cattle. *Meat Sci* 81:731–737.

Pant, S. D., F. S. Schenkel, C. P. Verschoor et al. 2010. A principal component regression based genome wide analysis approach reveals the presence of a novel QTL on BTA7 for MAP resistance in holstein cattle. *Genomics* 95:176–182.

Pethick, D. W., W. Barendse, J. F. Hocquette, J. M. Thompson, and Y. H. Wang. 2007. Regulation of marbling and body composition—Growth and development, gene markers and nutritional biochemistry. In: *Energy and Protein Metabolism*. No. 124. I. Ortiques-Marty, (ed.), pp. 75–88. Wageningen, the Netherlands: Wageningen Academic Publishers.

Polkinghorne, R., J. Philpott, A. Gee, A. Doljanin, and J. Innes. 2008. Development of a commercial system to apply the Meat Standards Australia grading model to optimise the return on eating quality in a beef supply chain. *Aust J Exp Agric* 48:1451–1458.

Ponsuksili, S., E. Murani, C. Phatsara et al. 2008. Expression profiling of muscle reveals transcripts differentially expressed in muscle that affect water-holding capacity of pork. *J Agric Food Chem* 56:10311–10317.

Poso, A. R. and E. Puolanne. 2005. Carbohydrate metabolism in meat animals. *Meat Sci* 70:423–434.

Pryce, J. E., M. Haile-Mariam, K. Verbyla et al. 2010. Genetic markers for lactation persistency in primiparous Australian dairy cows. *J Dairy Sci* 93:2202–2214.

Reardon, W., A. M. Mullen, T. Sweeney, and R. M. Hamill. 2010. Association of polymorphisms in candidate genes with colour, water-holding capacity, and composition traits in bovine *M. longissimus* and *M. semimembranosus*. *Meat Sci.* doi: 10.1016/j.meatsci.2010.04.013

Renaville, R., M. Hammadi, and D. Portetelle. 2002. Role of the somatotropic axis in the mammalian metabolism. *Domest Anim Endocrinol* 23:351–360.

Renou, J.-P., G. Bielicki, C. Deponge et al. 2004. Characterization of animal products according to geographic origin and feeding diet using nuclear magnetic resonance and isotope ratio mass spectrometry. Part II: Beef meat. *Food Chem* 86:251–256.

Renou, J. P., G. Monin, and P. Sellier. 1985. Nuclear magnetic resonance measurements on pork of various qualities. *Meat Sci* 15:225–233.

Rothschild, M. F. and D. C. Ciobanu. 2003. Novel alleles characterized by polymorphism in calpastatin gene, which are useful to genetically type animals. United States Patent 7625703.

Ryu, Y. C. and B. C. Kim. 2005. The relationship between muscle fiber characteristics, postmortem metabolic rate, and meat quality of pig longissimus dorsi muscle. *Meat Sci* 71:351–357.

Scheffler, T. L. and D. E. Gerrard. 2007. Mechanisms controlling pork quality development: The biochemistry controlling postmortem energy metabolism. *Meat Sci* 77:7–16.

Schellander, K. 2007. Drip loss and water holding capacity of porcine meat. *J Anim Breed Genet* 124:1. [This is the preface page.]

Schenkel, F., S. Miller, Z. Jiang et al. 2006. Association of a single nucleotide polymorphism in the calpastatin gene with carcass and meat quality traits of beef cattle. *J Anim Sci* 84:291–299.

Schenkel, F. S., S. P. Miller, X. Ye et al. 2005. Association of single nucleotide polymorphisms in the leptin gene with carcass and meat quality traits of beef cattle. *J Anim Sci* 83:2009–2020.

Scollan, N. D., I. Richardson, S. De Smet et al. 2005. Enhancing the content of beneficial fatty acids in beef and consequences for meat quality. In: *Indicators of Milk and Beef Quality*, J. F. Hocquette and S. Gigli (eds.), pp. 151–162. Wageningen, the Netherlands: Academic Publishers.

Settles, M., R. Zanella, S. D. McKay et al. 2009. A whole genome association analysis identifies loci associated with Mycobacterium avium subsp paratuberculosis infection status in US holstein cattle. *Anim Genet* 40:655–662.

Shendure, J. 2008. The beginning of the end for microarrays? *Nat Methods* 5:585–587.

Shintu, L., S. Caldarelli, and B. M. Franke. 2007. Pre-selection of potential molecular markers for the geographic origin of dried beef by HR-MAS NMR spectroscopy. *Meat Sci* 76:700–707.

Sieczkowska, H., M. Kocwin-Podsiadla, A. Zybert et al. 2010. The association between polymorphism of PKM2 gene and glycolytic potential and pork meat quality. *Meat Sci* 84:180–185.

Simm, G., N. Lambe, L. Buenger, E. Navajas, and R. Roehe. 2009. Use of meat quality information in breeding programmes. In: *Improving the Sensory and Nutritional Quality of Fresh Meat*, J. Kerry and D. A. Ledward (eds.), pp. 264–291. Cambridge, U.K.: Woodhead Publishing Ltd.

Sinclair, K. D., G. E. Lobley, G. W. Horgan et al. 2001. Factors influencing beef eating quality—1. Effects of nutritional regimen and genotype on organoleptic properties and instrumental texture. *Anim Sci* 72:269–277.

Skrlep, M., M. Candek-Potokar, T. Kavar et al. 2010. Association of PRKAG3 and CAST genetic polymorphisms with traits of interest in dry-cured ham production: Comparative study in France, Slovenia and Spain. *Livest Sci* 128:60–66.

Snelling, W. M., M. F. Allan, J. W. Keele et al. 2010. Genome-wide association study of growth in crossbred beef cattle. *J Anim Sci* 88:837–848.

Sorheim, O., J. Idland, E. C. Halvorsen et al. 2001. Influence of beef carcass stretching and chilling rate on tenderness of *m. longissimus dorsi. Meat Sci* 57:79–85.

Stoop, W. M., A. Schennink, M. Visker et al. 2009. Genome-wide scan for bovine milk-fat composition. I. Quantitative trait loci for short- and medium-chain fatty acids. *J Dairy Sci* 92:4664–4675.

Straadt, I. K., M. Rasmussen, H. J. Andersen, and H. C. Bertram. 2007. Aging-induced changes in microstructure and water distribution in fresh and cooked pork in relation to water-holding capacity and cooking loss—A combined confocal laser scanning microscopy (CLSM) and low-field nuclear magnetic resonance relaxation study. *Meat Sci* 75:687–695.

Suzuki, K., K. Inomata, K. Katoh, H. Kadowaki, and T. Shibata. 2009. Genetic correlations among carcass cross-sectional fat area ratios, production traits, intramuscular fat, and serum leptin concentration in Duroc pigs. *J Anim Sci* 87:2209–2215.

Sybesma, W. and G. Eikelenboom. 1969. Malignant hyperthermia syndrome in pigs. *Neth J Vet Sci* 2:155–160.

Taniguchi, M., T. Utsugi, K. Oyama et al. 2004. Genotype of stearoyl-CoA desaturase is associated with fatty acid composition in Japanese Black cattle. *Mamm Genome* 15:142–148.

Tatsuda, K., A. Oka, E. Iwamoto et al. 2008. Relationship of the bovine growth hormone gene to carcass traits in Japanese black cattle. *J Anim Breed Genet* 125:45–49.

Terentyev, D., A. E. Belevych, R. Terentyeva et al. 2009. miR-1 overexpression enhances Ca2+ release and promotes cardiac arrhythmogenesis by targeting PP2A regulatory subunit B56 alpha and causing CaMKII-dependent hyperphosphorylation of RyR2. *Circ Res* 104:514–521.

Thaller, G., C. Kuhn, A. Winter et al. 2003. DGAT1, a new positional and functional candidate gene fopr intramuscular fat deposition in cattle. *Anim Genet* 34:354–357.

Thompson, J. M., D. Perry, B. Daly et al. 2006. Genetic and environmental effects on the muscle structure response post-mortem. *Meat Sci* 74:59–65.

van de Wiel, D. F. M., X. Zeng, and W. L. Zhang. 2006. Proteomics for improved meat quality. In: *Forum of Scholars from Home & Abroad*, on the occasion of the Centenary, China.

van de Wiel, D. F. M. and W. L. Zhang. 2007. Identification of pork quality parameters by proteomics. *Meat Sci* 77:46–54.

van der Steen, H., G. Prall, and G. Plastow. 2005. Application of genomics to the pork industry. *J Anim Sci* 83(e-supplement):E1–E8.

van der Wal, P. G., B. Engel, G. van Beek, and C. H. Veerkamp. 1995. Chilling pig carcasses: Effects on temperature, weight loss and ultimate meat quality. *Meat Sci* 40:193–202.

Van Eenennaam, A. L., J. Li, R. M. Thallman et al. 2007. Validation of commercial DNA tests for quantitative beef quality traits. *J Anim Sci* 85:891–900.

Van Tassell, C. P., T. P. L. Smith, L. K. Matukumalli et al. 2008. SNP discovery and allele frequency estimation by deep sequencing of reduced representation libraries. *Nat Methods* 5:247–252.

VanRaden, P. M., C. P. Van Tassell, G. R. Wiggans et al. 2009. Invited review: Reliability of genomic predictions for North American Holstein bulls. *J Dairy Sci* 92:16–24.

Verbeke, W., F. J. A. Perez-Cueto, M. D. de Barcellos, A. Krystallis, and K. G. Grunert. 2009. European citizen and consumer attitudes and preferences regarding beef and pork. *Meat Sci* 84:284–292.

Vogel, H. J., P. Lundberg, S. Fabiansson et al. 1985. Post-mortem energy metabolism in bovine muscles studied by non-invasive phosphorus-31 nuclear magnetic resonance. *Meat Sci* 13:1–18.

Wang, Y. H., N. I. Bower, A. Reverter et al. 2009a. Gene expression patterns during intramuscular fat development in cattle. *J Anim Sci* 87:119–130.

Wang, Z., M. Gerstein, and M. Snyder. 2009b. RNA-Seq: A revolutionary tool for transcriptomics. *Nat Rev Genet* 10:57–63.

Wang, Z., M. Sargolzaei, D. Kolbehdari et al. 2009c. Whole genome association analysis for mapping QTL affecting economically important trais in North American Holstein cattle. *Can J Anim Sci* 89:126.

Watkins, P. J., G. Rose, L. Salvatore et al. 2010. Age and nutrition influence the concentrations of three branched chain fatty acids in sheep fat from Australian abattoirs. *Meat Sci* 86:594–599.

Watson, R., R. Polkinghorne, and J. M. Thompson. 2008. Development of the Meat Standards Australia (MSA) prediction model for beef palatability. *Aust J Exp Agric* 48:1368–1379.

Wheeler, T. L., L. V. Cundiff, S. D. Shackelford, and M. Koohmaraie. 2004. Characterization of biological types of cattle (Cycle VI): Carcass, yield, and *longissimus* palatability traits. *J Anim Sci* 82:1177–1189.

White, S., E. Casas, T. L. Wheeler et al. 2005. A new single nucleotide polymorphism in CAPN1 extends the current tenderness marker test to include cattle of *Bos indicus*, *Bos taurus* and crossbred descent. *J Anim Sci* 83:2001–2008.

Wibowo, T., C. Gaskins, R. Newberry et al. 2008. Genome assembly anchored QTL map of bovine chromosome 14. *Int J Biol Sci* 4:406–414.

Wiggans, G. R., T. S. Sonstegard, P. M. Vanraden et al. 2009. Selection of single-nucleotide polymorphisms and quality of genotypes used in genomic evaluation of dairy cattle in the United States and Canada. *J Dairy Sci* 92:3431–3436.

Wilhelm, B. T. and J.-R. Landry. 2009. RNA-Seq-quantitative measurement of expression through massively parallel RNA-sequencing. *Methods* 48:249–257.

Wilkins, M. R., C. Pasquali, R. D. Appel et al. 1996. From proteins to proteomes: Large scale protein identification by two-dimensional electrophoresis and amino acid analysis. *Biotechnology* 14:61–66.

Wimmers, K., E. Murani, M. Pas et al. 2007. Associations of functional candidate genes derived from gene-expression profiles of prenatal porcine muscle tissue with meat quality and muscle deposition. *Anim Genet* 38:474–484.

Wimmers, K., N. T. Ngu, D. G. J. Jennen et al. 2008. Relationship between myosin heavy chain isoform expression and muscling in several diverse pig breeds. *J Anim Sci* 86:795–803.

Wind, R. A. and J. Z. Hu. 2006. In vivo and ex vivo high-resolution $^1$H NMR in biological systems using low-speed magic angle spinning. *Prog Nucl Magn Reson Spectrosc* 49:207–259.

Wood, J. D., M. Enser, A. V. Fisher et al. 2008. Fat deposition, fatty acid composition and meat quality: A review. *Meat Sci* 78:343–358.

Yang, A., T. Larson, S. Smith, and R. Tume. 1999. Δ9 desaturase activity in bovine subcutaneous adipose tissue of different fatty acid composition. *Lipids* 34:971–978.

Yang, H., Z. Y. Xu, M. G. Lei et al. 2010. Association of 3 polymorphisms in porcine troponin I genes (TNNI1 and TNNI2) with meat quality traits. *J Appl Genet* 51:51–57.

Young, J. F., H. C. Bertram, K. Rosenvold, G. Lindahl, and N. Oksbjerg. 2005. Dietary creatine monohydrate affects quality attributes of Duroc but not Landrace pork. *Meat Sci* 70:717–725.

Yu, J., S. Tang, E. Bao et al. 2009. The effect of transportation on the expression of heat shock proteins and meat quality of *M. longissimus dorsi* in pigs. *Meat Sci* 83:474–478.

Zapata, I., H. N. Zerby, and M. Wick. 2009. Functional proteomic analysis predicts beef tenderness and the tenderness differential. *J Agric Food Chem* 57:4956–4963.

Zhang, S., T. J. Knight, J. M. Reecy, and D. C. Beitz. 2008. DNA polymorphisms in bovine fatty acid synthase are associated with beef fatty acid composition. *Anim Genet* 39:62–70.

# 12 Functional Genomics to Improve Meat Quality in Pigs

*Roberta Davoli, Paolo Zambonelli,*
*and Silvia Braglia*

## CONTENTS

## 12.1   INTRODUCTION

For the meat industry, one of the major goals is to focus on breeding and selection of animals to produce meat of high quality. The most significant change in biological science during the last decades has been the development of "genomics." Since the 1990s, genomic studies in livestock have stressed on the identification of quantitative trait loci (QTL) and candidate genes and their application for selective breeding, gene mapping, and association studies (Andersson et al. 1994, Haley and Visscher 1998, Rothschild and Plastow 2008, Rothschild et al. 2007). These approaches allowed to successfully identify a number of genes that have a great importance in meat production: for instance, insulin-like growth factor 2 (*IGF2*), melanocortin 4 receptor (*MC4R*), ryanodine receptor 1 (*RYR1*), and protein kinase, AMP-activated, gamma 3 noncatalytic subunit (*PRKAG3*). These genes can affect meat production and meat quality traits in pigs. Briefly, the p.Arg615Cys mutation in *RYR1* results in pale, soft, and exudative meat (Fujii et al. 1991) and the p.Arg200Gln substitution of *PRKAG3* is responsible for acid meat in Hampshire and Hampshire-synthetic lines (Milan et al. 2000); the p.Asp298Asn mutation in *MC4R* has been associated with fatter, higher-feed consuming, and faster-growing animals (Kim et al. 2000); and the intron 3 mutation g.3072G > A in *IGF2* increases muscle mass and reduces backfat thickness (Van Laere et al. 2003).

Approaches to large-scale gene polymorphism analysis and expression evaluation made it possible to combine information coming from genome sequences or cDNA libraries with powerful recent chip technologies to integrate analysis of gene characteristics and expression. Thanks to these techniques, it was possible to develop data bank containing a large amount of molecular information related to the biological function of several gene networks or to discover new key genes involved in a specific physiological function. Combined with classical physiology using modeling tools, genome-wide approaches are expected to advance our knowledge of cell biology and in particular for meat production and muscle cell biology. One of the main challenges of postgenomics era is the possibility to mine the huge amount of the farm animals' DNA data already available to find the genetic basis of the phenotypic differences in multifactorial trait–identifying markers that will be used to genetically improve the reared breeds.

## 12.2   WHAT IS GENOMICS?

Genomics is the study of an organism's entire genome. The genome includes both genes and DNA sequences presently classified as non-coding. Whereas the term "genome" appeared in the literature in 1920–1930, the term "genomics" only appeared in the 1980s and took off in the 1990s with the initiation and development of genome projects in different species. The advent of genome-wide techniques was realized quite recently thanks to the development of high-throughput techniques allowing the study of the genome of organisms as a whole.

Genomics can be divided into functional genomics, structural genomics, and comparative genomics.

Structural genomics studies the genome sequence and its variations. From the beginning of DNA sequencing (at the end of the 1970s), the amount of nucleotide sequences in the databases has increased logarithmically (source GenBank database http://www.ncbi.nlm.nih.gov/genbank/genbankstats.html, release note 180, October 15, 2010.) due to different technical innovations. Moreover, on a per-nucleotide basis, sequencing fees also has been impressively lowered from 1986 to date (Robert 2008).

The lowering of the sequencing price and the improvement of sequencing techniques allowed to strongly improve data production and more than 1100 complete genomes have been sequenced so far (http://genomesonline.org/gold_statistics.htm; Liolios et al. 2010). The rate-limiting steps are likely nowadays to be connected with necessity to constantly develop powerful new bioinformatics tools able to manage the huge amount of data coming from sequencing projects (Hutchison 2007). Up to now many projects (http://www.genomesonline.org/) aimed at completely sequencing genomes of some animals have been undertaken: over 90% of mouse genome is available (http://genome.wustl.edu/projects/mouse/index.php), chicken sequence was available since 2004 (Burt 2006, http://www.ensembl.org/Gallus_gallus/Info/Index, International Chicken Genome Sequencing Consortium 2004), and bovine complete genome was recently published (Elsik et al. 2009, Gibbs et al. 2009, Liu et al. 2009). As for the pig, the paper on complete porcine genomic sequence is in preparation by the Wellcome Trust Sanger Institute that coordinates an international consortium (http://www.piggenome.org/) working on deciphering the sequence of the pig chromosomes http://www.animalgenome.org/pigs/community/WhitePaper/2010.pdf).

Thanks to the possibility of applying functional genomics approaches, scientists have the opportunity to analyze interactions between genes (and between their products) at the genome level, and therefore to understand the interactions between the various systems of a cell on a large-scale basis, including the interrelationship of its DNA, RNA, and synthesized proteins as well as metabolites, and to learn how these interactions are regulated.

Comparative genomics analyses the differences between different organisms. This aspect is of fundamental importance as rich sources of genome information from human (or mouse) could be helpful in annotating livestock genomes, to improve livestock maps and to identify new genes. On the other hand, identifying functional sequences in livestock genomes helps in predicting genes and regulatory elements in biological pathways in human and other species.

## 12.3   FUNCTIONAL GENOMICS: FROM DNA TO RNA

Functional genomics refers to the analysis that uses global approaches to understand the functions of genes and proteins. The goal of functional genomics is to identify pathways and gene networks underlying the genetic control of phenotypes under study with the final aim to identify the candidate genes. A fundamental prerequisite of these studies is the knowledge of the genes expressed in specific tissues. For the researches aimed at identifying the mechanisms determining meat quality, the knowledge of the expression level of the genes in skeletal muscle and adipose tissues is of primary importance. This knowledge will supply fundamental tools to explore the molecular mechanisms regulating pork quality and will be useful to improve meat production.

In biology, it had been proposed a well-known "dogma": genes are encoded in DNA, the DNA is copied into RNA, and the RNA molecules are used to synthesize proteins. In general, a gene is the stretch of DNA, including regulatory elements, that specifies a protein. Nowadays this dogma has been widely revised by a deeper knowledge of some events like alternative splicing (AS) and/or epigenetics.

Functional genomics seeks to contribute to the elucidation of some fundamental questions about how the exact sequence of DNA differs between individuals or how proteins interact to perform the pathways required for life or how differential gene expression results in different types of cells and tissues in a multicellular organism (Fields et al. 1999).

After the sequencing of a great number of genomes, genomics is thus now shifting to the study of gene expression and function. RNA is the core of biological complexity that cannot be explained only by the analysis of DNA sequence alone. Functional genomics allows the detection of genes that are turned on or off at any given time and in any physiological or nutritional situation.

Although the genetic information, the genome, is the same in every cell, the mRNA and protein content vary between cells. The number of genes expressed in a cell depends, in part, on both the environmental and developmental conditions. In general, only a fraction of the genes are expressed (transcribed) at a certain time in any cell type or tissue. Thus, gene expression studies detect the abundance of certain messenger RNA (mRNA) molecules produced in a cell or a collection of cells at a specific time or in specific circumstances.

Transcriptomics is the study of the transcriptome, which means the complete set of RNA transcripts produced by the genome at any time. Similarly, proteomics is the large-scale study of proteins, in particular their structures and functions. In addition, functional genomics focuses on the dynamic aspects such as gene transcription and translation and also on the molecular mechanisms regulated by noncoding sequences.

In addition to sequencing, epigenomics promises novel insights into the genome because of its potential to detect quantitative alterations, multiplex modifications, and regulatory sequences outside of genes. Epigenomics is thus the study of factors surrounding DNA that affect gene expression. In this context, epigenetics may aid in identification and detecting the function of DNA regulatory sequences within the mammalian genome.

Several genome-wide studies have also demonstrated that DNA polymorphisms influence gene expression at the mRNA level. Loci influencing transcripts levels have been termed "eQTL" for QTL (Quantitative Trait Laci) of expression. The combination of association analyses and expression profiling is called "genetical genomics." The merging of these two terms into a single definition indicates the importance of both structural and functional analyses to decipher the molecular mechanisms that regulate the phenotypic expression of polygenic traits.

In the last 25 years, techniques for evaluating gene expression have progressed from methods developed for the analysis of single specific genes (northern, slot and dot blotting, semiquantitative polymerase chain reaction, PCR) to those focused on identifying a range of genes that differ in expression between experimental samples. Broad spectrum approaches to identify differences in gene expression (described later on) include suppression subtractive hybridization (SSH), differential display (DD), sequence analysis, gene expression, and microarray hybridization. One of the useful aspects of these techniques is that they may be applied without need of any prior knowledge of genomic information on the living organism being studied. At the beginning of the application of these techniques as there was a lack of information on genomics of livestock species, it was useful to have the possibility to use genomic approaches without previous information on genes and genomes.

With the development of high-throughput sequencing techniques, many projects were set up to develop expressed sequence tag (EST) libraries in plant but also in animal field (Burt and White 2007, Colecchia et al. 2009, Couture et al. 2009, Grosse et al. 2000, Hu et al. 2005, Kim et al. 2006b, Lee et al. 2009, Liang and Pardee 2001, Moody 2001, Uenishi et al. 2004, 2007). These libraries were produced picking up clones from cDNA libraries and generating a single sequence per clone. Differences of gene expression were estimated counting how many times a sequence occurred in EST libraries from different sources.

Several gene expression surveys from human and mouse studies have demonstrated important applications of gene expression analyses obtained from different organs and tissues (Saito-Hisaminato et al. 2002, Shyamsundar et al. 2005, Su et al. 2004, Zhang et al. 2004). Compendiums of gene expression, such as human gene expression (HuGE) index (Haverty et al. 2002, Hsiao et al. 2001), gene normal tissue expression (GeneNote, updated version October 2008; Shmueli et al. 2003), and SymAtlas (Su et al. 2004), have also been created as early publicly available web resources derived from extensive gene expression surveys. Finally, the availability of such a large amount of data in human and mice have been used to predict functions of previously uncharacterized genes, that is, by comparing the expression pattern of genes with unknown functions with those of already characterized ones. Much of the data obtained in such species could be applied to livestock studies to help in understanding farm animals RNA expression profiles of farm animals in order to improve knowledge of livestock species (e.g., increased livestock productivity, meat and milk quality, prevention of diseases) as it will be described later on, in Section 12.5.

The way followed by biologists to study gene expression and cell biology is fast changing. Messenger RNA is revealing a high level of complexity and different kinds of small RNA molecules playing an important role in the control of gene expression and cellular function began to be discovered with the most recent genomic technologies.

### 12.3.1 MicroRNA

In 1993, the first small noncoding RNA (ncRNA) was discovered in nematode (Lee et al. 1993) and this discovery provided the first example of a novel regulatory mechanism that is mediated by small, ncRNAs.

These ncRNAs, termed microRNA (miRNA), comprise a class of small RNAs (18–26 nucleotides long), the majority of which are found either in the introns of protein coding genes or in intergenic regions where they are under the control of their own promoters (reviewed in Ying and Lin 2009).

Hundreds of miRNAs have been found to be encoded in most eukaryotic genomes, and it is likely that many miRNAs are yet to be discovered. miRNAs regulate many biological processes, such as cell proliferation and differentiation, and are particularly important in gene regulation during development (reviewed in Carthew and Sontheimer 2009). In livestock in particular, these small RNAs act as regulatory factors affecting development and growth of tissues such as skeletal muscle and adipose tissue. This technology could find application in improvement of pig genetics through the identification of genomic variation controlling an economically important phenotypes. MicroRNAs were initially reported to have a role in skeletal muscle development utilizing mouse, *Drosophila*, and zebrafish models. Three muscle-specific miRNAs (miR-1, miR-133, and miR-206) that undergo an increase during muscle cell differentiation and at the same time modulate skeletal muscle cell differentiation and proliferation were identified (Brennecke et al. 2005, Chen et al. 2006b, Nguyen and Frasch 2006). Furthermore, miRNA have been reported to regulate different stages of myogenesis (Anderson et al. 2006, McCarthy and Esser 2007, Nakajima et al. 2006), and muscle-specific miRNA were reported to regulate genes that directly affect economic traits in livestock (Clop et al. 2006).

Most miRNAs are expressed in a spatiotemporal manner, suggesting that they have very specific functions even if their role in biological processes has not been yet fully described (McDaneld 2009). Comparative analysis of miRNA sequences indicates that they are highly conserved among species as diverse as nematodes and mammals supporting the hypothesis that they are of central importance to biology and developmental processes (reviewed in McDaneld 2009). Many progresses in understanding miRNA biogenesis have been made, nevertheless the posttranscriptional regulation mechanism remains unclear, and the role of specific miRNA in biological functions is just now becoming established. MicroRNA genes are predominately located in intergenic regions, but they have also been identified in introns (reviewed in Brown et al. 2008) and exons of protein-coding genes (Saini et al. 2007). Their transcription is differentially regulated among tissues in all analyzed species (McDaneld 2009) by multiple mechanisms including transcriptional factors (Liu et al. 2007) and other miRNA (Tuccoli et al. 2006). For example, muscle-specific transcription factors, myocyte-enhancing factor-2, and myoblast-determining protein have been identified as activators of muscle-specific miRNA transcription through an intragenic enhancer (Liu et al. 2007).

miRNA biogenesis is an almost completely known and well-described process. Briefly, biogenesis of functional miRNA sequences begins in the nucleus with transcription of the miRNA gene by RNA polymerase II, generating the long primary miRNA that contains the mature miRNA as an RNA hairpin. Once transcribed, the primary miRNA is cleaved by Drosha, an endonuclease, to create an approximately 70-bp precursor miRNA. The precursor miRNA is then exported to the cytoplasm by exportin-5 for further processing by a second endonuclease, Dicer. This second step excises the miRNA:miRNA-complementary strand duplex by cutting near the hairpin loop. This duplex contains the miRNA strand identified by the RNA-induced silencing complex (RISC) and the miRNA complementary strand that is generally degraded (for a review, see Liu et al. 2010, McDaneld 2009).

MicroRNAs regulate gene expression through the recognition of the respective miRNA target sites. The majority of miRNA target sites lie within the 3'UTR of the mRNA of the targeted gene. There are three main regulations of mRNA: degradation of the mRNA sequence, block of initiation of protein translation, translocation of processing bodies (for a review, see McDaneld 2009).

Repression of translation via miRNA is a result of deadenylation of the poly-A tail and subsequent decapping of the mRNA sequence. As a result, the mRNA sequence becomes unstable and is susceptible to degradation, resulting in decreased mRNA abundance and subsequent decrease in translation. An alternative mechanism of posttranscriptional control by miRNA began to emerge as research revealed that mRNA abundance did not always decrease with gene translation, suggesting that miRNA regulate translation through multiple mechanisms (McDaneld 2009). A third proposed mechanism of miRNA action involves posttranscriptional regulation by translocation of the miRNA:mRNA complex to cytoplasmic foci in the cell, known as processing bodies (P-bodies), after the miRNA:RISC complex binds the mRNA target.

Despite extensive effort in cataloguing miRNAs, novel miRNAs continue to be discovered, showing that the current list of miRNAs is incomplete and more miRNAs remain to be revealed. Novel miRNAs are most often identified using either homology searching of known miRNAs in other species or small RNA library sequencing or a combination of both. In vertebrates, miRNAs have been extensively studied in the mouse and human, but less so in other species, as reflected by the number of miRNAs identified in each species present in the official miRNA database, miRBase (Release 18, November 2010; http://www.mirbase.org/; Kozomara and Griffiths-Jones 2010): this database counts 18,226 entries expressing 21,643 mature miRNA products, in 168 species. Currently the number of annotated porcine miRNAs is relatively small. This is because the pig genome assembly is not yet complete, which impedes both bioinformatics prediction and experimental verification of miRNAs. Nevertheless, recently several studies have been developed in different pig tissues to improve this number (Cho et al. 2010, Zhou et al. 2010, Zhou and Liu 2010), providing useful information for further investigation of miRNA biological functions associated with growth and development of skeletal muscle or adipose tissue in the pig.

## 12.3.2 ALTERNATIVE SPLICING

Alternative splicing is a cellular mechanism in eukaryotes first described at the beginning of the 1980s (Alt et al. 1980) that greatly increases the diversity of gene products: a very surprising example reported in the cited paper is the *Drosophila melanogaster* gene *Down syndrome cell adhesion molecule* (*Dscam*), which can generate 38,016 distinct mRNA isoforms starting from 95 exons. Basically, there are different ways that a gene can be alternatively spliced (Liang Zhang et al. 2007, McKeown 1992).

For a particular gene, more than one AS possibility may apply simultaneously, and the combination gives birth to tremendous variations of gene products. About 95% of human genes are estimated to have two or more AS products (Li et al. 2008a). Different AS forms have been associated with different physiological conditions and biological phenotypes (Norris and Whan 2008), and such kind of regulation can be tissue specific or determined by development signals (Sánchez 2008).

Splicing of pre-mRNAs occurs in a two-step reaction. In the first step, the message is cleaved at the 5' end of an intron, and this 5' end is linked to the branch point, which is typically in close proximity upstream of the 3' end of the intron. In the second step, the mRNA intermediate is cleaved at the 3' splice site, exons are ligated, and the intron lariat is released. This important task is executed in the nucleus by the spliceosome, a large ribonucleoprotein (RNP) complex that involves five small nuclear RNAs and potentially hundreds of proteins, the core components of which are highly conserved across metazoan genomes (Black 2003).

As alternative splicing is a process leading to complex aspect of gene expression, experimental and computational large-scale studies have started to illuminate the extent, structure, and regulatory consequences of AS and its differential usages in mammalian genomes (Hu et al. 2010, Mollet et al. 2010, Phang 2009, Turro et al. 2010). The principal computational approach to identifying AS genes, and to infer individual alternative exon events or complete alternative isoform structures, relies on the comparison of available transcript data to assembled genomes and known gene loci. To date, some databases have been generated (Sinha et al. 2010, Takeda et al. 2010) to collect the huge amount of information coming from AS complexity.

## 12.4    METHODS AND NEW TECHNOLOGIES TO ANALYZE TRANSCRIPTOME AND RNA COMPLEXITY

Understanding the relationship between DNA sequence variation, transcript abundance variability, and phenotypic variation for quantitative or complex traits will yield important insights for the prediction of productive aptitude of an animal to obtain high-quality productions (meat, milk, eggs) and for increasing the efficiency of breeding programs in selected populations. The process of detecting and localizing quantitative trait nucleotides (QTNs) of the causative genes will be possible through intermediate steps, taking into account not only the knowledge of DNA sequence variation and its association with variation in phenotypes but also the molecular phenotypes such as transcript abundance that can be considered like an intermediate trait in the chain of causation from gene variation to phenotypic variation. Genetical genomics or systems genetics approaches integrate DNA sequence variation, variation in transcript abundance and variation in phenotypes allowing to interpret quantitative genetic variation in terms of biologically meaningful causal networks of correlated transcripts (Jansen and Nap 2001). These approaches have been allowed by the development of new transcriptional profiling methods to define the correlations between gene expression and phenotypes. Next-generation sequence technologies are bringing this opportunity closer to reality (Mackay et al. 2009, Wang et al. 2009).

## 12.4.1 TRANSCRIPTOMICS AND RNA COMPLEXITY

Gene expression is a "quantitative trait" finely regulated by numerous proteins that modulate in its turn the RNA content and its spatial–temporal expression to ensure that the correct complement of RNA and proteins is present in the right cell at the correct time. The "omic" science that considers and analyses gene expression on a genome-wide level is called transcriptomics. Transcriptome is the complete set of transcripts in a cell, and their quantity, for a specific developmental stage of physiological condition (Jacquier 2009). Understanding the transcriptome is essential for interpreting the functional elements of the genome and revealing the molecular constituents of cells and tissues and also for understanding developmental and genetic factors responsible for modified performance level of an animal.

Until recently, the description of a transcriptome was essentially limited to the characterization of the transcription products of known annotated genes. These products were mainly mRNAs and known stable non-coding RNAs (ncRNAs), such as transfer RNAs (tRNAs) and small nucleolar RNAs (snoRNAs). The identification and quantification of mRNA species under different conditions or in different cell types have long been of interest to biologists. Unexpected levels of RNA complexity began to emerge, firstly with the discovery of interfering RNAs, such as small interfering RNAs (siRNAs) and microRNAs (Jacquier 2009). Methodological advances, including bioinformatics, microarray-based, biochemical and deep-sequencing studies, are producing new insights into the roles that the regulation of RNA complexity has. In consideration of these recently described functional features of the animal genomes, trancriptomics has new key aims concerning the characterization of all species of transcripts, including mRNAs, ncRNAs, and small RNAs; the definition of the transcriptional structure of genes, in terms of their start sites, 5' and 3' ends, splicing patterns, and other posttranscriptional modifications and the quantification and the variation of expression levels for each transcript during growth and development and under different conditions (Zhao et al. 2009).

## 12.4.2 METHODS AND TECHNOLOGIES FOR TRANSCRIPT PROFILING

### 12.4.2.1 Suppression Subtractive Hybridization and Differential Display

Suppression subtractive hybridisation (SSH) or subtractive hybridization (Diatchenko et al. 1996) is a technique used in animal genetics to analyze cDNA to determine the difference between two genomes, that is, two samples are otherwise identical except for a differentially transcribed region. These difference can be detected using this technique that relies on the removal of dsDNA formed by hybridization between a control and test sample, thus eliminating cDNAs or gDNAs of similar abundance and retaining differentially expressed, or variable in sequence, transcripts or genomic sequences.

Another technology, differential display (DD) (Liang and Pardee 1992, 2001) has been used in the past few years in animal genetics to identify differentially expressed genes allowing to compare simultaneously multiple samples and to identify changes in gene expression between and within individuals. The assumption at the basis of the DD method is the use of a limited number of short arbitrary primers in combination with the anchored oligo-dT primers to systematically amplify and visualize most of the mRNA in a cell. Since its invention in the early 1990s, DD has been used by different research groups to detect differentially expressed genes at the mRNA level.

One of the major disadvantages of both these techniques is the fact that SSH and DD are not fully quantitative and especially DD may produce a high rate of false-positive and PCR-associated errors; for this reason, they are almost given up.

### 12.4.2.2 SAGE

Various technologies have been developed to deduce and quantify the transcriptome and different approaches to high-throughput gene expression profiling have been considered in the past decade to allow the simultaneous interrogation of gene expression levels on a genome-wide scale. Serial Analysis of Gene Expression (SAGE) is the first sequencing-based technique developed by Velculescu et al. (1995) to estimate transcript abundance and the relative amounts of expressed sequences in the genome of interest. This approach was applied to analyze transcriptomes by sequencing of cDNA fragments followed by counting the number of times a particular fragment has been observed. In SAGE, restriction enzymes are used to obtain short sequence fragments (tags) of 10–20 bp, usually derived from the 3′end of an mRNA; the tags are concatenated and sequenced to determine the expression profiles of their corresponding mRNAs. These tags can be mapped back to known cDNA sequence and the resulting data is analyzed for relative abundance (Tuggle et al. 2007). This early technique revealed some unexpected disadvantages because a large proportion of transcripts did not correspond to protein-coding genes that did not match with any annotated feature in the genome of reference. As at the time of the technique, setting up deep sequencing of the tags was not an available technology, no specific pattern could be recognized for these putative transcripts, and it was not clear whether they represented random transcriptional noise or some degree of experimental noise.

### 12.4.2.3 Microarrays

Systematic effort to analyze RNA and RNA changes began with an approach represented by a group of methods based on microarray in which cDNA is hybridized to an array of complementary oligonucleotide probes corresponding to genes of interest, and the abundance of a particular mRNA species is estimated from its hybridization intensity to the relevant probe (Ness 2007, Schena et al. 1995). Array technology has facilitated the development of rapid and comprehensive approaches to characterizing genomes and has enabled whole-genome gene expression studies of tens of thousands of genes across a single sample. DNA microarrays are a collection of DNA probes that are arrayed on a solid support and are used to assay, through hybridization, the presence of complementary DNA that is present in a sample. DNA microarrays are made either by chemically synthesizing DNA probes on a solid surface or by attaching premade DNA probes to a solid surface. A variety of microarray-based platforms (custom-made microarrays or commercial high-density oligo microarrays) and techniques have been developed in recent years to elucidate RNA complexity and to analyze splice variants (Wang et al. 2009). Moreover the availability of high-density microarrays has facilitated the development of rapid and comprehensive approaches to characterizing genomes. Since their development little more than a decade ago, DNA microarrays have provided scientists with the capacity to simultaneously investigate thousands of genes in a single experiment. A distinction is between microarrays that provide truly comprehensive coverage of the genome (whole genome) and those that provide partial coverage across the genome (genome scale). The microarray technology is broadly adopted also in animal science generating relevant advances of knowledge in this field and creating entirely new themes of research: microarrays forever changed the way in which high-throughput tissue gene expression profiling is done. Microarray studies have been applied in many species to obtain a better knowledge and to understand the changes in gene expression, that is, during muscle growth and development in farm animals, and the pig is no exception (Tuggle et al. 2007). In this specie, different platforms for porcine expression profiling have been used and annotations of DNA elements on the array are an important and growing area of research. Specialized microarrays have also been designed and genome tiling microarrays have been constructed to obtain the mapping of transcribed regions to a very high resolution (Wang et al. 2009). As an example, in tiling arrays technology, cDNA probes are hybridized to DNA microarrays that carry overlapping oligonucleotides that cover the complete genome or a fraction of a genome conferring resolution from several base pairs to 100 bp. In these arrays, the DNA probes are chosen from contiguous stretches of the genome (Gresham et al. 2008). Additional specialized microarrays have been utilized mainly in humans more than in animals, for example, exon-junction microarrays used to interrogate RNA populations from different tissues led to the recognition that a large number of multi-exon genes are alternatively spliced or microarrays used to identify tissue-restricted patterns of alternative mRNA expression provided insights into their regulation by specific RNA-binding proteins.

Microarray studies produce data that are usually submitted to validation and confirmation by real-time quantitative PCR (q-PCR) technique that can also be used to measure gene expression independently of microarray confirmation. q-PCR is traditionally not viewed as a high-throughput screening tool due to the lack of large sets of specific assays available for some species like pig transcripts as well as the relatively high cost per gene and biological sample assayed. Many reports of q-PCR have been produced to measure the abundance of porcine transcripts and many groups have used a significant number of q-PCR assays to validate results from microarrays or different transcript-profiling methods (Tuggle et al. 2007).

The ability to quantitatively survey the global behavior of transcriptomes has been a key milestone in the field of systems biology, enabled by the advent of DNA microarray. Key applications of microarrays have included transcriptome analysis, profiling of protein–DNA interactions, and characterization of both small-scale (SNP) and large-scale (i.e., Copy Number Variation, CNV) genetic variation (Shendure 2008). Microarray technology analysing large-scale data sets provided opportunities to link molecular profiling of animal genomes (in normal physiological conditions or determined by specific treatments or breeding systems) with the metabolic and biochemical patterns of animals, producing a relevent scientific and cultural impact. Although this approach has literally transformed our vision and approach to cellular physiology and provided valuable data on alternative RNA processing and diversity in different biological contexts, the use of microarray technology showed some limitations due to several factors (Licatalosi and Darnell 2010). One of these factors, the incomplete nature of gene annotation and limited microarray density, continually improved over time but others such as the need to predefine targets (such as alternative exons) preclude the identification of novel alternative mRNA isoforms. This is one of the elements that have represented a relevant constraint and disadvantage for a more efficient utilization of new technologies to identify genetic basis of production traits in animals and to know the genes responsible for qualitative characteristics of foods derived from animal productions. One of the main limitations presented by these methods is that they are dependent on nucleic acid hybridization, and researchers need to consider signal-to-noise ratios that can vary owing to the differences in base composition and annealing properties between individual probes. The levels of background signal owing to cross-hybridizations can be high and it is possible to have a limited range of detection owing to both background and saturation of signals. In these conditions, the confident detection and quantification of low-abundance species is difficult.

Moreover, comparing expression levels across different experiments is often not easy and can require complicated normalization methods: Microarray users have encountered major challenges with respect to the reproducibility of results between laboratories and across platforms. These limitations are being addressed with a new technology: direct high-throughput sequencing.

### 12.4.2.4  RNA-Seq

Advances in sequencing technology with the so-called next-generation sequencing technologies have had impressive impact on genomic research. The recent development of sequencing technologies applied to functional genomics research allowed transcriptome characterization that was not biased by previous genome annotations. These new methodologies based on RNA deep-sequencing revealed that the transcription landscape in higher eukaryotes is much more complex than it had been anticipated, with a high proportion of transcripts originating from intergenic regions that were previously thought to be silent. These innovative transcriptional profiling techniques promise a wealth of new data that can be used to develop a more complete understanding of gene function, regulation, and interactions.

The next-generation sequencing approaches allow the characterization of transcriptomes with remarkable depth and resolution and are beginning to revolutionize our ability to understand the complexity of eukaryotic transcriptomes, including the study of small ncRNA. Transcription that does not refer to genes has also been found in some organisms and the elevated and unexpected high level of RNA complexity has led to the notion of extensive transcription, which refers to the fact that the transcripts are not restricted to well-defined functional features, such as genes. ncRNA are RNA molecules that are not translated into a protein product. This class of RNAs includes tRNA, ribosomal RNA (rRNA) small nuclear and small nucleolar RNAs (siRNAs) and microRNAs. Recent research has considered misRNAs, approximately 20–30 nucleotides long RNA molecules, as crucial posttranscriptional regulators of gene expression, in both animals and plants (Morozova and Marra 2008, Rajewsky 2006). The basic approach of shotgun transcriptome sequencing with short-read technology has been widely called "RNA-Seq." In contrast to microarray methods, sequence-based approaches directly determine the cDNA sequence, and sequencing-based characterization of a transcriptome appeared immediately as an appealing technology because it effectively overcomes the limitations of microarrays. The term "RNA-Seq" applies to any of the several different high-throughput (next-generation) sequencing methods used to obtain transcriptome-wide RNA profile. Typically RNA from two samples that are to be compared is sheared, converted to cDNA, and sequenced. The use of current sequencing technologies yield million sequence reads that are upto 100 nucleotide in length (Wang et al. 2009). The sequence technology is rapidly evolving and in the near future new approaches recently developed will increase the output and decrease the cost of the analysis opening new opportunities for researches.

There is little dispute that array profiling methods have been a revolutionary tool in the postgenomic era, providing the means to survey gene expression and correlate gene activity with animal biological processes and physiological states. However, the extensive transcriptional complexity in many organisms means that transcriptomics content and dynamics cannot be effectively surveyed with current array technologies. Shotgun sequencing provides an effective alternative method for interrogating the transcriptome due to its open-ended scalability and the superior discriminatory power of sequence content over hybridization signals. Recently in pigs and in other farm animals, an increasing number of studies have been realized utilizing the innovative sequencing technology, and several studies utilizing RNA deep-sequencing applied to animal transcriptome analysis and characterization are in progress (for a review, see Liu et al. 2009, McDaneld et al. 2009, Turner et al. 2009).

A further advantage of RNA-Seq relative to DNA microarrays is that RNA-Seq has very low, if any, background signal because DNA sequences can been unambiguously mapped to unique regions of the genome. RNA-Seq has also been shown to be highly accurate for quantifying expression levels as determined using q-PCR and spike-in controls of known concentration. The results of RNA-Seq also show high levels of reproducibility for both technical and biological replicates. Taking all these advantages into account, RNA-Seq can be considered as the first sequencing-based method that allows the entire transcriptome to be surveyed in a very high-throughput and quantitative manner and often at a much lower cost than the most widely used methodology for transcriptome analysis (Wang et al. 2009, Wilhelm and Landry 2009).The ability of mRNA-Seq to detect previously uncharacterized mRNA isoforms and new classes of ncRNAs illustrates the use of this rapidly evolving technology, which is assuming an increasingly dominant role in RNA analyses.

Next-generation sequencing technologies afford many opportunities but will also pose considerable challenges. The major challenges of these technologies revolve around the management and analysis of the sequence data. Because every DNA sequencing runs on a next-generation sequencing platform generating many gigabytes of data that must be analyzed and archived, considerable computational resources are required. For this reason there is the need of computational resources to handle the amount of data that these technologies are capable of generating. There is likely to be an evolution in the software available for analyzing sequencing data, and just as it has occurred with microarray analysis, this will enhance the power of new sequencing technologies (Turner et al. 2009). Like other high-throughput sequencing technologies, RNA-Seq faces several informatics challenges including the development of efficient methods to store, retrieve, and process large amounts of data, which must be overcome to reduce errors in base calling and remove low-quality reads.

Bioinformatics has emerged as a powerful complement to current efforts to analyze the complexity of RNA. Advances in bioinformatics are ongoing and improvements are needed if these systems are to keep pace with the continuing developments in sequencing technologies. Therefore, bioinformatics is likely to become more powerful as a new technology that improves data set of sequences available (Licatalosi and Darnell 2010). RNA-Seq technologies that are in the early stages of use have clear advantages over previously developed transcriptomic methods and an impressive range of applications and more are being developed.

New technologies will allow to perform genotype–phenotype mapping studies on the scale of and with the density of molecular markers required to simultaneously identify many genes that affect variation of quantitative traits. We are beginning to interpret these associations in terms of genetic networks through the incorporation of information on whole genome variation in transcript abundance in the mapping populations (MacKay et al. 2009). This provides unprecedented insights into the biological underpinnings of complex traits like meat production and meat quality and the pleiotropic connections between traits.

The process of detecting and characterizing Quantitative Trait Nucleotides (QTNs) will be accelerated by the knowledge of complete DNA and RNA sequences. New technologies can now be applied to solve current challenges and can describe how a systems genetics approach for integrating genotype–phenotype relationship can uncover genetic pathways that affect variation of complex traits in livestock and can identify many genes controlling variation of quantitative traits.

## 12.5 MAIN APPLICATIONS BASED ON FUNCTIONAL GENOMICS APPROACHES FOR THE IMPROVEMENT OF MEAT PRODUCT QUALITY

Meat has a relevant importance among foods as it is a valuable source of nutrients of high biological value. Nevertheless, meat quality is a concept that is changing according to the necessities of the different operators involved in the meat production chain from farm to fork: pig breeders, slaughterers, transformers, distributors, and consumers (Table 12.1).

From Table 12.1, it is easy to see that there are relevant differences in the definitions of the most important meat quality attributes in the functioning of the requests of the different agents in the meat production chain. Several times the requests are quite different and it can be difficult to satisfy all needs. For these aspects, the improvement of meat quality is one of the main and most challenging goals of the breeders' association and is also characterized by traits (listed in Table 12.1) difficult to be measured. Helpfully, molecular biology can aid the genetic improvement efficiency by providing new tools to be integrated in the current selective scheme when genes underlying a quantitative trait are detected and an SNP changing the expression level or the gene product is found (Davoli 2004). Moreover the expression level of a highly variable gene in an individual is considered as the "phenotype," which is possibly influenced by genetic determinants (Schellander 2009). According to this idea genetic analysis can therefore be used to map and to identify also the genes and/or regulatory regions that control expression of meat trait phenotypes (Cheung and Spielman 2002).

**TABLE 12.1**

**Quality Parameters Required by the Different Operators Involved in the Pork Supply Chain**

| Pig Breeders | Slaughterers | Transformers | Distributors | Consumers |
|---|---|---|---|---|
| Growth rate | Carcass weight | Weight of cuts | Carcass weight | Healthiness |
| Feed conversion efficiency | Weight of cuts | Yield of production | Yield of production | Pleasant aspect |
| Carcass weight | The same requests of transformers and consumers | Seasoning attitude | Drip losses | Cooking losses |
| The same requests of slaughterers and transformers | | Drip losses | Shear force | Tastiness |
| | | Lean meat content | The same requests of consumers | Savoriness |
| | | The same requests of consumers | | Tenderness |
| | | | | Fat quantity and fat quality |

On the whole, these techniques may be used to address the selection scheme toward quality differentiation strategies for the use of pork to be sold directly (fresh meat) or to be seasoned to produce cured products like salamis and "Prosciutto" (dry cured ham) by selecting pig lines specifically addressed to a particular production system. Functional genomics approaches will be useful to know the genetic factors determining the specific attitudes of the breeds used to obtain these products and to improve the qualitative characteristics of the productions.

## 12.5.1 Discovery of Porcine Tissue-Specific Genes

Skeletal muscle is a tissue that serves as an important source of food (meat) through relevant and complex biochemical processes. The processes of change between muscle and meat involve metabolic, physical, and structural alterations. Moreover skeletal muscle and adipose tissue are the main elements in order of priority implicated in these processes. The structural and functional study of the genes expressed in these tissues represent the basic step to have a better and deeper knowledge on the processes that influences meat quality.

In humans, the identification of skeletal muscle–specific transcripts started with the works of Bortoluzzi et al. (1998) and Pallavicini et al. (1997), who identified and mapped several thousands of muscle-specific mRNAs producing a comprehensive transcript map of this tissue.

In pigs, the skeletal muscle gene discovery started in the late 1990s with the works of Davoli et al. (1999, 2002), Wang et al. (2006), and Yao et al. (2002), who sequenced many hundred ESTs obtained from unsubtracted or subtracted porcine skeletal muscle cDNA libraries. These researches allowed to define a first list of porcine muscular genes and to discover genes not yet described in any species. Furthermore, Bai et al. (2003) characterized 5500 cDNA clones from 2 skeletal muscles. This research allowed to identify and characterize a very high number of skeletal muscle genes isolated from different muscles, breeds, and developmental stages ensuring an adequate gene representation suitable for the construction of genome-wide arrays to be used in expression researches.

A first characterization of porcine ESTs obtained from adipose tissue was performed by Mikawa et al. (2004): these authors obtained 635 EST clones by sequencing more than 15,000 clones from a porcine backfat cDNA library and mapped 128 of these on porcine chromosomes. Chen et al. (2006a) sequenced 1527 different clones using a similar approach. Furthermore, Kim et al. (2006b) produced 5008 unique sequences of cloned derived from porcine backfat. The sequences generated in these studies providing a good coverage of the genes expressed in porcine fat are useful for functional studies intended to analyze the gene expression profiles of this tissue.

In recent years, Bonnet et al. (2008), Gorodkin et al. (2007), Hornshøj et al. (2007), and Lee et al. (2009) using high-throughput sequencing approaches obtained more than 100,000 EST contigs expressed in different tissues, including genes derived from skeletal muscle and adipose tissue libraries. These researches increased enormously the basic knowledge of the genes expressed in pigs including the characterization of genes expressed in different developmental stages and breeds. Among the identified genes, some were characterized to be ubiquitously expressed among tissues, while others showed a putative tissue-specific expression. A further step to expand the knowledge useful to facilitate the functional studies is to assess the expression level of the identified genes in the most important tissues involved in pig development and growth. With this aim, Hornshøj et al. (2007) established the transcriptional profile of about 20,000 genes in 23 porcine tissues producing a large catalogue of basic gene expression profiles. This knowledge is now available in pigs and can contribute also to the functional annotation of unknown genes considering that the attribution of a function to specific genes and their annotation on porcine genome are unresolved problems up to now and represent a limiting factor of the researches in this field. Other transcriptional profiles of several tissues, including different muscles and fat depots, were obtained by Ferraz et al. (2008) and Hornshøj et al. (2009).

Another important contribution to the characterization of porcine genes is the work performed by the research group of Uenishi who developed the pig EST/ Expression Data Explorer database (Uenishi et al. 2004, 2007) in order to produce high-quality ESTs and to sequence the full insert of cloned genes: These authors described the complete sequence for more than 10,000 genes allowing an easier exploration of pig genes influencing quantitative and qualitative traits such as those related to meat quality.

## 12.5.2 Functional Analysis of Genes Involved in Meat and Fat Traits

The application of functional genomic approaches to study genes involved in meat quality has already resulted in the identification of differentially expressed genes in porcine skeletal muscle. Postnatal muscle growth largely depends on the number and size of muscle fibers that develop during the fetal period. For this reason, a complete knowledge of the pathways involved in skeletal muscle differentiation and development can be achieved by analyzing the gene expression level in different stages during both pre- and postnatal growth. The porcine breeds show differences in the aptitude to muscle and fat growth, and the genomic analyses can be applied to discover at the gene level the factors responsible for the different breed characteristics. For example, among the European and Northern American widespread breeds, Pietrain animals show an extremely relevant muscular growth producing carcasses with a high content of lean meat, while Duroc pigs show a good growth rate but the carcass has more fat and muscles show a higher fat content compared to other breeds (Pietrain and Large White). Several researches were carried out by comparing a cosmopolite breed and a local one because the latter usually shows strong phenotypic differences such as slower growth rate and higher fat content on the carcass.

The pattern of expression in prenatal muscle tissue from Duroc and Pietrain pigs was investigated by Cagnazzo et al. (2006) and Te Pas et al. (2005) who reported the expression profiles in different stages of embryo development and the specificity of expression of the two analyzed breeds elucidating the role of some genes and network of genes on the development of prenatal skeletal muscles in pigs. Moreover, Te Pas et al. (2007) described a bioinformatics approach useful to combine the results of different microarray analyses in order to better define the pathways associated with myoblast and cytoskeleton formation and energy metabolism during myogenesis. On the whole, these authors observed that myogenic differentiation could be better described by a balance between activated and underexpressed genes rather than by the observation of the expression level of single genes affecting this trait. Muráni et al. (2007) used a DD approach to analyze the prenatal skeletal muscle development in different key stages of myogenesis in Pietrain and Duroc pigs, and Davoli et al. (2010) analyzed the expression level of 11 genes by real-time PCR on the same two breeds. In these researches, genes differentially expressed between developmental stages and also between the two breeds were observed. These studies revealed several genes associated with myogenesis and expanded the knowledge of genetic factors operating during skeletal muscle development. The most frequent functional categories were represented by genes encoding myofibrillar proteins; genes involved in cell adhesion, cell–cell signaling, and extracellular matrix synthesis/remodeling; genes regulating gene expression; and genes involved in metabolism. Tang et al. (2007) used long-SAGE to detect expression differences between Tongcheng and Landrace pigs in embryos at different ages post coitus. These authors detected several growth factors, antiapoptotic factors, and genes involved in the protein synthesis that were overexpressed in Landrace pigs suggesting their putative role to determine a higher attitude of animals of this breed in producing lean meat compared to Tongcheng pigs.

The postnatal gene transcription profile was characterized by Lin and Hsu (2005) who analyzed the differences in expression of skeletal muscles collected at different neonatal ages from Duroc and the local Taiwanese breed Taoyuan using a cDNA microarray. This analysis allowed to distinguish more than 100 differentially expressed genes among the two breeds. The genes overexpressed in Duroc includes some encoding myofibrillar proteins, ribosomal proteins, transcription regulatory proteins, and energy metabolic enzymes indicating which metabolic patterns may be involved in the higher postnatal muscle growth capacity of Duroc breed compared to the Taiwanese breed.

A particular study was carried out by Zhu et al. (2009) who revealed differences of expression among Tibetan pigs and the breeds Landrace and Meishan. Tibetan pigs are adapted to live in high-altitude conditions and are characterized by lower body weight compared to the two other breeds. The analysis of the expression profile of skeletal muscle and adipose tissue at various growth stages revealed that specific gene expression patterns characterized Tibetan pigs. These results indicated that peculiar gene networks seemed to influence the attitude of these animals to live in high-altitude areas likely reflecting specific physiological changes such as higher skeletal muscle growth and higher adipose metabolism, while the genes downregulated were associated with fat deposition. The comparison of gene expression profile in Tibetan pigs adapted to an extreme altitude with the profile observed in breeds derived from other environments may be useful to elucidate specific mechanisms used by pigs to modify body composition.

Some researchers used a genome-wide gene expression analysis to search candidate genes for quantitative traits in livestock, including eye muscle area (Ponsuksili et al. 2000), body composition (Ponsuksili et al. 2005), drip loss, and pH (Ponsuksili et al. 2008a, b, 2009, Srikanchai et al. 2010, Wimmers et al. 2010) in pigs. Among these traits, drip loss and pH are some of the most important measures utilized to assess meat quality and for this reason the improvement of knowledge of the physiologic pathways that influence their phenotypic expression is one of the main goals for pig meat production in the near future. In their studies, these authors described the successful identification of candidate genes for water-holding capacity traits (e.g., drip loss and pH) using gene expression profiling. Several pathways and genes were detected, both up- and downregulated, suggesting their role in the biological processes involved in the postmortem transformation of muscle to meat and the changes influencing drip loss and pH.

A microarray analysis comparing skeletal muscle gene expression profile of Italian Large White pigs divergent for glycolytic potential (GP) revealed that genes related to energy metabolism were differentially expressed between pigs with high and low level of GP in muscle (Davoli et al. 2007, 2008). GP of meat is a measure of the quantity of glucidic compounds that can be converted postmortem into lactic acid and is an important parameter of skeletal muscles affecting pork quality traits such as lower ultimate pH, meat color, water-holding capacity, drip loss, tenderness, and yield processing. Comparative expression profiling by hybridization of the Operon/Qiagen pig 11k Oligo set array (*Sus scrofa* (pig) AROS version 1.0—http://omad.operon.com/download/index.php; Zhao et al. 2005) showed significant overexpression in the pool with low GP for several energy metabolism and ATP synthesis genes (Davoli et al. 2008).

Muscle tenderness influences meat quality and the genetic control of this trait is poorly understood. Lobjois et al. (2008) analyzed by microarray the *Longissimus* muscle samples representing different levels of tenderness measured with Warner–Bratzler shear force of cooked meat. The samples with high shear force showed differentially expressed genes involved in three functional categories: cell cycle, energy metabolism, and muscle development. The genes with different levels of transcription, mapped in genomic regions where QTLs for this trait were found, can be considered as positional candidates for meat tenderness.

The effect of preslaughter stress treatment on meat quality traits in pigs of different breeds was analyzed after having studied the expression level of some genes and corresponding proteins using a proteomic approach. The expression level was generally not correlated with the level of the corresponding proteins. One of the most meaningful associations between gene expression/ protein level with meat quality traits was that a slower pH decline was observed in samples with lower levels of heat shock protein 72 mRNA and higher levels of the corresponding protein (Kwasiborski et al. 2009).

The fat content in carcass and muscles is among the main factors influencing the quality of meat products. One of the first research in this field was carried out by Gerbens et al. (2001) who analyzed the genes coding for adipocyte and hearth fatty acid binding proteins (*A-FABP*, *H-FABP*), two important proteins involved in fatty acid transport. These authors described the relationships between the gene expression level and some SNPs of the genes. These authors observed an association between the expression profiles of both *FABP* mRNAs and the intramuscular fat content in *Longissimus lumborum* muscle in barrows. Interestingly they did not find a similar association considering the content of the two FABP proteins: This discrepancy does not support the hypothesis of a direct involvement of these two genes in controlling the intramuscular fat content and the authors hypothesized that the intramuscular fat differences can be explained by a change in the protein functionality rather than in protein expression level.

A research aimed to discover differences in adipocyte functions among three fat depots—intramuscular, subcutaneous, perirenal—was conducted by Gardan et al. (2006). The authors described differences, among the three tissues, in the q-PCR expression pattern of genes coding for enzymes and hormones involved in fat synthesis. In particular the expression levels of these genes observed in adipocytes derived from muscle are quite different to those obtained from adipose cells derived by subcutaneous and abdominal fat, supporting the evidence that intramuscular fat displays specific biological features.

Microarray studies were performed to analyze the gene expression pattern in adipose tissue obtained from different depots and from fetuses, neonatal pigs, and gilts at different ages using custom arrays representing more than 600 pig genes involved in growth and reproduction (Hausman et al. 2006, 2007, 2008). These works described the expression of genes in pre- and postnatal porcine adipose tissue that may be involved in its growth and reported that the expression patterns of some genes are specific to the location of fat depots. Li et al. (2008) analyzed by pathway-focused oligo microarray the expression profiles of 140 genes related to meat quality and carcass traits during postnatal development of backfat in five growth stages of pigs from the lean Western breed Landrace and the fatty indigenous Chinese breed Tahiu. The authors described breed-specific pattern of expression. In particular, Landrace pigs overexpressed genes mainly related to the biosynthesis of fatty acids while in Tahiu breed they found that some genes mainly involved in cell growth were upregulated. These findings suggested that some possible candidate genes regulating fatty acid biosynthesis and degradation can explain the differences in fat deposition aptitude observed between the two breeds. The same research group investigated the developmental expression pattern of insulin-like growth factor 2 (*IGF2*) and insulin-like growth factor binding protein 3 (*IGFBP3*) in backfat tissue of Landrace and Tahiu pig breeds showing different patterns of expression between the two breeds and specific developmental changes of transcription (Guo et al. 2008).

A further study was carried out by Lee et al. (2009) who analyzed ESTs obtained by sequencing several thousand cDNA clones derived from full-length enriched cDNA libraries constructed from porcine abdominal fat, loin muscle, liver, and pituitary gland. The expression profile obtained by analyzing the sequence data discovered 12 genes involved in gluconeogenesis and translation elongation that were significantly more abundant in fat than in muscle tissue providing important insight into the discovery of the functional pathways and the specificity of the metabolism in these tissues.

The linking between changes in the diet and the transcription profile of tissues were also analyzed in order to gain insight into the signaling molecules that mediate the effects of dietary restriction. da Costa et al. (2004) analyzed the expression changes in skeletal muscles of pigs fed with restriction of dietary energy and protein performing a cDNA microarray experiment showing an upregulation of energy-related metabolic pathways but also an increase in substrate (protein, glycogen, and lipid) turnover rising the intramuscular fat deposition of diet-restricted pigs. The same behavior in the expression profile was observed in muscles differing in fiber-type composition. Lkhagvadorj et al. (2009) reported results from transcriptional profiling coupled with blood metabolite analyses comparing pigs fed ad libitum versus fasted animals belonging to different breeds to identify genes and pathways that respond to a fasting treatment. The results showed a transcriptional response to fasting in two key metabolic tissues of pigs: liver and fat. In animals subjected to fasting, 7029 genes were differentially expressed in fat tissue: overexpression was observed for genes involved in extracellular matrix pathway, while underexpression was reported for lipid and steroid synthesis.

Functional studies were also carried out to determine which genes were regulated by clenbuterol administration, a beta-adrenergic receptor agonist that induces skeletal muscle hypertrophy and reduces fat accumulation. This molecule was banned from the pig production chain because its residues contaminating pork poisoned some people eating it. Two papers searched for genes and physiological pathways that are important clenbuterol targets (Spurlock et al. 2006, Zhang et al. 2007). A specific knowledge of the clenbuterol target genes is useful in order to understand the metabolic pathways stimulated by this molecule and that induces muscle hypertrophy in order to obtain the same positive effect on muscle and lean meat deposition in pigs without any pharmacological treatment. In the first paper, the gene expression changes were determined using a microarray approach comparing pigs treated with clenbuterol and control animals not receiving this molecule. Some of the overexpressed genes found in treated pigs were involved in an early phase of protein synthesis (translational initiation) indicating a link with the increased level of protein. Other overexpressed genes were involved in myogenic differentiation suggesting a concordance with the observed muscle hypertrophy of the treated pigs. In the paper of Zhang et al. (2007) 82 differentially expressed genes belonging to functional categories related to lipid metabolism and signal transduction were described. Of particular relevance was the identification of changes in the expression for apolipoprotein D and R because their synthesis level increased in treated animals; therefore, these changes may be related to the decrease in fat accumulation observed in the same subjects.

### 12.5.3 Studies on Porcine MicroRNA Search and Their Role in Controlling Skeletal Muscle Development

As previously described (Section 12.3.1), miRNAs are small non-coding RNAs that negatively regulate gene expression at the posttranscriptional level. There is increasing evidence to suggest that miRNAs participate in muscle development and growth and adipocyte differentiation in humans and mice. Presently in literature are reported some recent papers aimed to detect and analyze miRNAs in porcine muscle tissue, and the researches aimed to identify miRNAs in adipose tissue are just at a nascent stage. All miRNAs detected are catalogued in a public database miRBase (http://microrna.sanger.ac.uk/). Despite the low number of porcine miRNAs included in this database compared to other animal species (Table 12.2), sequence comparisons indicate they are highly conserved supporting the hypothesis that they are fundamental in regulating biological pathways and cell development. The high similarity facilitates the analysis of these RNAs in pigs, which are not extensively described till date, using heterologous sequences.

#### 12.5.3.1 Identification of Porcine miRNAs and Expression Analysis in Skeletal Muscle

The identification of porcine-specific miRNAs started just 4 years ago (Kim et al. 2006a, 2008). The first work characterizing miRNA expressed in porcine skeletal muscle was performed by Feng et al. (2008) who isolated six miRNAs expressed in this porcine tissue by searching on genomic sequences available in databases.

**TABLE 12.2**
**Number of miRNAs for Some Animal Species Listed in miRBase Release 18 (Accessed November, 2011)**

| Species | Number of miRNAs |
|---|---|
| *Homo sapiens* | 1527 |
| *Mus musculus* | 741 |
| *Bos taurus* | 662 |
| *Gallus gallus* | 499 |
| *Rattus norvegicus* | 408 |
| *Equus caballus* | 341 |
| *Canis familiaris* | 323 |
| *Sus scrofa* | 228 |
| *Ovis aries* | 55 |

Using an in silico prediction approach, Huang et al. (2008) identified more than 700 candidate miRNAs on porcine genome and analyzed their expression profile by heterologous microarray in prenatal and adult skeletal muscles. The results obtained by these authors showed differences of expression among ages, suggesting a different role of these genes in biological processes associated with muscle growth in the different developmental stages. Another research analyzed the expression profile of miRNAs during fetal development of porcine skeletal muscles using a deep-sequencing approach (McDaneld et al. 2009). These authors found miR-206 as the most abundant transcript (about 60% of total reads) during the fetal development but was expressed at very low levels in proliferating satellite cells suggesting its role in the switch from precursor to mature muscle cells. Recently Xie et al. (2010) and Cho et al. (2010) isolated some tens of porcine miRNAs obtained from skeletal muscle and adipose tissue and used real-time PCR to demonstrate that some miRNAs were enriched in a tissue-specific manner and, in particular, ssc-miR-206 was expressed specifically in skeletal muscle. The identification of 212 miRNAs in porcine skeletal muscle was described by Nielsen et al. (2010): the majority of these miRNAs was discovered for the first time in pigs. These authors used a deep sequencing approach to identify the majority of the miRNAs expressed in this tissue and to determine their expression level. The most abundant one was miR-1 (87.1% of all reads) followed by miR-206, let-7, miR-133 (7.4% overall). The remaining 5.5% of the reads account for all other miRNAs detected demonstrating that deep sequencing allows also the uncovering of rare transcripts. Another important outcome of the deep sequencing approach is the identification of sequences variants, typically identified as different length of the 3' end of the molecule, that are useful to predict their target specificity. The target mRNA prediction was obtained for the 10 most abundant genes showing that the main pathway regulated by the considered miRNAs is the MAPK signaling pathway, which is involved in skeletal muscle differentiation and development (Keren et al. 2006), signal transduction, cell–cell and cell–extracellular matrix communication, and neural development and function. Li et al. (2010) contributed extensively toward a comprehensive knowledge of the whole set of miRNA of porcine skeletal muscle (microRNAome) with the identification of 777 unique miRNAs through an in silico search on the first release of porcine genomic sequence and on the whole data set of the porcine ESTs. Some of the miRNAs found were tested by q-PCR in order to confirm their tissue localization and information about development-specific expression and multiple variants of mature sequences.

The discovery of novel miRNAs and the characterization of the expression of porcine sequences grew quickly in the last few years and, in particular, the almost completed pig genome assembly was an important resource to perform bioinformatics prediction of miRNAs. The most challenging goal of future researches may be directed toward understanding the functional role and the importance of miRNAs in livestock species by discovering the target genes that are regulated by miRNAs (McDaneld 2009, Liu et al. 2010) and the contribution of these regulatory molecules to meat development. Furthermore, the miRNA species so far described in pigs are presently close to those described in humans, close to 1000, probably representing more or less the whole porcine set of miRNAs. For this reason now it is possible to analyze the regulatory map of the porcine miRNAome at the whole genome level and the outcomes of these researches can be of relevant importance for understanding complex phenotypes and networks of metabolic processes involved in growth and development in pigs but also the results obtained in porcine species can be useful and relevant to analyze complex human diseases using pig as a model (Li et al. 2010).

## 12.6 FUTURE PERSPECTIVES

The integration of different approaches of gene expression analysis is fundamental for identifying and validating the metabolic pathways and the network of genes controlling qualitative traits of pig meat. The final challenge of these researches will be to elucidate the role of individual genes and their casual QTNs in influencing the long list of traits defining the multiple aspects of meat quality. This goal should be met in the near future by applying the most powerful available technologies (deep sequencing, other approaches) that will integrate more efficiently the widely utilized microarray analysis. The technical improvement of the sequence-based approaches will allow a more and more efficient investigation of the transcripts accompanied by an expected continuous reduction of the costs. The technical development described in this chapter must be integrated with progresses in bioinformatics because the extraction of knowledge by such a great amount of information can be addressed only with adequate computational approaches useful to identify not only the role of single genes but also networks of genes allowing to interpret quantitative genetic variation in terms of biologically causal network of correlated transcripts. The different categories of operators of meat production chain and, in particular, the consumers can receive benefits from the application of results of these studies in order to improve efficiency of meat production and to satisfy the requirements of better quality.

## REFERENCES

Alt, F. W., A. L. Bothwell, M. Knapp et al. 1980. Synthesis of secreted and membrane-bound immunoglobulin mu heavy chains is directed by mRNAs that differ at their 3′ ends. *Cell* 20:293–301.

Anderson, C., H. Catoe, and R. Werner. 2006. MIR-206 regulates connexin43 expression during skeletal muscle development. *Nucleic Acids Res* 34:5863–5871.

Andersson, L., C. S. Haley, H. Ellegren et al. 1994. Genetic mapping of quantitative trait loci for growth and fatness in pigs. *Science* 263:1771–1774.

Bai, Q., C. McGillivray, N. da Costa et al. 2003. Development of a porcine skeletal muscle cDNA microarray: Analysis of differential transcript expression in phenotypically distinct muscles. *BMC Genom* 4:8.

Black, D. L. 2003. Mechanisms of alternative pre-messenger RNA splicing. *Annu Rev Biochem* 72:291–336.

Bonnet, A., E. Iannuccelli, K. Hugot et al. 2008. A pig multi-tissue normalised cDNA library: Large-scale sequencing, cluster analysis and 9 K micro-array resource generation. *BMC Genom* 9:17.

Bortoluzzi, S., L. Rampoldi, B. Simionati et al. 1998. A comprehensive, high-resolution genomic transcript map of human skeletal muscle. *Genome Res* 8:817–825.

Brennecke, J., A. Stark, and S. M. Cohen. 2005. Not miR-ly muscular: MicroRNAs and muscle development. *Genes Dev* 19:2261–2264.

Brown, J. W. S., D. F. Marshall, and M. Echeverria. 2008. Intronic noncoding RNAs and splicing. *Trends Plant Sci* 13:335–342.

Burt, D. W. 2006. The chicken genome. *Genome Dyn* 2:123–137.

Burt, D. W. and S. J. White. 2007. Avian genomics in the 21st century. *Cytogenet Genome Res* 117:6–13.

Cagnazzo, M., M. F. W. te Pas, J. Priem et al. 2006. Comparison of prenatal muscle tissue expression profiles of two pig breeds differing in muscle characteristics. *J Anim Sci* 84:1–10.

Carthew, R. W. and E. J. Sontheimer. 2009. Origins and mechanisms of miRNAs and siRNAs. *Cell* 136:642–655.

Chen, C. H., E. C. Lin, W. T. K. Cheng, H. S. Sun, H. J. Mersmann, and S. T. Ding. 2006a. Abundantly expressed genes in pig adipose tissue: An expressed sequence tag approach. *J Anim Sci* 84:2673–2683.

Chen, J.-F., E. M. Mandel, J. M. Thomson et al. 2006b. The role of microRNA-1 and microRNA-133 in skeletal muscle proliferation and differentiation. *Nat Genet* 38:228–233.

Cheung, V. G. and R. S. Spielman. 2002. The genetics of variation in gene expression. *Nat Genet* 32 (Suppl):522–525.

Cho, I. S., J. Kim, H. Y. Seo et al. 2010. Cloning and characterization of microRNAs from porcine skeletal muscle and adipose tissue. *Mol Biol Rep* 37:3567–3574.

Clop, A., F. Marcq, H. Takeda et al. 2006. A mutation creating a potential illegitimate microRNA target site in the myostatin gene affects muscularity in sheep. *Nat Genet* 38:813–818.

Colecchia, F., D. Kottwitz, M. Wagner et al. 2009. Tissue-specific regulatory network extractor (TS-REX): A database and software resource for the tissue and cell type-specific investigation of transcription factor-gene networks. *Nucleic Acids Res* 37:e82.

Couture, O., K. Callenberg, N. Koul et al. 2009. ANEXdb: An integrated animal ANnotation and microarray EXpression database. *Mamm Genome* 20:768–777.

da Costa, N., C. McGillivray, Q. Bai, J. D. Wood, G. Evans, and K.-C. Chang. 2004. Restriction of dietary energy and protein induces molecular changes in young porcine skeletal muscles. *J Nutr* 134:2191–2199.

Davoli, R. 2004. Molecular strategies to enhance and control meat quality. Beyond thinking—tomorrow. In *Proceedings of the International Food Conference*, Dublin, Ireland, June 17–18, 2004, pp. 108–119.

Davoli, R., S. Braglia, V. Russo, L. Varona, and M. F. W. te Pas. 2010. Expression profiling of functional genes in prenatal skeletal muscle tissue in Duroc and Pietrain pigs. *J Anim Breed Genet*. doi: 10.1111/j.1439–0388.2010.00867.x

Davoli, R., M. Colombo, S. Schiavina, L. Fontanesi, L. Buttazzoni, and V. Russo. 2007. Transcriptome analysis of porcine skeletal muscle: Differentially expressed genes in Italian Large White pigs with divergent values for glycolytic potential. In *Proceedings of the ASPA 17th Congress*, Alghero, Italy, May 29–June 1, 2007. *Ital J Anim Sci* 6 (Suppl 1):113.

Davoli, R., L. Fontanesi, P. Zambonelli et al. 2002. Isolation of porcine expressed sequence tags for the construction of a first genomic transcript map of the skeletal muscle in pig. *Anim Genet* 33:3–18.

Davoli, R., P. Zambonelli, D. Bigi, L. Fontanesi, and V. Russo. 1999. Analysis of expressed sequence tags of porcine skeletal muscle. *Gene* 233:181–188.

Davoli, R., P. Zambonelli, S. Braglia et al. 2008. Microarray analysis of skeletal muscle genes in pigs divergent for glycolytic potential. 2119. In *Proceedings of XXXI Conference of the International Society for Animal Genetics*, Amsterdam, the Netherlands, July 20–24, 2008.

Diatchenko, L., Y. F. Lau, A. P. Campbell et al. 1996. Suppression subtractive hybridization: A method for generating differentially regulated or tissue-specific cDNA probes and libraries. *Proc Natl Acad Sci USA* 93:6025–6030.

Elsik, C. G., R. L. Tellam, K. C. Worley et al. 2009. The genome sequence of taurine cattle: A window to ruminant biology and evolution. *Science* 324:522–528.

Feng, Y., T. H. Huang, B. Fan, and S. H. Zhao. 2008. Mapping of six miRNAs expressed in porcine skeletal muscle. *Anim Genet* 39:91–92.

Ferraz, A. L. J., A. Ojeda, M. López-Béjar et al. 2008. Transcriptome architecture across tissues in the pig. *BMC Genom* 9:173.

Fields, S., Y. Kohara, and D. J. Lockhart. 1999. Functional genomics. *Proc Natl Acad Sci USA* 96:8825–8826.

Fujii, J., K. Otsu, F. Zorzato et al. 1991. Identification of a mutation in porcine ryanodine receptor associated with malignant hyperthermia. *Science* 253:448–451.

Gardan, D., F. Gondret, and I. Louveau. 2006. Lipid metabolism and secretory function of porcine intramuscular adipocytes compared with subcutaneous and perirenal adipocytes. *Am J Physiol-Endocrinol Metab* 291:E372–E380.

Gerbens, F., F. J. Verburg, H. T. Van Moerkerk et al. 2001. Associations of heart and adipocyte fatty acid-binding protein gene expression with intramuscular fat content in pigs. *J Anim Sci* 79:347–354.

Gibbs, R. A., J. F. Taylor, C. P. Van Tassell et al. 2009. Genome-wide survey of SNP variation uncovers the genetic structure of cattle breeds. *Science* 324:528–532.

Gorodkin, J., S. Cirera, J. Hedegaard et al. 2007. Porcine transcriptome analysis based on 97 non-normalized cDNA libraries and assembly of 1,021,891 expressed sequence tags. *Genome Biol* 8:R45.

Gresham, D., M. J. Dunham, and D. Botstein. 2008. Comparing whole genomes using DNA microarrays. *Nat Rev Genet* 9:291–302.

Grosse, W. M., S. M. Kappes, and R. A. McGraw. 2000. Linkage mapping and comparative analysis of bovine expressed sequence tags (ESTs). *Anim Genet* 31:171–177.

Guo, Y.-J., G.-Q. Tang, X.-W. Li, L. Zhu, and M.-Z. Li. 2008. Developmental expression changes of IGF2 and IGFBP3 genes in adipose tissue of two pig breeds. *Yi Chuan = Hereditas/Zhongguo Yi Chuan Xue Hui Bian Ji* 30:602–606.

Haley, C. S. and P. M. Visscher. 1998. Strategies to utilize marker-quantitative trait loci associations. *J Dairy Sci* 81:85–97.

Hausman, G. J., C. R. Barb, and R. G. Dean. 2007. Patterns of gene expression in pig adipose tissue: Transforming growth factors, interferons, interleukins, and apolipoproteins. *J Anim Sci* 85:2445–2456.

Hausman, G. J., C. R. Barb, and R. G. Dean. 2008. Patterns of gene expression in pig adipose tissue: Insulin-like growth factor system proteins, neuropeptide Y (NPY), NPY receptors, neurotrophic factors and other secreted factors. *Domest Anim Endocrinol* 35:24–34.

Hausman, G. J., S. P. Poulos, R. L. Richardson et al. 2006. Secreted proteins and genes in fetal and neonatal pig adipose tissue and stromal-vascular cells. *J Anim Sci* 84:1666–1681.

Haverty, P. M., Z. Weng, N. L. Best et al. 2002. HugeIndex: A database with visualization tools for high-density oligonucleotide array data from normal human tissues. *Nucleic Acids Res* 30:214–217.

Hornshøj, H., E. Bendixen, L. N. Conley et al. 2009. Transcriptomic and proteomic profiling of two porcine tissues using high-throughput technologies. *BMC Genom* 10:30.

Hornshøj, H., L. N. Conley, J. Hedegaard, P. Sørensen, F. Panitz, and C. Bendixen. 2007. Microarray expression profiles of 20.000 genes across 23 healthy porcine tissues. *PLoS ONE* 2:e1203.

Hsiao, L. L., F. Dangond, T. Yoshida et al. 2001. A compendium of gene expression in normal human tissues. *Physiol Genom* 7:97–104.

Hu, Z.-L., K. Glenn, A. M. Ramos, C. J. Otieno, J. M. Reecy, and M. F. Rothschild. 2005. Expeditor: A pipeline for designing primers using human gene structure and livestock animal EST information. *J Hered* 96:80–82.

Hu, Y., K. Wang, X. He, D. Y. Chiang, J. F. Prins, and J. Liu. 2010. A probabilistic framework for aligning paired-end RNA-seq data. *Bioinformatics* 26:1950–1957.

Huang, T.-H., M.-J. Zhu, X.-Y. Li, and S.-H. Zhao. 2008. Discovery of porcine microRNAs and profiling from skeletal muscle tissues during development. *PLoS ONE* 3:e3225.

Hutchison, C. A. 2007. DNA sequencing: Bench to bedside and beyond. *Nucleic Acids Res* 35:6227–6237.

International Chicken Genome Sequencing Consortium. 2004. Sequence and comparative analysis of the chicken genome provide unique perspectives on vertebrate evolution. *Nature* 432:695–716.

Jacquier, A. 2009. The complex eukaryotic transcriptome: Unexpected pervasive transcription and novel small RNAs. *Nat Rev Genet* 10:833–844.

Jansen, R. C. and J. P. Nap. 2001. Genetical genomics: The added value from segregation. *Trends Genet* 17:388–391.

Keren, A., Y. Tamir, and E. Bengal. 2006. The p38 MAPK signaling pathway: A major regulator of skeletal muscle development. *Mol Cell Endocrinol* 252:224–230.

Kim, J., I. S. Cho, J. S. Hong, Y. K. Choi, H. Kim, and Y. S. Lee. 2008. Identification and characterization of new microRNAs from pig. *Mamm Genome* 19:570–580.

Kim, H.-J., X.-S. Cui, E.-J. Kim, W.-J. Kim, and N.-H. Kim. 2006a. New porcine microRNA genes found by homology search. *Genome* 49:1283–1286.

Kim, T.-H., N.-S. Kim, D. Lim et al. 2006b. Generation and analysis of large-scale expressed sequence tags (ESTs) from a full-length enriched cDNA library of porcine backfat tissue. *BMC Genom* 7:36.

Kim, K. S., N. Larsen, T. Short, G. Plastow, and M. F. Rothschild. 2000. A missense variant of the porcine melanocortin-4 receptor (MC4R) gene is associated with fatness, growth, and feed intake traits. *Mamm Genome* 11:131–135.

Kozomara, A. and S. Griffiths-Jones. 2011. miRBase: Integrating microRNA annotation and deep-sequencing data. *Nucleic Acids Res.* 39 (suppl 1):D152–D157 doi: 10.1093/nar/gkq1027

Kwasiborski, A., D. Rocha, and C. Terlouw. 2009. Gene expression in large white or Duroc-sired female and castrated male pigs and relationships with pork quality. *Anim Genet* 40:852–862.

Lee, K.-T., M.-J. Byun, D. Lim et al. 2009. Full-length enriched cDNA library construction from tissues related to energy metabolism in pigs. *Mol Cells* 28:529–536.

Lee, R. C., R. L. Feinbaum, and V. Ambros. 1993. The *C. elegans* heterochronic gene lin-4 encodes small RNAs with antisense complementarity to lin-14. *Cell* 75:843–854.

Li, M., X. Li, L. Zhu, Y. Jiang, and G. Tang. 2008a. Developmental expression changes of specific genes in adipose tissue for different pig breeds by using pathway-focused microarray. *Sheng Wu Gong Cheng Xue Bao = Chin J Biotechnol* 24:665–672.

Li, M., Y. Xia, Y. Gu et al. 2010. MicroRNAome of porcine pre- and postnatal development. *PLoS ONE* 5:e11541.

Li, M., L. Zhu, X. Li et al. 2008b. Expression profiling analysis for genes related to meat quality and carcass traits during postnatal development of backfat in two pig breeds. *Sci China Ser C-Life Sci China Acad Sci* 51:718–733.

Liang, P. and A. B. Pardee. 1992. Differential display of eukaryotic messenger RNA by means of the polymerase chain reaction. *Science* 257:967–971.

Liang, P. and A. B. Pardee. 2001. Differential display of mRNA by PCR. In *Current Protocols in Molecular Biology*, Chapter 25, Unit B3, F. M. Ausubel, R. Brent, R. E. Kingston et al. (eds.), Hoboken, NJ: John Wiley & Sons, pp. 1–10.

Licatalosi, D. D. and R. B. Darnell. 2010. RNA processing and its regulation: Global insights into biological networks. *Nat Rev Genet* 11:75–87.

Lin, C. S. and C. W. Hsu. 2005. Differentially transcribed genes in skeletal muscle of Duroc and Taoyuan pigs. *J Anim Sci* 83:2075–2086.

Liolios, K., I.-M. A. Chen, K. Mavromatis et al. 2010. The Genomes On Line Database (GOLD) in 2009: Status of genomic and metagenomic projects and their associated metadata. *Nucleic Acids Res* 38:D346–D354.

Liu, H.-C., J. A. Hicks, N. Trakooljul, and S.-H. Zhao. 2010. Current knowledge of microRNA characterization in agricultural animals. *Anim Genet* 41:225–231.

Liu, Y., X. Qin, X.-Z. H. Song et al. 2009. *Bos taurus* genome assembly. *BMC Genom* 10:180.

Liu, N., A. H. Williams, Y. Kim et al. 2007. An intragenic MEF2-dependent enhancer directs muscle-specific expression of microRNAs 1 and 133. *Proc Natl Acad Sci USA* 104:20844–20849.

Lkhagvadorj, S., L. Qu, W. Cai et al. 2009. Microarray gene expression profiles of fasting induced changes in liver and adipose tissues of pigs expressing the melanocortin-4 receptor D298N variant. *Physiol Genom* 38:98–111.

Lobjois, V., L. Liaubet, M. SanCristobal et al. 2008. A muscle transcriptome analysis identifies positional candidate genes for a complex trait in pig. *Anim Genet* 39:147–162.

Mackay, T. F. C., E. A. Stone, and J. F. Ayroles. 2009. The genetics of quantitative traits: Challenges and prospects. *Nat Rev Genet* 10:565–577.

McCarthy, J. J. and K. A. Esser. 2007. MicroRNA-1 and microRNA-133a expression are decreased during skeletal muscle hypertrophy. *J Appl Physiol* 102:306–313.

McDaneld, T. G. 2009. MicroRNA: Mechanism of gene regulation and application to livestock. *J Anim Sci* 87:E21–E28.

McDaneld, T. G., T. P. L. Smith, M. E. Doumit et al. 2009. MicroRNA transcriptome profiles during swine skeletal muscle development. *BMC Genom* 10:77.

McKeown, M. 1992. Alternative mRNA splicing. *Annu Rev Cell Biol* 8:133–155.

Mikawa, A., H. Suzuki, K. Suzuki et al. 2004. Characterization of 298 ESTs from porcine back fat tissue and their assignment to the SSRH radiation hybrid map. *Mamm Genome* 15:315–322.

Milan, D., J. T. Jeon, C. Looft et al. 2000. A mutation in PRKAG3 associated with excess glycogen content in pig skeletal muscle. *Science* 288:1248–1251.

Mollet, I. G., C. Ben-Dov, D. Felício-Silva et al. 2010. Unconstrained mining of transcript data reveals increased alternative splicing complexity in the human transcriptome. *Nucleic Acids Res* 38:4740–4754.

Moody, D. E. 2001. Genomics techniques: An overview of methods for the study of gene expression. *J Anim Sci* 79:E128–E135.

Morozova, O. and M. A. Marra. 2008. Applications of next-generation sequencing technologies in functional genomics. *Genomics* 92:255–264.

Muráni, E., M. Murániová, S. Ponsuksili, K. Schellander, and K. Wimmers. 2007. Identification of genes differentially expressed during prenatal development of skeletal muscle in two pig breeds differing in muscularity. *BMC Dev Biol* 7:109.

Nakajima, N., T. Takahashi, R. Kitamura et al. 2006. MicroRNA-1 facilitates skeletal myogenic differentiation without affecting osteoblastic and adipogenic differentiation. *Biochem Biophys Res Commun* 350:1006–1012.

Ness, S. A. 2007. Microarray analysis: Basic strategies for successful experiments. *Mol Biotechnol* 36:205–219.

Nguyen, H. T. and M. Frasch. 2006. MicroRNAs in muscle differentiation: Lessons from *Drosophila* and beyond. *Curr Opin Genet Dev* 16:533–539.

Nielsen, M., J. H. Hansen, J. Hedegaard et al. 2010. MicroRNA identity and abundance in porcine skeletal muscles determined by deep sequencing. *Anim Genet* 41:159–168.

Norris, B. J. and V. A. Whan. 2008. A gene duplication affecting expression of the ovine ASIP gene is responsible for white and black sheep. *Genome Res* 18:1282–1293.

Pallavicini, A., R. Zimbello, N. Tiso et al. 1997. The preliminary transcript map of a human skeletal muscle. *Hum Mol Genet* 6:1445–1450.

Phang, T. 2009. R and Bioconductor solutions for alternative splicing detection. *Hum Genom* 4:131–135.

Ponsuksili, S., E. Jonas, E. Murani et al. 2008a. Trait correlated expression combined with expression QTL analysis reveals biological pathways and candidate genes affecting water holding capacity of muscle. *BMC Genom* 9:367.

Ponsuksili, S., E. Murani, C. Phatsara et al. 2008b. Expression profiling of muscle reveals transcripts differentially expressed in muscle that affect water-holding capacity of pork. *J Agric Food Chem* 56:10311–10317.

Ponsuksili, S., E. Murani, C. Phatsara, M. Schwerin, K. Schellander, and K. Wimmers. 2009. Porcine muscle sensory attributes associate with major changes in gene networks involving CAPZB, ANKRD1, and CTBP2. *Funct Int Genom* 9:455–471.

Ponsuksili, S., E. Murani, K. Schellander, M. Schwerin, and K. Wimmers. 2005. Identification of functional candidate genes for body composition by expression analyses and evidencing impact by association analysis and mapping. *Biochim Biophys Acta* 1730:31–40.

Ponsuksili, S., K. Wimmers, F. Schmoll, A. Robic, and K. Schellander. 2000. Porcine ESTs detected by differential display representing possible candidates for the trait 'eye muscle area'. *J Anim Breed Genet* 117:25–35.

Rajewsky, N. 2006. microRNA target predictions in animals. *Nat Genet* 38 (Suppl):S8–S13.

Robert, C. 2008. Challenges of functional genomics applied to farm animal gametes and pre-hatching embryos. *Theriogenology* 70:1277–1287.

Rothschild, M. F., Z. Hu, and Z. Jiang. 2007. Advances in QTL mapping in pigs. *Int J Biol Sci* 3:192–197.

Rothschild, M. F. and G.S. Plastow. 2008. Impact of genomics on animal agriculture and opportunities for animal health. *Trends Biotechnol* 26:21–25.

Saini, H. K., S. Griffiths-Jones, and A. J. Enright. 2007. Genomic analysis of human microRNA transcripts. *Proc Natl Acad Sci USA* 104:17719–17724.

Saito-Hisaminato, A., T. Katagiri, S. Kakiuchi, T. Nakamura, T. Tsunoda, and Y. Nakamura. 2002. Genome-wide profiling of gene expression in 29 normal human tissues with a cDNA microarray. *DNA Res* 9:35–45.

Sánchez, L. 2008. Sex-determining mechanisms in insects. *Int J Dev Biol* 52:837–856.

Schellander, K. 2009. Identifying genes associated with quantitative traits in pigs: Integrating quantitative and molecular approaches for meat quality. In *Proceedings of the ASPA 18th Congress*. Palermo, Italy, June 9–12, 2009. *Ital J Anim Sci* 8 (Suppl 2): 19–25.

Schena, M., D. Shalon, R. W. Davis, and P. O. Brown. 1995. Quantitative monitoring of gene expression patterns with a complementary DNA microarray. *Science* 270:467–470.

Shendure, J. 2008. The beginning of the end for microarrays? *Nat Methods* 5:585–587.

Shmueli, O., S. Horn-Saban, V. Chalifa-Caspi et al. 2003. GeneNote: Whole genome expression profiles in normal human tissues. *C R Biol* 326:1067–1072.

Shyamsundar, R., Y. H. Kim, J. P. Higgins et al. 2005. A DNA microarray survey of gene expression in normal human tissues. *Genome Biol* 6:R22.

Sinha, R., T. Lenser, N. Jahn et al. 2010. TassDB2—A comprehensive database of subtle alternative splicing events. *BMC Bioinform* 11:216.

Spurlock, D. M., T. G. McDaneld, and L. M. McIntyre. 2006. Changes in skeletal muscle gene expression following clenbuterol administration. *BMC Genom* 7:320.

Srikanchai, T., E. Murani, K. Wimmers, and S. Ponsuksili. 2010. Four loci differentially expressed in muscle tissue depending on water-holding capacity are associated with meat quality in commercial pig herds. *Mol Biol Rep* 37:595–601.

Su, A. I., T. Wiltshire, S. Batalov et al. 2004. A gene atlas of the mouse and human protein-encoding transcriptomes. *Proc Natl Acad Sci USA* 101:6062–6067.

Takeda, J.-I., Y. Suzuki, R. Sakate et al. 2010. H-DBAS: Human-transcriptome database for alternative splicing: Update 2010. *Nucleic Acids Res* 38:D86–D90.

Tang, Z., Y. Li, P. Wan et al. 2007. LongSAGE analysis of skeletal muscle at three prenatal stages in Tongcheng and Landrace pigs. *Genome Biol* 8:R115.

Te Pas, M. F. W., A. A. De Wit, J. Priem et al. 2005. Transcriptome expression profiles in prenatal pigs in relation to myogenesis. *J Muscle Res Cell Motil* 26:157–165.

Te Pas, M. F. W., I. Hulsegge, A. Coster, M. H. Pool, H. H. Heuven, and L. L. G. Janss. 2007. Biochemical pathways analysis of microarray results: Regulation of myogenesis in pigs. *BMC Dev Biol* 7:66.

Tuccoli, A., L. Poliseno, and G. Rainaldi. 2006. miRNAs regulate miRNAs: Coordinated transcriptional and post-transcriptional regulation. *Cell Cycle* 5:2473–2476.

Tuggle, C. K., Y. Wang, and O. Couture. 2007. Advances in swine transcriptomics. *Int J Biol Sci* 3:132–152.

Turner, D. J., T. M. Keane, I. Sudbery, and D. J. Adams. 2009. Next-generation sequencing of vertebrate experimental organisms. *Mamm Genome* 20:327–338.

Turro, E., A. Lewin, A. Rose, M. J. Dallman, and S. Richardson. 2010. MMBGX: A method for estimating expression at the isoform level and detecting differential splicing using whole-transcript Affymetrix arrays. *Nucleic Acids Res* 38:e4.

Uenishi, H., T. Eguchi, K. Suzuki et al. 2004. PEDE (Pig EST Data Explorer): Construction of a database for ESTs derived from porcine full-length cDNA libraries. *Nucleic Acids Res* 32:D484–D488.

Uenishi, H., T. Eguchi-Ogawa, H. Shinkai et al. 2007. PEDE (Pig EST Data Explorer) has been expanded into Pig Expression Data Explorer, including 10 147 porcine full-length cDNA sequences. *Nucleic Acids Res* 35:D650–D653.

Van Laere, A.-S., M. Nguyen, M. Braunschweig et al. 2003. A regulatory mutation in IGF2 causes a major QTL effect on muscle growth in the pig. *Nature* 425:832–836.

Velculescu, V. E., L. Zhang, B. Vogelstein, and K. W. Kinzler. 1995. Serial analysis of gene expression. *Science* 270:484–487.

Wang, Z., M. Gerstein, and M. Snyder. 2009. RNA-Seq: A revolutionary tool for transcriptomics. *Nat Rev Genet* 10:57–63.

Wang, X.-L., K.-L. Wu, N. Li et al. 2006. Analysis of expressed sequence tags from skeletal muscle-specific cDNA library of Chinese native Xiang pig. *Yi Chuan Xue Bao/Acta Genet Sin* 33:984–991.

Wilhelm, B. T. and J.-R. Landry. 2009. RNA-Seq-quantitative measurement of expression through massively parallel RNA-sequencing. *Methods* 48:249–257.

Wimmers, K., E. Murani, and S. Ponsuksili. 2010. Functional genomics and genetical genomics approaches towards elucidating networks of genes affecting meat performance in pigs. *Brief Funct Genom* 9:251–258.

Xie, S. S., T. H. Huang, Y. Shen et al. 2010. Identification and characterization of microRNAs from porcine skeletal muscle. *Anim Genet* 41:179–190.

Yao, J., P. M. Coussens, P. Saama, S. Suchyta, and C. W. Ernst. 2002. Generation of expressed sequence tags from a normalized porcine skeletal muscle cDNA library. *Anim Biotechnol* 13:211–222.

Ying, S.-Y. and S.-L. Lin. 2009. Intron-mediated RNA interference and microRNA biogenesis. *Method Mol Biol* 487:387–413.

Zhang, J., Q. He, Q. Y. Liu et al. 2007a. Differential gene expression profile in pig adipose tissue treated with/without clenbuterol. *BMC Genom* 8:433.

Zhang, W., Q. D. Morris, R. Chang et al. 2004. The functional landscape of mouse gene expression. *J Biol* 3:21.

Zhang, L., L. Tao, L. Ye et al. 2007b. Alternative splicing and expression profile analysis of expressed sequence tags in domestic pig. *Genom Proteom Bioinform* 5:25–34.

Zhao, E., M. P. Keller, M. E. Rabaglia et al. 2009. Obesity and genetics regulate microRNAs in islets, liver, and adipose of diabetic mice. *Mamm Genome* 20:476–485.

Zhao, S.-H., J. Recknor, J. K. Lunney et al. 2005. Validation of a first-generation long-oligonucleotide microarray for transcriptional profiling in the pig. *Genomics* 86:618–625.

Zhou, B. and H.-L. Liu. 2010. Computational identification of new porcine microRNAs and their targets. *Anim Sci J* 81:290–296.

Zhou, B., H. L. Liu, F. X. Shi, J. Y. Wang. 2010. MicroRNA expression profiles of porcine skeletal muscle. *Anim Genet* 41:499–508.

Zhu, L., M. Li, X. Li et al. 2009. Distinct expression patterns of genes associated with muscle growth and adipose deposition in Tibetan pigs: A possible adaptive mechanism for high altitude conditions. *High Alt Med Biol* 10:45–55.

# 13 Meat Science and Proteomics

*Kristin Hollung and Eva Veiseth-Kent*

## CONTENTS

## 13.1 INTRODUCTION

Quality traits of muscle foods are influenced by a number of different factors such as genetics, environmental factors, and processing conditions. While the genes remain more or less constant during the lifetime of the animal, the expression of the genes to mRNA and proteins is regulated by a large number of factors such as environmental and processing conditions, which may have an impact on different meat quality traits. However, the underlying molecular mechanisms determining these quality traits are far from understood. The proteome is the protein complement of the genome and consists of the total amount of proteins expressed at a certain time point and may thus be viewed as the mirror image of the gene activity (Wilkins et al. 1996). While the genome contains the information on genes and alleles that are present in the genome, the proteome contains information on genes that are actually being expressed and translated into proteins. In contrast to the genome, the proteome is continuously changing according to factors influencing either protein synthesis or degradation. Thus, analyzing the proteome can be viewed as analyzing snapshots of a system in constant change. In this regard, the proteome can be seen as the molecular link between the genome and the functional quality of the muscle or meat. Thus, understanding the variations and different components of the proteome with regard to certain quality or processing parameters will lead to knowledge that can be used in optimizing the conversion of muscles to meat (Bendixen 2005, Bendixen et al. 2005, Hollung et al. 2007, Mullen et al. 2006).

In contrast to traditional methods, studying one or a few specific genes or proteins at a time, studies can now be conducted without any a priori hypotheses on the mechanisms involved. Proteomics are the tools used to analyze the proteomes. Over the last decades, there have been significant improvements of methods. Basically, there are two analytical strategies used in proteomics. One is based on two-dimensional gel electrophoresis (2-DE) for separation of proteins, followed by identification of separated proteins by mass spectrometry (MS). The other is based on liquid chromatography (LC) in one or more dimensions, coupled with MS.

We will give a brief overview of the two strategies in the following sections. Although several attempts have been made, there is yet no single method spanning the whole proteome in one experiment (Li et al. 2005, Melchior et al. 2009, Patel et al. 2009).

## 13.2  MUSCLE PROTEIN SOLUBILIZATION AND FRACTIONATION

Based on the sequence of the *Bos taurus* genome, it has been estimated that the cattle genome contains a minimum of 22,000 genes (Elsik et al. 2009). Taking into account the possible posttranslational modifications, the number of different proteins is even higher. However, only a subset of the proteins is expressed in each cell type, tissue, or within a specific time frame. In muscle tissue, the proteins are localized in different compartments. Some proteins are part of large protein aggregates, like the myofibrillar proteins. Other proteins are localized in membranes and yet others are enzymes localized in the cytoplasm. The functional role and cellular localization will also affect the solubility of the protein. So far no single method has been able to separate and analyze all these different proteins in a single experiment. Thus, there is a need for fractionation of the muscle proteins to simplify the composition of different proteins.

The proteins one chooses to investigate in an experiment will determine the choice of prefractionation strategy. Using prefractionation techniques based on solubilization and extraction procedures on muscle, the enrichment of soluble sarcoplasmic or myofibrillar proteins can be achieved. These proteins have very different chemical properties that can be used to isolate the proteins in different fractions.

Several established protein and peptide fractionation techniques including stepwise extractions of proteins, immunodepletion, reverse phase or ion exchange chromatography, and gel filtration are being used, for a review see (Righetti et al. 2005). The choice of technique is greatly dependent on the subset of proteins that is of interest. To avoid protein losses, it is always advisable to keep sample preparation as simple as possible. However, if low-abundance proteins are of interest or if only a subset of the proteins in the tissues or cells is of interest, prefractionation can be employed during sample preparation. Depending on the project and hypothesis, different strategies for extraction and prefractionation of muscle proteins should be considered. Typically, approximately 1000 different proteins can be analyzed on one 2-DE image and one needs to assure that the most interesting proteins are among the proteins that are actually studied.

The presence of high-abundance proteins masks low-abundance proteins and thus generally prevents their detection and identification in proteome studies. Presence of actin and tubulin in a muscle tissue extract will typically mask the presence of sarcoplasmic enzymes of lower abundance or proteins with similar pI and molecular weight (MW). Prefractionation of the protein sample can lead to identification and detection of low-abundance proteins that may ultimately prove to be informative biomarkers. If the aim is to analyze the sarcoplasmic proteins, these are usually easy to solubilize without capturing the structural proteins. However, to enrich the structural proteins one might wish to remove the easily soluble proteins first and then solubilize the structural proteins in a second step using a urea buffer.

The protein solubility is also dependent on the pH of the extraction buffer and the internal muscle pH. During postmortem storage of meat, the muscle pH drops from neutral to a pH close to 5.5 depending on muscle and animal. We have observed a shift in the solubility of several proteins during postmortem storage of beef (Bjarnadottir et al. 2010, Jia et al. 2007a). In this study, proteins that are present in the sarcoplasmic easily soluble protein fraction early postmortem, like creatine kinase and glycerol-3-phosphate dehydrogenase, are becoming more abundant in the insoluble protein fraction after 2 days of storage. The same observation is done in other studies where easily soluble proteins are identified in the insoluble protein fraction of pork and beef (Boles et al. 1992, Laville et al. 2009a, Zapata et al. 2009). This may indicate a shift in protein solubility during postmortem storage of meat. It has been suggested that this shift is caused by changes in temperature and pH postmortem (Laville et al. 2009a, Pulford et al. 2008, Zapata et al. 2009). This may result in chemical modification or denaturation followed by aggregation of the proteins (Boles et al. 1992, Laville et al. 2009a). Probably, the shift in solubility depends on the protein and is most likely caused by several mechanisms.

For comprehensive proteome analysis by 2-DE, prefractionation is essential for several reasons. First, by partitioning the proteome into compartments, the complexity of each compartment is reduced, facilitating spot identification and quantitative analysis. Second, there is a pronounced bias inherent in 2-DE toward abundant proteins, which has the effect of masking low-abundance proteins. Prefractionation enriches low-abundance proteins. Third, the amount of any specific protein that can be resolved on a 2-DE is limited. Prefractionation allows the proteins present in a particular fraction to be loaded at high levels, further increasing the representation of low-abundance proteins. Finally, the number of proteins that are solubilized during the differential extraction procedures is greatly increased, yielding a more comprehensive representation of the proteome.

It is important to keep in mind that whatever method is chosen for prefractionation or proteome analysis, there is no protocol yet providing an analysis of the complete proteome of complex samples in one run. Several groups have tried to compare different strategies on the same samples, ending up with only partly overlapping results (Bodenmiller et al. 2007, Bodnar et al. 2003, Frohlich et al. 2006, Grove et al. 2006,

Li et al. 2005, McDonald et al. 2006, Melchior et al. 2009, Patel et al. 2009, Wu et al. 2006). This demonstrates that none of the methods are superior and that in most cases more information is obtained on the samples by combining different methods.

Usually, a few hundred to several thousand proteins are analyzed in one experimental setup. Choice of extraction method for the proteins is determining which proteins can be studied, and proteins that are not extracted will thus not be considered. It is necessary to bear in mind that this still is only a small part of the entire proteome. Thus it is important to draw conclusions based on the proteins that are actually under investigation and not extrapolate the results to the proteins that failed to be analyzed. Careful consideration should be made to choose the most optimal strategy for analysis of the data resulting from these experiments.

## 13.3 TOOLS FOR SEPARATION OF PROTEINS (2-DE AND MS)

### 13.3.1 Two-Dimensional Gel Electrophoresis

In meat science, the most common method for proteome analyses is based on separation of proteins using 2-DE followed by identification of specific proteins with MALDI-MS. Separation of proteins by 2-DE is an old method (O'Farrell 1975). However, major technical improvements such as the introduction of immobilized pH gradients have been important for the reproducibility of the method, for a review see (Gorg et al. 2000, 2004). In addition to semiquantitative information on the proteins that are present in the sample, 2-DE also provides information on modifications, as the same protein may occur in several spots in the gels. A schematic diagram of the workflow of a 2-DE-based proteome analysis is shown in Figure 13.1.

Following extraction and sample preparation, the proteins are first separated by charge using isoelectric focusing (IEF), and then the focused proteins are separated by mass using SDS-PAGE. For reproducible and comparable results, IEF is usually performed in immobilized pH gradients. Length and pH range of the gel strip determines the scale of separation. The gradients are usually between 7 and 24 cm long, with a pH range of wide gradients (e.g., 3–10), medium gradients (e.g., 4–7), or narrow gradients (e.g., 4.5–5.5) (Gorg et al. 2004). The protein composition and complexity of the sample determines which gradient will provide most information. Proteomes of low complexity can usually be separated on a wide gradient, while a narrow gradient is needed to separate more complex samples. A narrow gradient will reduce the number of overlapping protein spots. However, conclusions can only be drawn based on the separated proteins that are being analyzed. Thus the proteins having a pI outside the pH range or a high or low MW will not be part of the investigation, although they may be involved in the experimental response. In addition, very hydrophobic proteins,

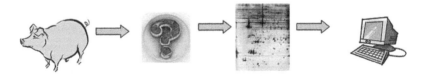

**FIGURE 13.1** Schematic overview of the workflow in a 2-DE proteomics experiment.

membrane proteins, and high MW proteins are often difficult to solubilize and to ana-lyze by 2-DE (Fey and Larsen 2001, Gorg et al. 2004). These are among the major limitations with 2-DE analyses compared to gel-free systems.

In addition to the separation, there is a need for a robust method for quantification of the protein spots to be able to compare the protein abundance profiles between samples. Because of the great differences in protein concentration in the different protein spots in the gel, this can be challenging. Thus the method must be highly sen-sitive to detect the low-abundance proteins, it must have a high and linear dynamic range, and finally it should be compatible with protein identification methods like MS. Although the protein stains are continuously improving, there are no methods meeting all of these demands (Grove et al. 2009, Lopez 2007, Patton 2000, 2002).

Basically, two different principles can be used to visualize the proteins on a 2-DE gel. Either the proteins are labeled with radioactivity or fluorescent tags prior to separation or the proteins are stained in the gel after separation using either fluo-rescent or nonfluorescent dyes. Fluorescent dyes have the advantage of a high linear dynamic range, but they are more expensive compared to traditional stains like silver or coomassie brilliant blue (CBB) and demand the use of a robot for spot picking as the spots are not visible by the eye.

The other principle is to label the proteins prior to electrophoresis of which the most common method is the difference gel electrophoresis (DIGE) (Unlu et al. 1997). A major advantage with DIGE is the simultaneous separation of samples in a single gel using different labels for each sample. Up to three samples are commonly separated on the same gel. An advantage of this is that comigration of the same proteins from different samples are secured, thus simplifying the analysis between the samples.

As in other -omics data, there is a need for a special attention to analysis and statistical validation of the results. In contrast to traditional experiments with few measurements/variables in many samples/animals, the opposite is true for pro-teomics data. In most -omics analyses, the number of samples are kept at a mini-mum due to costly and time-consuming analysis. However, the amount of data that is collected from each sample can be huge. This puts requirements on the statistical analysis. Several statistical approaches have been used to analyze proteomics data. Multivariate analyses such as principal component analysis (PCA) have proven to be a very useful tool for validation of data from 2-DE experiments and to identify and remove outliers from the analyses. Multivariate approaches have also been used for selection of significant changes in the 2-DE data according to the design parameters (Jessen et al. 2002, Jia et al. 2006a, Kjaersgard et al. 2006). Assessment of hierarchi-cal clustering methodologies, commonly used in transcriptomics studies, has also been performed on proteomics data (Meunier et al. 2007). The different statistical methods will shed light on different aspects of the proteomics data as has been dis-cussed in several papers (Jacobsen et al. 2007, Maurer et al. 2005).

In contrast to the gel-free methods, only the proteins that are changed accord-ing to the experimental design are identified. The most common MS protein iden-tification technique is called peptide mass fingerprinting (PMF) (Yates et al. 1993). The unknown protein is cleaved into peptides by a residue-specific enzyme such as trypsin. The absolute masses of the peptides are accurately measured with a mass

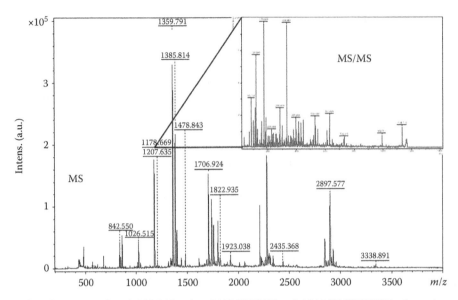

**FIGURE 13.2** MS and MS/MS using MALDI-TOF and MALDI-TOF/TOF of porcine malate dehydrogenase. Peak 1178 *m/z* is selected for MS/MS analysis.

spectrometer, and the matching of these absolute masses against theoretical peptide libraries generated from protein sequence databases is used to create a list of likely protein identifications. Matrix-assisted laser desorption ionization (MALDI) (Hillenkamp et al. 1991) is most common for analysis of peptides from 2-DE gels because of its robustness and ease of use. To confirm the PMF-based protein identification, MS/MS analysis and repeated MASCOT database searches of several precursor ions recognized in the PMF search can be performed, see Figure 13.2. However, several factors including both experimental and theoretical pI values, the number of peptide matches, as well as sequence coverage are used to evaluate the database search results. Hence PMF-based protein identification is greatly facilitated in organisms for which the genomes have been fully sequenced. In meat science, PMF analysis has been successfully applied to identify proteins from muscles of different species (Hamelin et al. 2006, 2007, Kwasiborski et al. 2008a,b, Lametsch et al. 2002, 2003, 2006, Laville et al. 2007, Morzel et al. 2004, 2008, Sayd et al. 2006).

### 13.3.2 Gel-Free Methods

Gel-free analyses of complex protein samples are based on different combinations of LC and MS. The proteins are usually digested with trypsin prior to LC for a prefractionation of the peptides. The different fractions resulting from one or two LC runs are then analyzed by MS. In some LC-MS approaches, a first separation is performed by SDS-PAGE. The lane containing the sample is then divided in areas that are excised and digested to release the peptides that are then used in LC for the next separation step. The mass analyzer separates the ions according to their mass-to-charge ratio. Several types of analyzers exist including time-of-flight (TOF), quadrupole ion trap, quadrupole (Q), and Fourier transform ion cyclotron resonance (FTICR) mass analyzers (Shen et al. 2001).

To obtain the amino acid sequence of the peptides, the peptides need to be fragmented and analyzed by a separate analyzer. The MS/MS instruments contain two analyzers that can be of the same or of different types, such as Q-TOF or TOF/TOF. The two analyzers are separated by a collision cell that has the function to fragment and activate the precursor ion from the first analyzer. The fragmentation spectrum can be recorded in the second analyzer and true sequence data can be achieved. The most commonly used tandem mass spectrometers for proteomics applications are the tandem quadrupole, Q-TOF, and TOF/TOF instruments (Aebersold and Mann 2003). As the MS instruments are becoming more common and also more robust and easy to use, they also gain more attention among meat scientists. A great challenge with these gel-free analyses is the huge amount of redundant and non-informative data generated in each experiment.

Several methods have been developed to assist in quantitative comparisons between samples using MS-based approaches, for a recent review see (Elliott et al. 2009). These include both selective labeling of the samples to create mass shifts for comparison of peaks such as stable isotope labeling by amino acids (SILAC) (Ong et al. 2002), isotope-coded affinity tag (ICAT) (Gygi et al. 1999), and iTRAQ (Ross et al. 2004). These methods are fundamentally different in the aspect of when the tag is introduced to the sample and thus at what time point in the procedure the samples being compared are mixed. Other methods are based on inclusion of internal standards such as multiple reaction monitoring (MRM) (Lange et al. 2008) and selected reaction monitoring (SRM) (Picotti et al. 2007, 2009, 2010). However, these techniques require that the target proteins selected for quantification are identified and have been applied on a selected number of proteins in each analysis. High-throughput SRM methods based on crude synthetic peptide libraries are being developed that will greatly improve this strategy for quantitative comparisons between samples (Picotti et al. 2010). Label-free approaches are also being used. These are either based on comparison of signal intensities of the most intense peptides from specific proteins in different samples or by counting and comparisons of the number of MS/MS spectra obtained from a single protein (Chen 2008).

## 13.4   INTRODUCTION TO MEAT/MUSCLE QUALITY

### 13.4.1   Meat Quality Parameters

Meat quality can be determined by multiple features, including palatability, color, water-holding capacity, and nutritional value, and the importance of these features for describing meat quality can vary both between muscles within a carcass and between different breeds and species. Of these features, palatability and water-holding capacity are the two that have received most attention in meat science, probably because these are considered the most critical traits describing beef and pork meat quality. Much has been revealed regarding the factors that contribute to variation in these traits. However, due to the complexity of the underlying mechanisms, it is necessary to improve the knowledge at a molecular level, and consequently one can observe a shift in meat science toward implementation of different -omics technologies.

Meat palatability is mainly determined by three traits: flavor, juiciness, and tenderness. However, these do not contribute equally toward overall palatability, and the importance of each trait varies depending on the type of meat and the consumer profile. While consumers in New Zealand and Australia find lamb odor and flavor attractive, American consumers dislike these traits (Field et al. 1983), and whereas Scandinavian consumers rank flavor as the most important trait of pork (Bryhni et al. 2002), German consumers select pork based on fat content and color (Bredahl et al. 1998). When it comes to beef quality, 50% of the consumers in the United States said that tenderness was the most important quality trait (Miller et al. 1995).

Although individual muscles within a carcass vary in function and design, the essential structural features remain similar. An innervating and vascular network pervades the muscle tissue along with a stabilizing network comprised of connective tissue. In skeletal muscles, the connective tissue network can be divided into three categories: the epimysium surrounding the entire muscle, the perimysium surrounding bundles of muscle fibers, and the endomysium surrounding individual muscle fibers (see Figure 13.3). The muscle fibers contain structures called myofibrils that form the foundation of the contractile system of muscles, and the basic unit of this system is the sarcomere. The sarcomere is formed by bundles of overlapping or interlaced actin and myosin filaments bracketed by Z-discs, and this unit is repeated throughout the entire length of the myofibrils. Individual myofibrils are connected to one another through a three-dimensional lattice of intermediate filaments around the Z-discs, and another structural lattice, the costamere, serve to attach myofibrils to the plasma membrane.

## 13.4.2 CHANGES OCCURRING AFTER SLAUGHTER

Skeletal muscle is a dynamic tissue that even after slaughter will seek to maintain a physiologically balanced internal environment, and many of the cellular events that occur postmortem are direct results of this effort to maintain homeostasis. After exsanguination, the transport of nutrients and waste products stops, and when the oxygen supply ceases, the energy metabolism will switch from aerobic to anaerobic and lead to production and accumulation of lactic acid. The production of lactic acid will continue until the muscle stores of glycogen are depleted and result in a pH decline in postmortem muscle typically from pH 7 to 5.6. This pH decline together with other biochemical changes and temperature decline during cooling of carcasses will lead to the development of *rigor mortis*.

*Rigor mortis* describes the stiffening of postmortem muscle and occurs due to *postmortem* changes affecting the contractile apparatus. The contractile apparatus of muscle is dependent upon adenosine triphosphate (ATP) and calcium for muscle contraction. In the living muscle, $Ca^{2+}$ ions are under strict control, and the sarcoplasmic reticulum (SR) and mitochondria constantly sequester and store $Ca^{2+}$ ions by means of ion pumps. Following death, declines in both pH and temperature lead to reduced ion pump efficiency (Whiting 1980), and additionally the reduced temperature causes the SR membrane to become permeable to calcium (Jaime et al. 1992,

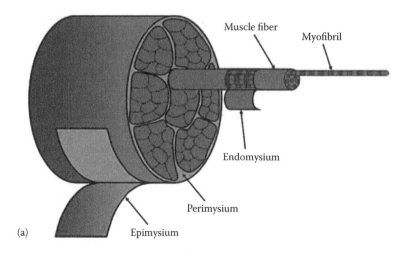

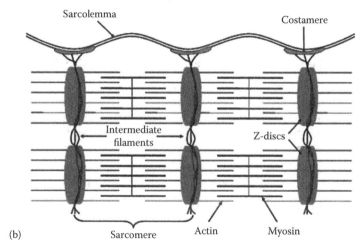

**FIGURE 13.3** Schematic drawing of skeletal muscle architecture at a macro- (a) and ultra-structural (b) level.

Jeacocke 1993). The net effect of these two changes is an increase in intracellular $Ca^{2+}$ concentration and formation of the tightly bound actin–myosin complex. If the muscle is depleted of ATP at this point, this complex cannot be released and the muscle becomes inextensible, that is, enters *rigor mortis*. However, it is very common to see a shortening of the muscle postmortem, and this is explained by the release of $Ca^{2+}$ ions while ATP concentrations remain sufficiently high for contraction (Honikel et al. 1983).

### 13.4.3 TENDERNESS

Since palatability, and particularly tenderness, is a central feature of meat quality, much research has been performed during the last decades in order to understand what contributes to the variation in meat tenderness. Significant variation in meat tenderness can be seen when comparing different muscles within an animal and when comparing the same muscle from different breeds and species (Arsenos et al. 2002, Ramsbottom et al. 1945, Shackelford et al. 1991, Strandine et al. 1949). The ultimate tenderness of meat is largely affected by three factors: the background toughness of meat, the toughening phase, and the tenderization phase. While the background toughness is thought to be a constant value established at slaughter, the opposing toughening and tenderization phases take place during postmortem storage.

Background toughness of meat results from the connective tissue component, and is defined as "the resistance to shearing of the unshortened muscle" (Marsh and Leet 1966). It is particularly the variation in composition, amount, and spatial organization of the connective tissue that is thought to affect background toughness (Purslow 2005). As mentioned earlier, the background toughness is not thought to change during postmortem storage; however, several groups have shown that the structural integrity and strength of the endo- and perimysium are weakened during aging of meat, and thus suggesting that these structures play a more active role in the tenderization phase (Hannesson et al. 2003, Nishimura et al. 1995).

The toughening phase is caused by the shortening of sarcomeres during rigor development (Wheeler and Koohmaraie 1994), and this usually occurs during the first 24 h postmortem, after which the sarcomere length does not change (Wheeler and Koohmaraie 1999). The relationship between sarcomere length and meat toughness is defined as curvilinear, with a strong negative relationship between sarcomere length and meat toughness when sarcomeres are shorter than 2 μm and a poor relationship when sarcomeres are longer than 2 μm (Bouton et al. 1973, Herring et al. 1967).

Meat tenderness is known to improve during cooler storage, and in 1917 it was suggested that these changes were mainly due to enzymatic activities (Hoagland et al. 1917). The tenderization phase has received much attention in meat science, and it is well known that tenderization is a result of degradation of key myofibrillar and associated proteins, whose main function is to maintain the structural integrity of the myofibrils (Taylor et al. 1995). Once some of these proteins are degraded, the rigid structure of the myofibrils is weakened and meat becomes more tender. There has been much debate regarding the proteolytic systems that take part in this degradation process; however, there is substantial evidence that the calpain proteolytic system plays a major role in this process (for reviews see Goll et al. 1991, Koohmaraie 1996).

## 13.5 CHANGES IN PROTEIN COMPOSITION DURING POSTMORTEM STORAGE

Studying postmortem changes in the proteome will lead to an increased understanding of the biochemical mechanisms behind meat quality traits, such as tenderness. A number of studies have described how postmortem degradation of myofibrillar protein may be involved in meat tenderness, and in particular, the degradation patterns of contractile proteins have been described in detail (Geesink and Koohmaraie 1999, Melody et al. 2004, Taylor et al. 1995).

Lately, proteomics has been used to study changes occurring in muscle during *postmortem* storage. Total protein extracts from pork *longissimus dorsi* samples collected at 0, 4, 8, 24, and 48 h after slaughter revealed that 15 proteins were changed, some increasing and some decreasing in abundance after slaughter (Lametsch and Bendixen 2001, Lametsch et al. 2002). Several of these proteins were identified as fragments of structural proteins such as actin, myosin heavy chain, and troponin T. Earlier studies using one-dimensional SDS-PAGE have concluded that actin is not degraded postmortem (Bandman and Zdanis 1988; Huff-Lonergan et al. 1995, Koohmaraie 1994). However, using 2-DE, the resolution allows for a better separation of the different actin fragments and demonstrates the potential of 2-DE. Some of the actin fragments observed in postmortem pork muscle were also significantly correlated with tenderness. In addition, several metabolic enzymes involved in energy metabolism were altered in the pork muscle.

During postmortem storage, the calpain system is believed to be important for degradation of myofibrillar proteins and development of tenderness (Goll et al. 1991, Koohmaraie 1994, 1996). In a proteome study in pork *longissimus dorsi* muscle, several of the myofibrillar substrates for μ-calpain were identified (Lametsch et al. 2004). Among the substrates that were degraded by *in vitro* incubation with μ-calpain were desmin, actin, myosin heavy chain, myosin light chain I, troponin T, tropomyosin α1, tropomyosin α4, thioredoxin, and CapZ.

Changes in metabolic protein composition in biopsies from live animals to *postmortem* samples collected shortly after slaughter in bovine *longissimus dorsi* muscle revealed that 24 protein spots were changed (Jia et al. 2006a). This reflects the contribution of several factors such as transportation, lairage, stunning, exsanguination, and dehiding on the *longissimus dorsi* muscle proteome. Identification of the proteins by MALDI-TOF/TOF MS revealed that a wide range of metabolic enzymes and stress proteins increased in abundance after slaughter. Several of these proteins were glycolytic enzymes such as enolase, aldehyde dehydrogenase, phosphoglycerate kinase, or enzymes involved in oxidative metabolism such as ATP-specific succinyl-CoA synthetase and isocitrate dehydrogenase. This supports an expected shift in energy metabolism in the muscle postmortem via the glycolytic pathway and also an increase in aerobic energy metabolism the first hour after slaughter.

In a comparative study, comparing the soluble and insoluble protein fraction from bovine *longissimus thoracis* muscle, four out of six metabolic enzymes were found in both protein fractions (Bjarnadottir et al. 2010, Jia et al. 2007). These were adenylate kinase 1, creatine kinase (two fragments), and glycerol-3-phosphate dehydrogenase 1. In both fractions, glycerol-3-phosphate dehydrogenase decreased in abundance postmortem, while the other three enzymes increased in abundance. A total of six proteins from the group of cellular defense/stress proteins were found in both protein fractions. All of them were HSP 27, and four were found to increase in abundance shortly after slaughter and then decrease over longer time period postmortem. In the group of cell structure proteins, only actin was identified in both of the protein fractions. However, only one spot was identified as actin in the soluble protein fraction while five were found in the insoluble protein fraction. Even though actin is, in theory, a component of the insoluble protein fraction, some copies have been found to be extracted with soluble proteins (Jia et al. 2006b). There were many proteins that were only changed in abundance in either the soluble or the insoluble protein fraction. It might be that the proteins that were detected in both of the protein fractions are more exposed to changes in solubility than those that were only found in the soluble protein fraction.

Changes in the muscle proteome between slaughter and 24 h storage in bovine *longissimus dorsi* and *semitendinosus* muscles were observed both between the sampling times and between the *longissimus dorsi* and *semitendinosus* muscles (Jia et al. 2006b). In this study, five proteins were changed in both muscles, namely, cofilin, lactoylglutathione lyase, substrate protein of mitochondrial ATP-dependent proteinase SP-22, HSP 27, and HSP 20. However, 15 proteins were changed in either *longissimus dorsi* or *semitendinosus* muscles. These differences reflect distinct metabolic and physiological functions of the different muscles.

## 13.6   MOLECULAR UNDERSTANDING OF MEAT QUALITY

Meat quality is comprised of many different features; however, tenderness is the trait that has been studied most extensively with the use of proteomics. Studies have been undertaken to unravel the underlying mechanisms behind this trait and to find potential protein biomarkers that can be used for prediction of meat tenderness. By using 1-DE for protein fingerprinting, seven protein bands were found from bovine *longissimus dorsi* muscles sampled at 36 h postmortem that together could explain 82% of the variation in Warner-Bratzler shear force (WBSF) observed in these muscles after 7 d of storage (Sawdy et al. 2004). Two of these bands were identified as fragments of myosin heavy chain, and the levels of these fragments at 36 h postmortem were elevated in the tender muscles. Similarly, several protein bands from the myofibrillar fraction of bovine *longissimus dorsi* muscle at 36 h postmortem were reported to correlate with WBSF measured at 72 h or 14 d postmortem and the difference in WBSF between these timepoints (Zapata et al. 2009). After identification of the proteins in these bands, several interesting trends were observed such as the occurrence of several structural proteins and enzymes involved in energy metabolism and the presence of heat shock and chaperone proteins. Since these protein bands were composed of a mixture of proteins, no conclusion could be made regarding which of these proteins were playing a direct role in the mechanisms underlying meat tenderness (Zapata et al. 2009).

However, by applying the more detailed 2-DE approach, succinate dehydrogenase (SDH), a mitochondrial enzyme of the TCA cycle, was identified as an early predictor (1 h postmortem) of bovine *longissimus thoracis* sensory tenderness at 14 d postmortem (Morzel et al. 2008). The abundance of the SDH protein spot was able to explain 66% and 58% of the variation in initial and overall tenderness, respectively. The major result of this study was however the significant positive correlation observed between initial levels of HSP 27 and both initial ($r = 0.89$) and overall tenderness ($r = 0.97$). The initial levels of HSP 27 were related to more actin fragmentation during storage, and it was suggested that HSP 27 would prevent actin aggregation and thereby facilitate proteolytic degradation of this protein during postmortem storage (Morzel et al. 2008). In a different comparative study of tough and tender bovine *longissimus thoracis* muscle, 20 protein spots in the insoluble protein fraction differed in abundance between these groups at the time of slaughter (Laville et al. 2009a). Six of these were proteins located in the inner and outer membrane of the mitochondria, and all were more abundant in the tender group. According to Laville et al. (2009a), the increased extractability of these proteins in the tender group indicates a more extensive degradation of the mitochondrial membranes very early postmortem, which again suggests a role of apoptosis during the development of meat tenderness. While all of the aforementioned studies were performed with postmortem muscle samples, we analyzed bovine *longissimus thoracis* biopsies taken 4 d prior to slaughter by 2-DE to identify protein markers for WBSF measured 7 d postmortem (Jia et al. 2009). This study revealed seven protein spots that differed antemortem between the tough and tender muscles, however, only one protein, peroxiredoxin-6, was confirmed with Western blotting. Peroxiredoxin-6 is an enzyme that plays a role in protection against oxidative stress, and the elevated level of this enzyme in the tender group was also found in samples taken 1 h postmortem from the same animals.

While the quality-related proteomic studies on beef have mainly focused on meat tenderness, the studies in pork have often had a broader meat quality focus including traits such as water-holding capacity, color, and pH. By applying SELDI-TOF analysis of *longissimus dorsi* muscle from Yorkshire and Duroc pigs stored for different lengths postmortem and comparing these with measurements of WBSF and drip loss, several potential biomarkers for these two quality traits were found (te Pas et al. 2009). Similarly, 27 candidate proteins whose postmortem changes coincided with either WBSF, drip loss, and/or hunter $L*$ values during storage were found in *longissimus dorsi* muscle from Landrace pigs (Hwang et al. 2005). Specifically, 16 out of 25 protein spots, which were related to WBSF, were also associated with hunter $L*$ value, including several structural proteins in addition to metabolic enzymes and chaperone proteins, while only 3 protein spots were related to drip loss. The connection between structural proteins and tenderness in pork had also been reported in an earlier study, where three actin fragments and one myosin heavy chain fragment were significantly correlated with WBSF (Lametsch et al. 2003). In addition, the level of triose phosphate isomerase I was correlated with WBSF, indicating that postmortem glycolysis could play an important role in postmortem tenderization. Moreover, 14 protein spots with differential expression were identified in 2 groups of pigs differing with respect to several quality traits of the *longissimus lumborum* muscle (Laville et al. 2007). The largest relative difference in expression between the two groups was found for the fatty acid carrier A-FABP, a protein that plays a role in the deposit of triacylglycerol. The overexpression of this protein in the tender group corresponded with the higher level of intramuscular fat in this group. The tender animals also had a higher ultimate pH compared to the tough animals, which was interpreted to be a result of a more lipid-oriented energy metabolism in the tender animals (Laville et al. 2007). Interestingly, a four and a half LIM domain protein, whose proteolysis is correlated with weakening of the Z-line during meat storage, was found to be overexpressed in the tough group as shown for tough beef muscles (Laville et al. 2009a).

Water-holding capacity and pH decline are central quality traits especially in pork. Using 2-DE to develop models that could explain some of these traits showed that one or two protein spots could explain between 24% and 85% of the variability in pH decline, color, and water-holding capacity (Kwasiborski et al. 2008b). Proteins identified by the models for ultimate pH, lightness, and drip loss were related to glycolysis, phosphate transfer, and muscle fiber type, while a model for thawing loss contained proteins involved in denaturation of myofibrils. Thus, the proteins included in the models were often related to known postmortem mechanisms related to the different traits. Likewise, pork muscles giving rise to dark meat had high levels of enzymes involved in oxidative metabolism, while muscles giving rise to light meat had high levels of glycolytic enzymes (Sayd et al. 2006).

In summary, proteomics has proven to be a valuable tool to study the underlying mechanisms behind different meat quality traits. Many of the observed changes have been supportive of existing hypotheses regarding the development of meat quality. This includes the link between muscle pH decline and meat tenderness, which is apparent by the finding of several enzymes involved in glycolysis or the TCA cycle that correlates with tenderness, and the importance of postmortem degradation of structural proteins, seen as the occurrence of structural protein fragments and solubility changes. In addition, other findings have led to the suggestion of new mechanisms, such as the involvement of chaperone proteins and the possible role of apoptosis in the development of meat quality.

## 13.7  PRE-SLAUGHTER CONDITIONS AND EFFECTS ON MOLECULAR MECHANISMS

In addition to genetic and slaughter treatment effects, meat quality can also be affected by different pre-slaughter factors, including rearing conditions such as feed and feeding strategies in addition to handling, mixing, and transport of animals. Currently, proteomics has been used most extensively in relation to effects of feed and feeding strategies. Administration of clenbuterol and other $\beta_2$-agonists has been illegally used to promote growth in meat-producing animals by increasing protein deposition and decreasing body fat accumulation, and proteomics have been used in combination with gene expression analysis to study the mechanism by which clenbuterol reduces fat accumulation in pig adipose tissue (Zhang et al. 2007). The clenbuterol treatment resulted in about 10% increase in lean meat percentage, and histological analysis revealed that adipose cells became smaller, while muscle fibers became thicker. From the 2-DE, two protein spots were found to be only expressed in the treated group, and one of these were identified as apolipoprotein R (apoR). The gene expression analysis showed that 16 genes related to cellular metabolism were differentially expressed between the groups, and one of these was the gene encoding the apoR protein. Based on these findings, it was concluded that apoR could be one of the critical molecules responsible for the reduced fat accumulation in treated animals (Zhang et al. 2007). Tetracycline (TC) administration is another treatment that is known to have growth-promoting effects, and its effect on protein expression in pig *longissimus dorsi* muscle has been studied by 2-DE and MS (Gratacos-Cubarsi et al. 2008). Over 50 protein spots were found to differ as a result of the treatment, and 3 of these were only present in the TC group. Based on this, the authors concluded that proteomics could be a valuable tool to reveal illegal treatments with TC.

In chicken, proteomics has been applied to study effect of dietary methionine status on protein expression in the *pectoralis major* muscle (Corzo et al. 2006). Broilers were fed either a methionine-deficient (MD) or methionine-adequate (MA) diet, and the MD birds showed reduced carcass yield, increased abdominal fat, and reduced yield of boneless–skinless breast meat. Muscle proteins were extracted and subjected to trypsin treatment before analysis by LC-ESI-MS. Peptides from three proteins were exclusively present in the breast muscle of MD chickens: the glycolytic enzyme pyruvate kinase, the structural protein myosin alkali light chain-1, and ribosomal protein L-29. However, Corzo et al. (2006) felt it was premature to label any of these proteins as biomarkers for methionine deficiency, but the results illustrate the potential for use of proteomics in such studies. In another study of feed effects, the difference in *semitendinosus* muscle protein expression between grass-fed and grain-fed cattle was investigated (Shibata et al. 2009). The muscle proteins were separated into a sarcoplasmic and a myofibrillar fraction and 20 and 9 protein spots were found to differ in intensity with feeding in these fractions, respectively. The changes observed in the myofibrillar fraction indicated a conversion from fast-twitch to slow-twitch muscle tissue in the grass-fed cattle. The sarcoplasmic protein fraction supported this by showing higher levels of several enzymes involved in aerobic metabolism in the grass-fed group and increased levels of enzymes of anaerobic metabolism in the grain-fed group. Moreover, myoglobin levels were also increased in the grass-fed group, illustrating the greater need for oxygen to support the increased aerobic metabolism in these muscles. In a comparative study of control and compensatory growth in pigs, improved tenderness in the *longissimus dorsi* muscle was observed in the compensatory growth group, and seven proteins were found to have reduced levels in this group at the time of slaughter (Lametsch et al. 2006). The reduced levels of enolase 3 and glycerol-3-phosphate dehydrogenase, two glycolytic enzymes, were interpreted to indicate a decrease in the glycolytic potential in the muscle due to compensatory growth. Moreover, the increased levels of myosin light chain II and III seen in the compensatory growth group after 7 d postmortem was suggested to be a result of greater proteolytic activity during postmortem storage in these pigs (Lametsch et al. 2006).

## 13.8 INFLUENCE OF GENETICS ON MUSCLE BIOCHEMISTRY

It is well known that genetic variations among animals may have a large impact on both growth performance and different meat qualities (Boccard 1981, Koohmaraie et al. 1995, Shackelford et al. 1991, Whipple et al. 1990), and application of proteomics has recently gained interest as a tool to unravel the molecular mechanisms underlying these genetic effects. Several groups have used proteomics to study changes in protein expression between different pig breeds. By applying SELDI-TOF analysis, the effect of breed and muscle types on the expression of muscle proteins in pigs were evaluated (Mach et al. 2010). Although the number of peaks per spectrum was not affected by the different pig breeds (Landrace, Duroc, Large White, Pietrain, Belgian Landrace) or muscle types (LM and SM), differences were seen in the average intensity of the peaks. While four potential protein biomarkers were found to distinguish between the two muscle types, two potential protein biomarkers were found to differentiate between the different pure pig breeds. A disadvantage of this study from a biological perspective is the lack of identification of these potential protein biomarkers. However, several groups have applied 2-DE in combination with MS to study differences in muscle protein expression between different pig breeds, and thereby gained knowledge regarding which proteins are affected by breed. In a comparative study of protein expression in *longissimus* muscle from Meishan and Large White pigs, 14 proteins were found to differ between the 2 breeds (Xu et al. 2009). These included several metabolism-related proteins, myofibrillar regulatory proteins, and stress-related proteins. The observed changes in metabolic proteins indicated that the Large White pigs relied more heavily on glycolytic metabolism than the Meishan pigs (Xu et al. 2009). Moreover, two isoforms of cytosolic glycerol phosphate dehydrogenase, an enzyme that plays a central role in triglyceride synthesis, were upregulated in *longissimus* muscle of Meishan pigs. This breed-related difference is in accordance with the increased intramuscular fat of the Meishan pigs. Similarly, both breed- and age-related changes in protein expression were observed in the *adductor* muscle of Norwegian Landrace and Duroc pigs, which indicated a higher glycolytic activity in the Norwegian Landrace than in the Duroc pigs (Hollung et al. 2009).

Proteomics has also been used to study the effect of gene deletions and quantitative trait loci (QTLs) related to muscle hypertrophy. Myostatin is a protein that negatively controls myoblast proliferation and differentiation, and a loss of myostatin function results in a large and widespread increase in skeletal muscle mass. The effect of an 11bp deletion in the *myostatin* gene in Belgian blue bulls on protein expression in the *semitendinosus* muscle has been investigated (Bouley et al. 2005). Comparing bulls that were both homozygote and heterozygote for the deletion and bulls without the deletion revealed that the changes in protein expression were more significant in the homozygote than in the heterozygote bulls. Several structural and metabolic proteins were affected by the myostatin deletion, and these changes indicated a shift from oxidative to glycolytic metabolism, which was coherent with the observed shift toward a higher proportion of fast-twitch muscle fibers in animals with the myostatin deletion. Proteomics has also been used as a tool to identify alternative candidate genes that could be responsible for the QTL for muscle hypertrophy in Belgian strains of Texel sheep (Hamelin et al. 2006). By comparing protein expression in 4 hypertrophied or nonhypertrophied muscles, 63 protein spots were differentially expressed between the genotypes. In the two muscles prone for hypertrophy (i.e., *longissimus dorsi* and *semimembranosus*), the expression of proteins associated with glycolytic metabolism was greater in the Texel sheep. Moreover, actin alpha 1, HSP 27, and HSC 70 were upregulated in the hypertrophied muscles, which was interpreted to indicate an increased need for proteins essential to promote myofibril assembly in the hypertrophied muscles.

In pigs, two major genes are known to have a negative effect on water-holding capacity of the meat. Halothane (HAL)-positive pigs have a hastened postmortem glycolysis, while Rendement Napole (RN) mutant pigs have an increased capacity for extended glycolysis and pH decline giving an abnormal low ultimate pH. In a comparative proteomics study of the RN gene effect, alterations in the expression of 13 protein spots were observed in the *longissimus dorsi* muscle (Hedegaard et al. 2004). Two isoforms of UDP-glucose pyrophosphorylase (UDPGP) were upregulated in the carriers of the RN⁻ mutation, and based on the observed 2-DE patterns, it was suggested that these were differentially phosphorylated isoforms of UDPGP (Hedegaard et al. 2004). Earlier studies have indicated that the RN⁻ mutation may either be a loss-of-function mutation leading to reduced degradation of glycogen or a gain-of-function mutation resulting in increased glycogen synthesis (Milan et al. 2000). The results presented by Hedegaard et al. (2004) indicate that the RN⁻ mutation is a gain-of-function mutation, since the hyperaccumulation of glycogen is a result of increased glycogen synthesis. Effects of the HAL genotype have also been studied by proteomics, and in a comparative study of pigs that were homozygous normal (NN), heterozygous (Nn), and homozygous (nn) for the mutation, protein expression in *lungissimus lomborum* muscle was investigated by 2-DE (Laville et al. 2009b). Out of 300 matched spots, 55 protein spots showed a significant difference between the genotypes. The accelerated postmortem pH decline in nn muscles was not reflected in higher abundance of glycolytic enzymes. Moreover, the nn muscles were less oxidative and had reduced antioxidative and repair capacities compared to the other groups. Together, all these studies illustrate the power of proteomics to reveal the molecular mechanisms underlying different genetic effects on meat quality.

## 13.9 EFFECTS OF DRY CURING OF MEAT ON PROTEIN COMPOSITION

Proteolysis is a major factor affecting flavor and texture in long-aged dry-cured hams (Arnau et al. 1998, Parolari et al. 1994, Rosell and Toldra 1998, Virgili et al. 1998). A number of proteomics strategies have been applied lately to investigate proteolysis and protein changes in dry-cured hams. Using simple lab-on-a-chip technology, it has been shown that the different steps in Bayonne ham processing have a diagnostic protein pattern when separated in only one dimension providing potential markers for muscle and dry curing (Theron et al. 2009). This is a simple method to distinguish between different processing steps without prior knowledge on the affected proteins in the samples. Based on published results, some of the protein peaks are assigned to known muscle proteins; however, due to poor separation, each peak probably contains more than one protein. As would be expected, if proteolysis were to occur, there is a shift from more protein in the peaks of high-molecular-weight to the peaks of lower-molecular-weight proteolytic peptides.

Proteome analyses have also been used to study protein changes in dry-cured hams, an example is shown in Figure 13.4. In one study, the myofibrillar proteins of raw meat and dry-cured hams after 6, 10, and 14 months of ripening were analyzed by 2-DE (Di Luccia et al. 2005). Actin, tropomyosin, and myosin light chains

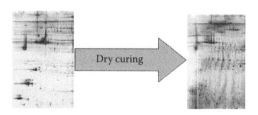

**FIGURE 13.4** Illustration of differences in protein composition between pork muscles before and after dry curing.

disappeared during the ripening period and were almost completely hydrolyzed after 12 months. In a pilot study of Norwegian dry-cured hams, we have earlier observed a variation in the protein degradation pattern between hams ripened for 6 months from different producers (Sidhu et al. 2005).

While the nature of the free amino acids in mature dry-cured hams is well established, the identity of the peptides present at the end of curing is poorly characterized. In a recent poster, three endogenous peptides resulting from degradation of myosin heavy chain were identified in Spanish Serrano dry-cured ham (Sentandreu et al. 2009). These peptides were identified in a deproteinated meat sample separated and identified using an LC-MALDI and ESI-ion trap MS approach. Although separated as three distinct peptides, they appeared to be overlapping spanning the amino acid region 371–387 and all sharing the same N-terminal end. This finding supports the involvement of cathepsin D as the cleavage site K-Q observed in the N-terminal end of these peptides are reported to result from cathepsin D cleavage in other proteins (Hasan et al. 2006). The same authors have previously reported the finding of four actin-derived oligopeptides in Spanish Serrano dry-cured ham using a similar protocol (Sentandreu et al. 2007). Two peptides with overlapping sequences originate from the C-terminal end of actin, and two peptides, also with overlapping sequences, originate from an internal region of actin. One of these peptides has been generated from bovine F-actin after *in vitro* digestion with cathepsin D, suggesting that cathepsin D may also be involved in the digestion of actin during processing of dry-cured hams.

Supportive evidence for the involvement of dipeptidyl peptidases in the generation of dipeptides in Spanish Serrano dry-cured hams was reported in another study using a proteomics approach (Mora et al. 2009b). Small peptides from myosin light chain I were identified, differing in the loss of one or two amino acids in the N-terminal end of the peptide. A similar observation was done for fragments of titin in the same experiment. Both myosin and titin are major myofibrillar proteins important for the texture of meat. Probably, the degradation and release of dipeptides from these proteins also contribute to flavor characteristics of these dry-cured hams. In a similar study of deproteinized samples from Spanish dry-cured ham, eight peptides corresponding to creatine kinase were identified using LC-MS/MS (Mora et al. 2009a). Creatine kinase is a sarcoplasmic enzyme involved in energy metabolism in muscles and is also used as an indicator of pre-slaughter stress or muscle damage in blood. In the first hours after slaughter, it has important functions related to the conversion of muscle to meat. Interestingly, all the identified peptides in this study correspond to the amino acid sequence between position 52 and 68 in the native protein, but the ends are somewhat different, suggesting that several proteases might have been involved in the degradation of this protein.

Using a proteomics approach, these studies have created a breakthrough in the understanding of development of flavor and texture properties in dry-cured products. These results were obtained due to the nature of the proteomics tools that make it possible to analyze and search for peptides without prior knowledge on the sequences to look for. Knowledge of these processes at the molecular level will in turn provide us with the tools needed to improve the production of dry-cured hams of superior quality, not only in the finished product but also during processing.

## 13.10 CONCLUSIONS

Proteomics has proven to be a valuable tool to study the underlying mechanisms behind different meat quality traits. Many of the observed changes have been supportive of existing hypotheses regarding the development of meat quality, while other observations have expanded the knowledge. Further studies using proteomics alone and in combination with other -omics methods will lead to an increased understanding of the biochemical mechanisms behind meat quality traits, such as tenderness. A number of studies have described how postmortem degradation of myofibrillar protein may be involved in meat tenderness and, in particular, the degradation of structural proteins, seen as the occurrence of structural protein fragments and solubility changes. In addition, other findings have led to the suggestion of new mechanisms, such as the involvement of chaperone proteins and the possible role of apoptosis in the development of meat quality. These results were obtained due to the nature of the proteomics tools that make it possible to analyze and search for peptides without prior knowledge.

Future methodological improvements will follow the developments in human proteomics. This will also include improved throughput, so many samples can be analyzed with less cost, leading to more robust methods. Combined -omics analyses and tools will further expand the knowledge on molecular mechanisms involved in complex samples of biological origin such as meats and other foods.

## REFERENCES

Aebersold, R. and M. Mann. 2003. Mass spectrometry-based proteomics. *Nature* 422:198–207.

Arnau, J., L. Guerrero, and C. Sarraga. 1998. The effect of green ham pH and NaCl concentration on cathepsin activities and the sensory characteristics of dry-cured hams. *J Sci Food Agric* 77:387–392.

Arsenos, G., G. Banos, P. Fortomaris et al. 2002. Eating quality of lamb meat: Effects of breed, sex, degree of maturity and nutritional management. *Meat Sci* 60:379–387.

Bandman, E. and D. Zdanis. 1988. An immunological method to assess protein-degradation in post-mortem muscle. *Meat Sci* 22:1–19.

Bendixen, E. 2005. The use of proteomics in meat science. *Meat Sci* 71:138–149.

Bendixen, E., R. Taylor, K. Hollung, K. I. Hildrum, B. Picard, and J. Bouley. 2005. Proteomics, an approach towards understanding the biology of meat quality. In *Indicators of Milk and Beef Quality*, J. F. Hocquette and S. Gigli (eds.), pp. 81–94. Wageningen, the Netherlands: Academic Publishers.

Bjarnadottir, S. G., K. Hollung, E. M. Færgestad, and E. Veiseth-Kent. 2010. Proteome changes in bovine *Longissimus thoracis* muscle during the first 48 h postmortem: Shifts in energy status and myofibrillar stability. *J Agric Food Chem* 58:7408–7414.

Boccard, R. 1981. Facts and reflections on muscular hypertrophy in cattle: Double muscling or culard. In *Developments in Meat Science-2*, R. Lawrie (ed.), pp. 1–28. London, U.K.: Applied Science Publishers Ltd.

Bodenmiller, B., L. N. Mueller, M. Mueller, B. Domon, and R. Aebersold. 2007. Reproducible isolation of distinct, overlapping segments of the phosphoproteome. *Nat Methods* 4:231–237.

Bodnar, W. M., R. K. Blackburn, J. M. Krise, and M. A. Moseley. 2003. Exploiting the complementary nature of LC/MALDI/MS/MS and LC/ESI/MS/MS for increased proteome coverage. *J Am Soc Mass Spectrom* 14:971–979.

Boles, J. A., F. C. Parrish, T. W. Huiatt, and R. M. Robson. 1992. Effect of porcine stress syndrome on the solubility and degradation of myofibrillar cytoskeletal proteins. *J Anim Sci* 70:454–464.

Bouley, J., B. Meunier, C. Chambon, S. De Smet, J. F. Hocquette, and B. Picard. 2005. Proteomic analysis of bovine skeletal muscle hypertrophy. *Proteomics* 5:490–500.

Bouton, P. E., P. V. Harris, W. Shorthos, and R. I. Baxter. 1973. Comparison of effect of aging, conditioning and skeletal restraint on tenderness of mutton. *J Food Sci* 38:932–937.

Bredahl, L., K. G. Grunert, and C. Fertin. 1998. Relating consumer perceptions of pork quality to physical product characteristics. *Food Qual Prefer* 9:273–281.

Bryhni, E. A., D. V. Byrne, M. Rodbotten et al. 2002. Consumer perceptions of pork in Denmark, Norway and Sweden. *Food Qual Prefer* 13:257–266.

Chen, C. H. 2008. Review of a current role of mass spectrometry for proteome research. *Anal Chim Acta* 624:16–36.

Corzo, A., M. T. Kidd, W. A. Dozier 3rd, L. A. Shack, and S. C. Burgess. 2006. Protein expression of pectoralis major muscle in chickens in response to dietary methionine status. *Br J Nutr* 95:703–708.

Di Luccia, A., G. Picariello, G. Cacace et al. 2005. Proteomic analysis of water soluble and myofibrillar protein changes occurring in dry-cured hams. *Meat Sci* 69:479–491.

Elliott, M. H., D. S. Smith, C. E. Parker, and C. Borchers. 2009. Current trends in quantitative proteomics. *J Mass Spectrom* 44:1637–1660.

Elsik, C. G., R. L. Tellam, K. C. Worley et al. 2009. The genome sequence of taurine cattle: A window to ruminant biology and evolution. *Science* 324:522–528.

Fey, S. J. and P. M. Larsen. 2001. 2D or not 2D. Two-dimensional gel electrophoresis. *Curr Opin Chem Biol* 5:26–33.

Field, R. A., J. C. Williams, and G. J. Miller. 1983. The effect of diet on lamb flavor. *Food Technol* 37:258–263.

Frohlich, T., D. Helmstetter, M. Zobawa et al. 2006. Analysis of the HUPO Brain Proteome reference samples using 2-D DIGE and 2-D LC-MS/MS. *Proteomics* 6:4950–4966.

Geesink, G. H. and M. Koohmaraie. 1999. Postmortem proteolysis and calpain/calpastatin activity in callipyge and normal lamb biceps femoris during extended postmortem storage. *J Anim Sci* 77:1490–1501.

Goll, D. E., R. G. Taylor, J. A. Christiansen, and V. F. Thompson. 1991. Role of proteinases and protein turnover in muscle growth and meat quality. In *44th Annual Reciprocal Meat Conference*, pp. 25–33, Kansas State University, Manhattan, KS.

Gorg, A., C. Obermaier, G. Boguth et al. 2000. The current state of two-dimensional electrophoresis with immobilized pH gradients. *Electrophoresis* 21:1037–1053.

Gorg, A., W. Weiss, and M. J. Dunn. 2004. Current two-dimensional electrophoresis technology for proteomics. *Proteomics* 4:3665–3685.

Gratacos-Cubarsi, M., M. Castellari, M. Hortos, J. A. Garcia-Regueiro, R. Lametsch, and F. Jessen. 2008. Effects of tetracycline administration on the proteomic profile of pig muscle samples (*L. dorsi*). *J Agric Food Chem* 56:9312–9316.

Grove, H., E. M. Faergestad, K. Hollung, and H. Martens. 2009. Improved dynamic range of protein quantification in silver-stained gels by modelling gel images over time. *Electrophoresis* 30:1856–1862.

Grove, H., K. Hollung, A. K. Uhlen, H. Martens, and E. M. Faergestad. 2006. Challenges related to analysis of protein spot volumes from two-dimensional gel electrophoresis as revealed by replicate gels. *J Proteome Res* 5:3399–3410.

Gygi, S. P., B. Rist, S. A. Gerber, F. Turecek, M. H. Gelb, and R. Aebersold. 1999. Quantitative analysis of complex protein mixtures using isotope-coded affinity tags. *Nat Biotechnol* 17:994–999.

Hamelin, M., T. Sayd, C. Chambon et al. 2006. Proteomic analysis of ovine muscle hypertrophy. *J Anim Sci* 84:3266–3276.

Hamelin, M., T. Sayd, C. Chambon et al. 2007. Differential expression of sarcoplasmic proteins in four heterogeneous ovine skeletal muscles. *Proteomics* 7:271–280.

Hannesson, K. O., M. E. Pedersen, R. Ofstad, and S. O. Kolset. 2003. Breakdown of large proteoglycans in bovine intramuscular connective tissue early postmortem. *J Muscle Foods* 14:301–318.

Hasan, L., L. Mazzucchelli, M. Liebi et al. 2006. Function of liver activation-regulated chemokine/CC chemokine ligand 20 is differently affected by cathepsin B and cathepsin D processing. *J Immunol* 176:6512–6522.

Hedegaard, J., P. Horn, R. Lametsch et al. 2004. UDP-glucose pyrophosphorylase is upregulated in carriers of the porcine RN⁻ mutation in the AMP-activated protein kinase. *Proteomics* 4:2448–2454.

Herring, H. K., R. G. Cassens, G. G. Suess, V. H. Brungardt, and E. J. Briskey. 1967. Tenderness and associated characteristics of stretched and contracted bovine muscles. *J Food Sci* 32:317–323.

Hillenkamp, F., M. Karas, R. C. Beavis, and B. T. Chait. 1991. Matrix-assisted laser desorption ionization mass-spectrometry of biopolymers. *Anal Chem* 63:A1193–A1202.

Hoagland, R., C. N. McBryde, and W. C. Powick. 1917. Changes in fresh beef during cold storage above freezing. *USDA Bull* 433:1–100.

Hollung, K., H. Grove, E. M. Færgestad, M. S. Sidhu, and P. Berg. 2009. Comparison of muscle proteome profiles in pure breeds of Norwegian Landrace and Duroc at three different ages. *Meat Sci* 81:487–492.

Hollung, K., E. Veiseth, X. Jia, E. M. Færgestad, and K. I. Hildrum. 2007. Application of proteomics to understand the molecular mechanisms behind meat quality. *Meat Sci* 77:97–104.

Honikel, K. O., P. Roncales, and R. Hamm. 1983. The influence of temperature on shortening and rigor onset in beef muscle. *Meat Sci* 8:221–241.

Huff-Lonergan, E., F. C. J. Parrish, and R. M. Robson. 1995. Effects of postmortem aging time, animal age, and sex on degradation of titin and nebulin in bovine longissimus muscle. *J Anim Sci* 73:1064–1073.

Hwang, I. H., B. Y. Park, J. H. Kim, S. H. Cho, and J. M. Lee. 2005. Assessment of postmortem proteolysis by gel-based proteome analysis and its relationship to meat quality traits in pig longissimus. *Meat Sci* 69:79–91.

Jacobsen, S., H. Grove, K. N. Jensen et al. 2007. Multivariate analysis of 2-DE protein patterns—Practical approaches. *Electrophoresis* 28:1289–1299.

Jaime, I., J. A. Beltran, P. Cena, P. Lopezlorenzo, and P. Roncales. 1992. Tenderization of lamb meat—Effect of rapid postmortem temperature droop on muscle conditioning and aging. *Meat Sci* 32:357–366.

Jeacocke, R. E. 1993. The concentration of free magnesium and free calcium-ions both increase in skeletal-muscle fibers entering rigor-mortis. *Meat Sci* 35:27–45.

Jessen, F., R. Lametsch, E. Bendixen, I. V. Kjærsgard, and B. M. Jorgensen. 2002. Extracting information from two-dimensional electrophoresis gels by partial least squares regression. *Proteomics* 2:32–35.

Jia, X., M. Ekman, H. Grove et al. 2007. Proteome changes in bovine *longissimus thoracis* muscle during the early postmortem storage period. *J Proteome Res* 6:2720–2731.

Jia, X., K. I. Hildrum, F. Westad, E. Kummen, L. Aass, and K. Hollung. 2006a. Changes in enzymes associated with energy metabolism during the early post mortem period in *longissimus thoracis* bovine muscle analyzed by proteomics. *J Proteome Res* 5:1763–1769.

Jia, X., K. Hollung, M. Therkildsen, K. I. Hildrum, and E. Bendixen. 2006b. Proteome analysis of early post-mortem changes in two bovine muscle types: *M. longissimus dorsi* and *M. semitendinosis. Proteomics* 6:936–944.

Jia, X., E. Veiseth-Kent, H. Grove et al. 2009. Peroxiredoxin-6-A potential protein marker for meat tenderness in bovine *longissimus thoracis* muscle. *J Anim Sci* 87:2391–2399.

Kjaersgard, I. V. H., M. R. Norrelykke, and F. Jessen. 2006. Changes in cod muscle proteins during frozen storage revealed by proteome analysis and multivariate data analysis. *Proteomics* 6:1606–1618.

Koohmaraie, M. 1994. Muscle proteinases and meat aging. *Meat Sci* 36:93–104.

Koohmaraie, M. 1996. Biochemical factors regulating the toughening and tenderization processes of meat. *Meat Sci* 43:S193–S201.

Koohmaraie, M., S. D. Shackelford, T. L. Wheeler, S. M. Lonergan, and M. E. Doumit. 1995. A muscle hypertrophy condition in lamb (callipyge): Characterization of effects on muscle growth and meat quality traits. *J Anim Sci* 73:3596–3607.

Kwasiborski, A., T. Sayd, C. Chambon, V. Sante-Lhoutellier, D. Rocha, and C. Terlouw. 2008a. Pig *Longissimus lumborum* proteome: Part I. Effects of genetic background, rearing environment and gender. *Meat Sci* 80:968–981.

Kwasiborski, A., T. Sayd, C. Chambon, V. Sante-Lhoutellier, D. Rocha, and C. Terlouw. 2008b. Pig *Longissimus lumborum* proteome: Part II. Relationships between protein content and meat quality. *Meat Sci* 80:982–996.

Lametsch, R. and E. Bendixen. 2001. Proteome analysis applied to meat science: Characterizing postmortem changes in porcine muscle. *J Agric Food Chem* 49:4531–4537.

Lametsch, R., A. Karlsson, K. Rosenvold, H. J. Andersen, P. Roepstorff, and E. Bendixen. 2003. Postmortem proteome changes of porcine muscle related to tenderness. *J Agric Food Chem* 51:6992–6997.

Lametsch, R., L. Kristensen, M. R. Larsen, M. Therkildsen, N. Oksbjerg, and P. Ertbjerg. 2006. Changes in the muscle proteome after compensatory growth in pigs. *J Anim Sci* 84:918–924.

Lametsch, R., P. Roepstorff, and E. Bendixen. 2002. Identification of protein degradation during post-mortem storage of pig meat. *J Agric Food Chem* 50:5508–5512.

Lametsch, R., P. Roepstorff, H. S. Moller, and E. Bendixen. 2004. Identification of myofibrillar substrates for mu-calpain. *Meat Sci* 68:515–521.

Lange, V., P. Picotti, B. Domon, and R. Aebersold. 2008. Selected reaction monitoring for quantitative proteomics: A tutorial. *Mol Syst Biol* 4:222.

Laville, E., T. Sayd, M. Morzel et al. 2009a. Proteome changes during meat aging in tough and tender beef suggest the importance of apoptosis and protein solubility for beef aging and tenderization. *J Agric Food Chem* 57:10755–10764.

Laville, E., T. Sayd, C. Terlouw et al. 2007. Comparison of sarcoplasmic proteomes between two groups of pig muscles selected for shear force of cooked meat. *J Agric Food Chem* 55:5834–5841.

Laville, E., T. Sayd, C. Terlouw et al. 2009b. Differences in pig muscle proteome according to HAL genotype: Implications for meat quality defects. *J Agric Food Chem* 57:4913–4923.

Li, X. H., Y. Gong, Y. Wang et al. 2005. Comparison of alternative analytical techniques for the characterisation of the human serum proteome in HUPO Plasma Proteome Project. *Proteomics* 5:3423–3441.

Lopez, J. L. 2007. Two-dimensional electrophoresis in proteome expression analysis. *J Chromatogr B Anal Technol Biomed Life Sci* 849:190–202.

Mach, N., E. Keuning, L. Kruijt, M. Hortos, J. Arnau, and M. te Pas. 2010. Comparative proteomic profiling of 2 muscles from 5 different pure pig breeds using surface-enhanced laser desorption/ionization time-of-flight proteomics technology. *J Anim Sci* 88:1522–1534.

Marsh, B. B. and N. G. Leet. 1966. Studies in meat tenderness. III. The effects of cold shortening on tenderness. *J Food Sci* 31:450–459.

Maurer, M. H., R. E. Feldmann Jr., J. O. Bromme, and A. Kalenka. 2005. Comparison of statistical approaches for the analysis of proteome expression data of differentiating neural stem cells. *J Proteome Res* 4:96–100.

McDonald, T., S. Sheng, B. Stanley et al. 2006. Expanding the subproteome of the inner mitochondria using protein separation technologies: One- and two-dimensional liquid chromatography and two-dimensional gel electrophoresis. *Mol Cell Proteomics* 5:2392–2411.

Melchior, K., A. Tholey, S. Heisel et al. 2009. Proteomic study of human glioblastoma multiforme tissue employing complementary two-dimensional liquid chromatography- and mass spectrometry-based approaches. *J Proteome Res* 8:4604–4614.

Melody, J. L., S. M. Lonergan, L. J. Rowe, T. W. Huiatt, M. S. Mayes, and E. Huff-Lonergan. 2004. Early postmortem biochemical factors influence tenderness and water-holding capacity of three porcine muscles. *J Anim Sci* 82:1195–1205.

Meunier, B., E. Dumas, I. Piec, D. Bechet, M. Hebraud, and J. F. Hocquette. 2007. Assessment of hierarchical clustering methodologies for proteomic data mining. *J Proteome Res* 6:358–366.

Milan, D., J. T. Jeon, C. Looft et al. 2000. A mutation in PRKAG3 associated with excess glycogen content in pig skeletal muscle. *Science* 288:1248–1251.

Miller, M. F., K. L. Huffman, S. Y. Gilbert, L. L. Hamman, and C. B. Ramsey. 1995. Retail consumer acceptance of beef tenderized with calcium chloride. *J Anim Sci* 73:2308–2314.

Mora, L., M. A. Sentandreu, P. D. Fraser, F. Toldra, and P. M. Bramley. 2009a. Oligopeptides arising from the degradation of creatine kinase in Spanish dry-cured ham. *J Agric Food Chem* 57:8982–8988.

Mora, L., M. A. Sentandreu, K. M. Koistinen, P. D. Fraser, F. Toldra, and P. M. Bramley. 2009b. Naturally generated small peptides derived from myofibrillar proteins in serrano dry-cured ham. *J Agric Food Chem* 57:3228–3234.

Morzel, M., C. Chambon, M. Hamelin, V. Sante-Lhoutellier, T. Sayd, and G. Monin. 2004. Proteome changes during pork meat ageing following use of two different pre-slaughter handling procedures. *Meat Sci* 67:689–696.

Morzel, M., C. Terlouw, C. Chambon, D. Micol, and B. Picard. 2008. Muscle proteome and meat eating qualities of *Longissimus thoracis* of "Blonde d'Aquitaine" young bulls: A central role of HSP27 isoforms. *Meat Sci* 78:297–304.

Mullen, A. M., P. C. Stapleton, D. Corcoran, R. M. Hamill, and A. White. 2006. Understanding meat quality through the application of genomic and proteomic approaches. *Meat Sci* 74:3–16.

Nishimura, T., A. Hattori, and K. Takahashi. 1995. Structural weakening of intramuscular connective tissue during conditioning of beef. *Meat Sci* 39:127–133.

O'Farrell, P. H. 1975. High resolution two-dimensional electrophoresis of proteins. *J Biol Chem* 250:4007–4021.

Ong, S. E., B. Blagoev, I. Kratchmarova et al. 2002. Stable isotope labeling by amino acids in cell culture, SILAC, as a simple and accurate approach to expression proteomics. *Mol Cell Proteomics* 1:376–386.

Parolari, G., R. Virgili, and C. Schivazappa. 1994. Relationship between cathepsin-B activity and compositional parameters in dry-cured hams of normal and defective texture. *Meat Sci* 38:117–122.

Patel, V. J., K. Thalassinos, S. E. Slade et al. 2009. A comparison of labeling and label-free mass spectrometry-based proteomics approaches. *J Proteome Res* 8:3752–3759.

Patton, W. F. 2000. A thousand points of light: The application of fluorescence detection technologies to two-dimensional gel electrophoresis and proteomics. *Electrophoresis* 21:1123–1144.

Patton, W. F. 2002. Detection technologies in proteome analysis. *J Chromatogr B Anal Technol Biomed Life Sci* 771:3–31.

Picotti, P., R. Aebersold, and B. Domon. 2007. The implications of proteolytic background for shotgun proteomics. *Mol Cell Proteomics* 6:1589–1598.

Picotti, P., B. Bodenmiller, L. N. Mueller, B. Domon, and R. Aebersold. 2009. Full dynamic range proteome analysis of *S. cerevisiae* by targeted proteomics. *Cell* 138:795–806.

Picotti, P., O. Rinner, R. Stallmach et al. 2010. High-throughput generation of selected reaction-monitoring assays for proteins and proteomes. *Nat Methods* 7:43–45.

Pulford, D. J., S. F. Vazquez, D. F. Frost, E. Fraser-Smith, P. Dobbie, and K. Rosenvold. 2008. The intracellular distribution of small heat shock proteins in post-mortem beef is determined by ultimate pH. *Meat Sci* 79:623–630.

Purslow, P. P. 2005. Intramuscular connective tissue and its role in meat quality. *Meat Sci* 70:435–447.

Ramsbottom, J. M., E. J. Strandine, and C. H. Koonz. 1945. Comparative tenderness of representative beef muscles. *Food Res* 10:497–509.

Righetti, P. G., A. Castagna, P. Antonioli, and E. Boschetti. 2005. Prefractionation techniques in proteome analysis: The mining tools of the third millennium. *Electrophoresis* 26:297–319.

Rosell, C. M. and F. Toldra. 1998. Comparison of muscle proteolytic and lipolytic enzyme levels in raw hams from Iberian and White pigs. *J Sci Food Agric* 76:117–122.

Ross, P. L., Y. L. N. Huang, and J. N. Marchese et al. 2004. Multiplexed protein quantitation in *Saccharomyces cerevisiae* using amine-reactive isobaric tagging reagents. *Mol Cell Proteomics* 3:1154–1169.

Sawdy, J. C., S. A. Kaiser, N. R. St-Pierre, and M. P. Wick. 2004. Myofibrillar 1-D fingerprints and myosin heavy chain MS analyses of beef loin at 36h postmortem correlate with tenderness at 7 days. *Meat Sci* 67:421–426.

Sayd, T., M. Morzel, C. Chambon et al. 2006. Proteome analysis of the sarcoplasmic fraction of pig semimembranosus muscle: Implications on meat color development. *J Agric Food Chem* 54:2732–2737.

Sentandreu, M. A., M. Armenteros, J. J. Calvete, A. Ouali, M. C. Aristoy, and F. Toldra. 2007. Proteomic identification of actin-derived oligopeptides in dry-cured ham. *J Agric Food Chem* 55:3613–3619.

Sentandreu, M. A., J. J. Calvete, M. Armenteros, A. Ouali, M. C. Aristoy, and F. Toldra. 2009. Identification of myosin peptides in Spanish dry-cured ham by tandem mass spectrometry. In *3rd EuPA Congress Clinical Proteomics*, pp. 481–483, Stockholm, Sweden.

Shackelford, S. D., M. Koohmaraie, M. F. Miller, J. D. Crouse, and J. O. Reagan. 1991. An evaluation of tenderness of the longissimus muscle of angus by Hereford versus Brahman crossbred heifers. *J Anim Sci* 69:171–177.

Shen, Y. F., N. Tolic, R. Zhao et al. 2001. High-throughput proteomics using high efficiency multiple-capillary liquid chromatography with on-line high-performance ESI FTICR mass spectrometry. *Anal Chem* 73:3011–3021.

Shibata, M., K. Matsumoto, M. Oe et al. 2009. Differential expression of the skeletal muscle proteome in grazed cattle. *J Anim Sci* 87:2700–2708.

Sidhu, M. S., K. Hollung, and P. Berg. 2005. Proteolysis in Norwegian dry-cured hams; preliminary results. In *51st ICOMST—The International Congress of Meat Science and Technology*, Baltimore, MD.

Strandine, E. J., C. H. Koonz, and J. M. Ramsbottom. 1949. A study of variations in muscles of beef and chicken. *J Anim Sci* 8:483–494.

Taylor, R. G., G. H. Geesink, V. F. Thompson, M. Koohmaraie, and D. E. Goll. 1995. Is Z-disk degradation responsible for postmortem tenderization? *J Anim Sci* 73:1351–1367.

te Pas, M., J. Jansen, K. Broekman, H. Reimert, and H. C. M. Heuven. 2009. Postmortem proteome degradation profiles of longissimus muscle in Yorkshire and Duroc pigs and their relationship with pork quality traits. *Meat Sci* 83:744–751.

Theron, L., L. Chevarin, N. Robert, C. Dutertre, and V. Sante-Lhoutellier. 2009. Time course of peptide fingerprints in semimembranosus and biceps femoris muscles during Bayonne ham processing. *Meat Sci* 82:272–277.

Unlu, M., M. E. Morgan, and J. S. Minden. 1997. Difference gel electrophoresis: A single gel method for detecting changes in protein extracts. *Electrophoresis* 18:2071–2077.

Virgili, R., C. Schivazappa, G. Parolari, C. S. Bordini, and M. Degni. 1998. Proteases in fresh pork muscle and their influence on bitter taste formation in dry-cured ham. *J Food Biochem* 22:53–63.

Wheeler, T. L. and M. Koohmaraie. 1994. Prerigor and postrigor changes in tenderness of ovine longissimus muscle. *J Anim Sci* 72:1232–1238.

Wheeler, T. L. and M. Koohmaraie. 1999. The extent of proteolysis is independent of sarcomere length in lamb longissimus and psoas major. *J Anim Sci* 77:2444–2451.

Whipple, G., M. Koohmaraie, M. E. Dikeman, J. D. Crouse, M. C. Hunt, and R. D. Klemm. 1990. Evaluation of attributes that affect longissimus muscle tenderness in *Bos taurus* and *Bos indicus* cattle. *J Anim Sci* 68:2716–2728.

Whiting, R. C. 1980. Calcium-uptake by bovine muscle mitochondria and sarcoplasmic-reticulum. *J Food Sci* 45:288–292.

Wilkins, M. R., C. Pasquali, R. D. Appel et al. 1996. From proteins to proteomes: Large scale protein identification by two-dimensional electrophoresis and amino acid analysis. *Biotechnology* 14:61–65.

Wu, W. W., G. Wang, S. J. Baek, and R. F. Shen. 2006. Comparative study of three proteomic quantitative methods, DIGE, cICAT, and iTRAQ, using 2D gel- or LC-MALDI TOF/TOF. *J Proteome Res* 5:651–658.

Xu, Y. J., M. L. Jin, L. J. Wang et al. 2009. Differential proteome analysis of porcine skeletal muscles between Meishan and Large White. *J Anim Sci* 87:2519–2527.

Yates, J. R., S. Speicher, P. R. Griffin, and T. Hunkapiller. 1993. Peptide mass maps—A highly informative approach to protein identification. *Anal Biochem* 214:397–408.

Zapata, I., H. N. Zerby, and M. Wick. 2009. Functional proteomic analysis predicts beef tenderness and the tenderness differential. *J Agric Food Chem* 57:4956–4963.

Zhang, J., Q. He, Q. Y. Liu et al. 2007. Differential gene expression profile in pig adipose tissue treated with/without clenbuterol. *BMC Genomics* 8:433.

# 14 Wine-Omics

## *New Platforms for the Improvement of Yeast Strains and Wine Quality*

Corine S.C. Ting, Anthony R. Borneman,
and Isak S. Pretorius

## CONTENTS

## 14.1  WINEMAKING AND SYSTEMS BIOLOGY: HISTORIC ART MEETS THE FUTURE OF BIOLOGICAL SCIENCE

The yeast *Saccharomyces cerevisiae* has long been used in the food and beverage industries of winemaking, baking, and brewing. During winemaking, *S. cerevisiae* is indispensible for converting grape juice into the complex aromatic beverage that is wine. Wine fermentation represents one of the world's oldest biotechnological processes, with wine production being reported as far back as 7000–5000 BCE in the region of Asia Minor, between the Black and Caspian Seas (Pretorius 2000). Historically, a lack of understanding of the primary factors that regulate wine fermentation confined wine production to the spontaneous fermentation of grape juices, a process with a highly variable success rate. These production inefficiencies relegated fine wine to becoming an expensive beverage the consumption of which was restricted to the wealthy. Today, the image of wine has changed completely. The highly controlled, large-scale production methods of modern winemaking allow wine to be supplied at high quality and low cost. This significant progress in wine production has been catalyzed by the continuous scientific research that has sought to progressively unravel the mysteries of wine fermentation.

The identification of *S. cerevisiae* as the agent responsible for the fermentation of grape sugars into ethanol and carbon dioxide by Louis Pasteur in 1863 represents the most momentous scientific discovery in the field of winemaking. The subsequent introduction of the concept of inoculating fermentations with pure cultures of *S. cerevisiae* has vastly improved the quality and efficiency of wine production (Henschke 1997). Consequently, the use of yeast starter cultures is almost ubiquitous in large-scale wine production to drive rapid and predictable fermentations to produce wines of consistent quality. This has resulted in hundreds of commercial wine yeast strains that have been selected for their superior fermentative capacities through both human intervention and natural selection pressures (Querol et al. 2003). While all these commercial wine yeast strains provide reliable fermentative performance, they are often phenotypically diverse in terms of their winemaking attributes, such as sensorial impact on the finished wine. Indeed, very distinct results can be achieved from an organoleptic point of view when different yeast strains are used to ferment identical grape musts (Swiegers and Pretorius 2005).

Given the increasing demands from consumers for newer and more distinctive wine styles, it would be beneficial if the biological principles behind the strain diversity could be understood at a level of detail that would allow the tailored development of optimized wine yeast strains. In the past, research into molecular biology of wine yeast, like most other fields of molecular biological research, applied classical single gene or so-called reductionist strategies to solve discrete biological questions (e.g., study the function of a single gene or protein) (Table 14.1). However, because many oenological properties are controlled by complex interactions between multiple genes, proteins, and metabolites, they are often not directly amenable to this type of research. Recent advances in molecular biotechnology have begun to provide the means to investigate these complex biological phenomena, with the field of wine research currently transitioning from reductionist studies to whole-cell methodologies, termed "systems biology." At its core, systems biology employs high-throughput -omic technologies to gather data on the cell in its

**TABLE 14.1**

**The Differences between Classical Reductionist and -Omic Technologies**

| Classical Reductionist Strategies | -Omic Technologies |
|---|---|
| Investigation of a single biological entity (e.g., single gene) in isolation | Global analysis of all possible components present within and between -omes |
| Hypothesis driven | Data driven |
| Data obtained are restricted to the object studied | High-throughput, able to yield a large amount of data |
| Cannot explain the dynamics and robustness of cellular functions | Systematic integration of -omic data with appropriate mathematical model enables the construction of a predictive computational model, which elucidates the behavior of a cell under different perturbations |

entirety and then uses bioinformatics and mathematical modeling to integrate these data to provide a predictive framework for the cell. These pioneering -omic studies promise to improve the winemaking process by generating a wealth of informative data on the physiology and metabolism of wine yeasts, which are of great value for downstream strain development. This chapter reviews the current state of -omic techniques available to yeast researchers and discusses how these cutting-edge methods can be integrated to provide a systems-level insight into the historic artisanal craft of winemaking.

## 14.2   -OMES AND SYSTEMS BIOLOGY

A phenotype is generally not a single-entity-dependent event. Instead, it is built on the complex interplay between a myriad of cellular and environmental constituents. This is especially true for winemaking-related traits, which are often determined by the complex interplay between multiple genes, proteins, and metabolites, as well as the prevailing environmental conditions. For example, it has been shown that one of most important oenological characteristics of wine yeast, resistance to ethanol stress, is the result of synergistic interactions between more than 250 genes and proteins (Auesukaree et al. 2009, Boulton et al. 1996, Fujita et al. 2006, Stanley et al. 2010). Therefore, in order to fully understand the cellular behavior of *S. cerevisiae* in winemaking, systems biology is required for the systematic and unbiased investigation of the wine yeast cell during the wine fermentation process.

The first steps in any true systems-level investigation is to gather whole-cell data from each level of the cellular hierarchy from genome through interactome (the -omes), identify all possible interactions between -omes on a global scale, and then integrate them into a web of interaction networks that explains the structure and function of a living cell (Figure 14.1) (Borneman et al. 2007). This systematic exploitation, when combined with mathematical modeling, provides the basis for in silico predictions regarding the expected phenotypic consequences of genetic or environmental perturbations (Borneman et al. 2007). This robust computational model will provide the key for the future of wine yeast strain development: It provides a firm basis for synthetic biology, which attempts in silico to design an artificial

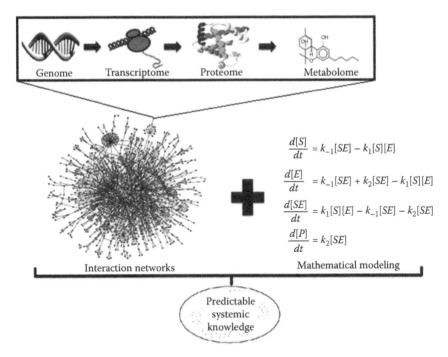

**FIGURE 14.1**    An overview of systems biology. Cell behavior is built on the complex inter-play between all relevant biological processes presented in the interacting metabolic networks. These networks are composed of many interconnected modules, each representing the func-tionally interacting -omes under a particular growth condition and time frame. Genome is the entire DNA nucleotide sequence content. Transcriptome represents the entire RNA comple-ment of the cell whose expression is dependent on genes being switched on and off. Proteome is the entire protein complement of the cell whose production is regulated by both genome and transcriptome. Metabolome is the most dynamic -ome that includes the entire complement of small chemicals and metabolites. In addition to genome, transcriptome, and proteome, its composition is also modulated by environment. Systems biology aims to capture the global -omic information provided by each collaborative modules and uses them to systematically reconstruct a network map that best resembles its native counterpart. The resulting interaction framework is then combined with mathematical modeling to yield a predictive computational model that elucidates the dynamic and robustness of a biological system.

biomolecular network for a phenotype of interest before engineering procedures are performed, thereby reducing both time and cost needed for prototype construction.

In order to build the predictive mathematical model for a wine yeast cell, a sig-nificant number of high-throughput technologies can be applied to interrogate and compile the information from each -omic category.

## 14.3    GENOMICS OF WINE YEASTS

Because dynamic cellular behavior ultimately relies upon specific portions of the genome being turned on or off, and because the genome sequence is the most static entity within the cell, investigation of yeast genomics is a logical starting point for understanding the molecular basis of desirable winemaking characteristics. With the advent of high-throughput whole-genome technologies, such as DNA microarrays and next-generation sequencing (NGS), it is now feasible to compare multiple strains of yeast at the whole-genome level, both computationally via comparative genomics and experimentally via functional genomics methodologies. This systems-level information is critical to link the genotypic variations to complex winemaking-related traits, which are the key for subsequent strain development.

## 14.3.1 COMPARATIVE GENOMICS

Traditional molecular methods used for wine yeast strain differentiation include DNA fingerprinting, chromosome fingerprinting, and polymerase chain reaction (PCR) (Pretorius 2000). Because these techniques rely heavily on the presence of specific subsets of genomic polymorphisms, they are confined to assaying small subsets of the genome, which may or may not be representative of the profile of variation across the whole genome (Pretorius 2000). However, with the publication of the entire nucleotide sequence of a lab strain of *S. cerevisiae*, S288c (Goffeau et al. 1996), the field of yeast research was profoundly revolutionized and has subsequently pushed relentlessly at the cutting edge of the whole-genome era. Since the completion of the S288c genome sequence, several comparative genomics analyses have taken advantage of this resource and have applied it to either microarray-based comparative genome hybridization (aCGH) or NGS to explore the genetic variations between yeast strains (Borneman et al. 2008, Carreto et al. 2008, Infante et al. 2003, Lashkari et al. 1997, Novo et al. 2009, Primig et al. 2000, Salinas et al. 2010, Schacherer et al. 2007, Steinmetz et al. 2006, Winzeler et al. 2003). These studies have tremendously improved our understanding of yeast from the whole-genome perspective and have paved the way for the subsequent functional analysis of the wine yeast genome.

### 14.3.1.1 Microarray-Based Comparative Genome Hybridization

By combining the complete sequence of the S288c reference strain with DNA microarrays, a high-throughput whole-genome comparative technique called aCGH emerged (Lashkari et al. 1997) (Figure 14.2). This method uses differences between microarray signals to detect copy number variations across the genomes, thereby indicating loci that have been either deleted or amplified relative to a reference strain (Winzeler et al. 2003).

Because aCGH provides a cost-effective and rapid analysis of yeast strain variation, a significant number of studies have employed this technique to compare yeast strains (Carreto et al. 2008, Dunn et al. 2005, Salinas et al. 2010, Winzeler et al. 2003). For example, Dunn et al. (2005) applied aCGH to investigate the genetic basis of phenotypic variation in four commercial wine *S. cerevisiae* strains with distinct fermentative and sensory qualities. This study unearthed several variations in the copy numbers of specific genes between the wine strains and the S288c lab strain that were then assigned as the "commercial wine yeast signature."

While aCGH is suited to identifying copy number changes between both genetically diverse and similar strains, it must be noted that aCGH studies are ultimately limited by the effective resolution of the microarray used. As such, most aCGH studies cannot accurately recognize single nucleotide polymorphisms (SNPs), which can

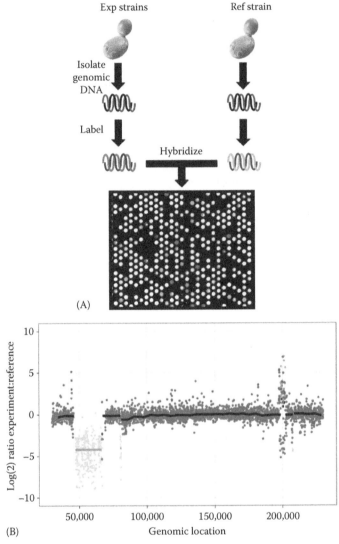

**FIGURE 14.2** Microarray-based comparative genome hybridization (aCGH). (A) In aCGH, genomic DNAs from an experimental strain (e.g., a wine yeast strain) and a wild-type reference strain (the sequenced laboratory *S. cerevisiae* strain S288c) are extracted and labeled with different fluorescent dyes (experimental strain is labeled as green whereas reference strain is red in this scenario). The two labeled samples are mixed, then competitively hybridized to a spotted DNA microarray in which each spot contains a PCR-amplified DNA probe corresponding to one gene of the reference S288c strain. The fluorescence intensities give an indication of which genes in the yeast strain assayed are amplified and deleted in relation to the S288c genes. (B) Tiling arrays can provide detailed information regarding the position and size of copy number variants (CNVs) when aCGH signals (log 2 ratios) from the large collection of probes are arranged in order of their position in the genome. This enables the identification and consolidation of signals from individual probes (small circles) to be consolidated into large regions of either normal copy number (black lines) or of potential CNV (light grey lines).

often be present at a high frequency throughout the yeast genome. "Tiling" DNA micro-arrays (TMAs) have sought to address this issue by employing large numbers of degen-erate, overlapping probes that "tile" the entire genome. While TMAs have been shown to be capable of detecting the location of SNPs between lab strains of *S. cerevisiae* and to map quantitative trait loci of industrial strains, this method for comparative genomic hybridization has yet to be applied to commercial wine yeasts (Argueso et al. 2009, Gresham et al. 2006, Hu et al. 2007, Katou et al. 2009, Marullo et al. 2007, Schacherer et al. 2007). Nevertheless, given their higher resolution, TMAs should enable the detec-tion of important variations between wine yeast strains and enable the identification of crucial genes relevant to wine fermentation at a single-base level.

In addition to the problem of SNPs, the other crucial drawback of aCGH (whether classical aCGH or by using TMAs) is that it provides no indication of novel sequences that are not present in the genome sequence used to design the DNA microarray. As a result, critical new genes that may be related to important phenotypic characteristics could not be discovered if we depended solely on aCGH.

### 14.3.1.2 Next-Generation Genome Sequencing

Next-generation sequencing (NGS) represents the latest advance in the genomic sci-ences and, due to its much higher resolution and improved cost effectiveness, NGS is poised to emerge as the dominant technology for comparative genome analysis (Bennett 2004, Margulies et al. 2005, Shendure et al. 2005). Unlike aCGH-based methods, NGS directly assays the nucleotide sequence of strains and is therefore able to track all genomic differences, including both SNPs and novel DNA sequences. In addition, NGS does not require prior knowledge of the query genome or a related reference genome, and provides absolute rather than relative data. Most importantly, since the genome is directly sequenced and not interrogated by hybridization to the reference sequences, NGS is capable of producing high-quality sequence output devoid of experimental bias and complications, such as cross-hybridization between similar but nonidentical sequences that are commonly found in microarray analysis.

Sequencing of different yeast strains not only provides a valuable resource for com-parative genomic studies of *S. cerevisiae,* it also forms the foundation for strain-specific systems-level studies. Borneman et al. (2008) were the first to apply NGS to the study of industrial yeast strains and were able to rapidly generate the first genome sequence of a wine yeast strain, AWRI1631. Comparison of this sequence with the existing genomes of S288c and a human pathogenic isolate YJM789 identified more than 100 kb of addi-tional genome sequence that was specific to the wine strain (Borneman et al. 2008, Goffeau et al. 1996, Wei et al. 2007). As more *S. cerevisiae* genome sequences are reported, the presence of strain-specific open reading frames (ORFs) has emerged as a general theme. The sequencing of two additional industrial strains, the wine strain EC1118 and the biofuel strain JAY291, also uncovered novel, strain-specific ORFs, which had not been found previously in the *S. cerevisiae* genome (Argueso et al. 2009, Novo et al. 2009). These ORFs may therefore provide the means for phenotypic diver-sification observed between yeast strains and suggest that the species-wide genome of *S. cerevisiae* may be much larger than that found in any single strain—a situation that has been observed in many phenotypically diverse species of bacteria such as *Streptococci* (Lefebure and Stanhope 2007). Further detailed characterization of these

ORFs is required to confirm their roles, thereby gaining more insights into the genetic basis for the fermentative and sensory characteristics found exclusively in wine strains.

## 14.3.2 FUNCTIONAL GENOMICS

While sequencing is extremely useful for identifying novel candidate genes that may be relevant to the winemaking process, the sequence information derived from the bioinformatics analyses must often be verified experimentally by functional genomics approaches in order to understand the actual phenotypic consequences of these nucleotide variations.

### 14.3.2.1 High-Throughput Functional Profiling

Gene disruption represents a powerful method to elucidate gene function through the study of loss-of-function phenotypes. Several classical random mutagenesis

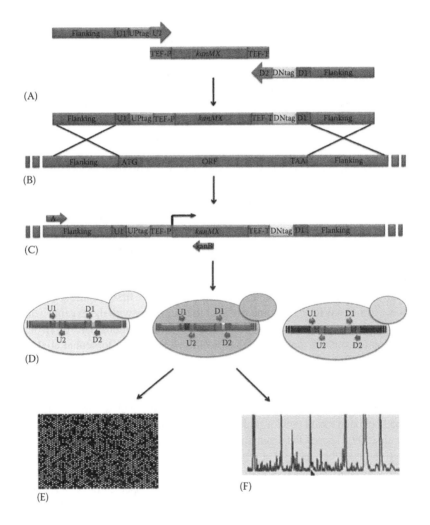

approaches such as transposon-mediated insertional mutagenesis have been used extensively for functional analysis in yeast (Kumar et al. 2000, 2002, 2004, Kumar 2008, Kumar and Snyder 2001, Lussier et al. 1997, Ross-Macdonald et al. 1999, Smith et al. 1995). However, as their names suggest, these approaches generate mutants at random and do not delete genes in a systematic and directed fashion. In yeast, this obstacle has been overcome by the development of PCR-based gene deletion (Baudin et al. 1993). This technique exploits the high rate of mitotic recombination that occurs in yeast such that the native ORF can be efficiently swapped with a selectable marker via homologous recombination between short, flanking repeats (Klinner and Schafer 2004, Wach et al. 1994).

By leveraging the information present in the genome sequence of S288c, an international consortium systematically deleted about 96% of the predicted ORFs of this strain using a high-throughput variant of the existing PCR deletion strategy (Giaever et al. 2002, Winzeler et al. 1999). In addition to deleting each ORF through the introduction of a common selectable marker (*kanMX*), each individual deletion also introduced a unique molecular barcode into that strain (Figure 14.3). This barcode approach allows for thousands of deletion strains to be assayed

---

**FIGURE 14.3** PCR-based deletion strategy and genome-wide competitive fitness assay. (A) To construct deletion strains, two oligonucleotide primers are synthesized, each containing approximately 50 bp of yeast genomic sequences that flank either the 5′ or 3′ end of the ORF to be deleted (Flanking), 18 or 17 bp of common sequences for subsequent PCR in the competitive fitness assay (U1 or D1), 20 bp of unique barcode sequences that track each deletion strain (UPtag or DNtag), and 18 or 19 bp of sequences complementary to the promoter or terminator of *TEF* gene obtained from the filamentous fungus *Ashbya gossypii* (U2 or D2, another common PCR priming site). These primers are then used to amplify the heterologous *kanMX* cassette, which confers resistance to geneticin (G418). (B) Transformation with the PCR product results in replacement of the target ORF (from start to stop codon, inclusively) with *kanMX* cassette via homologous recombination (indicated as crosses) at the flanking sequences. (C) The *kanMX* gene expressed from the constitutive *TEF* promoter allows for selection of transformants on G418 plate. To verify the correct integration of deletion cassette, two primers, A (positioned 250 bp away from the start codon of the ORF) and kanB (located within the coding region of *kanMX*) are used in PCR to amplify the genomic DNA extracted from the G418-resistant strain. Proper gene replacement event should yield a PCR product with expected size. (D) A pool of yeast deletion strains, each marked with unique molecular barcodes, is grown competitively in a condition of choice. If a gene is essential for growth under the condition tested, the strain carrying the corresponding deletion will grow more slowly and become underrepresented in the culture. To systematically quantify the relative abundance of each mutant strain, the unique UPtags and DNtags of all strains are simultaneously amplified by PCR using common primers (U1 and U2; D1 and D2) labeled with fluorescent dye. (E) The barcode PCR products can be analyzed in parallel by hybridization to a microarray bearing the homologous probes. The relative fitness of each gene is inferred by the fluorescent intensity measured by the microarray. As PCR is error prone, the tag sequences might carry mutations to interfere with hybridization; the use of two unique tags for each deletion strain could therefore increase the sensitivity of detection by adding redundancy. Alternatively, the fitness of individual deletion strains could be assessed systematically by NGS. In this case, barcode abundance is determined by counting the number of times each unique barcode is sequenced. This method is able to identify those barcodes with sequence errors that render them undetectable by the microarray hybridization. (F) Deletion strains can be further assayed by a variety of means including metabolomic screening, see Section 14.6.

simultaneously in competitive growth assays by applying either DNA microarray or NGS to score the fitness of individual strains via changes in the abundance of their specific barcode within the population (Figure 14.3) (Shoemaker et al. 1996, Smith et al. 2009, Winzeler et al. 1999). By applying this approach, Giaever et al. (2002) were able, quantitatively, to score the fitness contribution of each yeast gene for growth in five different environments (high salt, sorbitol, galactose, pH 8 minimal medium, and nystatin treatment). The results confirmed previously known genes that are required for growth and, more surprisingly, revealed new genes involved in the same process. Subsequent studies have been carried out using the similar strategy to systematically screen for the winemaking-related genes by exposing the deletion library to various stress and fermentation conditions (e.g., high ethanol and glucose concentrations) (Auesukaree et al. 2009, Fujita et al. 2006, Linderholm et al. 2008, Teixeira et al. 2009, 2010, Van Voorst et al. 2006, Yoshikawa et al. 2009).

This approach has also recently been combined with comparative genomics to produce the first whole-genome comparative functional genomics study (Dowell et al. 2010). The genomes of S288c and Σ1278b were compared both at the sequence level and also at the functional level through comparing the phenotypes of deletion strains in orthologous ORFs in the two species. It was shown that Σ1278b, like other yeast strains, contained ORFs that were not conserved across other yeast strains. However, the functional genomics work also showed that even for conserved genes, the phenotype of the orthologous deletion mutant in each strain could be very different, even to the point of displaying strain-dependent essentiality.

These profound strain-dependent differences stress the need for construction of a whole-genome deletion library in a sequenced wine strain. The construction of such a library is currently underway in the sequenced wine yeast AWRI1631. This will provide an invaluable resource for the downstream functional genomics analyses, enabling the discovery of all key genes participating in the winemaking process in a wine strain.

### 14.3.2.2 Genetic Interaction Map Construction

As demonstrated in S288c, functional profiling of a whole-genome deletion library is useful for grouping genes according to their fitness contribution in defined growth conditions. While assigning the relevant role to each individual gene is essential, it is of greater importance in understanding how these genes work together to regulate cellular processes, especially when dealing with industrial yeasts whose desirable properties are often polygenic in nature. This was addressed in the lab strain shortly after the yeast whole-genome deletion library became available through the development of several high-throughput techniques such as synthetic genetic array (SGA), epistatic miniarray profile (EMAP), and diploid-based synthetic lethality analysis on microarray (dSLAM), which map genetic interaction networks that link genes (Pan et al. 2004, Schuldiner et al. 2005, Tong et al. 2001). These methods harness the barcoded ORF-deletion resource for systematic construction of double mutants (under stringent genetic selections) and parallel analysis of the growth phenotypes of these mutants. By using these techniques, the functional relationship between a pair of nonessential genes (whose mutations act together to produce certain phenotypes such as lethality, while neither mutation by itself has pronounced effect) could be identified rapidly in a single experiment (Pan et al. 2004, Schuldiner et al. 2005, Tong et al. 2001). These high-throughput techniques have greatly accelerated the construction of a comprehensive genetic interaction map for yeast that, by a manual, one-at-a-time mating approach, would involve at least 25 million crosses for a thorough study of all yeast double mutants (Boone et al. 2007). Recently, a study has applied sophisticated computational modeling methods to quantitatively assemble 5.4 million gene–gene pairs based on the fitness profiles of double mutants determined by SGA, thereby constructing a global functional network of *S. cerevisiae* (Costanzo et al. 2010). This map can be used to predict the functions of previously uncharacterized genes according to their clustering positions, enabling a clear visualization of the link between genotype and phenotype.

## 14.4 TRANSCRIPTOMICS OF WINE YEASTS

The transcriptome represents the complete set of RNA species present in a cell at a specific time. Unlike the genome sequence, the transcriptome is dynamic and depends on genes being actively expressed or repressed in response to the prevailing environment. Changing the transcriptional levels of specific genes is the primary mechanism to initiate adaptive processes in a cell. Transcriptional regulation is crucial for wine yeast because winemaking is a dynamic process. During wine fermentation, *S. cerevisiae* is exposed to numerous stress conditions such as high osmotic pressure, acidity, nutrient deprivation, starvation, and high alcohol concentration. However, because wine production is a batch fermentation, the impact of these different stresses changes over time; for example, the osmotic stress present at the start of a fermentation is progressively replaced by ethanol stress as sugar is converted into alcohol (Attfield 1997, Bauer and Pretorius 2000). Therefore, the transcriptional machinery of yeast must be robust in order to withstand these stress factors while maintaining its ability to change in response to the environment.

Transcriptomics can be used to investigate the expression profile of mRNA molecules of wine yeasts by tracking and quantifying the changes in levels of each transcript at different stages during winemaking. As for the genome, the main tools for studying the transcriptome are microarrays and NGS.

### 14.4.1 EXPRESSION MICROARRAY

The DNA microarray was the very first high-throughput -omic technology that harnessed the knowledge present in the *S. cerevisiae* genome sequence. While also used for aCGH, DNA microarrays were initially used in yeast for transcriptomic studies via expression microarrays (EMA) by systematically printing each predicted ORF as an individual probe on the array. This allowed for the simultaneous and systematic detection of relative transcript levels for each and every ORF. Complementary DNAs (cDNA) were reverse transcribed from total mRNA to be analyzed, labeled fluorescently, and then hybridized with the probes on the DNA microarray. Global gene expression levels can then be deciphered by measuring the fluorescence intensities of the labeled cDNA that hybridized with the corresponding probes.

Given the utility of the transcriptomic microarray, several EMA studies of wine yeast have been undertaken (Beltran et al. 2006, Erasmus et al. 2003, Marks et al. 2003, Pizarro et al. 2008, Rossignol et al. 2003, Rossouw and Bauer 2009, Rossouw et al. 2009). As an example, Marks et al. (2003), analyzed the whole-genome expression of wine yeast during fermentation in grape juice and identified a group of genes that are dramatically induced at various points during fermentation. These genes were designated as fermentation stress response (FSR) genes, whose functions are related to the response to osmotic pressure change, nitrogen depletion, high ethanol concentration, and oxidative stress. These studies shed light on the adaptation and stress tolerance mechanisms of industrial wine yeast strains.

## 14.4.2   RNA Sequencing

As seen for aCGH, microarrays, while providing a powerful method for the analysis of the transcriptome, suffer from several drawbacks including cross-hybridization between homologous ORFs, limited dynamic range of detection of transcript levels (onefold to a few 100-fold) owing to the saturation of signals and an inability to detect sequences that are not present on the microarray (Wang et al. 2009). Recent advances in high-throughput sequencing have also provided the means to address many of the limitations of microarrays via a new method termed RNA sequencing (RNA-Seq). There are several RNA-Seq techniques that have been successfully applied to explore the transcriptome of *S. cerevisiae* (Lipson et al. 2009, Nagalakshmi et al. 2008, Ozsolak et al. 2009). Direct RNA-Seq (DRS) represents the most promising and reliable method because it is free of cDNA synthesis, adaptor ligation, and amplification steps. This enables a bias-free transcriptomic analysis and faithful quantification of transcripts to be made (Figure 14.4).

Regardless of the precise methodology, all RNA-Seq protocols share a significant advantage over microarrays: There is no upper limit for quantification as each transcript is subjected to sequencing, and the abundance of transcript therefore directly correlates with the number of sequences obtained. As a result, RNA-Seq has a much larger dynamic range for the quantification of gene expression levels. It was estimated that RNA-Seq displayed a greater than 9000-fold range over which *S. cerevisiae* transcripts can be detected (Nagalakshmi et al. 2008). In addition, RNA-Seq allows a direct characterization of total RNA by precisely revealing all RNA species (including mRNAs, noncoding RNAs, and small RNAs) and their transcriptional structures (e.g., 5' and 3' ends, transcriptional start sites, splicing patterns, and other posttranscriptional modifications). As such, RNA-Seq has been used in *S. cerevisiae* to identify 204 novel transcripts and refine its transcriptional landscape, such as exon boundaries (Nagalakshmi et al. 2008). Due to its unbiased nature, RNA-Seq is also able to detect novel sequences in RNA-Seq experiments through de novo assembly of sequences that do not match the reference strain genome (Nagalakshmi et al. 2008). This is vital if experiments are performed using industrial strains for which genome sequencing information is available.

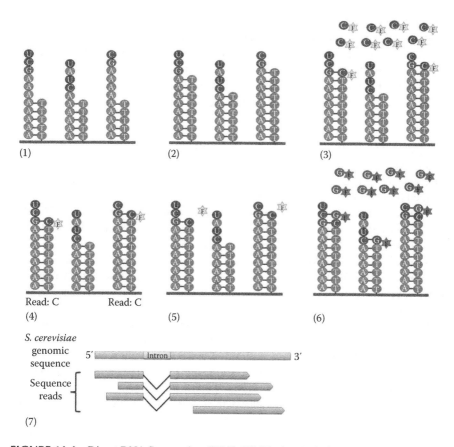

**FIGURE 14.4**   Direct RNA Sequencing (DRS). DRS is the newly innovated RNA sequencing technology, which allows a parallel high-throughput sequencing of RNA molecules directly without the need for cDNA conversion, adaptor ligation, and amplification steps, allowing a comprehensive and bias-free understanding of transcriptomes. (1) DRS begins with the hybridization of total transcripts to the flow cell surfaces coated with dT(50) oligonucleotide via their 3′ polyadenylated tails. (2) A 3′ end blocking is performed by filling the poly-A tails with natural dTTP to ensure that the sequencing begins at the true RNA sequences rather than the poly-A tails. (3) Each nucleotide carries a unique and chemically cleavable fluorescent dye enabling a step-wise sequencing by synthesis. Sequencing starts with the incorporation of a single type of fluorescence-labeled nucleotide (cytosine is shown here). (4) After a washing step, any unincorporated nucleotides are removed and images are taken to deduce the RNA sequences. (5) The fluorescent dyes are chemically cleaved from the incorporated nucleotide after imaging. (6) Next round of sequencing begins with alternative fluorescent nucleotide (guanine is shown here). (7) Repeating cycle of nucleotide extension, washing, and imaging provides a set of nucleotide signals that are then aligned to the available *S. cerevisiae* genomic sequences to derive the transcriptomic profile of the yeast strain assayed.

## 14.5  PROTEOMICS AND WINE YEASTS

The proteome represents the entire protein complement of the cell. Like the transcriptome, the proteome is highly dynamic; however, because the proteome is subjected to several additional levels of posttranscriptional regulation, its dynamic range exceeds that of the transcriptome. Proteomic studies aim to resolve the complexity of the proteome through identification and characterization of every single protein at the whole-genome level, thereby uncovering the proteins associated with specific cellular functions.

Mass spectrometry (MS) is the leading proteomic tool that is used to discern the identity of unknown proteins. MS relies heavily on two major strategies for the separation and visualization of proteins from complex mixtures; two-dimensional (2D) gel electrophoresis and liquid chromatography (LC) (Zhang et al. 2010). Purified proteins are digested into peptide fragments that undergo electrospray ionization (Fenn et al. 1989) or matrix-assisted laser desorption ionization (MALDI) (Karas and Hillenkamp 1988). Mass spectrometers determine the identity of proteins on the basis of the time-of-flight (TOF) of ionized peptides (single-stage MS). However, the efficacy of MS does not end with peptide identification. Tandem mass spectrometry (MS/MS) is widely used to determine the amino acid sequence of proteins as well as to detect posttranslational modification of specific residues (Bachi and Bonaldi 2008).

The identification of proteins at the proteome level is associated with numerous challenges given the complexity and dynamic nature of even the yeast proteome. While DNA and RNA are each composed of essentially 4 main monomeric building blocks, proteins can be built from combinations of the 20 amino acids and are subject to numerous protein modifications. Superior resolution of complex protein mixtures using MudPIT (multidimensional protein identification technology) has aided high-throughput protein identification at the proteome level (Link et al. 1999). This approach relies on the proteolysis of total proteome extracts, which are then separated using a biphasic LC column directly coupled to tandem MS (Kolkman et al. 2005). Wei et al. (2005) have since refined MudPIT technology through the development of a 3D LC method, whereby they were able to identify 3109 proteins from the yeast proteome (Wei et al. 2005).

With the rapid development of systems biology, there is an increasing demand for quantitative proteomic approaches to determine the abundance of particular proteins within the proteome. Traditionally, determination of protein expression levels in complex samples containing thousands of proteins has been accomplished by comparing spot intensities from 2D gels (Kolkman et al. 2005). Unfortunately, 2D gel electrophoresis is notorious for gel-to-gel variation and poor reproducibility, making comparative analysis of whole proteomes a challenging task. To overcome these inherent issues, Unlu (1999) developed a quantitative approach termed "difference in gel electrophoresis" (DiGE), which involves pre-electrophoretic labeling of independent protein samples with different cyanide dyes. These protein samples are then mixed and separated on the same 2D gel to directly compare the ratio of signal from each spot (Unlu 1999). This strategy was employed to determine the effects on the *S. cerevisiae* proteome after the addition of 15 different metals to its growth media.

DiGE analysis identified significant changes in protein expression in approximately 20% of the yeast proteome upon metal treatment, providing a systems approach to determine the proteins involved in the eukaryotic cellular defense pathways (Hu et al. 2003). Other quantitative MS-based proteomic methodologies rely on stable isotope labeling of proteins or peptides, and these strategies include isotope-coded affinity tags (ICAT), isobaric tag for relative and absolute quantitation (iTRAQ), and stable isotope labeling with amino acids in cell culture (SILAC) (Figure 14.5) (Gygi et al. 1999, Ong et al. 2002, Yan et al. 2008). Nevertheless, protein species that are expressed at low abundance in complex mixtures are often omitted by these approaches due to limited sensitivity. To circumvent this problem, a novel MS-based assay called selective reaction monitoring (SRM) has been developed to enhance the detection of proteins with concentrations below 50 copies per yeast cell (Picotti et al. 2009). Due to its higher sensitivity and coverage, Picotti et al. (2010) recently

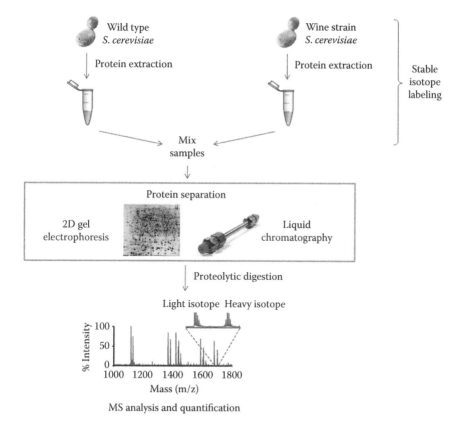

**FIGURE 14.5** Overview of the stable isotope labeling strategy to quantitatively identify differences in the proteome of *S. cerevisiae* strains. Proteins or peptide fragments are chemically or enzymatically labeled with stable isotopes using either ICAT or iTRAQ. Alternatively, proteins are cultured in growth media containing stable isotopes and metabolically labeled (SILAC). Both the unlabeled (light) and isotope labeled (heavy) samples are combined, separated using 2D gel electrophoresis or LC and analyzed by MS to quantify the ratio of "heavy" to "light" signal from each protein analyzed.

developed SRM into a high-throughput strategy, enabling a rapid and systematic assessment of entire *S. cerevisiae* protein species.

Several proteomic studies have been conducted in wine strain *S. cerevisiae* to analyze the changes in proteomic profiles during fermentation systematically. These studies have successfully identified proteins that are involved in different stress response and metabolism pathways according to their expression levels at different time points during the winemaking course (Braconi et al. 2008, Rossignol et al. 2009, Rowe et al. 2010, Salvado et al. 2008, Trabalzini et al. 2003a,b, Zuzuarregui et al. 2006). As an example of these, the proteome map of an industrial wine yeast strain compiled by Rossignol et al. (2009) displayed a strong representation of glycolysis and ethanol synthesis proteins, which are considered critical for fermentation capacity, thereby underlying the specific expression profile of wine strain *S. cerevisiae*.

## 14.6 METABOLOMICS AND WINE YEASTS

The metabolome represents the entire complement of small chemicals and metabolites found in the cell, excluding the DNA, RNA, and protein. The composition of the metabolome is extremely dynamic, exceeding that of both the transcriptome and proteome, because it is altered by the enzymatic action of the proteome in addition to being directly dependent on the composition of both the intra- and extracellular environments. Because the metabolome closely reflects the activities of a cell (i.e., phenotypes), it is now a rapidly expanding area of -omic research. In the context of winemaking, wine is essentially the combined metabolome of the grape, yeast, and bacteria that are present in the fermentation. So the investigation of wine style and quality is, at its heart, a metabolomic undertaking. Different yeast strains have distinct impacts on wine styles owing to discrete differences in their metabolism, which alter the levels of key aroma compounds (Romano et al. 2003, Swiegers and Pretorius 2005, Swiegers et al. 2005). Metabolomics thus represents another crucial niche that must be explored in order to gain a better understanding of how specific yeast strains affect wine attributes.

Like proteomics, metabolomics faces the problem of having to deal with a much higher diversity of chemical compounds than either genomics or transcriptomics and has likewise looked to MS as a means to identify these small molecules. However, the challenge of separating and characterizing the metabolome is far greater than even that of proteomics given the almost infinite number of chemically diverse small molecules that can exist in the cell at any one time. Therefore, in order to deal with this complexity, the field of metabolomics has sought systematically to divide the metabolome into smaller subsets that are defined both spatially and chemically.

Spatially, the yeast metabolome has been divided into both the compounds secreted by the cell into the growth medium (exometabolome) and the metabolites present within the cellular membrane (endometabolome). The exo- and endometabolomes can then either be further subdivided by chemical class (see below) or be studied using non-biased high-throughput MS approaches to produce metabolomic profiles (termed metabolomic fingerprinting or footprinting for the exometabolome and endometabolome, respectively) (Figure 14.6). While these metabolomic profiles

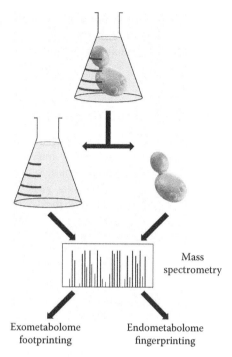

Mass
spectrometry

Exometabolome          Endometabolome
footprinting            fingerprinting

**FIGURE 14.6**   Metabolomic footprinting and fingerprinting.

do not provide exhaustive quantification of individual metabolites, they provide a
high-throughput means to classify cell types based on their metabolomic phenotype (Castrillo et al. 2003, Vijayendran et al. 2004). As such, fingerprinting and
footprinting have been applied to classify the yeast whole-genome collection and to
assist in the functional classifications of unknown ORFs based on the similarity of
their overall metabolic profile to proteins of known function (Castrillo et al. 2003,
Vijayendran et al. 2004).

Chemically, the metabolome can be subdivided and simplified through a variety
of separation and modification strategies, including the use of derivatization and
isotope labeling (dos Santos et al. 2003, Vijayendran et al. 2004, Villas-Bôas et al.
2003). While derivatization functions by altering specific subsets of the metabolome,
such as organic acids to enable their quantification, isotope labeling provides the
means to track the flux of specific metabolites (often $^{13}$C) and metabolic products
through various metabolic pathways (e.g., central carbon metabolism) in the cell.

Comparative metabolomic approaches have been applied to investigate the
impact of various wine strains of *S. cerevisiae* on the flavor profile of wines (Howell
et al. 2006, Son et al. 2009a,b, Swiegers et al. 2009, Vilanova and Sieiro 2006).
Strain-specific metabolite profiles were observed when identical musts and fermentation conditions were tested. These studies demonstrated that different wine
yeasts could produce distinct types of sensorially important metabolites at varying
levels, stressing the fact that the choice of yeast strain used for fermentation could
significantly affect wine style (Swiegers and Pretorius 2005, Swiegers et al. 2005).

In addition, the detected metabolite profiles of wine yeast also gave some insights into their fermentative behaviors: Yeast strains showing a higher yield of certain metabolites (e.g., glycerol and succinate) are associated with a faster fermentation (Son et al. 2009a,b).

## 14.7  INTERACTOMICS AND WINE YEASTS

The "interactome" refers to the entire complement of interactions between DNA, RNA, proteins, and metabolites within a cell. These interactions are readily influenced by genetic alterations or environmental stimuli, suggesting that studies are limited to examining the interactome of a particular yeast strain under particular growth conditions at a specific point in time. Despite the dynamic nature of the yeast interactome, numerous landmark studies have defined interaction networks for several of the -omic complexes.

### 14.7.1  THE DNA–PROTEIN INTERACTOME

Regulation of the transcriptome of the cell is achieved through systematic recruitment of transcription factors to the promoter regions of target genes to dictate transcript expression. Therefore, modulation of the DNA–protein interactome provides a novel avenue to manipulate the traits of *S. cerevisiae*. Transcription factor binding sites have been defined in *S. cerevisiae* through the use of genome-wide ChIP-chip (chromatin precipitation-on-chip) studies. ChIP-chip is a process that combines the traditional chromatin immunoprecipitation methodologies with cutting-edge microarray technologies. These DNA microarrays contain short genomic fragments that cover the cistrome of an organism and are used to map the physical recruitment of transcription factors to the promoters of target genes.

ChIP-chip technology was first successfully applied in *S. cerevisiae* a decade ago to define the DNA binding sites of GAL4 and Ste12 (Ren et al. 2000). Two years later, Lee et al. (2002) used a ChIP-chip-based systems approach to map the genomic DNA binding sites for 106 transcription factors (Lee et al. 2002). ChIP, followed by high-throughput sequencing (ChIP-Seq), is an alternative genome-wide strategy to map the physical binding sites of transcription factors. ChIP-Seq is not limited to predefined promoter sequences and therefore is replacing array-based ChIP-chip as the standard for transcription factor binding studies in higher eukaryotic organisms (Lefrancois et al. 2009). Nevertheless, ChIP-chip is still frequently used in yeast because it provides complete genome-wide coverage at a reduced cost in comparison to ChIP-Seq.

### 14.7.2  PROTEIN–PROTEIN INTERACTOME

Elucidation of the entire protein–protein interaction network in *S. cerevisiae* has been achieved over the past decade using several elegant genome-wide methodologies. These studies have evolved from the identification of individual paired interacting proteins to the quantification of large protein complexes.

### 14.7.2.1 Binary Interactomic Approaches

The yeast-two-hybrid assay system is the most widely used binary approach to explore the yeast protein interactome. This system relies on either the DNA binding domain or activator domain of a transcription factor (typically GAL4) tethered to two proteins being tested for interaction (Blow 2009). Upon interaction of these two proteins, the transcription factor will be regenerated and transcribe a reporter gene. Because the level of reporter gene expression indicates the strength of interaction, this high-throughput system can also provide information related to the dynamics of the protein–protein interaction.

With the knowledge of the *S. cerevisiae* genomic sequence (Goffeau et al. 1996), two independent research groups performed a yeast-two-hybrid screen involving a library of ORFs from the yeast genome (Ito et al. 2001, Uetz et al. 2000). Findings from these studies generated a comprehensive protein interactome network for *S. cerevisiae*.

Although two-hybrid approaches are informative and semiquantitative, they are limited to studying individual protein–protein interactions and do not have the ability to examine the formation of multi-protein complexes. Tertiary protein complexes are purified using immunoprecipitation followed by the use of proteomic tools such as MS to identify the associated interacting proteins. The success of this interactomic technology depends on the availability of an antibody that can effectively precipitate that native protein. Such limitations have been overcome through the use of epitope labeling of proteins. Furthermore, the use of yeast as a model system allows targeted integration of epitope tags in frame with gene products expressed from their natural chromosomal locations (Gavin et al. 2002). In particular, tandem affinity purification (TAP) coupled with MS has proven to be a powerful tool to identify the cellular binding partners of a protein (Rigaut et al. 1999). To further define the protein interactome network in yeast, *S. cerevisiae* strains with in-frame insertions of TAP tags at the 3′ end of each predicted ORF were generated (Krogan et al. 2006). Native protein complexes were affinity purified and the identities of associated binding partners determined using matrix-assisted laser desorption/ionization time-of-flight (MALDI-TOF) MS and liquid chromatography tandem mass spectrometry (LC-MS/MS) to increase coverage. This study provides superior coverage and accuracy over similar genome-wide studies identifying yeast interactome networks using purification of complexes following transient expression of bait proteins (Ho et al. 2002).

### 14.7.2.2 Protein Microarrays

Protein microarrays are powerful tools used to explore the protein interactome. Identification of all the protein-coding genes of an organism is a prerequisite for the generation of proteome microarrays (Kung and Snyder 2006). Therefore, *S. cerevisiae* provides an ideal model system for the development of proteome microarrays because the yeast genome was the first eukaryotic organism to be sequenced (Goffeau et al. 1996). *S. cerevisiae* whole-proteome microarrays are now commercially available and have been employed to define the yeast protein interactome (Blow 2009), kinase networks (Mok et al. 2009, Service 2005), and S-nitrosylation substrates (Foster et al. 2009). Unfortunately, complete proteome microarrays remain a costly and labor-intensive technology and therefore have had minimal impact in large-scale studies since their development.

## 14.8 INTEGRATION OF -OMIC DATA

While each -omic study of yeast is confined to a specific growth environment and time point, standing alone none of them can fully unravel the complexities of cellular functions. Hence, different -omic-scale datasets are required to be combined in order to provide a holistic view of the total cell system. Despite being a challenging task, several attempts have been made to bridge a subset of -omic data types in *S. cerevisiae* using different computational methods (Alberghina et al. 2009, Banks et al. 2008, Huang and Fraenkel 2009, Reimand et al. 2010, Rossouw et al. 2008, Seok et al. 2010, Usaite et al. 2009, Wang et al. 2009). Surprisingly, these studies have revealed many interaction and regulatory components that are not apparent in the single-omic assay, demonstrating the power of integrative -omic analysis in understanding the dynamics of cellular systems. While the research object is mainly the lab strain *S. cerevisiae*, four integrative -omic studies have been performed on wine yeasts, with particular focus on the correlation between transcriptome, proteome, and partial metabolome (Rossignol et al. 2009, Rossouw et al. 2008, 2010, Zuzuarregui et al. 2006).

However, a truly integrated -omic dataset covering the entire range of -omes is still lacking because the overlap between datasets is rather modest due to the diversity of the data types and the biases in experimental approaches and human interpretation. This stresses the need for a highly sophisticated computational analytic tool to normalize and compile the enormous amount of data generated across heterogeneous -omic experiments. The recent advent of "Robot Scientist," which harnesses artificial intelligence, has the ability to automate all aspects of the scientific process (including both "wet" benchwork and "dry" computational analysis), thereby enabling generation of reproducible and reusable datasets devoid of any potential biases (King et al. 2009, Sparkes et al. 2010). This state-of-art machine, when combined with high-throughput -omic assays, holds great potential to generate high-quality results and facilitate the integration of -omic datasets.

## 14.9 PREDICTIVE COMPUTATIONAL MODEL AS A PLATFORM FOR WINE YEAST STRAIN DEVELOPMENT

The wealth of dataset that has been generated by these high-throughput -omic approaches in yeast is astounding, not only in its amount but in its ever-increasing volume. While the data available specifically for wine yeast are still lacking in many areas, there are many studies currently underway that will provide large amounts of high-quality, coordinated -omic data on the wine yeast cell. Once available, these data will provide the building blocks for appropriate mathematic modeling to provide a prediction framework for the complex cellular functions of wine yeast. This will in turn enable the downstream development of ideal wine yeast strains that carry the ideal combinations of desirable genetic loci by a pioneering approach called synthetic biology. This next-level research tool carefully designs and constructs artificial biomolecular networks according to the robust model provided by system biology, such that the synergistic interactions of these networks would produce the phenotypes of interest (Cantone et al. 2009). As such, synthetic biology allows for precise engineering of a novel wine yeast strain with the desirable winemaking character-istics, such as increased or decreased ethanol production, improved fermentation robustness, and the modulation of flavor compounds. This is unattainable by conven-tional means, which are often associated with side effects (e.g., introduction of a new gene compromises the existing oenological properties) due to the lack of understand-ing the full intricacies of dynamic biological networks.

In conclusion, systems biology in combination with the growing body of syn-thetic biology data promises to improve the winemaking process by providing winemakers with more high-quality, customized wine yeast strains. The decoding and redesign of the building blocks of wine yeasts and the synthesis of large arti-ficial gene cassettes and perhaps even complete genomes are objectives that have a utilitarian purpose. However, it goes without saying that wine yeast strains without natural antecedents that have been designed on a computer will undoubtedly have to be thoroughly debated as part of the discussions surrounding genome-scale syn-thetic biology.

## ACKNOWLEDGMENTS

The Australian Wine Research Institute (AWRI), a member of the Wine Innovation Cluster in Adelaide, is supported by Australian grape growers and winemakers through their investment body, the Grape and Wine Research and Development Corporation, with matching funds from the Australian Government. Systems biol-ogy research at the AWRI is performed using resources provided as part of the National Collaborative Research Infrastructure Strategy (NCRIS), an initiative of the Australian Government, in addition to funds from the South Australian State Government. The AWRI's collaborating partners within this NCRIS-funded initiative, which is overseen by Bioplatforms Australia, are Genomics Australia, Proteomics Australia, Metabolomics Australia (of which the Microbial Metabolomics unit is housed at the AWRI), and Bioinformatics Australia.

## REFERENCES

Alberghina, L., T. Hofer, and M. Vanoni. 2009. Molecular networks and system-level proper-ties. *J Biotechnol* 144:224–233.

Argueso, J. L., M. F. Carazzolle, and P. A. Mieczkowski. 2009. Genome structure of a *Saccharomyces cerevisiae* strain widely used in bioethanol production. *Genome Res* 19:2258–2270.

Attfield, P. V. 1997. Stress tolerance: The key to effective strains of industrial baker's yeast. *Nat Biotechnol* 15:1351–1357.

Auesukaree, C., A. Damnernsawad, M. Kruatrachue et al. 2009. Genome-wide identification of genes involved in tolerance to various environmental stresses in *Saccharomyces cere-visiae. J Appl Genet* 50:301–310.

Bachi, A. and T. Bonaldi. 2008. Quantitative proteomics as a new piece of the systems biology puzzle. *J Proteomics* 71:357–367.

Banks, E., E. Nabieva, B. Chazelle, and M. Singh. 2008. Organization of physical inter-actomes as uncovered by network schemas. *PLoS Comput Biol* 4:e1000203. http://www.ploscompbiol.org/article/info%3Adoi%2F10.1371%2Fjournal.pcbi.1000203 (Accessed: April 5, 2010).

Baudin, A., O. Ozier-Kalogeropoulos, A. Denouel, F. Lacroute, and C. Cullin. 1993. A simple and efficient method for direct gene deletion in *Saccharomyces cerevisiae*. *Nucleic Acids Res* 2:3329–3330.

Bauer, F. F. and I. S. Pretorius. 2000. Yeast stress response and fermentation efficiency: How to survive the making of wine. *S Afr J Enol* 21:27–51.

Beltran, G., M. Novo, V. Leberre et al. 2006. Integration of transcriptomic and metabolic analyses for understanding the global responses of low-temperature winemaking fermentations. *FEMS Yeast Res* 6:1167–1183.

Bennett, S. 2004. Solexa Ltd. *Pharmacogenomics* 5:433–438.

Blow, N. 2009. Systems biology: Untangling the protein web. *Nature* 460:415–418.

Boone, C., H. Bussey, and B. J. Andrews. 2007. Exploring genetic interactions and networks with yeast. *Nat Rev Genet* 8:437–449.

Borneman, A. R., P. J. Chambers, and I. S. Pretorius. 2007. Yeast systems biology: Modelling the winemaker's art. *Trends Biotechnol* 25:349–355.

Borneman, A. R., A. H. Forgan, I. S. Pretorius, and P. J. Chambers. 2008. Comparative genome analysis of a *Saccharomyces cerevisiae* wine strain. *FEMS Yeast Res* 8:1185–1195.

Boulton, B., V. L. Singleton, L. F. Bisson, and R. E. Kunkee. 1996. Yeast and biochemistry of ethanol fermentation. In *Principles and Practices of Winemaking*, Boulton, B., V. L. Singleton, L. F. Bisson, and R. E. Kunkee (eds.), pp. 139–172. New York: Chapman & Hall.

Braconi, D., G. Bernardini, S. Possenti et al. 2008. Proteomics and redox-proteomics of the effects of herbicides on a wild-type wine *Saccharomyces cerevisiae* strain. *J Proteome Res* 8:256–267.

Cantone, I., L. Marucci, F. Iorio et al. 2009. A yeast synthetic network for in vivo assessment of reverse-engineering and modeling approaches. *Cell* 137:172–181.

Carreto, L., M. F. Eiriz, A. C. Gomes, P. M. Pereira, D. Schuller, and M. A. Santos. 2008. Comparative genomics of wild type yeast strains unveils important genome diversity. *BMC Genomics* 9:524.

Castrillo, J. I., A. H. Shabaz Mohammed, S. J. Gaskell, and S. G. Oliver. 2003. An optimized protocol for metabolome analysis in yeast using direct infusion electrospray mass spectrometry. *Phytochemistry* 62:929–937.

Costanzo, M., A. Baryshnikova, J. Bellay et al. 2010. The genetic landscape of a cell. *Science* 327:425–431.

dos Santos, M., A. K. Gombert, B. Christensen, L. Olsson, and J. Nielsen. 2003. Identification of in vivo enzyme activities in the cometabolism of glucose and acetate by *Saccharomyces cerevisiae* by using 13C-labeled substrates. *Eukaryot Cell* 2:599–608.

Dowell, R. D., O. Ryan, A. Jansen et al. 2010. Genotype to phenotype: A complex problem. *Science* 328:469.

Dunn, B., R. P. Levine, and G. Sherlock. 2005. Microarray karyotyping of commercial wine yeast strains reveals shared, as well as unique, genomic signatures. *BMC Genom* 6:53.

Erasmus, D. J., G. K. van der Merwe, and H. J. J. van Vuuren. 2003. Genome-wide expression analyses: Metabolic adaptation of *Saccharomyces cerevisiae* to high sugar stress. *FEMS Yeast Res* 3:375–399.

Fenn, J. B., M. Mann, C. K. Meng, S. F. Wong, and C. M. Whitehouse. 1989. Electrospray ionization for mass spectrometry of large biomolecules. *Science* 246:64–71.

Foster, M. W., M. T. Forrester, and J. S. Stamler. 2009. A protein microarray-based analysis of S-nitrosylation. *Proc Natl Acad Sci USA* 106:18948–18953.

Fujita, K., A. Matsuyama, Y. Kobayashi, and H. Iwahashi. 2006. The genome-wide screening of yeast deletion mutants to identify the genes required for tolerance to ethanol and other alcohols. *FEMS Yeast Res* 6:744–750.

Gavin, A. C., M. Bosche, R. Krause et al. 2002. Functional organization of the yeast proteome by systematic analysis of protein complexes. *Nature* 415:141–147.

Giaever, G., A. M. Chu, L. Ni et al. 2002. Functional profiling of the *Saccharomyces cerevisae* genome. *Nature* 418:387–391.

Goffeau, A., B. G. Barrell, H. Bussey et al. 1996. Life with 6000 genes. *Science* 274:563–577.

Gresham, D., D. M. Ruderfer, S. C. Pratt et al. 2006. Genome-wide detection of polymorphisms at nucleotide resolution with a single DNA microarray. *Science* 311:1932–1936.

Gygi, S. P., B. Rist, S. A. Gerber, F. Turecek, M. H. Gelb, and R. Aebersold. 1999. Quantitative analysis of complex protein mixtures using isotope-coded affinity tags. *Nat Biotechnol* 17:994–999.

Henschke, P. A. 1997. Wine yeast. In *Yeast Sugar Metabolism*, F. K. Zimmermann and K.-D. Entian (eds.), pp. 527–560. Lancaster, PA: Technomic Publishing.

Ho, Y., A. Gruhler, A. Heilbut et al. 2002. Systematic identification of protein complexes in *Saccharomyces cerevisiae* by mass spectrometry. *Nature* 415:180–183.

Howell, K. S., D. Cozzolino, E. J. Bartowsky, G. H. Fleet, and P. A. Henschke. 2006. Metabolic profiling as a tool for revealing *Saccharomyces cerevisiae* interactions during wine fermentation. *FEMS Yeast Res* 6:91–101.

Hu, Z., P. J. Killion, and V. R. Iyer. 2007. Genetic reconstruction of a functional transcriptional regulatory network. *Nat Genet* 39:683–687.

Hu, Y., G. Wang, G. Y. Chen, X. Fu, and S. Q. Yao. 2003. Proteome analysis of *Saccharomyces cerevisiae* under metal stress by two-dimensional differential gel electrophoresis. *Electrophoresis* 24:1458–1470.

Huang, S. S. and E. Fraenkel. 2009. Integrating proteomic, transcriptional, and interactome data reveals hidden components of signaling and regulatory networks. *Sci Signal* 2:40.

Infante, J. J., K. M. Dombek, L. Rebordinos, J. M. Cantoral, and E. T. Young. 2003. Genome-wide amplifications caused by chromosomal rearrangements play a major role in the adaptive evolution of natural yeast. *Genetics* 165:1745–1759.

Ito, T., T. Chiba, R. Ozawa, M. Yoshida, M. Hattori, and Y. Sakaki. 2001. A comprehensive two-hybrid analysis to explore the yeast protein interactome. *Proc Natl Acad Sci USA* 98:4569–4574.

Karas, M. and F. Hillenkamp. 1988. Laser desorption ionization of proteins with molecular masses exceeding 10,000 daltons. *Anal Chem* 60:2299–2301.

Katou, T., M. Namise, H. Kitagaki, T. Akao, and H. Shimoi. 2009. QTL mapping of sake brewing characteristics of yeast. *J Biosci Bioeng* 107:383–393.

King, R. D., J. Rowland, S. G. Oliver et al. 2009. The automation of science. *Science* 324:85–89.

Klinner, U. and B. Schafer. 2004. Genetic aspects of targeted insertion mutagenesis in yeasts. *FEMS Microbiol Rev* 28:201–223.

Kolkman, A., M. Slijper, and A. J. Heck. 2005. Development and application of proteomics technologies in *Saccharomyces cerevisiae*. *Trends Biotechnol* 23:598–604.

Krogan, N. J., G. Cagney, H. Yu et al. 2006. Global landscape of protein complexes in the yeast *Saccharomyces cerevisiae*. *Nature* 440:637–643.

Kumar, A. 2008. Multipurpose transposon insertion libraries for large-scale analysis of gene function in yeast. *Methods Mol Biol* 416:117–129.

Kumar, A., S. A. des Etages, P. S. Coelho, G. S. Roeder, and M. Snyder. 2000. High-throughput methods for the large-scale analysis of gene function by transposon tagging. *Methods Enzymol* 328:550–574.

Kumar, A., M. Seringhaus, C. M. Biery et al. 2004. Large-scale mutagenesis of the yeast genome using a Tn7-derived multipurpose transposon. *Genome Res* 14:1975–1986.

Kumar, A. and M. Snyder. 2001. Genome-wide transposon mutagenesis in yeast. *Curr Protoc Mol Biol* Chapter 13:Unit13.3.

Kumar, A., S. Vidan, and M. Snyder. 2002. Insertional mutagenesis: Transposon-insertion libraries as mutagens in yeast. *Methods Enzymol* 350:219–229.

Kung, L. A. and M. Snyder. 2006. Proteome chips for whole-organism assays. *Nat Rev Mol Cell Biol* 7:617–622.

Lashkari, D. A., J. L. DeRisi, J. H. McCusker et al. 1997. Yeast microarrays for genome wide parallel genetic and gene expression analysis. *Proc Natl Acad Sci USA* 94:13057–13062.

Lee, T. I., N. J. Rinaldi, F. Robert et al. 2002. Transcriptional regulatory networks in *Saccharomyces cerevisiae*. *Science* 298:799–804.

Lefebure, T. and M. J. Stanhope. 2007. Evolution of the core and pan-genome of *Streptococcus*: Positive selection, recombination, and genome composition. *Genome Biol* 8:R71. http://genomebiology.com/2007/8/5/R71

Lefrancois, P., G. Euskirchen, R. Auerbach et al. 2009. Efficient yeast ChIP-Seq using multiplex short-read DNA sequencing. *BMC Genom* 10:37.

Linderholm, A. L., C. L. Findleton, G. Kumar, Y. Hong, and L. F. Bisson. 2008. Identification of genes affecting hydrogen sulfide formation in *Saccharomyces cerevisiae*. *Appl Environ Microbiol* 74:1418–1427.

Link, A. J., J. Eng, D. M. Schieltz et al. 1999. Direct analysis of protein complexes using mass spectrometry. *Nat Biotechnol* 17:676–682.

Lipson, D., T. Raz, A. Kieu et al. 2009. Quantification of the yeast transcriptome by single-molecule sequencing. *Nat Biotechnol* 27:652–658.

Lussier, M., A. M. White, J. Sheraton et al. 1997. Large scale identification of genes involved in cell surface biosynthesis and architecture in *Saccharomyces cerevisiae*. *Genetics* 147:435–450.

Margulies, M., M. Egholm, W. E. Altman et al. 2005. Genome sequencing in microfabricated high-density picolitre reactors. *Nature* 437:376–380.

Marks, V. D., G. K. van der Merwe, and H. J. J. van Vuuren. 2003. Transcriptional profiling of wine yeast in fermenting grape juice: Regulatory effect of diammonium phosphate. *FEMS Yeast Res* 3:269–287.

Marullo, P., M. Aigle, M. Bely et al. 2007. Single QTL mapping and nucleotide-level resolution of a physiologic trait in wine *Saccharomyces cerevisiae* strains. *FEMS Yeast Res* 7:941–952.

Mok, J., H. Im, and M. Snyder. 2009. Global identification of protein kinase substrates by protein microarray analysis. *Nat Protoc* 4:1820–1827.

Nagalakshmi, U., Z. Wang, K. Waern et al. 2008. The transcriptional landscape of the yeast genome defined by RNA sequencing. *Science* 320:1344–1349.

Novo, M., F. Bigey, E. Beyne et al. 2009. Eukaryote-to-eukaryote gene transfer events revealed by the genome sequence of the wine yeast *Saccharomyces cerevisiae* EC1118. *Proc Natl Acad Sci USA* 106:16333–16338.

Ong, S. E., B. Blagoev, I. Kratchmarova et al. 2002. Stable isotope labeling by amino acids in cell culture, SILAC, as a simple and accurate approach to expression proteomics. *Mol Cell Proteomics* 1:376–386.

Ozsolak, F., A. R. Platt, D. R. Jones et al. 2009. Direct RNA sequencing. *Nature* 461:814–818.

Pan, X., D. S. Yuan, D. Xiang et al. 2004. A robust toolkit for functional profiling of the yeast genome. *Mol Cell* 16:487–496.

Picotti, P., B. Bodenmiller, L. N. Mueller, B. Domon, and R. Aebersold. 2009. Full dynamic range proteome analysis of *Saccharomyces cerevisiae* by targeted proteomics. *Cell* 138:795–806.

Picotti, P., O. Rinner, R. Stallmach, F. Dantel, T. Farrah, B. Doman, H. Wenschuh, and R. Aebersold. 2010. High-throughput generation of selected reaction-monitoring assays for proteins and proteomos. *Nat Methods*. 7:43–46.

Pizarro, F. J., M. C. Jewett, J. Nielsen, and E. Agosin. 2008. Growth temperature exerts differential physiological and transcriptional responses in laboratory and wine strains of *Saccharomyces cerevisiae*. *Appl Environ Microbiol* 74:6358–6368.

Pope, G. A., D. A. MacKenzie, M. Defernez et al. 2007. Metabolic footprinting as a tool for discriminating between brewing yeasts. *Yeast* 24:667–679.

Pretorius, I. S. 2000. Tailoring wine yeast for the new millennium: Novel approaches to the ancient art of winemaking. *Yeast* 16:675–729.

Primig, M., R. M. Williams, E. A. Winzeler et al. 2000. The core meiotic transcriptome in budding yeasts. *Nat Genet* 26:415–423.

Querol, A., M. T. Fernandez-Espinar, M. del Olmo, and E. Barrio. 2003. Adaptive evolution of wine yeast. *Int J Food Microbiol* 86:3–10.

Reimand, J., J. M. Vaquerizas, A. E. Todd, J. Vilo, and N. M. Luscombe. 2010. Comprehensive reanalysis of transcription factor knockout expression data in *Saccharomyces cerevisiae* reveals many new targets. *Nucleic Acids Res.* doi:10.1093/nar/gkq232

Ren, B., F. Robert, J. J. Wyrick et al. 2000. Genome-wide location and function of DNA binding proteins. *Science* 290:2306–2309.

Rigaut, G., A. Shevchenko, B. Rutz, M. Wilm, M. Mann, and B. Seraphin. 1999. A generic protein purification method for protein complex characterization and proteome exploration. *Nat Biotechnol* 17:1030–1032.

Romano, P., C. Fiore, M. Paraggio, M. Caruso, and A. Capece. 2003. Function of yeast species and strains in wine flavour. *Int J Food Microbiol* 86:169–180.

Ross-Macdonald, P., P. S. Coelho, T. Roemer et al. 1999. Large-scale analysis of the yeast genome by transposon tagging and gene disruption. *Nature* 402:413–418.

Rossignol, T., L. Dulau, A. Julien, and B. Blondin. 2003. Genome-wide monitoring of wine yeast gene expression during alcoholic fermentation. *Yeast* 20:1369–1385.

Rossignol, T., D. Kobi, L. Jacquet-Gutfreund, and B. Blondin. 2009. The proteome of a wine yeast strain during fermentation, correlation with the transcriptome. *J Appl Microbiol* 107:47–55.

Rossouw, D. and F. F. Bauer. 2009. Comparing the transcriptomes of wine yeast strains: Toward understanding the interaction between environment and transcriptome during fermentation. *Appl Microbiol Biotechnol* 84:937–954.

Rossouw, D., T. Naes, and F. F. Bauer. 2008. Linking gene regulation and the exo-metabolome: A comparative transcriptomics approach to identify genes that impact on the production of volatile aroma compounds in yeast. *BMC Genom.* 9:530.

Rossouw, D., R. Olivares-Hernandes, J. Nielsen, and F. F. Bauer. 2009. Comparative transcriptomic approach to investigate differences in wine yeast physiology and metabolism during fermentation. *Appl Environ Microbiol* 75:6600–6612.

Rossouw, D., A. H. van den Dool, D. Jacobson, and F. F. Bauer. 2010. Comparative transcriptomic and proteomic profiling of industrial wine yeast strains. *Appl Environ Microbiol* 76:3911–3923.

Rowe, J. D., J. F. Harbertson, J. P. Osborne, M. Freitag, J. Lim, and A. T. Bakalinsky. 2010. Systematic identification of yeast proteins extracted into model wine during aging on the yeast lees. *J Agric Food Chem* 58:2337–2346.

Salinas, F., D. Mandakovic, U. Urzua et al. 2010. Genomic and phenotypic comparison between similar wine yeast strains of *Saccharomyces cerevisiae* from different geographic origins. *J Appl Microbiol* 108:1850–1858.

Salvado, Z., R. Chiva, S. Rodriguez-Vargas, F. Randez-Gil, A. Mas, and J. M. Guillamon. 2008. Proteomic evolution of a wine yeast during the first hours of fermentation. *FEMS Yeast Res* 8:1137–1146.

Schacherer, J., D. M. Ruderfer, D. Gresham, K. Dolinski, D. Botstein, and L. Kruglyak. 2007. Genome-wide analysis of nucleotide-level variation in commonly used *Saccharomyces cerevisiae* strains. *PLoS ONE* 2:e322.

Schuldiner, M., S. R. Collins, N. J. Thompson et al. 2005. Exploration of the function and organization of the yeast early secretory pathway through an epistatic miniarray profile. *Cell* 123:507–519.

Seok, J., A. Kaushal, R. W. Davis, and W. Xiao. 2010. Knowledge-based analysis of microarrays for the discovery of transcriptional regulation relationships. *BMC Bioinform* 11 Suppl 1:S8. http://www.biomedcentral.com/1471–2105/11/S1/S8

Service, R. F. 2005. Proteomics. Protein chips map yeast kinase network. *Science* 307:1854–1855.

Shendure, J., G. J. Porreca, N. B. Reppas et al. 2005. Accurate multiplex polony sequencing of an evolved bacterial genome. *Science* 309:1728–1732.

Shoemaker, D. D., D. A. Lashkari, D. Morris, M. Mittmann, and R. W. Davis. 1996. Quantitative phenotypic analysis of yeast deletion mutants using a highly parallel molecular barcoding strategy. *Nat Genet* 14:450–456.

Smith, V., D. Botstein, and P. O. Brown. 1995. Genetic footprinting: A genomic strategy for determining a gene's function given its sequence. *Proc Natl Acad Sci USA* 92:6479–6483.

Smith, A. M., L. E. Heisler, J. Mellor et al. 2009. Quantitative phenotyping via deep barcode sequencing. *Genome Res* 19:1836–1842.

Son, H. S., G. S. Hwang, K. M. Kim et al. 2009a. $^1$H NMR-based metabolomic approach for understanding the fermentation behaviors of wine yeast strains. *Anal Chem* 81:1137–1145.

Son, H. S., G. S. Hwang, W. M. Park, Y. S. Hong, and C. H. Lee. 2009b. Metabolomic characterization of malolactic fermentation and fermentative behaviors of wine yeasts in grape wine. *J Agric Food Chem* 57:4801–4809.

Sparkes, A., W. Aubrey, E. Byrne et al. 2010. Towards robot scientists for autonomous scientific discovery. *Autom Exp* 2:1.

Stanley, D., S. Fraser, G. Stanley, and P. J. Chambers. 2010. Retrotransposon expression in ethanol-stressed *Saccharomyces cerevisiae*. *Appl Microbiol Biotechnol* 87:1447–1454.

Steinmetz, E., C. Warren, J. Kuehner, B. Panbehi, A. Ansari, and D. Brow. 2006. Genome-wide distribution of yeast RNA polymerase II and its control by Sen1 helicase. *Mol Cell* 24:735–746.

Swiegers, J. H., E. J. Bartowsky, P. A. Henschke, and I. S. Pretorius. 2005. Yeast and bacterial modulation of wine aroma and flavour. *Aust J Grape Wine Res* 11:139–173.

Swiegers, J. H., R. L. Kievit, T. Siebert et al. 2009. The influence of yeast on the aroma of Sauvignon Blanc wine. *Food Microbiol* 26:204–211.

Swiegers, J. H. and I. S. Pretorius. 2005. Yeast modulation of wine flavor. *Adv Appl Microbiol* 57:131–175.

Teixeira, M. C., L. R. Raposo, N. P. Mira, A. B. Lourenco, and I. Sa-Correia. 2009. Genome-wide identification of *Saccharomyces cerevisiae* genes required for maximal tolerance to ethanol. *Appl Environ Microbiol* 75:5761–5772.

Teixeira, M. C., L. R. Raposo, M. Palma, and I. Sa-Correia. 2010. Identification of genes required for maximal tolerance to high-glucose concentrations, as those present in industrial alcoholic fermentation media, through a chemogenomics approach. *OMICS* 14:201–210.

Tong, A. H., H. Evangelista, A. B. Parsons et al. 2001. Systematic genetic analysis with ordered arrays of yeast deletion mutants. *Science* 294:2364–2368.

Trabalzini, L., A. Paffetti, E. Ferro et al. 2003a. Proteomic characterization of a wild-type wine strain of *Saccharomyces cerevisiae*. *Ital J Biochem* 52:145–153.

Trabalzini, L., A. Paffetti, A. Scaloni et al. 2003b. Proteomic response to physiological fermentation stresses in a wild-type wine strain of *Saccharomyces cerevisiae*. *Biochem J* 370:35–46.

Uetz, P., L. Giot, G. Cagney et al. 2000. A comprehensive analysis of protein–protein interactions in *Saccharomyces cerevisiae*. *Nature* 403:623–627.

Unlu, M. 1999. Difference gel electrophoresis. *Biochem Soc Trans* 27:547–549.

Usaite, R., M. C. Jewett, A. P. Oliveira, J. R. Yates, L. Olsson, and J. Nielsen. 2009. Reconstruction of the yeast Snf1 kinase regulatory network reveals its role as a global energy regulator. *Mol Syst Biol* 5:319.

Van Voorst, F., J. Houghton-Larsen, L. Jønson, M. C. Kielland-Brandt, and A. Brandt. 2006. Genome-wide identification of genes required for growth of *Saccharomyces cerevisiae* under ethanol stress. *Yeast* 23:351–359.

Vijayendran, R., A. Gombert, B. Christensen, P. Kötter, and J. Nielsen. 2004. Phenotypic characterization of glucose repression mutants of *Saccharomyces cerevisiae* using experiments with $^{13}$C-labelled glucose. *Yeast* 21:769–779.

Vilanova, M. and C. Sieiro. 2006. Contribution by *Saccharomyces cerevisiae* yeast to fermentative flavour compounds in wines from cv. Albariño. *J Ind Microbiol Biotechnol* 33:929–933.

Villas-Bôas, S. G., D. G. Delicado, M. Åkesson, and J. Nielsen. 2003. Simultaneous analysis of amino and nonamino organic acids as methyl chloroformate derivatives using gas chromatography–mass spectrometry. *Anal Biochem* 322:134–138.

Wach, A., A. Brachat, R. Pohlmann, and P. Philippsen. 1994. New heterologous modules for classical or PCR-based gene disruptions in *Saccharomyces cerevisiae*. *Yeast* 10:1793–1808.

Wang, H., B. Kakaradov, S. R. Collins et al. 2009. A complex-based reconstruction of the *Saccharomyces cerevisiae* interactome. *Mol Cell Proteomics* 8:1361–1381.

Wei, W., J. H. McCusker, R. W. Hyman et al. 2007. Genome sequencing and comparative analysis of *Saccharomyces cerevisiae* strain YJM789. *Proc Natl Acad Sci USA* 104:12825–12830.

Wei, J., J. Sun, W. Yu et al. 2005. Global proteome discovery using an online three-dimensional LC-MS/MS. *J Proteome Res* 4:801–808.

Winzeler, E. A., C. I. Castillo-Davis, G. Oshiro et al. 2003. Genetic diversity in yeast assessed with whole-genome oligonucleotide arrays. *Genetics* 163:79–89.

Winzeler, E. A., D. D. Shoemaker, A. Astromoff et al. 1999. Functional characterization of the *Saccaromyces cerevisiae* genome by gene deletion and parallel analysis. *Science* 285:901–906.

Yan, W., D. Hwang, and R. Aebersold. 2008. Quantitative proteomic analysis to profile dynamic changes in the spatial distribution of cellular proteins. *Methods Mol Biol* 432:389–401.

Yoshikawa, K., T. Tanaka, C. Furusawa, K. Nagahisa, T. Hirasawa, and H. Shimizu. 2009. Comprehensive phenotypic analysis for identification of genes affecting growth under ethanol stress in *Saccharomyces cerevisiae*. *FEMS Yeast Res* 9:32–44.

Zhang, W., F. Li, and L. Nie. 2010. Integrating multiple 'omics' analysis for microbial biology: Application and methodologies. *Microbiology* 156:287–301.

Zuzuarregui, A., L. Monteoliva, G. Concha, and M. del Olmo. 2006. Transcriptomic and proteomic approach for understanding the molecular basis of adaptation of *Saccharomyces cerevisiae* to wine fermentation. *Appl Environ Microbiol* 72:836–847.

# 15 *Aspergillus flavus* Genetics and Genomics in Solving Mycotoxin Contamination of Food and Feed

*Jiujiang Yu, Deepak Bhatnagar,*
*Thomas E. Cleveland, Gary Payne,*
*William C. Nierman, and Joan W. Bennett*

## CONTENTS

## 15.1 *ASPERGILLUS* AND SECONDARY METABOLITES

In the fungal kingdom, *Aspergilli* belong to the class of imperfect filamentous fungi. Among the roughly 250 known species, many are capable of producing a broad array of beneficial secondary metabolites (Du'Lock 1965), such as antibiotics and other pharmaceuticals (Brakhage et al. 2008). For example, *Aspergillus terreus* produces lovastatin, a potent cholesterol-lowering drug. Other *Aspergilli* are used to produce antibiotics (penicillin and cephalosporin), antifungals (griseofulvin), and antitumor drugs (terrequinone A) (Hoffmeister and Keller 2007, Keller et al. 2005). There are many more uncharacterized compounds produced by *Aspergilli* through various metabolic pathways. These compounds include pathway end products and pathway intermediates or shunt metabolites formed along these pathways and may also have beneficial pharmaceutical properties that can be a potential source of new drugs.

## 15.2 MYCOTOXINS

The secondary metabolites produced by *Aspergillus* species, however, are not always beneficial. Some of them are toxic and carcinogenic. These compounds are called mycotoxins. The term "mycotoxin" is derived from the Greek words *mykhe* (or "myco" meaning fungus) and *to elkon* (meaning arrow poisons or toxins). Mycotoxins are a class of low-molecular-weight organic compounds. Structurally, mycotoxins are synthesized from amino acids, shikimic acid, or malonyl CoA through special pathways (Ehrlich 2007, Ehrlich et al. 1999a,b, Sweeney and Dobson 1999). They may accumulate in specialized structures such as mycelia, conidia, and sclerotia (Wicklow and Shotwell 1983) or be secreted into the surrounding environments. Mycotoxins have very diverse chemical structures, diverse toxic effects, and a variety of biological activities (Sweeney and Dobson 1998). Some mycotoxins are produced by a single species or even by one specific strain; others are made by a number of species.

Some mycotoxins have acute toxic effects leading to death while others have toxic effects from long-term exposure (chronic effects) resulting in chronic illness, such as suppressed immune response, malnutrition, or induction of cancer (Hsieh 1989, Van Egmond 1989).

## 15.3 AFLATOXINS

Aflatoxins produced by *Aspergillus flavus* are the most toxic and most potent natural carcinogen among the known mycotoxins (Jelinek et al. 1989). In addition to aflatoxin, *A. flavus* is known to produce over 14 mycotoxins (www.aspergillus.org.uk) such as cyclopiazonic acid (CPA), kojic acid, beta-nitropropionic acid, aspertoxin, aflatrem, and aspergillic acid (Goto et al. 1996). The aflatoxins, CPA, and aflatrem are the top three well-studied and better characterized mycotoxins. Aflatoxins were first identified as food poison after a mysterious "Turkey X" disease that killed more than 10,000 turkey poults in hatcheries in England 50 years ago after being fed with *A. flavus*–infested peanut meal (Allcroft et al. 1961, Asplin and Carnaghan 1961, Blount 1961, Lancaster et al. 1961). This incident was also the initial driving force to attract scientists worldwide to mycotoxin research centered on aflatoxins. The name aflatoxin was abbreviated from the species that it was first isolated, *A. flavus* toxin, i.e., *A-fla-toxin* (Diener et al. 1987). *A. flavus* and *Aspergillus parasiticus* are the two major species that produce aflatoxins (Cleveland et al. 2003). *Aspergillus tamarii, Aspergillus nomius* (Goto et al. 1996), and a few other species also make aflatoxins, but are less common (Cary and Ehrlich 2006, Ehrlich et al. 1999a,b, Kurtzman et al. 1987). *A. parasiticus* makes the four major aflatoxins: $B_1$, $B_2$, $G_1$, and $G_2$ (AFB$_1$, AFB$_2$, AFG$_1$, AFG$_2$, respectively) and *A. flavus* makes only AFB$_1$ and AFB$_2$ in most cases (Kurtzman et al. 1987). The B-type toxins show blue fluorescence under long-wave UV light and the G-type toxins show green fluorescence (Davis et al. 1987). The *A. flavus* species can be classified into two types of strains. The S strains produce numerous small sclerotia (average diameter is $<400\,\mu m$) and high levels of aflatoxins, but the L strains produce fewer but larger sclerotia and produce relatively less aflatoxins (Cotty 1989, Hesseltine et al. 1970, Saito et al. 1986). Within the S strains, some isolates produce only B-type of aflatoxins and so are termed $S_B$, while those S strains that produce both B-type and G-type of aflatoxins are termed SBG (Egel et al. 1994, Hesseltine et al. 1970, Saito et al. 1986). Most of the *A. flavus* strains isolated from West African countries, such as Nigeria and Republic of Benin, are S strains and produce not only AFB$_1$ but also AFG$_1$ (Cotty and Cardwell 1999). Some S strains of *A. flavus* are reported to produce both B-aflatoxins and G$_1$ and G$_2$ as well (Geiser et al. 2000).

The aflatoxin M$_1$ and M$_2$ are mammalian bioconversion products of AFB$_1$ and AFB$_2$, respectively, and were originally isolated and identified from bovine milk (Garrido et al. 2003, Hsieh et al. 1985, 1986, Huang and Hsieh 1988, Rice and Hsieh 1982). After entering the mammalian body (human or animals), aflatoxins are metabolized by the liver cytochrome P450 enzymes to a reactive epoxide intermediate, which becomes more carcinogenic, or are hydroxylated and become the less harmful aflatoxin M$_1$ and M$_2$.

### 15.3.1 Toxicology of Aflatoxins

The toxicity of aflatoxins exhibits both acute and chronic toxic effects. The liver is the primary target of aflatoxins (Scholl and Groopman 1995). Acute aflatoxicosis in humans is characterized by vomiting, abdominal pain, pulmonary edema, convulsions, coma, and death with cerebral edema of the liver, kidney, and heart (Richard and Payne 2003) if consumed in large quantity. Chronic effect can result in suppressed immune response, malnutrition, proliferation of the bile duct, centrilobular necrosis, and fatty infiltration of the liver, hepatomas, and hepatic lesions if exposed at low dose for a long period. $AFB_1$ also affects other organs and tissues, such as the lungs and the entire respiratory system (Kelly et al. 1997). In animal models, activation of $AFB_1$ by microsomal cytochrome P450 is required for its carcinogenic effect (Eaton and Gallagher 1994, Hsieh 1989, Lewis et al. 2005, Ngindu et al. 1982). The liver enzyme, cytochrome P450 monooxygenase, converts $AFB_1$ to a variety of metabolites of increased polarity including $AFB_1$-8, 9-epoxide, the ultimate carcinogen that binds covalently to N7 position of guanine in DNA. This results in a defective repair of DNA damages in the cells, which leads to mutations and ultimately carcinomas in many animal species (Busby and Wogan 1981). The role of aflatoxins in human carcinogenesis is complicated by hepatitis B virus (HBV) and C virus (HCV) infections, which are also associated with human hepatocarcinoma (Hsieh 1989, Peers et al. 1987, Wild et al. 1992). Multiple factors may be involved in carcinogenesis (Arsura and Cavin 2005, Chen et al. 1996a,b, McGlynn et al. 2003). Many children in developing countries are exposed to aflatoxin during pregnancy (Turner et al. 2007), nursing (Polychronaki et al. 2007), and after weaning (Gong et al. 2004). An association between hepatocellular carcinoma and dietary exposure to aflatoxins has been established from patients living in high-risk areas of People's Republic of China, Kenya, Mozambique, Philippines, Swaziland, Thailand, and Transkei of South Africa (Eaton and Gallagher 1994, Hsieh et al. 1985, Huang and Hsieh 1988, Lancaster et al. 1961, Lewis et al. 2005, Wilson 1989, Wogan 1992, Wong et al. 1977, Zhu et al. 1987, Zuckerman et al. 1967). The presence of DNA–aflatoxin adducts in urine is considered an indication of the transversion of guanine to thymine at the third base of codon 249, a mutation hot spot, in the tumor suppressor gene p53. The p53 gene is a transcription factor involved in the regulation of the cell cycle that is commonly mutated in human cancers (Groopman et al. 1994).

### 15.3.2 Food Safety and Economic Consequence of Aflatoxin Contamination

Aflatoxin contamination in food and feed is a significant food safety issue in the developing countries sometimes due to lack of detection, monitoring, and regulating measures to safeguard the food supply. It is estimated that approximately 4.5 billion people living in developing countries are chronically exposed to largely uncontrolled amounts of aflatoxin that severely results in changes in immunity and nutrition (Williams et al. 2004).

Major outbreaks of acute aflatoxicosis from contaminated food in humans have been documented in developing countries (CDC 2004, Lewis et al. 2005).

For example, in western India in 1974, 108 persons among 397 people infected died from aflatoxin poisoning (Krishnamachari et al. 1975). A more recent incident of aflatoxin poisoning occurred in Kenya in July 2004 leading to the death of 125 people among the 317 reported illnesses due to consumption of aflatoxin-contaminated maize (corn) (CDC 2004, Krishnamachari et al. 1975, Lewis et al. 2005). Acute toxicosis is not the only concern. The world health authorities warn that low doses with long-term dietary exposure to aflatoxins is also a major risk, as they can lead to hepatocellular carcinoma (Bressac et al. 1991, Fung and Clark 2004, Hsu et al. 1991, Wogan 1992). International Agency for Research on Cancer (IARC) has designated aflatoxin as a human liver carcinogen (Wogan 1992, 2000). This food poisoning problem is rarely observed in the United States in humans but does occasionally occur in animals. The most notable recent case involved the reported deaths of over 100 dogs that had consumed tainted dog feed.

Because there is no effective control method to prevent aflatoxin contamination of food and feed resulting in adverse effects in human and animals (Brown et al. 1998, Eaton and Gallagher 1994, Eaton and Groopman 1994, Robens 2001, Robens and Cardwell 2005), the concentrations of aflatoxin in food and feed is carefully regulated in developed countries such as the United States and many European countries. Over 100 countries have established limits on the content of allowable concentrations of aflatoxin (Magan and Olsen 2004). Regulatory guidelines of the U.S. Food and Drug Administration (FDA) have set limits of 20 ppb total aflatoxins for interstate commerce of food and feedstuff and 0.5 ppb $AFM_1$ for milk. The European Commission has set the limits on groundnuts subject to further processing at 15 ppb for total aflatoxins and 8 ppb for aflatoxin $B_1$, and for nuts and dried fruits subject to further processing at 10 ppb for total aflatoxins and 5 ppb for $AFB_1$. The aflatoxin standards for cereals, dried fruits, and nuts intended for direct human consumption are even more stringent, and the limit for total aflatoxins is 4 and 2 ppb for $AFB_1$ (Otsuki et al. 2001). Thus the threat of aflatoxin poisoning is low in most developed countries, but it incurs a significant economic loss to farmers and producers, since contaminated products are destroyed due to regulations. Thus aflatoxin contamination is more of an economic issue in developed countries. Due to the significant impact on human and animal health and on economy, an understanding of the biological and genetic mechanisms of aflatoxin formation and regulation is needed in an attempt to devise effective control strategies to solve aflatoxin contamination of food and feed.

### 15.3.3 AFLATOXIN BIOSYNTHETIC PATHWAY

Extensive research efforts have been focused on deciphering the pathway of aflatoxin biosynthesis shortly after the structure of these toxins was established (Bennett and Christensen 1983, Bennett and Klich 2003, Cleveland et al. 1990, 2009, Goldblatt 1969a,b, Yabe et al. 2003, Yu 2004, Yu et al. 2004a–c, 2010a,b). The establishment of aflatoxin biosynthetic pathway was attributed to the hallmark discovery of a color mutant that accumulates brick-red pigment, norsolorinic acid (NOR), in *A. parasiticus* (Bennett et al. 1976, 1971, 1997). NOR is the earliest and the first stable aflatoxin precursor (Bennett et al. 1997). This discovery led the way to identify all of the aflatoxin pathway steps and intermediates by scientists all over the world.

Significant progress has been made thus far in elucidating this pathway (Bennett and Klich 2003, Bennett et al. 1976, 1981, 1992 Bennett and Lee 1979, Bhatnagar et al. 1992, Cary et al. 2007, Chang 2004, Chang et al. 1993, 1995a,b, 1999a,b, 2010, Cleveland et al. 1987, Cotty 1988, Crawford et al. 2008, Ehrlich et al. 1999a,b, Keller et al. 1993, Payne and Brown 1998, Yabe et al. 2003, Yu et al. 1995, 2004a–c). At least 23 enzymatic steps have been characterized or proposed to be involved in the bioconversion of aflatoxin intermediates. To date, this aflatoxin biosynthetic pathway is one of the best studied fungal secondary metabolic pathways.

Aflatoxins are synthesized from malonyl CoA, first with the formation of hexanoyl CoA, followed by formation of a decaketide anthraquinone (Bhatnagar et al. 1992, Ehrlich et al. 1999a,b, Minto and Townsend 1997). There are two fatty acid synthases (FAS) and a polyketide synthase (PKS) involved in the synthesis of the polyketide from acetyl CoA (Watanabe and Townsend 2002). Aflatoxins are formed after a series of highly organized oxidation–reduction reactions (Townsend 1997, Yabe et al. 2003, 2004a,b,c). The established aflatoxin biosynthetic pathway scheme is a hexanoyl CoA precursor $\rightarrow$ norsolorinic acid, NOR $\rightarrow$ averantin, AVN $\rightarrow$ hydroxyaverantin, HAVN $\rightarrow$ oxoaverantin, OAVN $\rightarrow$ averufin, AVF $\rightarrow$ hydroxyversicolorone, HVN $\rightarrow$ versiconal hemiacetal acetate, VHA $\rightarrow$ versiconal, VAL $\rightarrow$ versicolorin B, VERB $\rightarrow$ versicolorin A, VERA $\rightarrow$ demethyl-sterigmatocystin, DMST $\rightarrow$ sterigmatocystin, ST $\rightarrow$ O-methylsterigmatocystin, OMST $\rightarrow$ aflatoxin $B_1$, AFB$_1$ and aflatoxin $G_1$, AFG$_1$. After the VAL step, there is a branch point in the pathway that leads from VERB to dihydro-DMST, DHOMST $\rightarrow$ dihydro-ST, DHST $\rightarrow$ dihydro-OMST, DHOMST $\rightarrow$ to AFB$_2$ and AFG$_2$ (Yabe et al. 2003, Yu et al. 1998).

Sterigmatocystin (ST) and dihydrosterigmatocystin (DHST), the penultimate precursors of aflatoxins, are produced by several species including *Aspergillus versicolor* and *Aspergillus nidulans*. ST and DHST are toxic and carcinogenic as well. They share common biochemical pathways, homologous genes, and regulatory mechanisms to aflatoxin synthesis in *A. flavus* and *A. parasiticus* (Brown et al. 1996, Yu et al. 2004a–c).

### 15.3.4 AFLATOXIN BIOSYNTHETIC PATHWAY GENES

The aflatoxin pathway genes and corresponding enzymes have been extensively studied (Bennett et al. 1971, Lee et al. 1971, Yabe and Nakajima 2004, Yu et al. 2004a–c). A comprehensive review on the complete aflatoxin pathway genes in *A. parasiticus* and *A. flavus* with a revised gene naming scheme that conforms to the naming convention in *Aspergillus* was reported (Yu et al. 2004a–c). The first aflatoxin pathway gene *aflD* (*nor-1*) was identified in *A. parasiticus* by the genetic complementation approach that selected for transformants with the loss of the characteristic red color of NOR. This gene encodes a reductase necessary for the conversion of NOR to averantin (AVN) (Bennett et al. 1997, Chang et al. 1992). Consistently, disruption or deletion of the *aflD* (*nor-1*) gene led to the accumulation of a brick-red pigment in the hyphae and blocked the synthesis of all aflatoxins and their intermediates beyond NOR (Bennett et al. 1971, 1981, Lee et al. 1971). The *aflM* (*ver-1*) gene, encoding a ketoreductase required for the conversion of versicolorin A (VERA) to demethylsterigmatocystin (DMST) and versicolorin B (VERB) to demethyldihydrosterigmatocystin (DMDHST), was the second gene cloned in *A. parasiticus* (Liang et al. 1996, Skory et al. 1992, 1993). The third gene named *aflP* (*omtA*) encoding an *O*-methyltransferase for the conversion of ST to OMST and DMST to dihydro-*O*-methylsterigmatocystin (DHOMST) was cloned by antibody screening of a cDNA expression library of *A. parasiticus* (Yu et al. 1993). A regulatory gene named *aflR*, present in *A. parasiticus* and *A. flavus* (originally named *afl-2* and *apa-2*), as well as in *A. nidulans*, was also cloned shortly thereafter (Chang et al. 1993). This is a positive regulatory gene involved in both the aflatoxin pathway gene expression in *A. flavus* and *A. parasiticus* and ST pathway gene expression in *A. nidulans*. The four genes were the cornerstones that led to the discovery of the entire aflatoxin gene cluster by aligning overlapping cosmid clones (Yu et al. 1995).

Genes involved in the early stages of aflatoxin biosynthesis include two large genes (7.5 kb transcripts), *aflB* (*fas-1*) and *aflA* (*fas-2*), encoding beta-(FASβ) and alpha-subunit (FASα) of a FAS, respectively (Mahanti et al. 1996, Trail et al. 1995a,b). Another large gene in early aflatoxin synthesis is the 7 kb *aflC* (*pksA*) gene encoding a PKS for the synthesis of the polyketides skeleton (Chang et al. 1995a,b). Disruption of the *aflC* (*pksA*) gene results in nonproduction of aflatoxin or any of its intermediates (Feng and Leonard 1995). The predicted amino acid sequence of this PKS reveals four typical conserved domains common to other known PKS proteins: beta-ketoacyl synthase (KS), acyltransferase (AT), acyl carrier protein (ACP), and thioesterase (TE) (Chang et al. 1995a,b). To recapitulate, *aflA*, *aflB*, and *aflC* genes are directly involved in the conversion of acetate to NOR.

The cloning of *aflQ* (*ordA*) and *aflU* (*cypA*) solved the major puzzle in later steps of aflatoxin biosynthesis especially the synthesis of the G-type aflatoxins (Ehrlich et al. 2004, Yu et al. 1998). There are two separate pathways leading to B-type (AFB$_1$ and AFB$_2$) and G-type (AFG$_1$ and AFG$_2$) aflatoxins (Yabe et al. 1988a,b). The gene named *aflQ* (*ordA*), encoding a cytochrome P450 monooxygenase, was demonstrated to be responsible for the conversion of OMST to AFB$_1$ and AFG$_1$, and DMDHST to AFB$_2$ and AFG$_2$ (Prieto and Woloshuk 1997, Yu et al. 1998). Expression and substrate feeding, using a yeast system, demonstrated that an additional enzyme was required for the formation of G-type aflatoxins (Yu et al. 1998). Functional studies demonstrated that the *aflU* (*cypA*) gene, encoding a cytochrome P450 monooxygenase, was responsible for the conversion of OMST to AFG$_1$ and DHOMST to AFG$_2$ (Ehrlich et al. 2004). The inability of *A. flavus* to produce G-type aflatoxins is thought to be due to a partial deletion of this gene during the evolution (Ehrlich et al. 2004). Recently, the *nadA* gene was shown by microarray studies to be a member of the aflatoxin gene cluster (Price et al. 2006) rather than belonging to the adjoining sugar utilization cluster as originally proposed (Yu et al. 2000).

As mentioned earlier, *A. flavus* produces AFB$_1$ and AFB$_2$, whereas *A. parasiticus* produces all four aflatoxins, AFB$_1$, AFB$_2$, AFG$_1$, and AFG$_2$. Coincidently, only the G-type aflatoxin producer, *A. parasiticus*, has intact *nadA* and *norB* genes. Further investigation by gene disruption experiments into the possible involvement of *nadA* and *norB* in AFG$_1$/AFG$_2$ formation demonstrated that both genes play a role in AFG$_1$ formation. The *nadA* encodes an OYE (old yellow enzyme) FMN-binding domain reductase for the conversion of cypA oxidation product, a 386 Da compound to a 362 Da compound (*nadA* reduction product). The 362 Da compound is further converted to a 360 Da compound by aryl alcohol dehydrogenase encoded by the *norB* gene (Ehrlich et al. 2008). NadA is a cytosolic enzyme and was reported to convert a new aflatoxin intermediate named NADA, which is between OMST and $AFG_1$ (Cai et al. 2008). NADA is likely the 386 Da compound. Most recently, the *norA* gene encoding an aryl alcohol dehydrogenase was shown to be involved in the final step of aflatoxin biosynthesis from deoxyAFB$_1$ to AFB$_1$ (Ehrlich et al. 2010). It is evidenced that the *norA* and *norB* genes are involved in later steps of aflatoxin formation rather than in the early step in the reduction of NOR as previously presumed based purely on DNA sequence alignment.

### 15.3.5 AFLATOXIN BIOSYNTHETIC PATHWAY GENE CLUSTER

In *A. flavus* and *A. parasiticus*, a complete aflatoxin pathway gene cluster consisting 29 genes or open reading frames (ORFs) have been confirmed to be involved in aflatoxin formation (Yu et al. 1995, 2004a–c). Initially, it was found that the *aflD (nor-1)* and *aflM (ver-1)* genes were linked with the regulatory gene *aflR* in a common cosmid clone (Skory et al. 1993, Trail et al. 1995a,b). This provided the first evidence indicating that aflatoxin pathway genes are clustered. The aflatoxin pathway gene cluster was established when nine cloned genes, including *aflD (nor-1)*, *aflR*, *aflM (ver-1)*, and *aflP (omtA)*, were mapped to a 75 kb DNA region by overlapping cosmid clones in *A. parasiticus* and *A. flavus* (Yu et al. 1995). Later, a completed aflatoxin pathway gene cluster was established when a 75 kb DNA sequence was determined (Yu et al. 2004a–c). Based on genome sequence data, this aflatoxin gene cluster is located on chromosome III near subtelomeric region (Yu et al. 2008, 2010a,b). The primary evolutionary advantage of gene clustering may be for the purpose of coordinated gene expression. Interestingly, a partially duplicated aflatoxin gene cluster was identified in *A. parasiticus* (Liang et al. 1996). This gene cluster consists of seven duplicated genes, named *aflR2*, *aflJ2*, *adhA2*, *estA2*, *norA2*, *ver1B*, and *omtB2* (Chang and Yu 2002). The number "2" denotes the second copy of the gene. The genes within this partially duplicated cluster are likely nonfunctional under normal conditions, although some of the gene sequences are intact. Lack of expression may be due to the chromosome location (Chiou et al. 2002).

### 15.3.6 GENETIC REGULATION OF AFLATOXIN BIOSYNTHESIS

#### 15.3.6.1 Positive Regulatory Gene *aflR*

The gene *aflR* is a positive regulatory gene in both the aflatoxin and ST gene clusters. Disruption of *aflR* results in the loss of aflatoxin pathway gene expression and aflatoxin production. Inclusion of an additional copy of *aflR* or elevated expression leads to overproduction of aflatoxin biosynthetic intermediates (Chang et al. 1995a,b, Flaherty and Payne 1997). The *aflR* gene, encoding a sequence-specific zinc binuclear DNA-binding protein, is required for transcriptional activation of most, if not all, of the aflatoxin pathway genes (Chang et al. 1995a,b, 1999a,b, Ehrlich et al. 1999a,b, Woloshuk et al. 1994). The AflR protein has major domains typical of fungal and yeast Gal4-type transcription factors: a *N*-terminal cysteine-rich stretch, $(Cys_6\text{-}Zn_2)$

DNA-binding domain (Chang et al. 1995a,b); an arginine-rich (RRARK) nuclear localization domain; and a transcription activation domain in the C-terminus (Chang et al. 1999a,b). Aflatoxin pathway gene transcription is activated when the AflR protein binds to the palindromic sequence 5'-TCGN5CGA-3' (also called AflR binding motif) in the promoter region of structural genes (Ehrlich et al. 1999a,b, Fernandes et al. 1998) in *A. parasiticus*, *A. flavus*, and *A. nidulans*. *Aspergillus sojae*, a nontoxigenic species used in industrial fermentations, was found to contain a defective AflR transcription activation domain due to the early termination of 62 amino acids from its C-terminus (Matsushima et al. 2001, Takahashi et al. 2002). Thus, in the absence of the functional AflR regulatory protein, no aflatoxin can be produced by this food grade *Aspergillus*.

Gene expression studies on an *aflR* disruptant mutant compared with wild type using microarrays in *A. parasiticus* SRRC 143 (SU-1) identified 23 highly expressed genes in the wild type. Eighteen of the genes are known as aflatoxin biosynthetic genes; three of these genes (*hypB*, *aflY*, and *nadA*) are in or adjacent to the established aflatoxin gene cluster (Yu et al. 2004a–c), and the last two genes (*hlyC* and *niiA*) are located outside the aflatoxin gene cluster. All of the aflatoxin biosynthetic genes have a putative consensus AflR-binding site (5'-TCGSWNNSCGR-3') from a typical 100–300 bp (Ehrlich et al. 1999a,b, Fernandes et al. 1998) up to 2.3 kb upstream in their promoter regions, except for *aflR*. The *niiA* gene is a member of the nitrogen assimilation gene cluster that is divergently transcribed with *niaD*.

### 15.3.6.2 Co-Regulatory Gene *aflS* (Old Name *aflJ*)

Adjacent to the *aflR* gene in the aflatoxin gene cluster, a divergently transcribed gene, *aflS* (*aflJ*), was also found to be involved in the regulation of transcription (Meyers et al. 1998). The AflJ protein binds to the carboxy terminal region of AflR and may affect AflR activity (Chang and Todd 2003). Disruption of *aflS* in *A. flavus* resulted in a failure to produce any aflatoxin pathway metabolites (Meyers et al. 1998).

### 15.3.6.3 Global Regulatory Gene *laeA*

A global regulatory gene, *laeA* (named such for lack of *aflR* expression), was identified initially in *A. nidulans* to reside outside of the ST/aflatoxin pathway gene cluster (Bok and Keller 2004, Butchko et al. 1999). The *laeA* encodes a nuclear protein containing an S-adenosylmethionine (SAM) binding motif. A homologue of this regulatory gene, *laeA*, was also found in *A. flavus* (EST ID: NAGEM53TV) (Bok and Keller 2004, Kim et al. 2006). Disruption of *laeA* resulted in loss not only of *aflR* gene expression for ST synthesis, but also expression of genes involved in penicillin biosynthesis in *A. nidulans*, as well as genes involved in gliotoxin biosynthesis in *Aspergillus fumigatus* (Bok and Keller 2004). Thus *laeA* appears to be involved in the global regulation of a number of different secondary metabolic pathways in several fungal species. Genes for CPA production are separated from the aflatoxin cluster by only two genes, and both CPA and aflatoxin gene clusters were shown to be regulated by LaeA (Duran et al. 2007). The exact mechanism of LaeA in regulating secondary metabolite gene expression is not well understood. However, transcriptional profiling of wild-type and *laeA* deletion mutants of *A. fumigatus* reveals that LaeA positively controls the biosynthesis of 20%–40% of major secondary metabolites (Perrin et al. 2007). Studies on *aflR* gene expression within and outside the ST gene cluster indicate that the LaeA regulates only genes that are within the cluster (Bok et al. 2006). This result led to a hypothesis that LaeA differentially affects histone proteins associated with clusters for secondary metabolism and makes the region more accessible to gene transcription (Bok et al. 2006).

#### 15.3.6.4 Developmental Regulatory Gene *veA*

A gene named *veA* was identified to function in light-dependent conidiation in *A. nidulans* (Mooney et al. 1990, Mooney and Yager 1990). Deletion of *veA* abolishes light dependence and results in the complete loss of ST and aflatoxin production under both light and dark conditions in *A. nidulans* and in *A. flavus* (Duran et al. 2007, Stinnett et al. 2007). Subsequent studies have shown that *veA* modulates expression of *aflR* in *A. flavus*, *A. parasiticus*, and *A. nidulans* (Calvo et al. 2004, Duran et al. 2007, Kato et al. 2003). The *veA* was also found to be necessary for the formation of sclerotia and to regulate the synthesis of the mycotoxins CPA and aflatrem. A *veA* deletion mutant of *A. flavus* was completely blocked in the production of aflatrem and showed greater than a twofold decrease in CPA production. Northern hybridization analysis showed that *veA* is required for the expression of *A. flavus* aflatrem genes *atmC*, *atmG*, and *atmM* (Duran et al. 2007).

### 15.3.7 FACTORS AFFECTING AFLATOXIN BIOSYNTHESIS

Aflatoxin biosynthesis is influenced by many biotic and abiotic environmental factors (Bennett and Papa 1988, Demain 1998, Kale and Bennett 1992, Kale et al. 1996, Yabe et al. 1988a,b) including nutritional factors such as carbon and nitrogen sources, environmental effects such as water activity and temperature, physiological conditions such as pH (Cotty 1988) and bioreactive agents (Guo et al. 2005, Payne and Brown 1998), and the subject matter is under intensive study. These studies would offer promise of devising control strategies to shut down aflatoxin production in aflatoxigenic *A. flavus* species through manipulations of environmental conditions for the fungal response to these factors.

#### 15.3.7.1 Carbon

Nutritional factors such as carbon, nitrogen, amino acid, lipid, and trace elements have long been observed to affect aflatoxin production (Cuero et al. 2003, Feng and Leonard 1998, Payne and Brown 1998). The best-known nutritional factors affecting aflatoxin biosynthesis are carbon and nitrogen sources (Adye and Mateles 1964, Bennett et al. 1979, Luchese and Harrigan 1993). The relationship between carbon source and aflatoxin formation has been well established. Simple sugars such as glucose, sucrose, fructose, and maltose support aflatoxin formation, while peptone, sorbose, and lactose do not (Buchanan and Lewis 1984, Payne and Brown 1998). Woloshuk et al. (1997) reported the connection between alpha amylase activity and aflatoxin production in *A. flavus*. Yu et al. (2000) identified a gene cluster related to sugar utilization in *A. parasiticus* next to the aflatoxin gene cluster. The expression of the *hxtA* gene, encoding a hexose transporter protein, was found to be concurrent with the aflatoxin pathway genes in aflatoxin-conducive medium. A close physical linkage between the two gene clusters could point to a relationship between the clusters in the processing of carbohydrates leading to the induction of aflatoxin biosynthesis. Lipid substrate is a good carbon source to support aflatoxin production (Fanelli and Fabbri 1989, Fanelli et al. 1983, 1995). A lipase gene, *lipA*, was cloned in *A. parasiticus* and *A. flavus* (Yu et al. 2003). The expression of *lipA* and subsequent aflatoxin production are induced by lipid substrate. The addition of 0.5% soybean oil to nonaflatoxin-conducive peptone medium induces lipase gene expression and leads to aflatoxin formation (Yu et al. 2003). However, the molecular mechanism by which a carbon source is involved in the regulation of aflatoxin pathway gene expression is poorly understood.

### 15.3.7.2  Nitrogen

Nitrogen source plays an important role in aflatoxin production (Payne and Brown 1998). Asparagine, aspartate, alanine, ammonium nitrate, ammonium nitrite, ammonium sulfate, glutamate, glutamine, and proline-containing media support aflatoxin production, while sodium nitrate and sodium nitrite containing media do not (Davis et al. 1967, Reddy et al. 1971, 1979). It was also suggested that nitrate represses averufin and aflatoxin formation (Kachholz and Demain 1983, Niehaus and Jiang 1989). Nitrate was reported to have a suppressive effect on aflatoxin production, and overexpression of *aflR* gene by additional copies of *aflR* overcomes the negative regulatory effect on aflatoxin pathway gene transcription (Chang et al. 1995a,b). Nitrogen utilization genes and a nitrogen regulator gene, *areA* from *A. parasiticus*, were cloned (Chang et al. 1996, 2000). In the intergenic region between *aflR* and *aflS* (*aflJ*), several AreA binding motifs have been identified (Chang et al. 1996, 2000). The AreA binding could prevent AflR binding. It seems that the aflatoxin formation and nitrogen metabolism are linked through a to-be-identified regulatory circuit. Certain amino acids can have opposing effects on aflatoxin production (Payne and Hagler 1983). Recent studies show that tryptophan inhibits aflatoxin formation while tyrosine enhances aflatoxin production in *A. flavus* (Wilkinson et al. 2007a,b).

### 15.3.7.3  Temperature

Temperature has long been documented to affect aflatoxin formation (Diener and Davis 1970, OBrian et al. 2007, Roy and Chourasia 1989, Schroeder and Hein 1968). Optimal aflatoxin production is observed at temperatures near 30°C (28°C–35°C) (OBrian et al. 2007). When temperature increases to above 36°C, aflatoxin production is nearly completely inhibited. Genome-wide gene profiling using microarray and RT-PCR verification (OBrian et al. 2007) indicated that high temperature is associated with a decrease in the expression of the aflatoxin pathway genes. RT-PCR detected ample amount of transcripts of both regulatory genes *aflR* and *aflS* (*aflJ*) (OBrian et al. 2007). So it was hypothesized that temperature may affect the activity of AflR or some other unknown regulatory element. High-resolution studies using next-generation sequencing technologies on aflatoxin pathway gene expression in response to temperature clearly showed that temperature affects the level of *aflR* and *aflS* transcripts (J. Yu et al., unpublished data). High temperature affects *aflS* more than *aflR*. Change in the ratio of *aflS* to *aflR* renders *aflR* unfunctional for transcription activation.

#### 15.3.7.4 Water Activity

High water activity favors spore germination and mycelial growth. Severe aflatoxin outbreaks in corn have been documented to occur under hot weather and drought conditions (Cotty and Jaime-Garcia 2007, Sanders et al. 1984). The mechanism of *A. flavus* infestation in corn under these conditions is not well understood. The possible scenarios may include a combination of these factors: (a) the plant defense mechanism is weakened under water stress conditions; (b) higher insect feeding and associated injuries to plant tissues, thus providing entry opportunities for fungal invasion; and (c) more fungal spores dispersed in the air under drier climate conditions.

#### 15.3.7.5 Culture pH

Ambient pH is also an important factor affecting aflatoxin formation (Cotty 1988). Aflatoxin biosynthesis in *A. flavus* occurs in acidic media, but is inhibited in alkaline media (Cotty 1988). The *pacC* gene is a major transcriptional regulatory factor for pH homeostasis (Keller et al. 1997). In the *aflR* promoter region, at least one PacC binding site has been identified (Ehrlich et al. 1999a,b). The presence of a putative PacC-binding site close to the *aflR* transcription start site may play some role in pH regulation on aflatoxin production (Keller et al. 1997, Tilburn et al. 1995). In the nonaflatoxin-conducive peptone medium, this site was shown to be inhibitory to aflatoxin formation (Cotty 1988). The regulatory mechanism might be due to the binding of *pacC* to this site at alkaline conditions to repress the transcription of acid-expressed gene *aflR* and thus aflatoxin formation (Espeso and Arst 2000, Espeso et al. 1993). The PacC and AreA (Chang et al. 2000) binding sites in the *aflR-aflS* (*aflJ*) intergenic region suggest that gene expression is regulated by environmental signals (pH and nitrate).

#### 15.3.7.6 Developmental Stage

Many fungal developmental stages such as sporulation and sclerotial formation are associated with secondary metabolism (Bennett et al. 1986, Calvo et al. 2002, Chang et al. 2002, Hicks et al. 1997). Spore formation and secondary metabolite formation occur at about the same time (Hicks et al. 1997, Trail et al. 1995a,b). Some mutants that are deficient in sporulation are unable to produce aflatoxins (Bennett and Papa 1988) and some compounds that inhibit sporulation in *A. parasiticus* also inhibit aflatoxin formation (Reib 1982). Moreover, chemicals that inhibit polyamine biosynthesis in *A. parasiticus* and *A. nidulans* inhibit both sporulation and aflatoxin/ST biosynthesis (Guzman-de-Pena et al. 1998). A more recent finding reveals that the regulation of sporulation and ST production is through a shared G-protein-mediated signaling pathway in *A. nidulans* (Hicks et al. 1997, Yu and Keller 2005). Mutations in *A. nidulans flbA* and *fadA* genes, early acting members of a G-protein signal transduction pathway, result in loss of ST gene expression, ST production, and sporulation (Hicks et al. 1997, Shimizu and Keller 2001, Yu et al. 1996). The regulation is partially mediated through protein kinase A (Shimizu and Keller 2001, Yu et al. 1996). This G-protein signaling pathway involving FadA in the regulation of aflatoxin production also exists in *A. parasiticus* and *A. flavus* (Hicks et al. 1997).

### 15.3.7.7 Oxidative Stress

The relationship between oxidative stress and aflatoxin biosynthesis in *A. parasiticus* has long been reported (Jayashree et al. 2000, Kim et al. 2006, Mahoney and Molyneux 2004, Reverberi et al. 2006). Oxidative stress was reported to induce aflatoxin biosynthesis in *A. parasiticus* (Jayashree and Subramanyam 2000). Treatment of *A. flavus* with *tert*-butyl hydroperoxide and gallic acid induced significant increases in aflatoxin production (Kim et al. 2006). Similar treatment of *A. parasiticus* also induced aflatoxin production (Reverberi et al. 2005, 2006). Hydrolysable tannins significantly inhibit aflatoxin biosynthesis, with the main antiaflatoxigenic constituents in these tannins being gallic acid (Mahoney and Molyneux 2004). Gallic acid reduces expression of structural genes within the aflatoxin biosynthetic cluster, but surprisingly not the aflatoxin pathway gene regulator, *aflR*. It appears that gallic acid disrupts signal transduction pathway(s) for aflatoxigenesis. When certain phenolics or other antioxidants, such as ascorbic acid, are added to oxidatively stressed *A. flavus*, aflatoxin production significantly declines, with no effect on fungal growth (Kim et al. 2006). Caffeic acid is another antioxidant that inhibits aflatoxigenesis. Microarray analysis of *A. flavus* treated with caffeic acid identified a gene, named *ahpC2*, an alkyl hydroperoxide reductase that is potentially involved in quelling the signal for aflatoxin production. However, no notable effect on expression of *laeA*, a gene encoding a global regulator for secondary metabolism in *Aspergillus* (Bok and Keller 2004), was observed when under caffeic acid treatment. It is obvious that many different regulatory mechanisms affect regulation of aflatoxin production.

### 15.3.7.8 Plant Metabolites

Plant metabolites also play some role in aflatoxin formation (Greene-McDowelle et al. 1999, Zeringue 2002, Zeringue and Bhatnagar 1993, Zeringue et al. 1996). Wright et al. (2000) reported that, in certain conditions, *n*-decyl aldehyde reduces not only fungal growth of *A. parasiticus* but also aflatoxin production by over 95% compared with control. Octanal reduces fungal growth by 60%; however, it increases aflatoxin production by 500%, while hexanal reduces fungal growth by 50%, but it has no effect on aflatoxin production. The 13(*S*)-hydroperoxide derivative of linoleic acid, the reaction product of lipoxygenase (encoded by L2 LOX gene from maize), is reported to reduce aflatoxin production (Wilson et al. 2001). Therefore, besides routine detection and screening, management of aflatoxin contamination in commodities must include preharvest as well as postharvest control measures.

### 15.3.8 Control of Aflatoxin Contamination

The economic implications of aflatoxins and their potential health threat to humans have clearly created a need to eliminate or at least minimize its contamination in food and feedstuff. Efforts include monitoring, managing, and controlling their levels in agricultural products from the farm to the market place. While an association between aflatoxin contamination and inadequate storage conditions has long been recognized, studies have revealed that seeds are contaminated with aflatoxins prior to harvest (Lillehoj et al. 1980).

### 15.3.8.1 Detection and Screening

Surveillance programs have been established to reduce the risk of aflatoxin consumption by humans and animals. Analytical testing methods for rapid detection of a large number of samples of food stuffs have been developed (Wilson 1989). Current analytical techniques for accurate characterization and quantitation of aflatoxins include thin layer chromatography (TLC), high-pressure liquid chromatography (HPLC), and gas chromatography (GC). Rapid immunoassay (RIA) and serum assay (ELISA) formats based on sera developed for major aflatoxins (Chu et al. 1987, Wilson 1989, Xiulan et al. 2005) are also available for rapid detection of aflatoxins at levels as low as one-tenth of a nanogram per milliliter (Malloy and Marr 1997). A dozen commercial test kits have been developed for field testing of various agricultural commodities.

### 15.3.8.2 Preharvest Control

Preharvest aflatoxin contamination can be reduced somewhat by appropriate cultural practices such as irrigation, control of insect pests, etc. In some cases, changes in cultural practices to minimize aflatoxin contamination are not feasible. For example, inclusion of extra irrigation regimes in desert cotton fields is not feasible because it would add significant cost to the grower even if they were available. However, significant control of aflatoxin contamination is expected to be dependent on a detailed understanding of the physiological and environmental factors that affect the biosynthesis of the toxin, the biology and ecology of the fungus, and the parameters of the host plant–fungal interactions. Efforts are underway to study these parameters, primarily by functional genomics approaches (Yu and Cleveland 2007, Yu et al. 2005).

Application of nonaflatoxigenic, biocompetitive, native *A. flavus* strains to outcompete toxigenic isolates in the fields has been effective in significantly reducing aflatoxin contamination (Cotty et al. 1994). Biocompetition may be most feasible in crops such as cotton where resistance against fungal infections is not available due to limited genetic diversity in the cotton germplasm. In the long term, however, significant control of the aflatoxin problem will likely be linked to introduction of resistant germplasms, which are resistant either to fungal invasion or toxin production or both. Naturally resistant germplasms are available and the identification of specific biochemical factors linked to resistance against *A. flavus* will assist in enhancing the observed resistance levels in the existing germplasms. Identification of a novel pool of germplasm that demonstrates the desired characteristics is also critical to the success of the current marker-assistance breeding programs. However, because the aflatoxin contamination process is so complex (Payne 1998), a combination of approaches will be required to control the preharvest contamination problem.

### 15.3.8.3 Postharvest Control

Postharvest aflatoxin contamination is prevalent in most tropical countries due to hot, wet climates coupled with subadequate methods of harvesting, handling, and storage practices, which often lead to severe fungal growth and thus contamination of food and feed (Cleveland et al. 1997, 2005). Significant emphasis has been placed on detoxification of contaminated lots to at least reduce the levels under the acceptable limits. Detoxification of aflatoxins has been extensively investigated, particularly in corn and peanuts (Goldblatt 1969a,b, Lillehoj and Wall 1986).

## 15.4 CYCLOPIAZONIC ACID

CPA is an indole tetramic acid that inhibits sarcoplasmic reticulum $Ca^{2+}$-ATPases by binding to calcium-free conformations of the ATPase enzyme (Soler et al. 1998) and blocking calcium channel access (Moncoq et al. 2007). Inhibition of these ATPases by CPA results in cell death as a result of stress response and activation of apoptotic pathways (Venkatesh and Vairamuthu 2005, Vinokurova et al. 2007). In mice, CPA has an $LD_{50}$ of approximately 13 mg/kg (Nishie et al. 1985) making consumption of a lethal dose unlikely, especially as there is no evidence that CPA accumulates in animal tissue. However, side effects of low doses have not been ruled out as its pharmacological properties are similar to classical antipsychotic drugs like reserpine and chlorpromazine (Nishie et al. 1985). These side effects include hyperkinesias, hypothermia, Parkinson-like tremors, catalepsy, and convulsions.

Strains of *A. flavus*, *Aspergillus minisclerotigenes* (Pildain et al. 2008), and *Aspergillus pseudotamarii* (Ito et al. 2001) can produce both CPA and aflatoxin. *Aspergillus oryzae*, which is thought to be a domesticated species of *A. flavus* and is important in industrial food fermentations, does not produce aflatoxin although some strains have the complete aflatoxin biosynthetic cluster and produce CPA. Interestingly, *A. parasiticus*, the other aflatoxin-producing species commonly found on agricultural commodities, is not reported to produce CPA. CPA production has been reported in *A. fumigatus*, but it is not typical. However a close relative, *Aspergillus lentulus*, does produce CPA (Larsen et al. 2007, Vinokurova et al. 2007). CPA contamination of food and feed has been reported, possibly because it is difficult to detect and thus overlooked. It can be a problem on Kodo millet, a food staple in regions of India. Consumption of moldy grain (usually attributed to *A. tamarii* or *A. flavus*) is associated with Kodo poisoning in humans and animals. Nausea, vomiting, delirium, depression, intoxication, and unconsciousness characterize Kodo poisoning. Kodo poisoning was originally thought to be caused by the mycotoxin fumigaclavin A but was later attributed to CPA (Antony et al. 2003, Janardhanan et al. 1984, Lalitha Rao and Husain 1985). CPA toxicity also has been linked to Turkey X disease. Turkey X disease was responsible for bringing *A. flavus* to notoriety with the discovery of aflatoxin (Nesbitt et al. 1962). However, some of the symptoms of Turkey X disease are consistent with CPA poisoning, and it is now widely believed that Turkey X was the result of a synergistic affect of the consumption of both aflatoxin and CPA present in contaminated feed (Cole 1986, Richard 2008). Testing of groundnut cake responsible for the original outbreaks of Turkey X disease revealed both aflatoxin and CPA (Richard 2008). It is common for strains of *A. flavus* to produce both aflatoxin and CPA and for commodities to contain both mycotoxins (Chang et al. 2005, Gallagher et al. 1978, Martins and Martins 1999, Widiastuti et al. 1988).

Recent studies on CPA and aflatoxin regulation under several conducive and nonconducive conditions for aflatoxin production (Georgianna et al. 2010) demonstrated that both toxins are produced in developing corn kernels during infection in the field, appearing first at 48 h after infection by the fungus. In the culture conditions tested, CPA was produced under conditions conducive as well as conditions nonconducive for aflatoxin production, indicating that its production may not be regulated the same way as that for aflatoxin.

The genomic location of the CPA cluster is now known. Chang predicted that the CPA gene cluster was close to the aflatoxin gene cluster, as strains with partial deletions for the aflatoxin cluster failed to produce CPA. Further analysis of CPA production in *A. oryzae* identified a PKS-NRPS gene necessary for CPA production (Chang et al. 2009, Georgianna et al. 2010, Tokuoka et al. 2008) working independently disrupted the dimethylallyl tryptophan synthase in *A. flavus* and showed that it was necessary for CPA production. The essential role for the predicted FAD oxidoreductase in CPA biosynthesis was described and its gene was named *maoA* (Chang et al. 2009). These genes reside in cluster 55, which spans a 20 kb DNA region near the telomere of chromosome 3, with only 2 genes predicted to separate the aflatoxin cluster from the CPA cluster.

## 15.5   AFLATREM

Aflatrem is a tremorgenic mycotoxin that has profound effects on the central nervous system, causing tremors, mental confusion, seizures, and death (Gallagher and Wilson 1979, Valdes et al. 1985). Aflatrem also has been found to cause significant histopathological changes in the heart, liver, and brain tissues of chicks (Rafiyuddin et al. 2006). The genes necessary for aflatrem biosynthesis have been identified and are located in two gene clusters located on chromosomes 5 and 7 (Nicholson et al. 2009, Zhang et al. 2004). *A. flavus* is the most widely described producer of aflatrem, but aflatrem also can be produced by *A. minisclerotigenes*, a species that resembles *A. flavus* in its ability to produce aflatoxins B1, B2, CPA, kojic and aspergillic acid (Pildain et al. 2008). In addition, *A. minisclerotigenes* also produces aflatoxins G1, G2 (Pildain et al. 2008). No other fungal genera are known to produce aflatrem; however, structurally related tremorgenic mycotoxins, such as penitrem from *Penicillium* spp., are prevalent in other fungi and likely share common enzymes for aflatrem production. There is no reported evidence for aflatrem contamination of any food or feed; however, this may be the result of a lack of testing.

The cloning and characterization of genes and gene products for paxilline biosynthesis in *Penicillium paxilli* has enabled studies on aflatrem biosynthesis in *A. flavus* (Zhang et al. 2004). Using degenerate primers for conserved domains of fungal geranylgeranyl diphosphate synthase, the gene *atmG* required for aflatrem biosynthesis in *A. flavus* was cloned (Zhang et al. 2004). Two other genes, *atmC* and *atmM*, were identified adjacent to *atmG*. These three genes were observed to be coordinately expressed, with transcript levels dramatically increasing at the onset of aflatrem biosynthesis. The genes also were found to have 64%–70% amino acid sequence similarity and conserved synteny with a cluster of orthologous genes, *paxG*, *paxC*, and *paxM*, from *P. paxilli*, which are required for paxilline biosynthesis. Because a genomic copy of *atmM* could complement a *paxM* deletion mutant of *P. paxilli*, *atmM* is a functional homolog of *paxM*. This provided the first genetic evidence for the biosynthetic pathway of aflatrem in *A. flavus*. More recently, another gene *atmP* was identified as coding for a cytochrome P450 monooxygenase, which may be involved in aflatrem synthesis (Nicholson et al. 2009). A search of the complete genome sequence of *A. flavus* identified the presence of a putative aflatrem gene cluster, with the genes for aflatrem synthesis being split between two discrete regions (Nicholson et al. 2009). The first cluster was found to be telomere proximal on chromosome 5, while the second was telomeric distal on chromosome 7. Although the expression of aflatoxin biosynthetic genes correlated well with the onset of aflatrem production, low-level expression of genes in the telomere-distal region was detected prior to the onset of aflatrem synthesis.

## 15.6 OTHER TOXIC COMPOUNDS

A lesser characterized mycotoxin produced by *A. flavus* is 3-nitropropionic acid (3-NPA). This secondary metabolite can be found in several species of both plants (Burdock et al. 2001) and fungi (El-Shanawany et al. 2005, Johnson et al. 2000). Endophytic fungi may be responsible for the production of 3-NPA in some legumes (Chomeheon et al. 2005). Exposure to 3-NPA produces a range of toxicological effects and consumption of food contaminated with 3-NPA leads to health risks. A safety assessment reported that the risk associated with consumption of 3-NPA is small (Burdock et al. 2001). However, cases of acute poisoning are known. For example, 217 cases were reported in China between 1972 and 1984, resulting in 88 deaths (Fu et al. 1995). 3-NPA irreversibly inactivates succinate dehydrogenase and impairs energy production within mitochondria (Johnson et al. 2000). Defects in mitochondrial energy productions play an important role in the pathology of neuro-degenerative diseases (Luchowski et al. 2002). Exposure to mitochondrial toxins in experimental animals produces neuropathologies resembling those seen in humans with Huntington's disease (Nony et al. 1999).

In addition to the known toxins produced by *A. flavus*, the fungus is predicted to synthesize several other toxic compounds as it colonizes seeds or grows on processed food and feed. Fungi have the capacity to produce an array of diverse secondary metabolites, and over 300 fungal secondary metabolites are described as mycotoxins (CAST 2003, Cole and Cox 1981, Richard and Payne 2003). Genes for secondary metabolism in fungi are usually arranged into specific clusters and found throughout the genome (Keller et al. 2005). An available genome sequence for *A. flavus* has allowed a bioinformatic prediction of the number of secondary metabolite clusters in the *A. flavus* genome. A genomic analysis by a software, Secondary Metabolite Unique Regions Finder (SMURF), available at http://jcvi.org/smurf/index.php, led to the prediction of 55 secondary metabolism gene clusters (Fedorova et al. 2008, Georgianna et al. 2010, Khaldi et al. 2010). Their predictive model identifies genes with a signature of genes known to be involved in secondary metabolism. This algorithm searches for multifunctional enzymes including nonribosomal peptide synthetases (NRPSs) for nonribosomal peptides, PKSs for polyketides, hybrid NRPS-PKS enzymes for hybrids, and prenyltransferases (PTRs) for terpenoids, all of which have been shown to be involved in secondary metabolism (Hoffmeister and Keller 2007, Keller et al. 2005). For example, the biosynthesis of aflatoxins requires a PKS, aflatrem requires a NRPS, and CPA biosynthesis involves a hybrid NRPS-PKS.

Once the program identifies these putative multifunctional enzymes, it next searches the surrounding genes for motifs of genes associated with secondary metabolism. The ability of *A. flavus* to produce a variety of products from one secondary metabolism cluster indicates that *A. flavus* has the potential to display a very diverse repertoire of secondary metabolites/mycotoxins.

## 15.7 ECOLOGY AND MEDICAL CONCERNS OF *ASPERGILLUS FLAVUS*

*A. flavus* is not only one of the most abundant, widely distributed, extremely competitive soil-borne fungal molds present worldwide, but is a saprobe capable of surviving on many organic nutrient sources like plant debris, tree leaves, decaying wood, animal fodder, cotton, compost piles, dead insects and animal carcasses, stored grains, and even human and animal patients (Klich 1998). The optimum temperature range for *A. flavus* growth is between 28°C and 37°C, but it can grow in a wide range of temperatures from 12°C to 48°C. The wide temperature range allows it to survive climatic region between latitudes 26° and 36° (Klich 2002). For most of its life cycle, the fungus exists in the form of mycelium or asexual spores known as conidia. Stress from adverse conditions, such as lack of adequate nutrients or water, causes the mycelium to form resistant structures called sclerotia. The fungus overwinters either as spores or as sclerotia or as mycelium in debris. Under favorable conditions, sclerotia germinates directly to produce new colonies or it can produce conidiophores with conidia (Bennett et al. 1986, Chang et al. 2002, Cotty 1988).

The ability of *A. flavus* to grow at relatively high temperatures contributes to its pathogenicity on humans and other warm blooded animals. After *A. fumigatus*, *A. flavus* is the second leading cause of invasive and noninvasive aspergillosis in humans and animals (Denning 1998, Denning et al. 1991, 2003, Mori et al. 1998). The incidence of aspergillosis is rising due to the increase of immunocompromised patients in the population (Denning 1998, Nierman et al. 2005, Ronning et al. 2005).

## 15.8 SEXUAL STAGE IN *ASPERGILLUS FLAVUS*

*A. flavus* populations are associated with agricultural environments. Traditionally, *A. flavus* is thought to have no sexual stage with asexual conidial spores, mycelia, or sclerotia, as means for reproduction. As an asexual fungus, it is broadly accepted that *A. flavus* has distinct clonal populations known as vegetative compatible groups (VCGs) (Horn et al. 1995). Bennett has long believed that sclerotia are a form of transitional sexual stage. From her early experiments, a sexual body-like structure was observed but short of observation under microscope by slicing dissection (J.W. Bennett, unpublished data). Dyer group has successfully demonstrated the formation of sexual spores after incubation for 4–6 months in the dark in oatmeal agar medium at 30°C in *A. fumigatus* (O'Gorman et al. 2009). Their studies demonstrated that *A. fumigatus* possesses a fully functional sexual reproductive cycle that leads to the production of cleistothecia and ascospores. Soon after, the sexual stages from both

*A. flavus* and *A. parasiticus* were reported (Horn et al. 2009a,b). It has been identified that there are two mating type loci, *Mat1-1* and *Mat1-2*, in nearly equal frequencies in the natural populations in *Aspergilli* (Ramirez-Prado et al. 2008).

This may imply that sexual recombination is occurring or has occurred in nature. Because *A. flavus* has the potential to undergo heterothallic recombination, it is an important issue to ponder as sexual recombination could have serious ramifications if an aggressive nonaflatoxigenic strain recombined with an aflatoxigenic strain. The ability of *Aspergillus* species to engage in sexual reproduction is highly significant in understanding the biology and evolution of the species. The presence of a sexual cycle provides an invaluable tool for classical genetic analyses and will facilitate research into the genetic basis of pathogenicity and fungicide resistance in *A. fumigatus* and *A. flavus* with the aim of improving methods for the control of aspergillosis.

## 15.9 GENOMICS OF *ASPERGILLUS FLAVUS*

Genomics is the process of revealing the entire genetic content of an organism by high-throughput sequencing of the DNA and bioinformatics identification of all of the ORFs. Recent technological breakthroughs allow scientists to sequence and annotate genomes in a very short time frame. A combination of expressed sequence tags (EST), whole genome sequencing, and microarray technologies provides high-throughput capabilities (Bennett and Arnold 2001, Kim et al. 2006, Payne et al. 2006, Yu et al. 2004a–c) that can be applied to the identification of genes involved in aflatoxin production and for studying the regulatory mechanisms of gene expression (i.e., functional genomics).

### 15.9.1 *Aspergillus flavus* Expressed Sequence Tags

The largest set of *A. flavus* ESTs was generated from a normalized cDNA library of wild-type strain NRRL 3357 (ATCC #20026) (Yu et al. 2004a–c). Over 26,110 cDNA clones from a normalized cDNA expression library were sequenced at the Institute for Genomic Research (TIGR, now named J. Craig Venter Institute [JCVI]). A total of 19,618 *A. flavus* ESTs were generated, from which 7,218 unique EST sequences were identified (Yu et al. 2004a–c). These EST sequences have been released to the public at the NCBI GenBank Database (http://www.ncbi.nlm.nih.gov/). The *A. flavus* Gene Index was constructed at TIGR (http://www.tigr.org), which is currently maintained and curated by the Dana Farber Cancer Institute (http://compbio.dfci.harvard.edu/tgi). From the EST database, an additional four new transcripts (*hypB*, *hypC*, *hypD*, and *hypE*) were identified in the aflatoxin biosynthetic gene cluster, which were not identified during chromosomal walking. In addition, several categories of other genes identified could potentially be involved, directly or indirectly, in aflatoxin production, such as those involved in global regulation, signal transduction, pathogenicity, virulence, and fungal development (Yu et al. 2004a–c). This collection of ESTs has been extremely valuable in the assembly of the genome of *A. flavus* as well as in the construction of whole genome DNA expression arrays.

## 15.9.2 Whole Genome Sequencing of *Aspergillus flavus*

The *A. flavus* whole genome sequencing project was funded by a USDA, National Research Initiative grant awarded to Professor Gary A. Payne and Ralph Dean, North Carolina State University, Raleigh, North Carolina. The Food and Feed Safety Research Unit of Southern Regional Research Center, USDA/ARS, provided funding for fine finishing and gene calling. The sequencing has been completed at TIGR (current name, JCVI) under the supervision of Dr. William C. Nierman by a shotgun approach and Sanger sequencing protocol. Primary assembly indicated that the *A. flavus* genome consists of eight chromosomes and the genome size is about 36.8 Mb. Aided with the *A. flavus* EST database, the *A. oryzae* EST database, and the *A. oryzae* whole genome sequence, annotation of the *A. flavus* genome sequence data has been almost completed. Preliminary results demonstrated that there are over 12,000 functional genes in the *A. flavus* genome, a number similar to those of other *Aspergillus* species (Galagan et al. 2005, Machida et al. 2005, Nierman et al. 2005, Yu and Cleveland 2007). Genes responsible for the biosynthesis of secondary metabolites such as aflatoxins have been identified. Other genes associated with secondary metabolism include those encoding PKSs, NRPSs, cytochrome P450 monooxygenases, FAS, carboxylases, dehydrogenases, reductases, oxidases, oxidoreductases, epoxide hydrolases, oxygenases, and methyltransferases (Galagan et al. 2005, Machida et al. 2005, Nierman et al. 2005, Yu et al. 2004a–c, Yu and Cleveland 2007). The availability of the *A. oryzae* whole genome sequence provided not only the sequence data but also the chromosomal structure for comparison with *A. flavus*. The sequence data have been deposited with the NCBI GenBank database (http://www.ncbi.nlm.nih.gov) and are also available through the *Aspergillus flavus* website (http://www.aspergillusflavus.org), *Aspergillus* Comparative Database of The Broad Institute at MIT (http://www.broadinstitute.org/annotation/genome/aspergillus_group/MultiHome.html), and Central Aspergillus Data Repository in the United Kingdom (http://www.cadre-genomes.org.uk/aspergillus_links.html).

## 15.9.3 Microarrays as Tools for Functional Genomics Studies

Microarrays are robust tools used for functional genomics studies. In recent years, several generations of *A. flavus* microarrays have been utilized including both amplicon- and oligo-based arrays. The first cDNA amplicon microarray, consisting of 753 gene features, including known aflatoxin pathway genes *aflD* (*nor-1*) and *aflP* (*omtA*) and regulatory gene *aflR*, was constructed at North Carolina State University. The unique ESTs identified from a cDNA library constructed using *A. flavus* RNA obtained under aflatoxin-producing conditions were spotted on Telechem SuperAldehyde glass slide using an Affymetrix 417 Arrayer (OBrian et al. 2003). A second generation 5002 gene elements *A. flavus* EST-based amplicon microarray was constructed by the Food and Feed Safety Research Unit, USDA/ARS/SRRC. This microarray has been updated to a 5031 gene-element array including genes of interest when their sequences became available. The Food and Feed Safety Research Unit, USDA/ARS/SRRC, has also constructed a comprehensive whole genome *A. flavus* oligo microarray. All of the 11,820 *A. flavus* unique genes, the unique genes present in *A. oryzae* but absent in *A. flavus*, and 10 corn genes that show resistance against *A. flavus* infection, have been represented by this whole genome microarray. A complete Affymetrix GeneChip microarray funded by USDA/NRI contains elements representing all of the *A. flavus* genes, a subset of *A. oryzae* genes not found in *A. flavus* NRRL 3357, approximately 9000 genes expressed in corn seed, and a few genes from *Fusarium* species, mouse and human genomes. Additionally, a peanut microarray, funded by Crop Protection and Management Laboratory, USDA/ARS, Tifton Georgia, has been constructed at JCVI.

These *A. flavus* microarray resources provide a platform for functional genomics to study how genetic, environmental, and nutritional factors influence aflatoxin production. Profiling of genes involved in aflatoxin formation using these microarrays, performed at USDA labs, the labs of North Carolina State University, and JCVI, has identified hundreds of genes that are significantly up- or downregulated under various growth conditions (Chang et al. 2007, 2010, Kim et al. 2006, OBrian et al. 2003, 2007, Price et al. 2005, 2006, Wilkinson et al. 2007a,b, Yu et al. 2007). Analysis of the gene expression data from Affymetrix microarray experiments confirmed 55 different secondary metabolism clusters predicted by SMURF. Hierarchical cluster analysis based on gene expression patterns for the multifunctional enzymes revealed four discernable expression patterns (called clades) (Georgianna et al. 2010). The aflatoxin pathway gene cluster, the CPA gene cluster, and additional six other predicted clusters were shown in similar expression patterns to be placed into the same clade. This clade had moderate to high levels of gene expression and contained clusters that are predicted to encode diverse array of secondary metabolites such as pigments and siderophores. Further studies using these microarray resources will surely reveal the mechanisms of aflatoxin production and how the process is regulated. The knowledge will empower researchers to find effective strategies for controlling aflatoxin contamination of food and feed.

### 15.9.4 NEXT-GENERATION SEQUENCING TECHNOLOGIES FOR GENOMICS AND FUNCTIONAL GENOMICS STUDIES

The National Human Genome Research Institute has put forth goals to reduce the cost of human genome sequencing to $100,000 in the short term and $1,000 in the long term to spur the innovative development of technologies that will permit the routine sequencing of human genomes for use as a diagnostic tool for disease (Hert et al. 2008). Technological breakthroughs in recent years have resulted in several platforms or instruments capable of producing millions of DNA sequence reads in a single run. These fast and low-cost next-generation DNA sequencing technologies include Roche (454) GS FLX sequencer using pyrosequencing chemistry, Illumina genome analyzer using polymerase-based sequencing-by-synthesis, and Applied Biosystems SOLid sequencer using ligation-based sequencing. The cost per reaction of DNA sequencing has fallen following Moore's law (Moore 1965). These technologies rapidly change the landscape of genetics and genomics research and provide the ability to answer questions with unimaginable speed. They have broad applications ranging from chromatin immunoprecipitation, mutation mapping, polymorphism discovery, genome comparisons, noncoding RNA discovery, antisense RNA, small RNA discoveries, and full-length cDNA analyses to serial analysis of gene expression (SAGE)-based methods. Next-generation sequencing has an astounding potential to bring enormous change in genetic and biological research and to enhance our fundamental biological knowledge. Unlike many microarray studies, RNA sequencing (RNA-Seq) can provide access to a cell's entire transcriptome with almost infinite resolution and reveal additional transcript complexity. The RNA-Seq technology was employed to characterize the *A. flavus* transcriptome and mapped to the majority of the known *A. flavus* genes. Further analysis revealed quantitative differences in gene expression between the conditions tested. It demonstrated that aflatoxin production is one of the most tightly regulated processes in a fungal cell. The transcript abundance for aflatoxin biosynthesis genes was 1000 times greater under conditions conducive to aflatoxin production. In addition, over 500 other genes were differentially expressed under the conditions tested. We anticipated that a high-resolution view of the entire fungal transcriptome will allow us to identify genes differentially expressed under conditions conducive and nonconducive to aflatoxin production.

## 15.10   FUTURE PERSPECTIVES

Studies by the traditional genetic methods, modern genetic cloning techniques, high-throughput genomic technologies, and the next-generation sequencing technologies have aided our understanding of the fungal biology, toxicology, and genetics of aflatoxin biosynthesis in *A. flavus*. With the rapid progress in fungal genomics, we will master a vast amount of new information on gene function, genetic regulation, and signal transduction within this fungal system as well as its interactions with the environment. It is now time to supplant the brute force, gene-by-gene strategy that has been so fruitful in the late twentieth and early twenty-first centuries with the cutting-edge whole genome approach including next-generation sequencing. In the genomic era, we must stop thinking about parts and start thinking about whole. New forms of systems analyses will allow us to understand the incredibly complex interactions between fungal secondary metabolism and an ever-changing environment. The genetic and genomic resources will significantly enhance our understanding of the mechanisms of aflatoxin production, pathogenicity of the fungus, and crop–fungus interactions. This information is vital for devising novel strategies to eliminate aflatoxin contamination resulting in a safer, nutritious, and sustainable food and feed supply.

## REFERENCES

Adye, J. and R. I. Mateles. 1964. Incorporation of labelled compounds into aflatoxins. *Biochim Biophys Acta* 86:418–420.
Allcroft, R., R. B. A. Carnaghan, K. Sargeant, and J. O'Kelly. 1961. A toxic factor in Brazilian groundnut meal. *Vet Rec* 73:428–429.
Antony, M., Y. Shukla, and K. K. Janardhanan. 2003. Potential risk of acute hepatotoxicity of kodo poisoning due to exposure to cyclopiazonic acid. *J Ethnopharmacol* 87:211–214.
Arsura, M. and L. G. Cavin. 2005. Nuclear factor-kappaB and liver carcinogenesis. *Cancer Lett* 229:157–169.

Asplin, F. D. and B. A. Carnaghan. 1961. The toxicity of certain groundnut meals for poultry with special reference to their effect on ducklings and chickens. *Vet Rec* 73:1215–1223.

Bennett, J. W. and J. Arnold. 2001. Genomics for fungi. In *The Mycota VIII, Biology of the Fungal Cell*. R. J. Howard and N. A. R. Gow (eds.), pp. 267–297. Berlin, Germany: Springer-Verlag, Heidelberg.

Bennett, J. W., P. K. Chang, and D. Bhatnagar. 1997. One gene to whole pathway: The role of norsolorinic acid in aflatoxin research. *Adv Appl Microbiol* 45:1–15.

Bennett, J. W. and S. B. Christensen. 1983. New perspectives on aflatoxin biosynthesis. *Adv Appl Microbiol* 29:53–92.

Bennett, J. W. and M. Klich. 2003. Mycotoxins. *Clin Microbiol Rev* 16:497–516.

Bennett, J. W., F. Kronberg, and G. Gougis. 1976. Pigmented isolates from anthraquinone-producing mutants of *Aspergillus parasiticus*. *Am Soc Microbiol* 76:6.

Bennett, J. W. and L. S. Lee. 1979. Mycotoxins—Their biosynthesis in fungi: Aflatoxins and other bisfuranoids. *J Food Prot* 42:805–809.

Bennett, J. W., L. S. Lee, and C. H. Vinnett. 1971. The correlation of aflatoxin and norsolorinic acid production. *J Am Oil Chem Soc* 48:368–370.

Bennett, J. W., P. M. Leong, S. J. Kruger, and D. Keyes. 1986. Sclerotial and low aflatoxigenic morphological variants from haploid and diploid *Aspergillus parasiticus*. *Experientia* 42:848–851.

Bennett, J. W. and K. E. Papa. 1988. The aflatoxigenic *Aspergillus* spp. *Adv Plant Pathol* 6:265–279.

Bennett, J. W., P. L. Rubin, L. S. Lee, and P. N. Chen. 1979. Influence of trace elements and nitrogen sources on versicolorin production by a mutant strain of *Aspergillus parasiticus*. *Mycopathologia* 69:61–66.

Bennett, J. W., R. B. Silverstein, and S. J. Kruger. 1981. Isolation and characterization of two nonaflatoxigenic classes of morphological variants of *Aspergillus parasiticus*. *J Am Oil Chem Soc* 58:952.

Bhatnagar, D., K. C. Ehrlich, and T. E. Cleveland. 1992. Oxidation–reduction reactions in biosynthesis of secondary metabolites. In *Mycotoxins in Ecological Systems*, Vol. 10. D. Bhatnagar, E. B. Lillehoj and D. K. Arora (eds.), pp. 255–285. New York: Marcel Dekker.

Blount, W. P. 1961. Turkey "X" disease. *Turkeys* 9:52–77.

Bok, J. W., D. Hoffmeister, L. A. Maggio-Hall, R. Murillo, J. D. Glasner, and N. P. Keller. 2006. Genomic mining for *Aspergillus* natural products. *Chem Biol* 13:31–37.

Bok, J.-W. and N. P. Keller. 2004. LaeA, a regulator of secondary metabolism in *Aspergillus* spp. *Eukaryot Cell* 3:527–535.

Brakhage, A. A., J. Schuemann, S. Bergmann, K. Scherlach, V. Schroeckh, and C. Hertweck. 2008. Activation of fungal silent gene clusters: A new avenue to drug discovery. *Prog Drug Res* 66:1:3–12.

Bressac, B., M. Kew, J. Wands, and M. Ozturk. 1991. Selective G to T mutations of p53 gene in hepatocellular carcinoma from southern Africa. *Nature* 350:429–431.

Brown, R. L., D. Bhatnagar, T. E. Cleveland, and J. W. Cary. 1998. Recent advances in preharvest prevention of mycotoxin contamination. In *Mycotoxin in Agriculture and Food Safety*. K. K. Sinha and D. Bhatnagar (eds.), pp. 351–379. New York: Marcel Dekkar, Inc.

Brown, D. W., J. H. Yu, H. S. Kelkar et al. 1996. Twenty-five coregulated transcripts define a sterigmatocystin gene cluster in *Aspergillus nidulans*. *Proc Natl Acad Sci USA* 93:1418–1422.

Buchanan, R. L. and D. F. Lewis. 1984. Regulation of aflatoxin biosynthesis: Effect of glucose on activities of various glycolytic enzymes. *Appl Environ Microbiol* 48:306–310.

Burdock, G. A., I. G. Carabin, and G. Soni-Madhusudan. 2001. Safety assessment of beta-nitropropionic acid: A monograph in support of an acceptable daily intake in humans. *Food Chem* 75:1–27.

Busby, W. F., Jr. and G. N. Wogan. 1981. Aflatoxins. In *Mycotoxins and N-nitrosocompounds*: *Environmental Risks*, Vol. 2. R. C. Shank (ed.), pp. 3–45. Boca Raton, FL: CRC Press.

Butchko, R. A., T. H. Adams, and N. P. Keller. 1999. *Aspergillus nidulans* mutants defective in *stc* gene cluster regulation. *Genetics* 153:715–720.

Cai, J., H. Zeng, Y. Shima et al. 2008. Involvement of the *nadA* gene in formation of G-group aflatoxins in *Aspergillus parasiticus*. *Fungal Genet Biol* 45:1081–1093.

Calvo, A. M., J.-W. Bok, W. Brooks, and N. P. Keller. 2004. VeA is required for toxin and sclerotial production in *Aspergillus parasiticus*. *Appl Environ Microbiol* 70:4733–4739.

Calvo, A. M., R. A. Wilson, J. W. Bok, and N. P. Keller. 2002. Relationship between secondary metabolism and fungal development. *Microbiol Mol Biol Rev* 66:447–459.

Cary, J. W. and K. C. Ehrlich. 2006. Aflatoxigenicity in *Aspergillus*: Molecular genetics, phylogenetic relationships and evolutionary implications. *Mycopathologia* 162:167–177.

Cary, J. W., G. R. OBrian, D. M. Nielsen et al. 2007. Elucidation of *veA*-dependent genes associated with aflatoxin and sclerotial production in *Aspergillus flavus* by functional genomics. *Appl Microbiol Biotechnol* 76:1107–1118.

CAST. 2003. *Mycotoxins: Risk in Plant, Animal, qnd Human Systems*. Ames, IA: Council for Agricultural Science and Technology.

CDC. 2004. Outbreak of aflatoxin poisoning—Eastern and central province, Kenya. *MMWR Morb Mortal Wkly Rep* 53:790–792.

Chang, P. K. 2004. Lack of interaction between AFLR and AFLJ contributes to nonaflatoxigenicity of *Aspergillus sojae*. *J Biotechnol* 107:245–253.

Chang, P. K., J. W. Bennett, and P. J. Cotty. 2002. Association of aflatoxin biosynthesis and sclerotial development in *Aspergillus parasiticus*. *Mycopathologia* 153:41–48.

Chang, P. K., J. W. Cary, D. Bhatnagar et al. 1993. Cloning of the *Aspergillus parasiticus apa-2* gene associated with the regulation of aflatoxin biosynthesis. *Appl Environ Microbiol* 59:3273–3279.

Chang, P. K., J. W. Cary, J. Yu, D. Bhatnagar, and T. E. Cleveland. 1995a. The *Aspergillus parasiticus* polyketide synthase gene *pksA*, a homolog of *Aspergillus nidulans wA*, is required for aflatoxin $B_1$ biosynthesis. *Mol Gen Genet* 248:270–277.

Chang, P. K., K. C. Ehrlich, J. E. Linz, D. Bhatnagar, T. E. Cleveland, and J. W. Bennett. 1996. Characterization of the *Aspergillus parasiticus niaD* and *niiA* gene cluster. *Curr Genet* 30:68–75.

Chang, P. K., K. C. Ehrlich, J. Yu, D. Bhatnagar, and T. E. Cleveland. 1995b. Increased expression of *Aspergillus parasiticus aflR*, encoding a sequence-specific DNA-binding protein, relieves nitrate inhibition of aflatoxin biosynthesis. *Appl Environ Microbiol* 61:2372–2377.

Chang, P. K., B. W. Horn, and J. W. Dorner. 2005. Sequence breakpoints in the aflatoxin biosynthesis gene cluster and flanking regions in nonaflatoxigenic *Aspergillus flavus* isolates. *Fungal Genet Biol* 42:914–923.

Chang, P. K., B. W. Horn, and J. W. Dorner. 2009. Clustered genes involved in cyclopiazonic acid production are next to the aflatoxin biosynthesis gene cluster in *Aspergillus flavus*. *Fungal Genet Biol* 46:176–182.

Chang, P. K., L. L. Scharfenstein, M. Luo, N. Mahoney, R. J. Molyneux, J. Yu, R. L. Brown, and B. C. Campbell. 2010. Loss of *msnA*, a putative stress regulatory gene, in *Aspergillus parasiticus* and *Aspergillus flavus* increased production of conidia, aflatoxins and kojic acid. Toxins, 3:82–104.

Chang, P. K., C. D. Skory, and J. E. Linz. 1992. Cloning of a gene associated with aflatoxin $B_1$ biosynthesis in *Aspergillus parasiticus*. *Curr Genet* 21:231–233.

Chang, P. K. and R. B. Todd. 2003. Metabolic pathway regulation. In *Handbook of Fungal Biotechnology*. D. K. Arora (ed.), pp. 25–37. New York: Marcel Dekker Inc.

Chang, P. K., J. W. Wilkinson, B. W. Horn, J. Yu, D. Bhatnagar, and T. E. Cleveland. 2007. Genes differentially expressed by *Aspergillus flavus* strains after loss of aflatoxin production by serial transfers. *Appl Microbiol Biotechnol* 77:917–925.

Chang, P. K. and J. Yu. 2002. Characterization of a partial duplication of the aflatoxin gene cluster in *Aspergillus parasiticus* ATCC 56775. *Appl Microbiol Biotechnol* 58:632–636.

Chang, P. K., J. Yu, D. Bhatnagar, and T. E. Cleveland. 1999a. The carboxy-terminal portion of the aflatoxin pathway regulatory protein AFLR of *Aspergillus parasiticus* activates *GAL1::lacZ* gene expression in *Saccharomyces cerevisiae*. *Appl Environ Microbiol* 65:2508–2512.

Chang, P. K., J. Yu, D. Bhatnagar, and T. E. Cleveland. 1999b. Repressor-AFLR interaction modulates aflatoxin biosynthesis in *Aspergillus parasiticus*. *Mycopathologia* 147:105–112.

Chang, P. K., J. Yu, D. Bhatnagar, and T. E. Cleveland. 2000. Characterization of the *Aspergillus parasiticus* major nitrogen regulatory gene, *areA*. *Biochim Biophys Acta* 1491:263–266.

Chen, C. J., L. Y. Wang, S. N. Lu et al. 1996a. Elevated aflatoxin exposure and increased risk of hepatocellular carcinoma. *Hepatology* 24:38–42.

Chen, C. J., M. W. Yu, Y. F. Liaw et al. 1996b. Chronic hepatitis B carriers with null genotypes of glutathione S transferase MI and TI polymorphisms who are exposed to aflatoxin are at increased risk of hepatocellular carcinoma. *Am J Human Genet* 59:128–134.

Chiou, C. H., M. Miller, D. L. Wilson, F. Trail, and J. E. Linz. 2002. Chromosomal location plays a role in regulation of aflatoxin gene expression in *Aspergillus parasiticus*. *Appl Environ Microbiol* 68:306–315.

Chomeheon, P., S. Wiyakrutta, N. Sriubolmas, N. Ngamrojanavanich, D. Isarangkul, and P. Kittakoop. 2005. 3-nitropropionic acid (3-NPA), a potent antimycobacterial agent from endophytic fungi: Is 3-NPA in some plants produced by endophytes? *J Nat Prod* 68:1103–1105.

Chu, F. S., T. S. Fan, G. S. Zhang, Y. C. Xu, S. Faust, and P. L. McMahon. 1987. Improved enzyme-linked immunosorbent assay for aflatoxin $B_1$ in agricultural commodities. *J Assoc Off Anal Chem* 70:854–857.

Cleveland, T. E., D. Bhatnagar, and P. Cotty. 1990. A perspective on aflatoxin in field crops and animal food products in the United States. A symposium of USDA/ARS, Washington D. C. 83:67–73.

Cleveland, T. E., D. Bhatnagar, and J. Yu. 2009. Elimination and control of aflatoxin contamination in agricultural crops through *Aspergillus flavus* genomics. In *Mycotoxin Provention and Control in Agriculture*. M. Apel, F. D. Kendra, and M. W. Trucksess (eds.), ACS Symposium Series 1031, pp. 93–106. Washington, DC: American Chemical Society.

Cleveland, T. E., J. W. Cary, R. L. Brown et al. 1997. Use of biotechnology to eliminate aflatoxin in preharvest crops. *Bull Inst Compr Agric Sci Kinki Univ* 5:75–90.

Cleveland, T. E., P. F. Dowd, A. E. Desjardins, D. Bhatnagar, and P. J. Cotty. 2003. United States Department of Agriculture-Agricultural Research Service research on pre-harvest prevention of mycotoxins and mycotoxigenic fungi in US crops. *Pest Manag Sci* 59:629–642.

Cleveland, T. E., A. R. Lax, L. S. Lee, and D. Bhatnagar. 1987. Appearance of enzyme activities catalyzing conversion of sterigmatocystin to aflatoxin B1 in late-growth-phase *Aspergillus parasiticus* cultures. *Appl Environ Microbiol* 53:1711–1713.

Cleveland, T. E., J. Yu, D. Bhatnagar et al. 2005. Progress in elucidating the molecular basis of the host plant–*Aspergillus flavus* interaction: A basis for devising strategies to reduce aflatoxin contamination in crops. In *Aflatoxin and Food Safety*. H. K. Abbas (ed.), pp. 167–193. Boca Raton, FL: CRC Press.

Cole, R. J. 1986. Etiology of turkey X disease in retrospect: A case for the involvement of cyclopiazonic acid. *Mycotoxin Res* 2:3–7.

Cole, R. J. and R. H. Cox. 1981. *Handbook of Toxic Fungal Metabolites*. New York: Academic Press.

Cotty, P. 1988. Aflatoxin and sclerotial production by *Aspergillus flavus*: Influence of pH. *Phytopathology* 78:1250–1253.

Cotty, P. J. 1989. Virulence and cultural characteristics of two *Aspergillus flavus* strains pathogenic on cotton. *Phytopathology* 79:808–814.

Cotty, P. J., D. S. Bayman, D. S. Egel, and K. S. Elias. 1994. Agriculture, aflatoxins and *Aspergillus*. In *The Genus Aspergillus*. K. Powell (ed.), pp. 1–27. New York: Plenum Press.

Cotty, P. J. and K. F. Cardwell. 1999. Divergence of West African and North American communities of *Aspergillus* section *Flavi*. *Appl Environ Microbiol* 65:2264–2266.

Cotty, P. J. and R. Jaime-Garcia. 2007. Influences of climate on aflatoxin producing fungi and aflatoxin contamination. *Int J Food Microbiol* 119:109–115.

Crawford, J. M., P. M. Thomas, J. R. Scheerer, A. L. Vagstad, N. L. Kelleher, and C. A. Townsend. 2008. Deconstruction of iterative multidomain polyketide synthase function. *Science* 320:243–246.

Cuero, R., T. Ouellet, J. Yu, and N. Mogongwa. 2003. Metal ion enhancement of fungal growth, gene expression and aflatoxin synthesis in *Aspergillus flavus*: RT-PCR characterization. *J Appl Microbiol* 94:953–961.

Davis, N. D., U. L. Diener, and V. P. Agnihotri. 1967. Production of aflatoxins $B_1$ and $G_1$ in chemically defined medium. *Mycopathol Mycol Appl* 31:251–256.

Davis, N. D., S. K. Iyer, and U. L. Diener. 1987. Improved method of screening for aflatoxin with a coconut agar medium. *Appl Environ Microbiol* 53:1593–1595.

Demain, A. L. 1998. Induction of secondary metabolism. *Int Microbiol* 1:259–264.

Denning, D. W. 1998. Invasive aspergillosis. *Clin Infect Dis* 26:781–805.

Denning, D. W., S. E. Follansbee, M. Scolaro, S. Norris, H. Edelstein, and D. A. Stevens. 1991. Pulmonary aspergillosis in the acquired immunodeficiency syndrome. *N Engl J Med* 324:654–662.

Denning, D. W., K. Riniotis, R. Dobrashian, and H. Sambatakou. 2003. Chronic cavitary and fibrosing pulmonary and pleural aspergillosis: Case series, proposed nomenclature and review. *Clin Infect Dis* 37(Suppl 3):S265–S280.

Diener, U. L., R. J. Cole, T. H. Sanders, G. A. Payne, L. S. Lee, and M. A. Klich. 1987. Epidemiology of aflatoxin formation by *Aspergillus flavus*. *Ann Rev Phytopathol* 25:249–270.

Diener, U. L. and N. D. Davis. 1970. Limiting temperature and relative humidity for aflatoxin production by *Aspergillus flavus* in stored peanuts. *J Am Oil Chem Soc* 47:347–351.

Du'Lock, J. D. 1965. The biosynthesis of natural product. London, U.K.: Magraw Hill.

Duran, R. M., J. W. Cary, and A. M. Calvo. 2007. Production of cyclopiazonic acid, aflatrem, and aflatoxin by *Aspergillus flavus* is regulated by *veA*, a gene necessary for sclerotial formation. *Appl Microbiol Biotechnol* 73:1158–1168.

Eaton, D. and E. Gallagher. 1994. Mechanisms of aflatoxin carcinogenesis. *Annu Rev Pharmacol Toxicol* 34:135–172.

Eaton, D. L. and J. D. Groopman. 1994. *The Toxicology of Aflatoxins: Human Health, Veterinary, and Agricultural Significance*. San Diego, CA: Academic Press.

Egel, D. S., P. J. Cotty, and K. S. Elias. 1994. Relationship among isolates of *Aspergillus* sect. *Flavi* that vary in aflatoxin production. *Phytopathology* 84:906–912.

Ehrlich, K. 2007. Polyketide biosynthesis in fungi. In *Polyketides Biosynthesis, Biological Activity, and Genetic Engineering*. A. M. Rimando and S. R. Baerson (eds.), 955: pp. 68–80. Washington, DC: American Chemical Society.

Ehrlich, K. C., J. W. Cary, and B. G. Montalbano. 1999a. Characterization of the promoter for the gene encoding the aflatoxin biosynthetic pathway regulatory protein AFLR. *Biochim Biophys Acta* 1444:412–417.

Ehrlich, K. C., P.-K. Chang, J. S. L. Scharfenstein, J. W. Cary, J. M. Crawford, and C. A. Townsend. 2010. Absence of the aflatoxin biosynthesis gene, *norA*, allows accumulation of deoxyaflatoxin B1 in *Aspergillus flavus* cultures. *FEMS Microbiol Lett* 305:65–70.

Ehrlich, K. C., P. K. Chang, J. Yu, and P. J. Cotty. 2004. Aflatoxin biosynthesis cluster gene *cypA* is required for G aflatoxin formation. *Appl Environ Microbiol* 70:6518–6524.

Ehrlich, K. C., B. G. Montalbano, and J. W. Cary. 1999b. Binding of the C6-zinc cluster protein, AFLR, to the promoters of aflatoxin pathway biosynthesis genes in *Aspergillus parasiticus*. *Gene* 230:249–257.

Ehrlich, K. C., J. S. L. Scharfenstein, B. G. Montalbano, and P.-K. Chang. 2008. Are the genes *nadA* and *norB* involved in formation of aflatoxin G1. *Int J Mol Sci* 9:1717–1729.

El-Shanawany, A. A., M. E. Mostafa, and A. Barakat. 2005. Fungal populations and mycotoxins in silage in Assiut and Sohag governorates in Egypt, with a special reference to characteristic Aspergilli toxins. *Mycopathologia* 159:281–289.

Espeso, E. A. and H. N. Arst, Jr. 2000. On the mechanism by which alkaline pH prevents expression of an acid-expressed gene. *Mol Cell Biol* 20:3355–3363.

Espeso, E. A., J. Tilburn, H. N. Arst, Jr., and M. A. Penalva. 1993. pH regulation is a major determinant in expression of a fungal penicillin biosynthetic gene. *EMBO J* 12:3947–3956.

Fanelli, C. and A. A. Fabbri. 1989. Relationship between lipids and aflatoxin biosynthesis. *Mycopathologia* 107:115–120.

Fanelli, C., A. A. Fabbri, S. Brasini, C. De Luca, and S. Passi. 1995. Effect of different inhibitors of sterol biosynthesis on both fungal growth and aflatoxin production. *Nat Toxins* 3:109–113.

Fanelli, C., A. A. Fabbri, E. Finotti, and S. Passi. 1983. Stimulation of aflatoxin biosynthesis by lipophilic epoxides. *J Gen Microbiol* 129:1721–1723.

Fedorova, N. D., N. Khaldi, V. S. Joardar et al. 2008. Genomic islands in the pathogenic filamentous fungus *Aspergillus fumigatus*. *PLoS Genet* 4:e1000046.

Feng, G. H. and T. J. Leonard. 1995. Characterization of the polyketide synthase gene (*pksL1*) aflatoxin biosynthesis in *Aspergillus parasiticus*. *J Bacteriol* 177:6246–6254.

Feng, G. H. and T. J. Leonard. 1998. Culture conditions control expression of the genes for aflatoxin and sterigmatocystin biosynthesis in *Aspergillus parasiticus* and *A. nidulans*. *Appl Environ Microbiol* 64:2275–2277.

Fernandes, M., N. P. Keller, and T. H. Adams. 1998. Sequence-specific binding by *Aspergillus nidulans* AflR, a C6 zinc cluster protein regulating mycotoxin biosynthesis. *Mol Microbiol* 28:1355–1365.

Flaherty, J. E. and G. A. Payne. 1997. Overexpression of *aflR* leads to upregulation of pathway gene expression and increased aflatoxin production in *Aspergillus flavus*. *Appl Environ Microbiol* 63:3995–4000.

Fu, Y. T., F. S. He, S. L. Zhang, and J. S. Zhang. 1995. Lipid-peroxidation in rats intoxicated with 3-nitropropionic acid. *Toxicon* 33:327–331.

Fung, F. and R. F. Clark. 2004. Health effects of mycotoxins: A toxicological overview. *J Toxicol Clin Toxicol* 42:217–234.

Galagan, J. E., S. E. Calvo, C. Cuomo et al. 2005. Sequencing of *Aspergillus nidulans* and comparative analysis with *A. fumigatus* and *A. oryzae*. *Nature* 438:1105–1115.

Gallagher, R. T., J. L. Richard, H. M. Stahr, and R. J. Cole. 1978. Cyclopiazonic acid production by aflatoxigenic and non-aflatoxigenic strains of *Aspergillus flavus*. *Mycopathologia* 66:31–36.

Gallagher, R. T. and B. J. Wilson. 1979. Aflatrem, the tremorgenic mycotoxin from *Aspergillus flavus*. *Mycopathologia* 66:183–185.

Garrido, N. S., M. H. Iha, M. R. Santos Ortolani, and R. M. Duarte Fávaro. 2003. Occurrence of aflatoxin M1 and aflatoxin M2 in milk commercialized in Ribeirão Preto-SP, Brazil. *J Food Addit Contam* 20:70–73.

Geiser, D. M., J. W. Dorner, B. W. Horn, and J. W. Taylor. 2000. The phylogenetics of myco-toxin and sclerotium production in *Aspergillus flavus* and *Aspergillus oryzae*. *Fungal Genet Biol* 31:169–179.

Georgianna, R. A., N. D. Fedorova, J. L. Burroughs et al. 2010. Beyond aflatoxin: Four distinct expression patterns and functional roles associated with *Aspergillus flavus* secondary metabolism gene clusters. *Mol Plant Pathol* 11:213–226.

Goldblatt, L. A. 1969a. *Aflatoxin-Scientific Background, Control and Implications*. New York: Academic Press.

Goldblatt, L. A. 1969b. Critical evaluation of aflatoxin detoxification in oilseeds. *Conference on Protein Food Prod Oilseeds*, New Orleans, LA, 1969.

Gong, Y., A. Hounsa, S. Egal et al. 2004. Postweaning exposure to aflatoxin results in impaired child growth: A longitudinal study in Benin, West Africa. *Environ Health Perspect* 112:1134–1138.

Goto, T., D. T. Wicklow, and Y. Ito. 1996. Aflatoxin and cyclopiazonic acid production by a sclerotium-producing *Aspergillus tamarii* strain. *Appl Environ Microbiol* 62:4036–4038.

Greene-McDowelle, D. M., B. Ingber, M. S. Wright, H. J. Zeringue, Jr., D. Bhatnagar, and T. E. Cleveland. 1999. The effects of selected cotton-leaf volatiles on growth, develop-ment and aflatoxin production of *Aspergillus parasiticus*. *Toxicon* 37:883–893.

Groopman, J. D., G. N. Wogan, B. D. Roebuck, and T. W. Kensler. 1994. Molecular bio-markers for aflatoxins and their application to human cancer prevention. *Cancer Res* 54:190–191.

Guo, B. Z., C. C. Holbrook, J. Yu, R. D. Lee, and R. E. Lynch. 2005. Application of technology of gene expression in response to drought stress and elimination of preharvest aflatoxin contamination. In *Aflatoxin and Food Safety*. H. K. Abbas (ed.), pp. 313–331. Boca Raton, FL: CRC Press.

Guzman-de-Pena, D., J. Aguirre, and J. Ruiz-Herrera. 1998. Correlation between the regula-tion of sterigmatocystin biosynthesis and asexual and sexual sporulation in *Emericella nidulans*. *Antonie Leeuwenhoek* 73:199–205.

Hert, D. G., C. P. Fredlake, and A. E. Barron. 2008 Advantages and limitations of next-generation sequencing technologies: A comparison of electrophoresis and non-electrophoresis meth-ods. *Electrophoresis* 29:4618–4626.

Hesseltine, C. W., O. Shotwell, M. Smith, J. J. Ellis, E. Vandegraft, and G. Shannon. 1970. Production of various aflatoxins by strains of the *Aspergillus flavus* series. *Proceedings of the First U.S.–Japan Conference on Toxic Microorganisms*, U.S. Government Printing Office, Washington, DC.

Hicks, J. K., J. H. Yu, N. P. Keller, and T. H. Adams. 1997. *Aspergillus* sporulation and myco-toxin production both require inactivation of the FadA G alpha protein-dependent sig-naling pathway. *EMBO J* 16:4916–4923.

Hoffmeister, D. and N. P. Keller. 2007. Natural products of filamentous fungi: Enzymes, genes, and their regulation. *Nat Prod Rep* 24:393–416.

Horn, B. W., R. L. Greene, and J. W. Dorner. 1995. Effect of corn and peanut cultivation on soil populations of *Aspergillus flavus* and *A. parasiticus* in southwestern Georgia. *Appl Environ Microbiol* 61:2472–2475.

Horn, B. W., J. H. Ramirez-Prado, and I. Carbone. 2009a. Sexual reproduction and recom-bination in the aflatoxin-producing fungus *Aspergillus parasiticus*. *Fungal Genet Biol* 46:169–175.

Horn, B. W., J. H. Ramirez-Prado, and I. Carbone. 2009b. The sexual state of *Aspergillus parasiticus*. *Mycologia* 101:275–280.

Hsieh, D. P. H. 1989. Potential human health hazards of mycotoxins. In *Mycotoxins and Phycotoxins*. S. Natori, H. Hashimoto and Y. Ueno (eds.), pp. 69–80. Amsterdam, the Netherlands: Elsevier.

Hsieh, D. P., L. M. Beltran, M. Y. Fukayama, D. W. Rice, and J. J. Wong. 1986. Production and isolation of aflatoxin $M_1$ for toxicological studies. *J Assoc Off Anal Chem* 69:510–512.

Hsieh, D. P., J. M. Cullen, L. S. Hsieh, Y. Shao, and B. H. Ruebner. 1985. Cancer risks posed by aflatoxin $M_1$. *Princess Takamatsu Symp* 16:57–65.

Hsu, I. C., R. A. Metcalf, T. Sun, J. A. Welsh, N. J. Wang, and C. C. Harris. 1991. Mutational hotspot in the p53 gene in human hepatocellular carcinomas. *Nature* 350:427–428.

Huang, J. H. and D. P. Hsieh. 1988. Comparative study of aflatoxins $M_1$ and $B_1$ production in solid-state and shaking liquid cultures. *Proc Natl Sci Counc Repub China* 12:34–42.

Ito, Y., S. W. Peterson, D. T. Wicklow, and T. Goto. 2001. *Aspergillus pseudotamarii*, a new aflatoxin producing species in *Aspergillus* section. *Flavi. Mycol Res* 105:233–239.

Janardhanan, K. K., A. Sattar, and A. Husain. 1984. Production of fumigaclavine A by *Aspergillus tamarii* Kita. *Can J Microbiol* 30:247–250.

Jayashree, T., J. Praveen Rao, and C. Subramanyam. 2000. Regulation of aflatoxin production by Ca(2+)/calmodulin-dependent protein phosphorylation and dephosphorylation. *FEMS Microbiol Lett* 183:215–219.

Jayashree, T. and C. Subramanyam. 2000. Oxidative stress as a prerequisite for aflatoxin production by *Aspergillus parasiticus*. *Free Radic Biol Med* 29:981–985.

Jelinek, C. F., A. E. Pohland, and G. E. Wood. 1989. Worldwide occurrence of mycotoxins in food and feeds—An update. *J Assoc Off Anal Chem* 72:223–230.

Johnson, J. R., B. L. Robinson, S. F. Ali, and Z. Binienda. 2000. Dopamine toxicity following long term exposure to low doses of 3-nitropropionic acid (3-NPA) in rats. *Toxicol Lett* 116:113–118.

Kachholz, T. and A. L. Demain. 1983. Nitrate repression of averufin and aflatoxin biosynthesis *Aspergillus parasiticus*. *J Nat Prod* 46:499–506.

Kale, S. and J. W. Bennett. 1992. Strain instability in filamentous fungi. In *Handbook of Applied Mycology*, Vol. 5. *Mycotoxins in Ecological Systems*, Vol. 5. D. Bhatnagar, E. B. Lillehoj, and D. K. Arora (eds.), pp. 311–332. New York: Marcel Dekker.

Kale, S. P., J. W. Cary, D. Bhatnagar, and J. W. Bennett. 1996. Characterization of experimentally induced, nonaflatoxigenic variant strains of *Aspergillus parasiticus*. *Appl Environ Microbiol* 62:3399–3404.

Kato, N., W. Brooks, and A. M. Calvo. 2003. The expression of sterigmatocystin and penicillin genes in *Aspergillus nidulans* is controlled by *veA*, a gene required for sexual development. *Eukaryot Cell* 2:1178–1186.

Keller, N. P., H. C. Dischinger, Jr., D. Bhatnagar, T. E. Cleveland, and A. H. Ullah. 1993. Purification of a 40-kilodalton methyltransferase active in the aflatoxin biosynthetic pathway. *Appl Environ Microbiol* 59:479–484.

Keller, N. P., C. Nesbitt, B. Sarr, T. D. Phillips, and G. B. Burow. 1997. pH regulation of sterigmatocystin and aflatoxin biosynthesis in *Aspergillus* spp. *Phytopathology* 87:643–648.

Keller, N. P., G. Turner, and J. W. Bennett. 2005. Fungal secondary metabolism—From biochemistry to genomics. *Nat Rev Microbiol* 3:937–947.

Kelly, J. D., D. L. Eaton, F. P. Guengerich, and R. A. Coulombe, Jr. 1997. Aflatoxin $B_1$ activation in human lung. *Toxicol Appl Pharmacol* 144:88–95.

Khaldi, N., F. T. Seifuddin, G. Turner et al. 2010. SMURF: Genomic mapping of fungal secondary metabolite clusters. *Fungal Genet Biol* 47(9):736–741.

Kim, J. H., B. C. Campbell, R. Molyneux et al. 2006. Gene targets for fungal and mycotoxin control. *Mycotoxin Res* 22:3–8.

Klich, M. A. 1998. Soil fungi of some low-altitude desert cotton fields and ability of their extracts to inhibit *Aspergillus flavus*. *Mycopathologia* 142:97–100.

Klich, M. A. 2002. Biogeography of *Aspergillus* species in soil and litter. *Mycologia* 94:21–27.

Krishnamachari, K. A., R. V. Bhat, V. Nagarajan, and T. B. Tilak. 1975. Hepatitis due to aflatoxicosis: An outbreak of hepatitis in parts of western India. *Lancet* 1:1061–1063.

Kurtzman, C. P., B. W. Horn, and C. W. Hesseltine. 1987. *Aspergillus nomius*, a new aflatoxin-producing species related to *Aspergillus flavus* and *Aspergillus tamarii*. *Antonie Leeuwenhoek* 53:147–158.

Lalitha Rao, B. and A. Husain. 1985. Presence of cyclopiazonic acid in kodo millet (*Paspalum scrobiculatum*) causing 'kodua poisoning' in man and its production by associated fungi. *Mycopathologia* 89:177–180.

Lancaster, M. D., F. P. Jenkins, and J. M. Philip. 1961. Toxicity associated with certain samples of ground nuts. *Nature* 192:1095–1096.

Larsen, T. O., J. Smedsgaard, K. F. Nielsen, M. A. Hansen, R. A. Samson, and J. C. Frisvad. 2007. Production of mycotoxins by *Aspergillus lentulus* and other medically important and closely related species in section Fumigati. *Med Mycol* 45:225–232.

Lee, L. S., J. W. Bennett, L. A. Goldblatt, and R. E. Lundin. 1971. Norsolorinic acid from a mutant strain of *Aspergillus parasiticus*. *J Am Oil Chem Soc* 48:93–94.

Lewis, L., M. Onsongo, H. Njapau et al. 2005. Aflatoxin contamination of commercial maize products during an outbreak of acute aflatoxicosis in eastern and central Kenya. *Environ Health Perspect* 113:1763–1767.

Liang, S. H., C. D. Skory, and J. E. Linz. 1996. Characterization of the function of the ver-1A and ver-1B genes, involved in aflatoxin biosynthesis in *Aspergillus parasiticus*. *Appl Environ Microbiol* 62:4568–4575.

Lillehoj, E. B., W. W. McMillian, W. D. Guthrie, and D. Barry. 1980. Aflatoxin-producing fungi in preharvest corn: Inoculum source in insects and soils. *J Environ Qual* 9:691–694.

Lillehoj, E. B. and J. H. Wall. 1986. Decontamination of aflatoxin-contaminated maize grain. *Proceedings of the workshop sponsored by CIMMYT (International Maize and Wheat Improvement Center), UNDP, and US-AID*, El Batan, Mexico, 1986, pp. 260–279.

Luchese, R. H. and W. F. Harrigan. 1993. Biosynthesis of aflatoxin—The role of nutritional factors. *J Appl Bacteriol* 74:5–14.

Luchowski, P., E. Luchowska, W. A. Turski, and E. M. Urbanska. 2002. 1-methyl-4-phenylpyridinium and 3-nitropropionic acid diminish cortical synthesis of kynurenic acid via interference with kynurenine aminotransferases in rats. *Neurosci Lett* 330:49–52.

Machida, M., K. Asai, M. Sano et al. 2005. Genome sequencing and analysis of *Aspergillus oryzae*. *Nature* 438:1157–1161.

Magan, N. and M. Olsen. 2004. Mycotoxins in food: Detection and control. Cambridge, U.K.: Woodhead Publishing Ltd.

Mahanti, N., D. Bhatnagar, J. W. Cary, J. Joubran, and J. E. Linz. 1996. Structure and function of *fas-1A*, a gene encoding a putative fatty acid synthetase directly involved in aflatoxin biosynthesis in *Aspergillus parasiticus*. *Appl Environ Microbiol* 62:191–195.

Mahoney, N. and R. J. Molyneux. 2004. Phytochemical inhibition of aflatoxigenicity in *Aspergillus flavus* by constituents of walnut (*Juglans regia*). *J Agric Food Chem* 52:1882–1889.

Malloy, C. D. and J. S. Marr. 1997. Mycotoxins and public health: A review. *J Public Health Manag Pract* 3:61–69.

Martins, M. L. and H. M. Martins. 1999. Natural and in vitro coproduction of cyclopiazonic acid and aflatoxins. *J Food Prot* 62:292–294.

Matsushima, K., P. K. Chang, J. Yu, K. Abe, D. Bhatnagar, and T. E. Cleveland. 2001. Pretermination in *aflR* of *Aspergillus sojae* inhibits aflatoxin biosynthesis. *Appl Microbiol Biotechnol* 55:585–589.

McGlynn, K. A., K. Hunter, T. LeVoyer et al. 2003. Susceptibility to aflatoxin $B_1$-related primary hepatocellular carcinoma in mice and humans. *Cancer Res* 63:4594–4601.

Meyers, D. M., G. Obrian, W. L. Du, D. Bhatnagar, and G. A. Payne. 1998. Characterization of *aflJ*, a gene required for conversion of pathway intermediates to aflatoxin. *Appl Environ Microbiol* 64:3713–3717.

Minto, R. E. and C. A. Townsend. 1997. Enzymology and molecular biology of aflatoxin biosynthesis. *Chem Rev* 97:2537–2556.

Moncoq, K., C. A. Trieber, and H. S. Young. 2007. The molecular basis for cyclopiazonic acid inhibition of the sarcoplasmic reticulum calcium pump. *J Biol Chem* 282:9748–9757.

Mooney, J. L., D. E. Hassett, and L. N. Yager. 1990. Genetic analysis of suppressors of the *veA1* mutation in *Aspergillus nidulans*. *Genetics* 126:869–874.

Mooney, J. L. and L. N. Yager. 1990. Light is required for conidiation in *Aspergillus nidulans*. *Genes Dev* 4:1473–1482.

Moore, G. 1965. Cramming more components onto integrated circuits. *Electronics* 38:114–117.

Mori, T., M. Matsumura, K. Yamada et al. 1998. Systemic aspergillosis caused by an aflatoxin-producing strain of *Aspergillus flavus*. *Med Mycol* 36:107–112.

Nesbitt, B. F., J. O'Kelly, K. Sargeant, and A. Sheridan. 1962. *Aspergillus flavus* and turkey X disease. Toxic metabolites of *Aspergillus flavus*. *Nature* 195:1062–1063.

Ngindu, A., B. K. Johnson, P. R. Kenya et al. 1982. Outbreak of acute hepatitis caused by aflatoxin poisoning in Kenya. *Lancet* 1:1346–1348.

Nicholson, M. J., A. Koulman, B. J. Monahan, B. L. Pritchard, G. A. Payne, and B. Scott. 2009. Identification of two aflatrem biosynthesis gene loci in *Aspergillus flavus* and metabolic engineering of Penicillium paxilli to elucidate their function. *Appl Environ Microbiol* 75:7469–7481.

Niehaus, W. G. J. and W. P. Jiang. 1989. Nitrate induces enzymes of the mannitol cycle and suppresses versicolorin synthesis in *Aspergillus parasiticus*. *Mycopathologia* 107:131–137.

Nierman, W. C., A. Pain, M. J. Anderson et al. 2005. Genomic sequence of the pathogenic and allergenic filamentous fungus *Aspergillus fumigatus*. *Nature* 438:1151–1156.

Nishie, K., R. J. Cole, and J. W. Dorner. 1985. Toxicity and neuropharmacology of cyclopiazonic acid. *Food Chem Toxicol* 23:831–839.

Nony, P. A., A. C. Scallet, R. L. Rountree, X. Ye, and Z. Binienda. 1999. 3-nitropropionic acid (3-NPA) produces hypothermia and inhibits histochemical labeling of succinate dehydrogenase (SDH) in rat brain. *Metab Brain Dis* 14:83–94.

OBrian, G. R., A. M. Fakhoury, and G. A. Payne. 2003. Identification of genes differentially expressed during aflatoxin biosynthesis in *Aspergillus flavus* and *Aspergillus parasiticus*. *Fungal Genet Biol* 39:118–127.

OBrian, G. R., D. R. Georgianna, J. R. Wilkinson et al. 2007. The effect of elevated temperature on gene transcription and aflatoxin biosynthesis. *Mycologia* 99:232–239.

O'Gorman, C. M., H. T. Fuller, and P. S. Dyer. 2009. Discovery of a sexual cycle in the opportunistic fungal pathogen *Aspergillus fumigatus*. *Nature* 457:471–474.

Otsuki, T., J. S. Wilson, and M. Sewadeh. 2001. What price precaution? European harmonization of aflatoxin regulations and African groundnuts exports. *Eur Rev Agric Econ* 28:263–284.

Payne, G. A. 1998. Process of contamination by aflatoxin-producing fungi and their impacts on crops. In *Mycotoxins in Agriculture and Food Safety*. K. K. Sinha and D. Bhatnagar (eds.), pp. 279–306. New York: Marcel Dekker.

Payne, G. A. and M. P. Brown. 1998. Genetics and physiology of aflatoxin biosynthesis. *Annu Rev Phytopathol* 36:329–362.

Payne, G. A. and W. M. Hagler, Jr. 1983. Effect of specific amino acids on growth and aflatoxin production by *Aspergillus parasiticus* and *Aspergillus flavus* in defined media. *Appl Environ Microbiol* 46:805–812.

Payne, G. A., W. C. Nierman, J. R. Wortman et al. 2006. Whole genome comparison of *Aspergillus flavus* and *A. oryzae*. *Med Mycol* 44(Suppl):9–11.

Peers, F., X. Bosch, J. Kaldor, A. Linsell, and M. Pluijmen. 1987. Aflatoxin exposure, hepatitis B virus infection and liver cancer in Swaziland. *Int J Cancer* 39:545–553.

Perrin, R. M., N. D. Fedorova, J. W. Bok et al. 2007. Transcriptional regulation of chemical diversity in *Aspergillus fumigatus* by LaeA. *PLoS Pathog* 3:e50.

Pildain, M. B., J. C. Frisvad, G. Vaamonde, D. Cabral, J. Varga, and R. A. Samson. 2008. Two novel aflatoxin-producing *Aspergillus* species from Argentinean peanuts. *Int J Syst Evol Microbiol* 58:725–735.

Polychronaki, N., R. M. West, P. C. Turner et al. 2007. A longitudinal assessment of afla-toxin M1 excretion in breast milk of selected Egyptian mothers. *Food Chem Toxicol* 45:1210–1215.

Price, M. S., J. Yu, D. Bhatnagar, T. E. Cleveland, W. C. Nierman, and G. A. Payne. 2005. The aflatoxin pathway regulatory gene *aflR* regulates genes outside of the aflatoxin biosyn-thetic cluster. PhD thesis, North Carolina State University, Raleigh, MC.

Price, M. S., J. Yu, W. C. Nierman et al. 2006. The aflatoxin pathway regulator AflR induces gene transcription inside and outside of the aflatoxin biosynthetic cluster. *FEMS Microbiol Lett* 255:275–279.

Prieto, R. and C. P. Woloshuk. 1997. *ord1*, an oxidoreductase gene responsible for conversion of *O*-methylsterigmatocystin to aflatoxin in *Aspergillus flavus*. *Appl Environ Microbiol* 63:1661–1666.

Rafiyuddin, M., N. J. Rao, S. Girisham, and S. M. Reddy. 2006. Toxicology of tremorgenic mycotoxins on chicks. *Natl Acad Sci Lett* (India) 29:311–315.

Ramirez-Prado, J. H., G. G. Moore, B. W. Horn, and I. Carbone. 2008. Characterization and population analysis of the mating-type genes in *Aspergillus flavus* and *Aspergillus para-siticus*. *Fungal Genet Biol* 45:1292–1299.

Reddy, T. V., L. Viswanathan, and T. A. Venkitasubramanian. 1971. High aflatoxin production on a chemically defined medium. *Appl Microbiol* 22:393–396.

Reddy, T. V., L. Viswanathan, and T. A. Venkitasubramanian. 1979. Factors affecting aflatoxin production by *Aspergillus parasiticus* in a chemically defined medium. *J Gen Microbiol* 114:409–413.

Reib, J. 1982. Development of *Aspergillus parasiticus* and formation of aflatoxin B1 under the influence of conidiogenesis affecting compounds. *Arch Microbiol* 133:236–238.

Reverberi, M., A. A. Fabbri, S. Zjalic, A. Ricelli, F. Punelli, and C. Fanelli. 2005. Antioxidant enzymes stimulation in *Aspergillus parasiticus* by Lentinula edodes inhibits aflatoxin production. *Appl Microbiol Biotechnol* 69:207–215.

Reverberi, M., S. Zjalic, A. Racelli, A. A. Fabbri, and C. Fanelli. 2006. Oxidant/antioxidant bal-ance in *Aspergillus parasiticus* affects aflatoxin biosynthesis. *Mycotoxin Res* 22:39–47.

Rice, D. W. and D. P. Hsieh. 1982. Aflatoxin $M_1$: In vitro preparation and comparative in vitro metabolism versus aflatoxin $B_1$ in the rat and mouse. *Res Commun Chem Pathol Pharmacol* 35:467–490.

Richard, J. L. 2008. Discovery of aflatoxins and significant historical features. *Toxin Rev* 27:171–201.

Richard, J. L. and G. A. Payne. 2003. *Mycotoxins: Risks in Plant, Animal and Human Systems.* Council for Agricultural Science and Technology (CAST), Ames, IA.

Robens, J. F. 2001. The costs of mycotoxin management to the USA: Management of aflatox-ins in the United States. *APSnet Feature*, pp. 2–8. http://www.apsnet.org/online/feature/mycotoxin/top.html (Accessed: 17 October 2010).

Robens, J. F. and K. Cardwell. 2005. The cost of mycotoxin management in the United States. In *Aflatoxin and Food Safety.* H. K. Abbas (ed.), pp. 1–12. Boca Raton, FL: CRC Press.

Ronning, C. M., N. D. Fedorova, P. Bowyer et al. 2005. Genomics of *Aspergillus fumigatus*. *Rev Iberoam Micol (RIAM)* 22:223–228.

Roy, A. K. and H. K. Chourasia. 1989. Effect of temperature on aflatoxin production in Mucuna pruriens seeds. *Appl Environ Microbiol* 55:531–532.

Saito, M., O. Tsuruta, P. Siriacha, S. Kawasugi, M. Manabe, and D. Buangsuwan. 1986. Distribution and aflatoxin productivity of the atypical strains of *Aspergillus flavus* isolated from soils in Thailand. *Proc Jpn Assoc Mycotoxicol* 24:41–46.

Sanders, T. H., P. D. Blankenship, R. J. Cole, and R. A. Hill. 1984. Effect of soil temperature and drought on peanut pod and stem temperatures relative to *Aspergillus flavus* invasion and aflatoxin contamination. *Mycopathologia* 86:51–54.

Scholl, P. and J. D. Groopman. 1995. Epidermiology of human exposures and its relationship to liver cancer. In *Molecular Approaches to Food Safety: Issues Involving Toxic Microorganisms*. M. Eklund, J. L. Richard and K. Mise (eds.), pp. 169–182. Fort Collins, CO: Alaken Inc.

Schroeder, H. W. and H. Hein, Jr. 1968. Effect of diurnal temperature cycles on the production of aflatoxin. *Appl Microbiol* 16:988–990.

Shimizu, K. and N. P. Keller. 2001. Genetic involvement of a cAMP-dependent protein kinase in a G protein signaling pathway regulating morphological and chemical transitions in *Aspergillus nidulans*. *Genetics* 157:591–600.

Skory, C. D., P. K. Chang, J. Cary, and J. E. Linz. 1992. Isolation and characterization of a gene from *Aspergillus parasiticus* associated with the conversion of versicolorin A to sterigmatocystin in aflatoxin biosynthesis. *Appl Environ Microbiol* 58:3527–3537.

Skory, C. D., P. K. Chang, and J. E. Linz. 1993. Regulated expression of the *nor-1* and *ver-1* genes associated with aflatoxin biosynthesis. *Appl Environ Microbiol* 59:1642–1646.

Soler, F., F. Plenge-Tellechea, I. Fortea, and F. Fernandez-Belda. 1998. Cyclopiazonic acid effect on Ca2+-dependent conformational states of the sarcoplasmic reticulum ATPase. Implication for the enzyme turnover. *Biochemistry* 37:4266–4274.

Stinnett, S. M., E. A. Espeso, L. Cobeno, L. Araujo-Bazan, and A. M. Calvo. 2007. *Aspergillus nidulans* VeA subcellular localization is dependent on the importin alpha carrier and on light. *Mol Microbiol* 63:242–255.

Sweeney, M. J. and A. D. Dobson. 1998. Mycotoxin production by *Aspergillus, Fusarium* and *Penicillium* species. *Int J Food Microbiol* 43:141–158.

Sweeney, M. J. and A. D. Dobson. 1999. Molecular biology of mycotoxin biosynthesis. *FEMS Microbiol Lett* 175:149–163.

Takahashi, T., P. K. Chang, K. Matsushima et al. 2002. Nonfunctionality of *Aspergillus sojae aflR* in a strain of *Aspergillus parasiticus* with a disrupted *aflR* gene. *Appl Environ Microbiol* 68:3737–3743.

Tilburn, J., S. Sarkar, D. A. Widdick et al. 1995. The *Aspergillus* PacC zinc finger transcription factor mediates regulation of both acid- and alkaline expressed genes by ambient pH. *EMBO J* 14:779–790.

Tokuoka, M., Y. Seshime, I. Fujii, K. Kitamoto, T. Takahashi, and Y. Koyama. 2008. Identification of a novel polyketide synthase-nonribosomal peptide synthetase (PKS-NRPS) gene required for the biosynthesis of cyclopiazonic acid in *Aspergillus oryzae*. *Fungal Genet Biol* 45:1608–1615.

Townsend, C. A. 1997. Progress towards a biosynthetic rationale of the aflatoxin pathway. *Pure Appl Chem* 58:227–238.

Trail, F., N. Mahanti, and J. Linz. 1995a. Molecular biology of aflatoxin biosynthesis. *Microbiology* 141:755–765.

Trail, F., N. Mahanti, M. Rarick et al. 1995b. Physical and transcriptional map of an aflatoxin gene cluster in *Aspergillus parasiticus* and functional disruption of a gene involved early in the aflatoxin pathway. *Appl Environ Microbiol* 61:2665–2673.

Turner, P. C., A. C. Collinson, Y. B. Cheung et al. 2007. Aflatoxin exposure in utero causes growth faltering in Gambian infants. *Int J Epidemiol* 36:1119–1125.

Valdes, J. J., J. E. Cameron, and R. J. Cole. 1985. Aflatrem: A tremorgenic mycotoxin with acute neurotoxic effects. *Environ Health Perspect* 62:459–463.

Van Egmond, H. P. 1989. Current situation on regulations for mycotoxins. Overview of toler-
ances and status of standard methods of sampling and analysis. *J Food Add Contam*
6:139–148.

Venkatesh, P. K. and S. Vairamuthu. 2005. Induction of apoptosis by fungal culture materials containing cyclopiazonic acid and T-2 toxin in primary lymphoid organs of broiler
chickens. *Mycopathologia* 159:393–400.

Vinokurova, N. G., N. E. Ivanushkina, I. I. Khmel'nitskaia, and M. U. Arinbasarov. 2007.
Synthesis of alpha-cyclopiazonic acid by fungi of the genus *Aspergillus*. *Prikl Biokhim
Mikrobiol* 43:486–489.

Watanabe, C. M. and C. A. Townsend. 2002. Initial characterization of a type I fatty acid
synthase and polyketide synthase multienzyme complex NorS in the biosynthesis of
aflatoxin $B_1$. *Chem Biol* 9:981–988.

Wicklow, D. T. and O. L. Shotwell. 1983. Intrafungal distribution of aflatoxins among conidia
and sclerotia of *Aspergillus flavus* and *Aspergillus flavus*. *Can J Microbiol* 29:1–5.

Widiastuti, R., R. Maryam, B. J. Blaney, Salfina, and D. R. Stoltz. 1988. Cyclopiazonic acid
in combination with aflatoxins, zearalenone and ochratoxin A in Indonesian corn.
*Mycopathologia* 104:153–156.

Wild, C. P., S. M. Shrestha, W. A. Anwar, and R. Montesano. 1992. Field studies of aflatoxin exposure, metabolism and induction of genetic alterations in relation to HBV
infection and hepatocellular carcinoma in The Gambia and Thailand. *Toxicol Lett*
64:455–461.

Wilkinson, J. R., J. Yu, H. K. Abbas et al. 2007a. Aflatoxin formation and gene expression in
response to carbon source media shift in *Aspergillus parasiticus*. *J Food Add Contam*
24:1051–1060.

Wilkinson, J. R., J. Yu, J. M. Bland, W. C. Nierman, D. Bhatnagar, and T. E. Cleveland. 2007b.
Amino acid supplementation reveals differential regulation of aflatoxin biosynthesis in
*Aspergillus flavus* NRRL 3357 and *Aspergillus parasiticus* SRRC 143. *Appl Microbiol
Biotechnol* 74:1308–1319.

Williams, J. H., T. D. Phillips, P. E. Jolly, J. K. Stiles, C. M. Jolly, and D. Aggarwal. 2004.
Human aflatoxicosis in developing countries: A review of toxicology, exposure, potential health consequences, and interventions. *Am J Clin Nutr* 80:1106–1122.

Wilson, D. M. 1989. Analytical methods for aflatoxins in corn and peanuts. *Arch Environ
Contam Toxicol* 18:308–314.

Wilson, R. A., H. W. Gardner, and N. P. Keller. 2001. Differentiation of aflatoxin-producing
and non-producing strains of *Aspergillus flavus* group. *Lett Appl Microbiol* 33:291–295.

Wogan, G. N. 1992. Aflatoxins as risk factors for hepatocellular carcinoma in humans. *Cancer
Res* 52:2114–2118.

Wogan, G. N. 2000. Impacts of chemicals on liver cancer risk. *Semin Cancer Biol* 10:201–210.

Woloshuk, C. P., J. R. Cavaletto, and T. E. Cleveland. 1997. Inducers of aflatoxin biosynthesis
from colonized maize kernels are generated by an amylase activity from *Aspergillus
flavus*. *Phytopathology* 87:164–169.

Woloshuk, C. P., K. R. Foutz, J. F. Brewer, D. Bhatnagar, T. E. Cleveland, and G. A. Payne.
1994. Molecular characterization of *aflR*, a regulatory locus for aflatoxin biosynthesis.
*Appl Environ Microbiol* 60:2408–2414.

Wong, J. J., R. Singh, and D. P. Hsieh. 1977. Mutagenicity of fungal metabolites related to
aflatoxin biosynthesis. *Mutat Res* 44:447–450.

Wright, M. S., D. M. Greene-McDowelle, H. J. Zeringue, D. Bhatnagar, and T. E. Cleveland.
2000. Effects of volatile aldehydes from *Aspergillus*-resistant varieties of corn on
*Aspergillus parasiticus* growth and aflatoxin biosynthesis. *Toxicon* 38:1215–1223.

Xiulan, S., Z. Xiaolian, T. Jian, J. Zhou, and F. S. Chu. 2005. Preparation of gold-labeled antibody probe and its use in immunochromatography assay for detection of aflatoxin $B_1$.
*Int J Food Microbiol* 99:85–94.

Yabe, K., Y. Ando, and T. Hamasaki. 1988a. Biosynthetic relationship among aflatoxins B₁, B₂, G₁, and G₂. *Appl Environ Microbiol* 54:2101–2106.

Yabe, K., N. Chihaya, S. Hamamatsu et al. 2003. Enzymatic conversion of averufin to hydroxy-versicolorone and elucidation of a novel metabolic grid involved in aflatoxin biosynthesis. *Appl Environ Microbiol* 69:66–73.

Yabe, K. and H. Nakajima. 2004. Enzyme reactions and genes in aflatoxin biosynthesis. *Appl Microbiol Biotechnol* 64:745–755.

Yabe, K., H. Nakamura, Y. Ando, N. Terakado, H. Nakajima, and T. Hamasaki. 1988b. Isolation and characterization of *Aspergillus parasiticus* mutants with impaired aflatoxin production by a novel tip culture method. *Appl Environ Microbiol* 54:2096–2100.

Yu, J. 2004. Genetics and biochemistry of mycotoxin synthesis. In *Fungal Biotechnology in Agricultural, Food, and Environmental Applications*. D. K. Arora (ed.), pp. 343–361. New York: Marcel Dekker.

Yu, J., D. Bhatnagar, and T. E. Cleveland. 2004a. Completed sequence of aflatoxin pathway gene cluster in *Aspergillus parasiticus*. *FEBS Lett* 564:126–130.

Yu, J., J. W. Cary, D. Bhatnagar, T. E. Cleveland, N. P. Keller, and F. S. Chu. 1993. Cloning and characterization of a cDNA from *Aspergillus parasiticus* encoding an *O*-methyltransferase involved in aflatoxin biosynthesis. *Appl Environ Microbiol* 59:564–571.

Yu, J., P. K. Chang, D. Bhatnagar, and T. E. Cleveland. 2000. Cloning of a sugar utilization gene cluster in *Aspergillus parasiticus*. *Biochim Biophys Acta* 1493:211–214.

Yu, J., P. K. Chang, J. W. Cary et al. 1995. Comparative mapping of aflatoxin pathway gene clusters in *Aspergillus parasiticus* and *Aspergillus flavus*. *Appl Environ Microbiol* 61:2365–2371.

Yu, J., P.-K. Chang, T. E. Cleveland, and J. W. Bennett. 2010a. Aflatoxins. In *Encyclopedia of Industrial Biotechnology: Bioprocess, Bioseparation, and Cell Technology*, Vol. 1. M. C. Flickinger (ed.), Hoboken, NJ: John Wiley & Sons, Inc., pp. 1–12 (Peer reviewed article).

Yu, J., P. K. Chang, K. C. Ehrlich et al. 1998. Characterization of the critical amino acids of an *Aspergillus parasiticus* cytochrome P-450 monooxygenase encoded by *ordA* that is involved in the biosynthesis of aflatoxins B₁, G₁, B₂, and G₂. *Appl Environ Microbiol* 64:4834–4841.

Yu, J., P. K. Chang, K. C. Ehrlich et al. 2004b. Clustered pathway genes in aflatoxin biosynthesis. *Appl Environ Microbiol* 70:1253–1262.

Yu, J. and T. E. Cleveland. 2007. *Aspergillus flavus* genomics for discovering genes involved in aflatoxin biosynthesis. In *Polyketides Biosynthesis, Biological Activity, and Genetic Engineering*, 955, A. M. Rimando and S. R. Baerson (eds.), pp. 246–260. Washington, DC: American Chemical Society.

Yu, J., T. E. Cleveland, W. C. Nierman, and J. W. Bennett. 2005. *Aspergillus flavus* genomics: Gateway to human and animal health, food safety, and crop resistance to diseases. *Rev Iberoam Micol* 22:194–202.

Yu, J. H. and N. Keller. 2005. Regulation of secondary metabolism in filamentous fungi. *Annu Rev Phytopathol* 43:437–458.

Yu, J., S. M. Mohawed, D. Bhatnagar, and T. E. Cleveland. 2003. Substrate-induced lipase gene expression and aflatoxin production in *Aspergillus parasiticus* and *Aspergillus flavus*. *J Appl Microbiol* 95:1334–1342.

Yu, J., W. C. Nierman, J. W. Bennett et al. 2010b. Genetics and genomics of *Aspergillus flavus*. In *Progress in Mycology*. M. K. Rai and G. Kovics (eds.), pp. 51–73. Kerala, India: Scientific Publishers.

Yu, J., G. A. Payne, W. C. Nierman et al. 2008. *Aspergillus flavus* genomics as a tool for studying the mechanism of aflatoxin formation. *J Food Add Contam* 25:1152–1157.

Yu, J., C. M. Ronning, J. R. Wilkinson et al. 2007. Gene profiling for studying the mechanism of aflatoxin biosynthesis in *Aspergillus flavus* and *A. parasiticus*. *J Food Add Contam* 24:1035–1042.

Yu, J., C. A. Whitelaw, W. C. Nierman, D. Bhatnagar, and T. E. Cleveland. 2004c. *Aspergillus flavus* expressed sequence tags for identification of genes with putative roles in aflatoxin contamination of crops. *FEMS Microbiol Lett* 237:333–340.

Yu, J. H., J. Wieser, and T. H. Adams. 1996. The *Aspergillus* FlbA RGS domain protein antagonizes G protein signaling to block proliferation and allow development. *EMBO J* 15:5184–5190.

Zeringue, H. J., Jr. 2002. Effects of methyl jasmonate on phytoalexin production and aflatoxin control in the developing cotton boll. *Biochem Syst Ecol* 30:497–503.

Zeringue, H. J. and D. Bhatnagar. 1993. Neem and control of aflatoxin contamination. In *Neem and Environment*. R. K. Singh, M. S. Chari, A. K. Raheja and W. Kraus (eds.), Vol. 2, pp. 713–727. Lebanon, New Hampshire: Science Publishers, Inc. USA.

Zeringue, H. J., Jr., R. L. Brown, J. N. Neucere, and T. E. Cleveland. 1996. Relationships between C6-C12 alkanal and alkenal volatile contents and resistance of maize genotypes to *Aspergillus flavus* and aflatoxin production. *J Agric Food Chem* 44:403–407.

Zhang, S., B. J. Monahan, J. S. Tkacz, and B. Scott. 2004. Indole-diterpene gene cluster from *Aspergillus flavus*. *Appl Environ Microbiol* 70:6875–6883.

Zhu, J. Q., L. S. Zhang, X. Hu et al. 1987. Correlation of dietary aflatoxin $B_1$ levels with excretion of aflatoxin $M_1$ in human urine. *Cancer Res* 47:1848–1852.

Zuckerman, A. J., K. R. Rees, D. Inman, and V. Petts. 1967. Site of action of aflatoxin on human liver cells in culture. *Nature* 214:814–815.

# Index